Updates on Pediatric Health and Diseases

(*Volume 1*)

Common Pediatric Diseases: an Updated Review

Edited by

Nima Rezaei

&

Noosha Samieefar

Network of Interdisciplinarity
in Neonates and Infants (NINI),
Universal Scientific Education
and Research Network (USERN),
Tehran, Iran

Updates on Pediatric Health and Diseases

Common Pediatric Diseases: an Updated Review

Volume # 1

Editors: Nima Rezaei & Noosha Samieefar

ISBN (Online): 978-981-5039-65-8

ISBN (Print): 978-981-5039-66-5

ISBN (Paperback): 978-981-5039-67-2

need for a court order if at any point you breach any terms of this License Agreement. In no event will any delay or failure by Bentham Science Publishers in enforcing your compliance with this License Agreement constitute a waiver of any of its rights.

3. You acknowledge that you have read this License Agreement, and agree to be bound by its terms and conditions. To the extent that any other terms and conditions presented on any website of Bentham Science Publishers conflict with, or are inconsistent with, the terms and conditions set out in this License Agreement, you acknowledge that the terms and conditions set out in this License Agreement shall prevail.

Bentham Science Publishers Pte. Ltd.
80 Robinson Road #02-00
Singapore 068898
Singapore
Email: subscriptions@benthamscience.net

BENTHAM SCIENCE

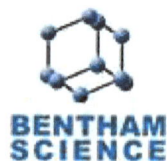

CONTENTS

PREFACE

Seeing the world through the eyes of a child/infant sounds inspirational. They are little, lovely, and defenseless. Pediatric is the science of taking care of these cute creations. Pediatric is a branch of medicine that focuses on the diagnosis and treatment of infants, children, and adolescents' diseases. As the medical sciences are getting more complex with the information explosion, interdisciplinarity is the essential tool to integrate different topics. Therefore, we established an interest group, entitled "Network of Interdisciplinarity in Neonates and Infants (NINI)" in the Universal Scientific Education and Research Network (USERN), and invited pediatricians and scientists in the field of pediatrics from all over the world to join this multidisciplinary network: https://usern.tums.ac.ir/Group/Info/NINI

The "Updates on Pediatric Health and Disease" series is a comprehensive text regarding childhood and adolescence health and diseases. Neonatology, as well as different diseases in all subspecialties of pediatrics, including pediatric allergy and immunology, pediatric cardiology, pediatric endocrinology, pediatric gastroenterology, pediatric hematology, pediatric infectious disease, pediatric nephrology, pediatric oncology, pediatric pulmonology, pediatric rheumatology, pediatric neurology, pediatric psychiatry, and pediatric dermatology, will be discussed in different volumes.

"Common Pediatric Diseases: An Updated Review" is the first volume of this book series; in this volume, after a rapid introduction to Pediatric diseases (Chapter 1), pediatric rheumatologic diseases are discussed (Chapter 2). Then, the book provides an update on common oral diseases (Chapter 3). Chapter 4 takes a specific view of Pediatric Metabolic Syndromes. The book also provides some chapters regarding neurologic diseases, including Pediatric Epilepsy Syndromes (Chapter 5), Pediatric Demyelinating Disorder (Chapter 7), and also a diagnostic algorithmic approach to Pediatric Genetic Epileptic Encephalopathies (Chapter 6). It contains several chapters concerning updates of Henoch-Schönlein purpura (Chapter 9), Atopic Dermatitis (Chapter 8), Childhood-Onset Systemic Lupus Erythematosus (Chapter 10), Severe Combined Immunodeficiency (Chapter 11), PFAPA- Periodic Fever, Aphthous Stomatitis, Pharyngitis, and Cervical Adenitis Syndrome (Chapter 12) and Pediatric Hepatoblastoma (Chapter 13).

Updates on Pediatric Health and Disease Book is the result of the valuable contribution of scientists and clinicians from well-known universities/institutes worldwide. I would like to hereby acknowledge the expertise of all contributors for generously devoting their time and considerable effort in preparing their respective chapters. I would also like to express my gratitude to the Bentham Science publication for providing me the opportunity to publish the book.

Finally, I hope that this timely book will be comprehensible, cogent, and of special value for researchers and clinicians who wish to extend their knowledge of Pediatrics.

Nima Rezaei
Network of Interdisciplinarity
in Neonates and Infants (NINI),
Universal Scientific Education
and Research Network (USERN),
Tehran, Iran

&

Noosha Samieefar
Network of Interdisciplinarity
in Neonates and Infants (NINI),
Universal Scientific Education
and Research Network (USERN),
Tehran, Iran

ACKNOWLEDGEMENT

I would like to express my gratitude to the Editorial Assistant of this book, Dr. Noosha Samieefar. Undoubtedly , the book would not have been completed without her contribution.

Nima Rezaei
Network of Interdisciplinarity
in Neonates and Infants (NINI),
Universal Scientific Education
and Research Network (USERN),
Tehran, Iran

DEDICATION

This book would not have been possible without the continuous encouragement by my family.

I wish to dedicate it to my daughters, Ariana and Arnika, with the hope that we learn enough from today to make a brighter future for the next generation.

List of Contributors

Ahmed Nugud Al Jalila Children's Specialty Hospital, Dubai, UAE

Alaa Nugud Latifa Women's and Children's Hospital, Dubai Health Authority, Dubai, UAE

Amit Agrawal Department of Pediatrics, Gandhi Medical College & Hamidia Hospital, Bhopal, MP 462030, India

Anju Gupta Department of Pediatrics, Postgraduate Institute of Medical Education and Research, Chandigarh, India

Assmaa Nugud Ras Al Khaimah Medical and Health Sciences University, Ras Al Khaimah, UAE

Ana Luisa Rodríguez-Lozano Immnunology Department, Instituto Nacional de Pediatría, Mexico City, Mexico

Beata Wolska-Kuśnierz Immunology Department, Children's Memorial Health Institute, Av. Dzieci Polskich 20 , 04-730 Warsaw, Poland

Bożena Mikołuć Department of Pediatrics, Rheumatology, Immunology and Metabolic Bone Diseases, Medical University of Bialystok, Waszyngtona 17 Str., 15-274 Bialystok, Poland

Caroline Brand Graduate Program in Health Promotion - University of Santa Cruz do Sul, Santa Cruz do Sul, Rio Grande do Sul, Brazil

Cézane P. Reuter Graduate Program in Health Promotion - University of Santa Cruz do Sul, Santa Cruz do Sul, Rio Grande do Sul, Brazil

Consolato M. Sergi Children's Hospital of Eastern Ontario (CHEO), University of Ottawa 401 Smyth Road Ottawa, ON, K1H8L1 Canada

Donya Alinejhad Department of Pediatric Dentistry, School of Dentistry, Tehran University of Medical Sciences, Tehran, Iran

Edna Morán-Villaseñor Department of Dermatology, National Institute of Pediatrics, Mexico City 04530, Mexico

Fausto Cossu Pediatric Clinic of University, "Antonio Cao" Hospital, Cagliari, Sardinia, Italy

Fernando Santos Division of Pediatric Nephrology. Hospital Universitario Central de Asturias, Oviedo, Asturias, Spain
Department of Medicine, University of Oviedo. Oviedo, Asturias, Spain

Francisco Eduardo Rivas-Larrauri Immnunology Service, Instituto Nacional de Pediatría, México City, México

Guillermo Santos-Simarro Department of Pediatrics, Hospital Universitario La Paz, Madrid, Spain

Heliya Ziaei Network of Immunity in Infection, Malignancy and Autoimmunity (NIIMA), Universal Scientific Education and Research Network (USERN, Tehran, Iran
Maxillofacial Surgery & Implantology & Biomaterial Research foundation, Tehran, Iran

María Teresa García-Romero — Department of Dermatology, National Institute of Pediatrics, Mexico City 04530, Mexico

Nima Rezaei — Network of Interdisciplinarity in Neonates and Infants (NINI), Universal Scientific Education and Research Network (USERN), Tehran, Iran
Research Center for Immunodeficiencies, Pediatrics Center of Excellence, Children's Medical Center, Tehran University of Medical Sciences, Tehran, Iran

Noosha Samieefar — Student Research Committee, School of Medicine, Shahid Beheshti University of Medical Sciences, Tehran, Iran
Network of Interdisciplinarity in Neonates and Infants (NINI), Universal Scientific Education and Research Network (USERN), Tehran, Iran
USERN Office, School of Advanced Technologies in Medicine, Shahid Beheshti University of Medical Sciences, Tehran, Iran

Patricia Morán-Álvarez — Department of Rheumatology, Hospital Universitario Ramón y Cajal, Madrid, Spain

Rajnarayan R. Tiwari — ICMR-National Institute for Research in Environmental Health (NIREH), Bhopal, Madhya Pradesh-462030, India

Ramesh Bhat. Y. — Department of Paediatrics Kasturba Medical College Manipal Academy of Higher Education University Manipal, Karnataka, India

Roya Kelishadi — Child Growth and Development Research Center, Research Institute for Primordial Prevention of Non-Communicable Disease, Isfahan University of Medical Sciences, Isfahan, Iran

Selma Cecilia Scheffler-Mendoza — Immnunology Service, Instituto Nacional de Pediatría, Mexico City, Mexico

Shahrzad Banan — School of Dentistry, Guilan University of Medical Sciences, Rasht, Iran

Shomous Nugud — University of Sharjah, Sharjah, UAE

Shwetha Chiplunkar — Department of Pediatrics, Maidstone and Tunbridge Wells NHS Trust, Kent county ME16 9QQ, United Kingdom

Umesh Pandwar — Department of Pediatrics, Gandhi Medical College & Hamidia Hospital, Bhopal, MP 462030, India

Vikas Dhiman — Department of Environmental Health and Epidemiology, ICMR-National Institute for Research in Environmental Health (NIREH), Bhopal, Madhya Pradesh-462030, India

CHAPTER 1

Introduction of Common Pediatric Diseases

Nima Rezaei[1,2,*] and **Noosha Samieefar**[3,1,4]

[1] *Network of Interdisciplinarity in Neonates and Infants (NINI), Universal Scientific Education and Research Network (USERN), Tehran, Iran*

[2] *Research Center for Immunodeficiencies, Pediatrics Center of Excellence, Children's Medical Center, Tehran University of Medical Sciences, Tehran, Iran*

[3] *Student Research Committee, School of Medicine, Shahid Beheshti University of Medical Sciences, Tehran, Iran*

[4] *USERN Office, School of Advanced Technologies in Medicine, Shahid Beheshti University of Medical Sciences, Tehran, Iran*

Abstract: Pediatric health has improved over the past decades and there is a decline in deaths caused by infectious diseases. Yet, the top three causes of disease in children younger than 10 years in 2019 include neonatal disorders, lower respiratory tract infections, and diarrheal diseases. While in the adolescence age group, the major causes are road injuries, headache disorders, and self-harm. Preterm birth complications, pneumonia, and birth asphyxia are the most leading cause of death in children under five years. While in the five to nine years of age group, injuries, including road traffic injuries, drowning, burns, and falls, are the leading causes of death.

Keywords: Communicable disease, Disease, Epidemiology, Health, Infectious disease, Integrated medicine, Inter-disciplinary, Medicine, Morbidity, Mortality, Multi-disciplinary, Non-Communicable disease, Pediatrics, Pediatrician.

INTRODUCTION

Pediatrics, a branch of clinical medicine that studies the diseases and health conditions associated with infants, children, and adolescents, is not just a profession but solicitude. Children should not be considered tiny adults, and their diseases must be studied and investigated professionally and specifically.

With information explosion and new advances in medical sciences, pediatrics is going to be a set of subspecialties rather than just a specialty.

* **Corresponding author Nima Rezaei:** Research Center for Immunodeficiencies, Children's Medical Center Hospital, Dr. Qarib St, Keshavarz Blvd, Tehran 14194, Iran; Tel: +9821-6692-9234; Fax: +9821-6692-9235; E-mail: rezaei_nima@tums.ac.ir

This emphasizes the need to develop multidisciplinary and inter-disciplinary approaches and researches. Care coordination could be defined as "a patient- and family-centered, assessment-driven, team-based activity designed to meet the needs of children and youth while enhancing the caregiving capabilities of families. Care coordination addresses interrelated medical, social, developmental, behavioral, educational, and financial needs to achieve optimal health and wellness outcomes". The results of such different disciplines coordination are efficient care coordination, cost efficiency, improvement of the team working, better communication with families, and finally better health outcomes [1].

Particularly, the mental health care of children is a neglected part of primary care settings. The integrated care models in multidisciplinary centers with psychiatric consults would result in better mental health outcomes [2].

Another condition in which integrated approaches are critical is the management of severe cases as they usually suffer from comorbidities simultaneously.

However, these integrated models demand a precise schedule and a well-designed set of collaborations. Additionally, all the medical services should not be directed in highly specialized pediatric centers that would reduce the local hospital referrals [3].

In this chapter, firstly, we review the epidemiology and trend of pediatric diseases. Then, a brief review of common pediatric diseases based on the organ involved is provided.

EPIDEMIOLOGY

The health status of children is improving over the years. The burden of diseases among children under 10 years has declined dramatically about 60 percent, during the years 1990-2019. The reason is better management of infectious diseases, mainly lower respiratory tract infections, diarrheal diseases, and meningitis. However, communicable diseases are still a leading cause of morbidity in children accounting for six of the top ten causes of burden in children. The main causes of disease burden in children younger than 10 years in 2019 include neonatal disorders, lower respiratory tract infections, diarrheal diseases, congenital birth defects, malaria, meningitis, dietary iron deficiency, protein-energy malnutrition, whooping cough, STIs (sexually transmitted infections excluding HIV), respectively.

In the 10-24 years age group, which include adolescents, the top ten causes of burden include road injuries, headache disorders, self-harm, depressive disorders, interpersonal violence, anxiety disorders, low back pain, dietary iron deficiency, HIV/AIDS, and diarrheal diseases, respectively [4].

The common causes of death among children could be categorized as follows: 1. Respiratory diseases like pneumonia, whooping cough, *etc*. 2. Gastrointestinal diseases like diarrhea, hepatitis, *etc*. 3. Malnutrition and nutritional disorders 4. Malaria 5. Chronic neurological diseases include hydrocephalus, cerebral palsy, and so on 6. Acute neurological diseases such as meningitis, encephalitis, *etc*. 7. Tuberculosis leading to pulmonary, extra-pulmonary, or disseminated involvements 8. Acute rash and fever/infection like Measles, dengue fever, *etc*. 9. HIV infection 10. Emergencies like bowel obstruction, trauma, poisoning, *etc*. 11. Renal diseases include urinary tract infection, acute renal failure, chronic renal failure, *etc*. 12. Endocrine diseases such as diabetes and thyroid diseases 13. Hematological disorders like anemia, bleeding disorders, *etc*. 14. Heart diseases 15. Cancer 16. Child protection problems like sexual and physical abuse, neglect, homicide, suicide, and so on 17. Low birth weight 18. Prematurity 19. Neonatal infections e cord sepsis, congenital infections (examples include syphilis, malaria, rubella), *etc* 20. Perinatal conditions such as birth asphyxia, respiratory distress syndrome, *etc*. 21. Congenital malformations like malrotations, gastroschisis, imperforate anus, *etc* [5].

Preterm birth complications, pneumonia, birth asphyxia, diarrhea, and malaria are reported to be the top five causes of death in children under five years. While in five to nine years of age group injuries, including road traffic injuries, drowning, burns, and falls, are the leading causes of death [6].

According to the United Nations Inter-agency Group for Child Mortality Estimation (UN IGME) report, 6.2 million deaths in children younger than 15 years were recorded only in 2018. Unfortunately, most of these deaths are from preventable causes, and most are in the youngest group, neonates [7].

Although there have been improvements in declining the death rate, there is much to do. The mortality rate has declined from 76 to 39 per 1000 from 2000 to 2018. Many of these deaths occur in sub-Saharan Africa [6].

PEDIATRIC DISEASES TREND

Overall, with increasing Socio-demographic Index or SDI (an index of social development evaluation), pediatric diseases are shifting from communicable to non-communicable [4]. Now, more attention is attracted to psychological and behavioral morbidities and mental health [8].

However, in low-income countries, infectious and communicable diseases are still life-threatening, especially in children below ten years of age. Malnutrition is another problem they are faced with [9].

In sub-Saharan Africa, around fifty percent of children do not have access to common vaccines like tetanus. In some areas of developing countries, the access rate to vaccination is less than 20 percent [10].

INTEGUMENTARY SYSTEM

In a study of skin diseases surveillance, the three most common causes of pediatric dermatology clinic referral were eczema, bacterial, and fungal infections [11].

Impetigo

Impetigo is a common bacterial skin infection caused by *Staphylococcus aureus* and *Streptococcus pyogenes*. The disease is categorized into Bullous or Non-Bollous forms. The typical key for clinicians that helps the diagnosis is the yellowish crusts surrounded by erythema [12, 13].

Folliculitis

Folliculitis is a superficial staphylococcal infection that results in inflammation of the hair follicles.

Furuncle (Boil)

Furuncle is a deep painful staphylococcal infection in which the adjacent soft tissue is involved, too. The collection of furuncles is named carbuncle [13].

Staphylococcal Scalded Skin Syndrome (SSSS)

SSSS or Ritter disease is a severe skin infection caused by *Staphylococcus aureus* exfoliative toxin. The presentation is erythroderma or bullae followed by diffuse epidermal exfoliation [14].

Molluscum Contagiosum

Molluscum Contagiosum is a viral skin infection caused by a poxvirus. The lesions are papules with a dimple in the center [13].

Rubella

Rubella, also called German measles or three-day measles, is a viral infection characterized by rash and fever. The rashes are spotty, erythematous, and maculopapular. Forchheimer spot is a petechial lesion on the soft palate that develops in 20% of cases [15].

Measles

Measles or Rubeola is caused by a virus of the Paramyxoviridae family. It is a highly contagious viral disease that is characterized by fever and generalized rash. Koplil's spot is a pathognomonic sign [12].

Herpes Simplex

It is a viral infection that results in grouped vesicles. Herpes Simplex Virus (HSV) type one is associated mainly with orofacial involvement, while HSV type 2 causes genital infections [16].

Varicella

Varicella or chickenpox, caused by varicella zoster virus (VZV), is a highly contagious disease. The presentation begins with flu-like symptoms followed by itchy rashes and teardrop vesicles [17].

Hand-Foot-Mouth Syndrome

Hand-Foot-Mouth Disease, mostly caused by a coxsackievirus, is a self-limited viral infection. The symptoms include oral ulcers and blisters, fever, and blisters on extremities [18].

Fifth Disease

Also known as slapped cheek disease or Erythema infectiosum, it is a viral infection characterized by reddish rashes. Human Parvovirus B19 has been identified as the causative agent [19].

Sixth Disease

Exanthem subitum, roseola infantum or Roseola is a viral illness. The causative agent is human herpesvirus 6 (HHV-6) and less frequently human herpesvirus 7 (HHV-7). The skin presentation is maculopapular pink rashes accompanied by high fever [20].

Tinea Capitis

Tinea capitis is a prevalent dermatophytic infection usually caused by *Trichophyton tonsurans* that presents with alopecia [12, 13].

Tinea Versicolor

Tinea Versicolor, caused by *Malassezia furfur*, is another common fungal infection that is characterized by hypo-pigmented macules.

Scabies

Scabies is a common skin infestation. The cause is a mite, the hominis variety of Sarcoptes. Pruritus and the subsequent irritability along with typical lesions in examination (burrows) are the key to diagnosis.

Pediculosis

Pediculosis is an infestation caused by lice, and transmission occurs *via* direct contact. The symptoms start with itching that might lead to secondary lesions like excoriation. The Nits or lice could be visible on the hair or scalp [13].

Sclerema Neonatorum

Sclerema neonatorum is a form of panniculitides that the subcutaneous tissue that becomes hard with wax-like changes. The prognosis is poor, and usually, the pediatrician should suspect a critical underlying health condition [12].

Acne Vulgaris

Acne is a chronic inflammatory skin disease with the involvement of sebaceous glands. The obstruction of the hair follicle results in lesions from comedones, papules, pustules, nodules to cysts [21].

Psoriasis

Psoriasis is a chronic skin condition with typical lesions: scaly erythematous patches resulting from hyperproliferation and inflammation [22].

Dermatitis

Dermatitis with different types is another common pediatric skin disease. Common pediatric types include Atopic, Seborrheic, Irritant Contact Diaper, and Candidal Diaper Dermatitis [12].

Pityriasis Rosea

It is a self-limited skin rash. The eruption begins with a herald patch, a single pink scaly rash that the center is clear. Days or weeks after, it is followed by generalized rashes, which is called the christmas-tree pattern [23].

Erythema Toxicum Neonatorum

Erythema Toxicum Neonatorum is another benign condition described as erythematous macules, papules, and pustules [12].

Erythema Multiforme

It is an acute hypersensitivity reaction in the skin that is triggered by infectious agents or medicines and is self-limited. The skin eruption typical presentation is target lesion (also called iris lesion) [24]. Toxic Epidermal Necrolysis (TEN) and Stevens-Johnson syndrome (SJS) are the severe and life-threatening forms when mucosal involvement is added [25].

Vitiligo

Vitiligo is a skin condition characterized by hypo or depigmented lesions. It is an autoimmune disorder and may be associated with a simultaneous autoimmune disease [13].

Pityriasis Alba

Hypo-pigmented scaly patches that are self-limited [12].

Dermal Melanosis

A congenital pigmented lesion occurs when melanocytes fail to complete their migration from the neural crest to the basal layer of the epidermis [26]. Most of them are found over the lumbosacral area named Mongolian spots [12].

Pyogenic Granuloma

Pyogenic Granuloma, lobular capillary hemangioma, or granuloma telangiectaticum is the reactive proliferation of capillary blood vessels resulting in small round reddish nodules [27].

Port-Wine Stain

Port-Wine Stain or nevus flammeus is one of the most common vascular malformations. It is a birthmark that the name resembles its appearance. The presence indicates the need for evaluation of an associated syndrome or defect [28].

Infantile Hemangioma

Infantile Hemangioma is a benign birthmark, and it is the most common vascular tumor among infants [29].

Nevus Simplex

Nevus Simplex, salmon patches, erythema nuchae, angel's kiss, or stork bite is another vascular birthmark that is formed by the dilation of the capillaries in the dermis [30].

Intertrigo

It is defined as the rashes on skin folds.

Milia

Milia is small yellow or white bump that are usually self-limited with no therapy [12].

Alopecia Areata

Alopecia Areata is a non-scarring type of hair loss, an autoimmune disorder characterized by circumscribed lesions [13].

RESPIRATORY SYSTEM

Respiratory diseases range from acute self-limited conditions like common cold to chronic involvements such as asthma or critical conditions like epiglottitis [31].

Choanal Stenosis (Atresia)

Choanal Stenosis is the congenital narrowing of the back of the nasal cavity connected with the nasopharynx. It is called Choanal Atresia when the connection is totally blocked [32].

Adenoid Hypertrophy

The hypertrophy of the pharyngeal tonsil is called Adenoid Hypertrophy. It leads to obstruction and congestion [33].

Laryngomalacia

Laryngomalacia, the most common cause of stridor in neonates, is the congenital softening of the laryngeal cartilage [34].

Rhinosinusitis

Pediatric Rhinosinusitis is another common health condition associated with the respiratory system that is the inflammation of the paranasal and nasal sinus mucosa. The underlying mechanism could be inflammatory or infectious agents [35].

Epiglottitis

Epiglottitis is inflammation of the epiglottis. The onset is rapid, and it is potentially life-threatening. The tripod positioning (sitting and leaning forward), drooling, dyspnea and tachypnea are the hallmarks for diagnosis [36].

Croup

Croup (Laryngotrachebronchitis) is the infection of the middle respiratory tract mostly caused by parainfluenza viruses. The most important manifestation is respiratory stridor [37].

Bronchiolitis

Bronchiolitis, the leading cause of infant hospitalization, is mostly caused by a viral lower respiratory tract infection. The symptoms include wheezing, dyspnea, and fever, which is usually similar to the common cold. Although it might lead to respiratory failure, the prognosis is good, and the treatment is mainly supportive.

Pneumonia

Pneumonia is defined as the lower respiratory tract infection and is a leading cause of morbidity and mortality among children [37].

Influenza

Influenza is a common respiratory infection that might be self-limited or life-threatening, and it is still a leading cause of mortality and morbidity. Most common symptoms include high fever, headaches, sore throat, diarrhea, runny nose, fatigue, and so on [31].

Asthma

Asthma is a chronic respiratory disease characterized by shortness of breath, cough and wheezing. The underlying etiology is inflammation that results in airway hyper-responsiveness and mucus thickening [37].

Acute Respiratory Distress Syndrome (ARDS)

ARDS is a respiratory failure with sudden onset of lung infiltration. The underlying etiology is inflammation [38].

Transient Tachypnea of the Newborn (TTN)

TTN is a benign and self-limited condition caused by delayed clearance of lung fluid that leads to respiratory distress [39].

Bronchopulmonary Dysplasia (BPD)

It is known as chronic lung disease of premature babies that is the result of a developmental disorder. It leads to a lung airway and vascular dysfunction. BPD is the most common complication among extremely preterm newborns [40].

Meconium Aspiration Syndrome

It is characterized by respiratory distress as the result of aspiration of the amniotic fluid that had been contaminated with the infant's fecal material called meconium [41].

Cystic Fibrosis

It is an autosomal recessive disease that can be life-threatening. Cystic Fibrosis Transmembrane Conductance Regulator (CFTR) gene mutation leads to the dysfunction of the chloride channels of the epithelial cells. The disease has various presentations, mostly respiratory and gastrointestinal symptoms [42].

Pneumothorax and Pneumomediastinum

Pneumothorax occurs when the air leaks to the pleural space. Pneumomediastinum or mediastinal emphysema is the presence of air within the mediastinum [43, 44].

Pleural Effusion

It is defined as excess fluid between two layers of the pleura. The presentation varies from asymptomatic to severe respiratory symptoms [45].

Pulmonary Edema

It is the condition that there is excess fluid in the lungs. The symptoms include cough, dyspnea, and tachypnea [46].

Cor Pulmonale

Cor Pulmonale is the result of right ventricular failure due to increases pulmonary hypertension. It can present with dyspnea or syncope [47].

CARDIAC SYSTEM

Despite many advances in medical science, Cardiovascular diseases are still among the leading cause of morbidity and mortality in children. Congenital Heart Diseases, the first cause of congenital malformations, are one of the most common types of birth defects.

Syncope

Syncope is the sudden and transient loss of consciousness and postural muscle tone resulting from autonomic dysfunction [48].

Arrhythmias

Although abnormal heart rhythm or rate occurs less frequently than in adults, they are critical to consider. Dysrhythmias can be atrial, ventricular, or heart blocks [49, 50].

Heart Failure

Heart Failure is a medical condition that the blood pumped by the heart does not meet the demand [51].

Rheumatic Fever

Acute Rheumatic Fever (ARF) is a cardiac disease sequenced by streptococcal infection through inflammatory, immunological reactions. Patients can further develop rheumatic heart disease [52].

Cardiomyopathies (CM)

It is a chronic heart condition that involves the myocardium. It is a group of different types, and the most frequent subtype is dilated CM [53, 54].

Pericarditis

Pericarditis is defined as the inflammation of the pericardium resulting in pericardial effusion [55].

Atrial Septal Defect (ASD)

ASD is one of the most common congenital cardiac anomalies in children resulting from the interruption in the formation of the septum between the two atria [56].

Endocardial Cushion Defect (ECD)

Also known as Atrioventricular Canal Defect or Atrioventricular Septal Defect is the abnormal endocardial cushion development and the atrioventricular valves [57].

Patent Ductus Arteriosus (PDA)

PDA is a congenital heart disease in which the ductus arteriosus fails to close after birth [58].

Ventricular Septal Defect (VSD)

VSD, the most common congenital heart defect in children, is a developmental defect. The defect occurs in the interventricular septum that makes a shunt between ventricles [59].

Tricuspid Atresia

It is a condition that the tricuspid valve is not formed completely or is absent [60].

Pulmonary or Aortic Stenosis

They are birth defects resulting in pulmonary valve obstruction or narrowing. They can be symptomatic or may present with severe symptoms [61].

Coarctation of the Aorta (COA)

COA is a congenital heart disease in the aorta that becomes narrower than usual. The most common site is the insertion of ductus artreiosus [62].

Tetralogy of Fallot

It is the combination of four structural abnormalities: VSD, pulmonary stenosis, right ventricular hypertrophy, and overriding aorta [63].

CIRCULATORY SYSTEM

Diseases related to the circulatory system consist of a wide spectrum of disorders involving the vascular structure and the hematologic system.

Anemia

Anemia is the lack of adequate normal blood cells. It is classified based on the size and amount of hemoglobin. Iron deficiency anemia is the most common form of pediatric anemia [64].

Hemostatic Diseases

Hemostatic Diseases are disorders characterized by impairment in coagulation. The common homeostatic diseases include hemophilia (A and B), von Willebrand disease, factor V leiden (activated protein c resistance), protein S or C deficiency, plasminogen deficiency, dysfibrinogenemia, antithrombin III deficiency, and vitamin K deficiency [65].

Immune Thrombocytopenia (ITP)

ITP, Autoimmune thrombocytopenic purpura (ATP) or Idiopathic thrombocytopenic purpura, is an immune disease that the number of platelet cells decreases, leading to bruising and bleeding [66].

Vasculitis

Henoch–Schonlein purpura (HSP) and Kawasaki disease (KD) are the commonest pediatric vasculitis [67].

Leukemia

Leukemia is cancer that involves the white blood cells precursors in the bone marrow. Acute Lymphoblastic Leukemia (ALL) is the most frequent form [68].

Lymphoma

Lymphoma, the cancer of lymphoid tissue, is classified as Hodgkin and non-Hodgkin [69].

DIGESTIVE SYSTEM

Gastrointestinal symptoms including diarrhea, constipation, reflux, and abdominal pain are among the most common complaints every physician/pediatrician faces.

Cleft Lip and Palate

Cleft lip and cleft palate, also known as orofacial cleft, can occur simultaneously or separately. They might be a part of a genetic syndrome or isolated finding [70].

Esophageal Atresia (EA) with or without tracheoesophageal fistula (TEF)

It is a congenital malformation of the structure of the esophagus. The continuity between the upper and lower pouches of the esophagus is disturbed, usually with a TEF [71].

Esophageal Reflux

Gastroesophageal Reflux (GER) is defined as the retrograde movement of the stomach content into the esophagus. However, when it becomes persistent and symptomatic, it is called Gastroesophageal Reflux Disease (GERD). Symptoms include regurgitation, cough, abdominal pain (heartburn), and it can lead to the child poor growth [72].

Peptic Ulcer Disease

It is defined as the sore or injury by acid secretion in the stomach or duodenum [73].

Gastrointestinal Bleeding (GIB)

GIB is a pediatric medical emergency. The parents could complain the presence of blood either in the emesis or stool of their child [74].

Pyloric Stenosis

Infantile hypertrophic pyloric stenosis (IHPS) is an acquired condition as the result of pylorus hypertrophy. The key presentation is forceful vomiting [75].

Intestinal Atresia

It is a congenital disease of the intestine that is partially or completely blocked [76].

Intestinal Obstruction (IO)

The partial or total blockage of the intestine, presenting with acute abdomen, is a surgical emergency [77].

Malrotation

Malrotation is an abnormally developed intestine when the rotation during fetal life is incomplete [76].

Meckel Diverticulum

It is a congenital defect in the gastrointestinal tract. It is a true diverticulum, an outpouching in the distal ileum [78].

Infantile Colic

Infantile colic is defined as a benign condition that the infant cry more than three hours of the day for more than three days of the week. Rome IV criteria define it as "recurrent and prolonged periods of infant crying, fussing or irritability reported by caregivers that occur without obvious cause and cannot be prevented or resolved" [79].

Gastroenteritis

Gastroenteritis is referred to the inflammation of the stomach and the intestine that results in diarrhea and emesis. It can be due to viral, bacterial, or parasitic infection [80].

Irritable Bowel Syndrome (IBS)

IBS in children usually manifests as abdominal pain and changes in bowel habits. The pediatrician cannot find any anatomical or para-clinical abnormalities in these patients [81].

Inflammatory Bowel Disease (IBD)

IBD is a chronic condition usually classified as Ulcerative Colitis (UC) and Crohn's Disease (CD). The most important clinical manifestations are abdominal pain, weight loss, fever, and rectal bleeding. UC involves the colon, while in CD, the perianal, ileal, and other parts of the gastrointestinal tract involvement occur, too. Strictures, skip lesions, Granulomas, and fistula are also frequent in CD [82, 83].

Intussusception

It is a medical condition in which a segment of the intestine folds into the section downstream, presenting with crampy abdominal pain [84].

Celiac Disease

It is an immunological disease that the gluten ingestion leads to damage in the small intestine [85].

Lactose Intolerance

Lactose is the main carbohydrate of dairy products. Lactose malabsorption or intolerance is the inability to digest lactose due to the lactase enzyme insufficiency [86].

Hirschsprung Disease (HSCR)

HSCR, also known as congenital aganglionic megacolon, is the congenital absence of ganglion cells in the intestine [87].

Constipation

Constipation is described by the North American Society of Gastroenterology, Hepatology, and Nutrition (NASPGHAN), as "a delay or difficulty in defecation, present for 2 weeks or more, and sufficient to cause significant distress to the patient" [88].

Encopresis

Encopresis is defined as the "repeated, voluntary or involuntary passage of feces, usually of normal or near-normal consistency, in places not appropriate for that purpose in the individual's own socio-cultural setting", by the International Classification of Diseases, 10th revision [89].

Imperforate Anus

Imperforate Anus is an anorectal malformation in which the anus has developed incompletely [90].

Gastroschisis

Gastroschisis is a serious abdominal wall defect in which the intestine is herniated and is free [91].

Omphalocele

Omphalocele or exomphalos is a congenital defect in the abdominal wall where the intestine is protruded through the umbilicus. However, the intestine is covered with peritoneum or amniotic membrane [92].

Cholestasis

It is a liver disease that the flow of bile is reduced, characterized by hyperbilirubinemia [93].

Hepatitis

It is the inflammatory condition of the liver, commonly caused by viral infections [94].

Wilson Disease

It is a genetic disorder that excess copper is stored in the liver and other tissues [95].

Pancreatitis

The inflammatory involvement and injury of the pancreas, Pancreatitis, is classified as Acute Pancreatitis (AP), Acute Recurrent Pancreatitis (ARP), and Chronic Pancreatitis (CP) [96].

Peritonitis

Peritonitis is referred to the inflammation of the peritoneum, usually caused by infections [97].

Appendicitis

It is the most common surgical emergency in children and presents with acute abdominal pain [98].

ENDOCRINE SYSTEM

Endocrine and metabolic disorders are among the major health problems of childhood referral to pediatricians. Growth retardation, precocious puberty, diabetes and obesity are among these disorders that can affect the future of a child's health.

Pubertal Delay

It is defined as the latency in the expected time of sexual development. In girls, the time for puberty is 8 to 13 years, while in boys, 9 to 14 years is considered [99].

Precocious Puberty

Precocious Puberty is referred to as the sexual maturation before the age of 8 years in girls and 9 years in boys [100].

Diabetes Mellitus (DM)

DM is a metabolic disease that the body is not able to use glucose properly. In childhood, DM type one is more frequent, which is an autoimmune disorder in which insulin production is impaired. However, with increasing obesity, the incidence of diabetes type II is also increasing, a type of DM in which the insulin receptor sensitivity is decreased.

Diabetic Ketoacidosis (DKA) is a medical emergency and complication of DM type one [101, 102].

Hypothyroidism

Hypothyroidism is defined as thyroid hormone deficiency. It can be due to thyroid gland insufficiency, which is called primary hypothyroidism. Secondary hypothyroidism is the condition of the pituitary gland that is responsible for the reduced thyroid hormone. When the pathology is in the hypothalamus, tertiary hypothyroidism occurs.

Congenital hypothyroidism is a preventable cause of mental retardation that defects the thyroid gland developmen.

Iodine deficiency also can cause acquired hypothyroidism named endemic cretinism [103, 104].

Autoimmune Thyroiditis (AIT)

AIT is an immunologic thyroid disorder that manifests as primary hypothyroidism.

Hashimoto's thyroiditis, also known as chronic lymphocytic thyroiditis, is the goitrous type that causes acquired hypothyroidism. The non-goitrous type is named atrophic thyroiditis or primary myxedema [105].

Hyperthyroidism

Most cases of hyperthyroidism in children are diagnosed with Grave's disease. Grave's disease, also called toxic diffuse goiter, is an autoimmune disease that autoantibodies called Thyroid Stimulating Immunoglobulin (TSI) against receptor for Thyroid-Stimulating Hormone (TSH) are the underlying mechanisms.

Congenital hyperthyroidism is the state that the maternal TSI that crosses the placenta in mothers with Grave's disease [106, 107].

Primary Adrenal Insufficiency (PAI)

Most cases of PAI are diagnosed with Addison's Disease. Addison's Disease is an autoimmune acquired PAI that results in hypo-cortisolism.

Congenital Adrenal Hyperplasia (CAH) is another type of PAI, a group of genetic disorders with the autosomal recessive inheritance that cortisol production is impaired. 21-hydroxylase deficiency is the most common form [108, 109].

Cushing Syndrome

Cushing Syndrome is the state of hypercortisolism. The source of excess cortisol could be endogenous or exogenous. It is called Cushing disease when the source is a micro-adenoma in the pituitary gland [110].

Metabolic Disorders

Inborn errors of metabolism (IEMs) are not among common pediatric disorders. They are genetic disorders that an enzyme dysfunction leads to impaired proteins, fats and carbohydrates metabolism or affects an organelle function [111].

SKELETAL SYSTEM

The normal function of the skeletal system guarantees normal gait and activity in a child. However, as children's bones are more elastic, they are prone to various problems. Skeletal problems can range from infections affecting bones and joints to structural problems such as scoliosis and different malignancies of childhood

Osteomyelitis (OM)

It is defined as the infection of bone [112].

Septic Arthritis

Septic Arthritis, joint infection, or infectious arthritis, is a critical condition and is referred to as the bacterial infection of joints [113].

Juvenile Idiopathic Arthritis (JIA)

JIA is the most common pediatric rheumatologic disease. It typically presents with joint inflammation, although life-threatening complications like macrophage activation syndrome may occur, too [114].

Scaphoid Fracture

It is the most frequent carpal fracture in pediatrics [115].

Nurse Maid's Elbow

Nurse Maid's Elbow is the radial head subluxation [116].

Glenohumeral Dislocation

Glenohumeral Dislocation is more prevalent in adolescents and usually happens anteriorly [117].

Little Leaguer's Shoulder

Proximal humeral epiphysiolysis is stress injury or fracture of the epiphyseal cartilage of the proximal humerus [118].

Metatarsus Adductus

Also called metatarsus varus, is a common foot deformity that metatarsal bones that turn inward [119].

Hypermobile Planus

Flatfoot or pes planus is a medical condition as the result of ligaments laxity. Flatfoot could be flexible (hypermobile) or secondary. Hypermobile Planus or Flexible Flatfoot makes no limitation in daily activities [120].

Cavus Foot

Cavus Foot or Pes Cavus is when the medial longitudinal arch of the foot is raised [121].

Talipes Equiovarus (TEV)

TEV also known as Clubfoot Deformity, is the foot deformity in which the foot points downward and inward [122].

Curly Deformity

Curly, underlapping or varus toe is caused by the contracture of the flexor digitorum longus and flexor digitorum brevis tendons [123].

Sever Disease

Calcaneal apophysitis is the common cause of inflammation and pain of heel [124].

Toddler's Fracture

Toddler's Fracture is the oblique non-displaced fracture in the distal part of the tibia [125].

Angular Variation (Genu Varum and Valgum)

Genu varum or bowlegs is the condition that the legs curve outward. Genu valgum or knock knees is the opposite [126].

Osteochondritis Dissecans

It is a condition that a small segment of the bone besides the articular cartilage separates from the surrounding area due to vascular deprivation [127].

Baker Cyst

A fluid-filled cyst, also called a popliteal cyst, develops at the back of the knee [128].

Osgood-Schlatter Disease (OSD)

It is a self-limiting condition, the inflammation in the insertion part of the patellar tendon on the tibial tuberosity [129].

Patellofemoral Pain Syndrome (PFPS)

PFPS or Idiopathic Anterior Knee Pain is common among adolescents. The pain increases with knee activity [130].

Developmental Dislocation of the Hip (DDH)

It is a spectrum of structural abnormalities that congenital dislocation of the hip occurs [131].

Leg-Length Discrepancy (LLD)

LLD is the result of femur or tibia differences. It affects the gait and posture of the patient [132].

Torsional Variation (In-toeing and Out-toeing)

Out-toeing is an outward twist to the leg, while in-toeing is the opposite [133].

Legg-Calve-Perthes Disease (LCPD)

LCPD involves the hip joint with idiopathic avascular necrosis in the proximal femoral head [134].

Slipped Capital Femoral Epiphysis (SCFE)

The slippage of the proximal femoral growth plate is an orthopedic emergency. SCFE is one of the important differential diagnoses to be considered in patients presenting with hip pain [135].

Transient Synovitis

Transient Synovitis, a common cause of acute hip pain, is a self-limited inflammatory condition of the hip synovium [136].

Scoliosis

Scoliosis is the abnormal sideways curve of the spine [137].

Kyphosis

Kyphosis is an abnormal forward rounding of the spine [138].

Torticollis

Wryneck is a dystonic condition in the neck tilts [139].

Diskitis

Diskitis is the inflammation of the intervertebral discs of the spine [140].

Salter Harris Fracture

Salter Harris Fracture is the physeal fracture and injury in the growth plate [141].

Osteoid Osteoma

It is a benign bone tumor. One specific finding that helps in diagnosis is that the pain is relieved by Non-Steroidal Anti-Inflammatory Drugs (NSAIDs) like aspirin [142].

Osteochondroma

Osteochondroma, also called osteocartilaginous exostosis or cartilage-capped exostosis is a benign tumor of the bone resulting from cartilage overgrowth [143].

Sarcoma

Sarcoma is a malignant tumor arising from soft tissue or bone [144].

NERVOUS SYSTEM

Nervous system diseases can affect the central or peripheral nervous system. Normal neurological function is a very important factor affecting a child's normal life and development. Neurological problems include numerous diagnoses ranging from migraines and other headaches to syncope, epileptic syndromes, sleep disorders, movement disorders, motor neuron disorders, and even neurometabolic disorders.

Stroke

Stroke is an ischemic cerebrovascular disease. Although uncommon, it is a critical condition [145].

Seizures

Seizure is a brain condition resulting from abnormal brain neurological activity [146].

Tension Headache

Headache is a commonest neurologic disorder. Tension Headaches are a mild type with no associated symptom.

Migraine

Migraine is a recurrent headache characterized by pounding pain and associated symptoms like vomiting or aura [147, 148].

Meningitis

Meningitis is the inflammation of the meningeal membrane [149].

Encephalitis

Encephalitis is defined as the inflammation of the brain [150].

Transverse Myelitis

Transverse Myelitis is the acute demyelinating inflammation of the spinal cord usually following an infection [151].

Spinal Muscular Atrophy (SMA)

SMA is an inherited disease that affects the anterior horn of the spinal cord [152].

Guillian-Barre Syndrome

It is an autoimmune post-infectious disease that causes inflammation in the peripheral nervous system [153].

Myasthenia Gravis

Myasthenia Gravis is a neuromuscular autoimmune disease. Antibodies block the nicotinic acetylcholine receptor (AChR) at the neuromuscular junction [154].

Duchenne Muscular Dystrophy

It is an X-linked disorder that the muscle tissue replaces with fibrotic tissue [155].

Pseudotumor Cerebri

It is also known as idiopathic intracranial hypertension, a condition in which the intracranial pressures increases [156].

Spina Bifida

It is a birth defect that the vertebral column is not closed properly. Myelomeningocele is the severe type in which the spinal cord and meninges protrude [157].

Holoprosencephaly (HPE)

HPE is the failure of the prosencephalon, and the hemispheres do not develop completely [158].

Hydrocephalus

It is the condition of excess Cerebrospinal Fluid (CSF) in the brain [159].

Neuroblastoma (NB)

It is the cancer of nerve tissue and the most common solid tumor of infancy [160].

GENITOURINARY SYSTEM

Dysfunction of the urogenital system and kidneys can interfere greatly with a child's normal living. These problems can affect a child from the very early stages of life till later in childhood or adolescence. Among these problems, nephrotic and nephritic syndromes, hypospadias, torsions, refluxes, *etc.*, can be named.

Hypertension

The increased blood pressure can be essential (primary) or secondary. The high prevalence of obesity has made essential hypertension more frequent [161].

Acute Renal Failure (AKI)

AKI is the condition in which a sudden reduction in renal function happens. It is classified to pre-renal (renal hypoperfusion), renal (intrinsic kidney injury) and post-renal (obstruction distal to the kidney) [162].

Chronic Renal Failure

A chronic condition in which the kidney's ability to filter waste and fluid from the blood decreases [163].

Nephrotic Syndrome

Nephrotic syndrome is diagnosed by heavy proteinuria, hypoalbuminemia, hypercholesterolemia and edema. Nephritic syndrome is characterized by hematuria and proteinuria [164].

Glomerulonephritis (GN)

GN is a group of kidney diseases that injury to Glumeruli occurs. Acute Post Streptococcal Glomerulonephritis (APSGN) is common in children that happens after a sore throat [165].

Hemolytic Uremic Syndrome (HUS)

HUS is a triad of non-immune microangiopathic hemolytic anemia, thrombocytopenia and AKI [166].

Vesicoureteral Reflux (VUR)

VUR is the backward return of urine from the bladder that might result in kidney scarring [167].

Nephrolithiasis

Nephrolithiasis or kidney stones is becoming more frequent. The presentation could be flank or abdominal pain and nausea/vomiting [168].

Wilms Tumor

Also known as nephroblastoma, it is kidney cancer and the most common one [169].

Undescended Testes (UDT)

Undescended testicle or cryptorchidism is the condition that the testicle has not moved down to its accurate position [170].

Testicular Torsion

It is a urology emergency when the spermatic cord twists and cuts off the testicle blood supply [171].

Epididymitis

It is the inflammation of the epididymis that presents with scrotal pain and might be associated with urinary symptoms [172].

Posterior Urethral Valve (PUV)

PUV or Congenital Obstructing Posterior Urethral Membranes (COPUM) is a developmental abnormality that there is an obstructing membrane in the posterior urethra [173].

Chordee

Chordee is the congenital abnormality of the penile curvature [174].

Paraphimosis

It is the condition in which foreskin of the penis (prepuce) becomes trapped behind the coronal sulcus [175].

Phimosis

Phimosis is the inability to pull back the prepuce [176].

Hypospadias

Hypospadias is a condition when the opening of the urethral meatus is located ventrally [177].

Labial Fusion

Labial adhesions, labial agglutination or labial fusion is the adhesion of labia minora. The patient may present with urinary tract infection or urinary symptoms like irritation or dribbling.

Vulvovaginitis

It is the inflammation of the vulva and vagina. Symptoms include discharge, tenderness, pruritus, vulvar irritation, or burning on urination.

Lichen Sclerosus

It is a chronic skin disease of genitalia. Patients develop itchy white patches]

IMMUNE SYSTEM

An intact immune system protects a child from being infected with the pathogens they encounter every day. When a part of the immune system fails to maintain its normal function and the normal baseline immune response is altered, various infections and problems are expected to be seen. In general, the most common immunological defects leading to infections include phagocyte defect, humoral defect, and combined defect. Alterations in the immune response can also manifest as autoimmune disorders or hyperactive responses and allergies

Autoimmune Disorders

Autoimmune diseases are abnormal immune responses to intrinsic antigens. Common autoimmune diseases among children are Systemic lupus erythematosus (SLE), celiac disease, ankylosing spondylitis, graves' disease, type one diabetes, juvenile idiopathic arthritis, crohn's disease, ulcerative colitis, multiple sclerosis, scleroderma, idiopathic thrombocytopenic purpura, and behcet's disease [179].

Allergies

Allergies are the results of immune system hyperresponsiveness. Common types among children are asthma, food allergy, allergic rhinitis (also known as hay fever), atopic dermatitis, urticaria, angioedema, anaphylaxis, serum sickness, adverse drug reaction, *etc* [180].

Immunodeficiencies

Immunodeficiencies are groups of diseases that the immune system function is impaired, so the patient is susceptible to infections. They are classified into primary and secondary (acquired). Primary Immunodeficiencies are results of B-cells, T cells, neutrophil, or complement defects. Each results in susceptibility in different micro-organisms infections [181, 182].

CONCLUSION

During the past years, the pattern of pediatric diseases has changed. Socioeconomic improvement, immunization and antibiotics, are leading to the reduction of communicable diseases burden. However, in developing countries due to limited resources, infectious diseases are still a great problem and a major cause of morbidity and mortality. The major health problems requiring more attention now are non-communicable diseases, chronic illnesses, mental health disorders, and injuries.

New advances in pediatric knowledge with developing transdisciplinary cooperation would help overcome the health problems and challenges.

CONSENT FOR PUBLICATION

Not applicable.

CONFLICT OF INTEREST

The authors declare no conflict of interest, financial or otherwise.

ACKNOWLEDGEMENT

Declared none.

REFERENCES

[1]   Antonelli RC, McAllister JW, Popp J. Making care coordination a critical component of the pediatric health system: a multidisciplinary framework 2009.

[2]   Burkhart K, Asogwa K, Muzaffar N, Gabriel M. Pediatric integrated care models: a systematic review. Clin Pediatr (Phila) 2020; 59(2): 148-53.
[http://dx.doi.org/10.1177/0009922819890004] [PMID: 31762297]

[3]   Ehrich JH, Kerbl R, Pettoello-Mantovani M, Lenton S. Opening the debate on pediatric subspecialties and specialist centers: opportunities for better care or risks of care fragmentation? The Journal of Pediatrics 2015; 167(5): 1177-8. e2.
[http://dx.doi.org/10.1016/j.jpeds.2015.07.060]

[4]   Vos T, Lim SS, Abbafati C, *et al.* Global burden of 369 diseases and injuries in 204 countries and territories, 1990-2019: a systematic analysis for the Global Burden of Disease Study 2019. Lancet 2020; 396(10258): 1204-22.

[http://dx.doi.org/10.1016/S0140-6736(20)30925-9] [PMID: 33069326]

[5]   World Health Organization https://www.who.int/ maternal_child_adolescent/documents /improving-maternal-newborn-care-quality/en2016.

[6]   World Health Organization https://www.who.int/data/maternal-newborn-child-adolescent-ageing /child-data/child---mortality-causes-of-death

[7]   World Health Organization https://www.who.int/maternal_child_ adolescent/documents/levels_trends _child_mortality_2019/en/

[8]   Robert M. Kliegman JSG Overview of Pediatrics Nelson Textbook of Pediatrics. Elsevier 2020.

[9]   World Health Organization https://www.who.int/teams/maternal-newborn-child-adolescent-health-and-ageing/child-health/integrated-management-of-childhood-illness/

[10]   World Health Organization. https://www.who.int/news/item/20-11-2002-low-investment-in -immunization-and-vaccines-threatens-global-health

[11]   Kelbore AG, Owiti P, Reid AJ, Bogino EA, Wondewosen L, Dessu BK. Pattern of skin diseases in children attending a dermatology clinic in a referral hospital in Wolaita Sodo, southern Ethiopia. BMC Dermatol 2019; 19(1): 5.
[http://dx.doi.org/10.1186/s12895-019-0085-5] [PMID: 30961561]

[12]   Anand P, Dhyani A. Common Skin Diseases in Pediatric Practice

[13]   Sethuraman G, Bhari N. Common skin problems in children. Indian J Pediatr 2014; 81(4): 381-90.
[http://dx.doi.org/10.1007/s12098-013-1271-9] [PMID: 24362956]

[14]   Leung AKC, Barankin B, Leong KF. Staphylococcal-scalded skin syndrome: evaluation, diagnosis, and management. World J Pediatr 2018; 14(2): 116-20.
[http://dx.doi.org/10.1007/s12519-018-0150-x] [PMID: 29508362]

[15]   Leung AKC, Hon KL, Leong KF. Rubella (German measles) revisited. Hong Kong Med J 2019; 25(2): 134-41.
[PMID: 30967519]

[16]   Thappa DM. Common skin problems. Indian J Pediatr 2002; 69(8): 701-6.
[http://dx.doi.org/10.1007/BF02722708] [PMID: 12356223]

[17]   Heininger U, Seward JF. Varicella. Lancet 2006; 368(9544): 1365-76.
[http://dx.doi.org/10.1016/S0140-6736(06)69561-5] [PMID: 17046469]

[18]   Repass GL, Palmer WC, Stancampiano FF. Hand, foot, and mouth disease: identifying and managing an acute viral syndrome. Cleve Clin J Med 2014; 81(9): 537-43.
[http://dx.doi.org/10.3949/ccjm.81a.13132] [PMID: 25183845]

[19]   Allmon A, Deane K, Martin KL. Common skin rashes in children. Am Fam Physician 2015; 92(3): 211-6.
[PMID: 26280141]

[20]   Mullins TB, Krishnamurthy K. Roseola Infantum (Exanthema Subitum, Sixth Disease). StatPearls 2020. [Internet]

[21]   Zaenglein AL. Acne Vulgaris. N Engl J Med 2018; 379(14): 1343-52.
[http://dx.doi.org/10.1056/NEJMcp1702493] [PMID: 30281982]

[22]   Napolitano M, Megna M, Balato A, *et al.* Systemic treatment of pediatric psoriasis: a review. Dermatol Ther (Heidelb) 2016; 6(2): 125-42.
[http://dx.doi.org/10.1007/s13555-016-0117-6] [PMID: 27085539]

[23]   Urbina F, Das A, Sudy E. Clinical variants of pityriasis rosea. World J Clin Cases 2017; 5(6): 203-11.
[http://dx.doi.org/10.12998/wjcc.v5.i6.203] [PMID: 28685133]

[24]   Lamoreux MR, Sternbach MR, Hsu WT. Erythema multiforme. Am Fam Physician 2006; 74(11):

1883-8.
[PMID: 17168345]

[25]   Daniel BS, Wheeler LR, Murrell DF. Erythema Multiforme, Stevens–Johnson Syndrome and Toxic Epidermal Necrolysis. Harper's Textbook of Pediatric Dermatology 2019; pp. 777-84.
[http://dx.doi.org/10.1002/9781119142812.ch66]

[26]   Stanford DG, Georgouras KE. Dermal melanocytosis: a clinical spectrum. Australas J Dermatol 1996; 37(1): 19-25.
[http://dx.doi.org/10.1111/j.1440-0960.1996.tb00989.x] [PMID: 8936066]

[27]   Pagliai KA, Cohen BA. Pyogenic granuloma in children. Pediatr Dermatol 2004; 21(1): 10-3.
[http://dx.doi.org/10.1111/j.0736-8046.2004.21102.x] [PMID: 14871318]

[28]   Updyke KM, Khachemoune A. Port-Wine Stains: A Focused Review on Their Management. J Drugs Dermatol 2017; 16(11): 1145-51.
[PMID: 29141064]

[29]   Leung AK, Lam JM, Leong KF, Hon KL. Infantile Hemangioma: An Updated Review. Curr Pediatr Rev 2020.
[PMID: 32384034]

[30]   Rozas-Muñoz E, Frieden IJ, Roé E, Puig L, Baselga E. Vascular stains: proposal for a clinical classification to improve diagnosis and management. Pediatr Dermatol 2016; 33(6): 570-84.
[http://dx.doi.org/10.1111/pde.12939] [PMID: 27456075]

[31]   Doyle JD, Campbell AP. Pediatric influenza and illness severity: what is known and what questions remain? Curr Opin Pediatr 2019; 31(1): 119-26.
[http://dx.doi.org/10.1097/MOP.0000000000000721] [PMID: 30531402]

[32]   Kurosaka H. Choanal atresia and stenosis: Development and diseases of the nasal cavity. Wiley Interdiscip Rev Dev Biol 2019; 8(1)e336
[http://dx.doi.org/10.1002/wdev.336] [PMID: 30320458]

[33]   Pereira L, Monyror J, Almeida FT, *et al.* Prevalence of adenoid hypertrophy: A systematic review and meta-analysis. Sleep Med Rev 2018; 38: 101-12.
[http://dx.doi.org/10.1016/j.smrv.2017.06.001] [PMID: 29153763]

[34]   Bedwell J, Zalzal G, Eds. Laryngomalacia Seminars in Pediatric Surgery. Elsevier 2016.

[35]   Badr DT, Gaffin JM, Phipatanakul W. Pediatric Rhinosinusitis. Curr Treat Options Allergy 2016; 3(3): 268-81.
[http://dx.doi.org/10.1007/s40521-016-0096-y] [PMID: 28042527]

[36]   Stroud RH, Friedman NR. An update on inflammatory disorders of the pediatric airway: epiglottitis, croup, and tracheitis. Am J Otolaryngol 2001; 22(4): 268-75.
[http://dx.doi.org/10.1053/ajot.2001.24825] [PMID: 11464324]

[37]   Choi J, Lee GL. Common pediatric respiratory emergencies. Emerg Med Clin North Am 2012; 30(2): 529-563, x.
[http://dx.doi.org/10.1016/j.emc.2011.10.009] [PMID: 22487117]

[38]   Shankar-Hari M, Fan E, Ferguson ND. Acute respiratory distress syndrome (ARDS) phenotyping. Intensive Care Med 2019; 45(4): 516-9.
[http://dx.doi.org/10.1007/s00134-018-5480-6] [PMID: 30519902]

[39]   Alhassen Z, Vali P, Guglani L, Lakshminrusimha S, Ryan RM. Recent advances in pathophysiology and management of transient tachypnea of newborn. J Perinatol 2020; •••: 1-11.
[PMID: 32753712]

[40]   Thébaud B, Goss KN, Laughon M, *et al.* Bronchopulmonary dysplasia. Nat Rev Dis Primers 2019; 5(1): 78.
[http://dx.doi.org/10.1038/s41572-019-0127-7] [PMID: 31727986]

[41]   Haakonsen Lindenskov PH, Castellheim A, Saugstad OD, Mollnes TE. Meconium aspiration syndrome: possible pathophysiological mechanisms and future potential therapies. Neonatology 2015; 107(3): 225-30.
[http://dx.doi.org/10.1159/000369373] [PMID: 25721501]

[42]   Farrell PM, White TB, Ren CL, Hempstead SE, Accurso F, Derichs N, *et al.* Diagnosis of cystic fibrosis: consensus guidelines from the Cystic Fibrosis Foundation. The Journal of pediatrics 2017; 181:S4-S15 e1.
[http://dx.doi.org/10.1016/j.jpeds.2016.09.064]

[43]   Imran JB, Eastman AL. Pneumothorax. JAMA 2017; 318(10): 974.
[http://dx.doi.org/10.1001/jama.2017.10476] [PMID: 28898380]

[44]   Kouritas VK, Papagiannopoulos K, Lazaridis G, *et al.* Pneumomediastinum. J Thorac Dis 2015; 7 (Suppl. 1): S44-9.
[PMID: 25774307]

[45]   Givan DC, Eigen H. Common pleural effusions in children. Clin Chest Med 1998; 19(2): 363-71.
[http://dx.doi.org/10.1016/S0272-5231(05)70083-6] [PMID: 9646987]

[46]   O'Brodovich H. Pulmonary edema in infants and children. Curr Opin Pediatr 2005; 17(3): 381-4.
[http://dx.doi.org/10.1097/01.mop.0000159780.42572.6c] [PMID: 15891430]

[47]   Rashid A, Ivy D. Severe paediatric pulmonary hypertension: new management strategies. Arch Dis Child 2005; 90(1): 92-8.
[http://dx.doi.org/10.1136/adc.2003.048744] [PMID: 15613526]

[48]   Runser LA, Gauer RL, Houser A. Syncope: Evaluation and differential diagnosis. Am Fam Physician 2017; 95(5): 303-12.
[PMID: 28290647]

[49]   Doniger SJ, Sharieff GQ. Pediatric dysrhythmias. Pediatr Clin North Am 2006; 53(1): 85-105, vi.
[http://dx.doi.org/10.1016/j.pcl.2005.10.004] [PMID: 16487786]

[50]   Rohit M, Kasinadhuni G. Management of arrhythmias in pediatric emergency. Indian J Pediatr 2020; 87(4): 295-304.
[http://dx.doi.org/10.1007/s12098-020-03267-2] [PMID: 32166608]

[51]   Hoffman TM. Chronic heart failure. Pediatr Crit Care Med 2016; 17(8) (Suppl. 1): S119-23.
[http://dx.doi.org/10.1097/PCC.0000000000000755] [PMID: 27490589]

[52]   Karthikeyan G, Guilherme L. Acute rheumatic fever. Lancet 2018; 392(10142): 161-74.
[http://dx.doi.org/10.1016/S0140-6736(18)30999-1] [PMID: 30025809]

[53]   Wilkinson JD, Landy DC, Colan SD, *et al.* The pediatric cardiomyopathy registry and heart failure: key results from the first 15 years. Heart Fail Clin 2010; 6(4): 401-413, vii.
[http://dx.doi.org/10.1016/j.hfc.2010.05.002] [PMID: 20869642]

[54]   Elmasry OA, Kamel TB, El-Feki NF. Pediatric cardiomyopathies over the last decade: a retrospective observational epidemiology study in a tertiary institute, Egypt. The Journal Of The Egyptian Public Health Association. 2011; 86: pp. (3 and 4)63-7.1

[55]   Perez-Brandão C, Trigo C, F Pinto F. Pericarditis - Clinical presentation and characteristics of a pediatric population. Rev Port Cardiol 2019; 38(2): 97-101.
[http://dx.doi.org/10.1016/j.repce.2018.05.014] [PMID: 30876791]

[56]   Menillo AM, Lee L, Pearson-Shaver AL. Atrial Septal Defect. ASD 2019.

[57]   Person AD, Klewer SE, Runyan RB. Cell biology of cardiac cushion development. Int Rev Cytol 2005; 243: 287-335.
[http://dx.doi.org/10.1016/S0074-7696(05)43005-3] [PMID: 15797462]

[58]   Gillam-Krakauer M, Reese J. Diagnosis and management of patent ductus arteriosus. Neoreviews

2018; 19(7): e394-402.
[http://dx.doi.org/10.1542/neo.19-7-e394] [PMID: 30505242]

[59]   Dakkak W, Oliver TI. Ventricular septal defect. StatPearls 2020. [Internet]

[60]   Minocha PK, Phoon C. Tricuspid atresia StatPearls. StatPearls Publishing 2020. Internet

[61]   Mack G, Silberbach M. Aortic and pulmonary stenosis. Pediatr Rev 2000; 21(3): 79-85.
[http://dx.doi.org/10.1542/pir.21.3.79] [PMID: 10702320]

[62]   Doshi AR, Chikkabyrappa S. Coarctation of aorta in children. Cureus 2018; 10(12)e3690
[PMID: 30761242]

[63]   Starr JP. Tetralogy of fallot: yesterday and today. World J Surg 2010; 34(4): 658-68.
[http://dx.doi.org/10.1007/s00268-009-0296-8] [PMID: 20091166]

[64]   Khan L. Anemia in Childhood. Pediatr Ann 2018; 47(2): e42-7.
[http://dx.doi.org/10.3928/19382359-20180129-01] [PMID: 29446792]

[65]   Lippi G, Franchini M, Montagnana M, Guidi GC, Eds. Coagulation testing in pediatric patients: the young are not just miniature adults. 2007.

[66]   Kayal L, Jayachandran S, Singh K. Idiopathic thrombocytopenic purpura. Contemp Clin Dent 2014; 5(3): 410-4.
[http://dx.doi.org/10.4103/0976-237X.137976] [PMID: 25191085]

[67]   Barut K, Sahin S, Kasapcopur O. Pediatric vasculitis. Curr Opin Rheumatol 2016; 28(1): 29-38.
[http://dx.doi.org/10.1097/BOR.0000000000000236] [PMID: 26555448]

[68]   Cooper SL, Brown PA. Treatment of pediatric acute lymphoblastic leukemia. Pediatr Clin North Am 2015; 62(1): 61-73.
[http://dx.doi.org/10.1016/j.pcl.2014.09.006] [PMID: 25435112]

[69]   Mauz-Körholz C, Metzger ML, Kelly KM, *et al.* Pediatric hodgkin lymphoma. J Clin Oncol 2015; 33(27): 2975-85.
[http://dx.doi.org/10.1200/JCO.2014.59.4853] [PMID: 26304892]

[70]   Leslie EJ, Marazita ML, Eds. Genetics of cleft lip and cleft palate American Journal of Medical Genetics Part C: Seminars in Medical Genetics. Wiley Online Library 2013.

[71]   Pinheiro PFM, Simões e Silva AC, Pereira RM. Current knowledge on esophageal atresia. World J Gastroenterol 2012; 18(28): 3662-72.
[http://dx.doi.org/10.3748/wjg.v18.i28.3662] [PMID: 22851858]

[72]   Savarino E, de Bortoli N, De Cassan C, *et al.* The natural history of gastro-esophageal reflux disease: a comprehensive review. Dis Esophagus 2017; 30(2): 1-9.
[PMID: 27862680]

[73]   Sierra D, Wood M, Kolli S, Felipez LM. Pediatric gastritis, gastropathy, and peptic ulcer disease 2018.
[http://dx.doi.org/10.1542/pir.2017-0234]

[74]   Scott AT, Shelton J. Gastrointestinal bleeding Pearls and Tricks in Pediatric Surgery. Springer 2020; pp. 227-31.

[75]   Peters B, Oomen MW, Bakx R, Benninga MA. Advances in infantile hypertrophic pyloric stenosis. Expert Rev Gastroenterol Hepatol 2014; 8(5): 533-41.
[http://dx.doi.org/10.1586/17474124.2014.903799] [PMID: 24716658]

[76]   Adams SD, Stanton MP. Malrotation and intestinal atresias. Early Hum Dev 2014; 90(12): 921-5.
[http://dx.doi.org/10.1016/j.earlhumdev.2014.09.017] [PMID: 25448782]

[77]   Shah M, Gallaher J, Msiska N, McLean SE, Charles AG. Pediatric intestinal obstruction in Malawi: characteristics and outcomes. Am J Surg 2016; 211(4): 722-6.
[http://dx.doi.org/10.1016/j.amjsurg.2015.11.024] [PMID: 26810940]

[78]   Lin XK, Huang XZ, Bao XZ, Zheng N, Xia QZ, Chen CD. Clinical characteristics of Meckel diverticulum in children: A retrospective review of a 15-year single-center experience. Medicine (Baltimore) 2017; 96(32)e7760
[http://dx.doi.org/10.1097/MD.0000000000007760] [PMID: 28796070]

[79]   Sung V. Infantile colic. Aust Prescr 2018; 41(4): 105-10.
[http://dx.doi.org/10.18773/austprescr.2018.033] [PMID: 30116077]

[80]   Rivera-Dominguez G, Castano G. Gastroenteritis. Pediatric 2018.

[81]   El-Matary W, Spray C, Sandhu B. Irritable bowel syndrome: the commonest cause of recurrent abdominal pain in children. Eur J Pediatr 2004; 163(10): 584-8.
[http://dx.doi.org/10.1007/s00431-004-1503-0] [PMID: 15290263]

[82]   Conrad MA, Rosh JR. Pediatric inflammatory bowel disease. Pediatr Clin North Am 2017; 64(3): 577-91.
[http://dx.doi.org/10.1016/j.pcl.2017.01.005] [PMID: 28502439]

[83]   Waugh N, Cummins E, Royle P, Kandala N, Shyangdan D, Arasaradnam R, *et al.* Faecal calprotectin testing for differentiating amongst inflammatory and non-inflammatory bowel diseases: systematic review and economic evaluation 2013.
[http://dx.doi.org/10.3310/hta17550]

[84]   Edwards EA, Pigg N, Courtier J, Zapala MA, MacKenzie JD, Phelps AS. Intussusception: past, present and future. Pediatr Radiol 2017; 47(9): 1101-8.
[http://dx.doi.org/10.1007/s00247-017-3878-x] [PMID: 28779197]

[85]   Green PH, Lebwohl B, Greywoode R. Celiac disease. J Allergy Clin Immunol 2015; 135(5): 1099-106.
[http://dx.doi.org/10.1016/j.jaci.2015.01.044] [PMID: 25956012]

[86]   Bayless TM, Brown E, Paige DM. Lactase non-persistence and lactose intolerance. Curr Gastroenterol Rep 2017; 19(5): 23.
[http://dx.doi.org/10.1007/s11894-017-0558-9] [PMID: 28421381]

[87]   Karina SM, Dwihantoro A. Outcomes in patients with Hirschsprung disease following definitive surgery. BMC Res Notes 2018; 11(1): 1-5.
[PMID: 29291749]

[88]   Evaluation and treatment of constipation in children: summary of updated recommendations of the North American Society for Pediatric Gastroenterology, Hepatology and Nutrition. J Pediatr Gastroenterol Nutr 2006; 43(3): 405-7.
[http://dx.doi.org/10.1097/01.mpg.0000232574.41149.0a] [PMID: 16954970]

[89]   Rutter M. Multiaxial classification of child and adolescent psychiatric disorders: the ICD-10 classification of mental and behavioural disorders in children and adolescents. Cambridge University Press 1996.

[90]   Brantberg A, Blaas HG, Haugen SE, Isaksen CV, Eik-Nes SH. Imperforate anus: A relatively common anomaly rarely diagnosed prenatally. Ultrasound Obstet Gynecol 2006; 28(7): 904-10.
[http://dx.doi.org/10.1002/uog.3862] [PMID: 17091530]

[91]   Holland AJ, Walker K, Badawi N. Gastroschisis: an update. Pediatr Surg Int 2010; 26(9): 871-8.
[http://dx.doi.org/10.1007/s00383-010-2679-1] [PMID: 20686898]

[92]   Frolov P, Alali J, Klein MD. Clinical risk factors for gastroschisis and omphalocele in humans: a review of the literature. Pediatr Surg Int 2010; 26(12): 1135-48.
[http://dx.doi.org/10.1007/s00383-010-2701-7] [PMID: 20809116]

[93]   Copple BL, Jaeschke H, Klaassen CD, Eds. Oxidative stress and the pathogenesis of cholestasis. 2010.
[http://dx.doi.org/10.1055/s-0030-1253228]

[94]   Nel E, Sokol RJ, Comparcola D, *et al.* Viral hepatitis in children. J Pediatr Gastroenterol Nutr 2012;

55(5): 500-5.
[http://dx.doi.org/10.1097/MPG.0b013e318272aee7] [PMID: 22983372]

[95] Członkowska A, Litwin T, Dusek P, *et al.* Wilson disease. Nat Rev Dis Primers 2018; 4(1): 21.
[http://dx.doi.org/10.1038/s41572-018-0018-3] [PMID: 30190489]

[96] Pohl JF, Uc A. Paediatric pancreatitis. Curr Opin Gastroenterol 2015; 31(5): 380-6.
[http://dx.doi.org/10.1097/MOG.0000000000000197] [PMID: 26181572]

[97] Ross JT, Matthay MA, Harris HW. Secondary peritonitis: principles of diagnosis and intervention.
BMJ 2018; 361: k1407.
[http://dx.doi.org/10.1136/bmj.k1407] [PMID: 29914871]

[98] Caruso AM, Pane A, Garau R, *et al.* Acute appendicitis in children: not only surgical treatment. J
Pediatr Surg 2017; 52(3): 444-8.
[http://dx.doi.org/10.1016/j.jpedsurg.2016.08.007] [PMID: 27612631]

[99] Tang C, Damian M. Delayed Puberty StatPearls. StatPearls Publishing 2019. Internet

[100] Latronico AC, Brito VN, Carel J-C. Causes, diagnosis, and treatment of central precocious puberty.
Lancet Diabetes Endocrinol 2016; 4(3): 265-74.
[http://dx.doi.org/10.1016/S2213-8587(15)00380-0] [PMID: 26852255]

[101] Bhatt M, Nahari A, Wang P-W, *et al.* The quality of clinical practice guidelines for management of
pediatric type 2 diabetes mellitus: a systematic review using the AGREE II instrument. Syst Rev 2018;
7(1): 193.
[http://dx.doi.org/10.1186/s13643-018-0843-1] [PMID: 30442196]

[102] Lopes CL, Pinheiro PP, Barberena LS, Eckert GU. Diabetic ketoacidosis in a pediatric intensive care
unit. J Pediatr (Rio J) 2017; 93(2): 179-84.
[http://dx.doi.org/10.1016/j.jped.2016.05.008] [PMID: 27770618]

[103] Wassner AJ. Pediatric hypothyroidism: diagnosis and treatment. Paediatr Drugs 2017; 19(4): 291-301.
[http://dx.doi.org/10.1007/s40272-017-0238-0] [PMID: 28534114]

[104] Agrawal P, Philip R, Saran S, *et al.* Congenital hypothyroidism. Indian J Endocrinol Metab 2015;
19(2): 221-7.
[http://dx.doi.org/10.4103/2230-8210.131748] [PMID: 25729683]

[105] Brown RS. Autoimmune thyroiditis in childhood. J Clin Res Pediatr Endocrinol 2013; 5 (Suppl. 1):
45-9.
[PMID: 23154164]

[106] Kaplowitz PB, Vaidyanathan P. Update on pediatric hyperthyroidism. Curr Opin Endocrinol Diabetes
Obes 2020; 27(1): 70-6.
[http://dx.doi.org/10.1097/MED.0000000000000521] [PMID: 31789723]

[107] Kurtoğlu S, Özdemir A. Fetal neonatal hyperthyroidism: diagnostic and therapeutic approachment.
Turkish Archives of Pediatrics/Türk Pediatri Arşivi 2017; 52(1) 1.
[http://dx.doi.org/10.5152/TurkPediatriArs.2017.2513]

[108] Trapp CM, Speiser PW, Oberfield SE. Congenital adrenal hyperplasia: an update in children. Curr
Opin Endocrinol Diabetes Obes 2011; 18(3): 166-70.
[http://dx.doi.org/10.1097/MED.0b013e328346938c] [PMID: 21494138]

[109] Kirkgoz T, Guran T. Primary adrenal insufficiency in children: Diagnosis and management. Best Pract
Res Clin Endocrinol Metab 2018; 32(4): 397-424.
[http://dx.doi.org/10.1016/j.beem.2018.05.010] [PMID: 30086866]

[110] Wagner-Bartak NA, Baiomy A, Habra MA, *et al.* Cushing syndrome: diagnostic workup and imaging
features, with clinical and pathologic correlation. AJR Am J Roentgenol 2017; 209(1): 19-32.
[http://dx.doi.org/10.2214/AJR.16.17290] [PMID: 28639924]

[111] Agana M, Frueh J, Kamboj M, Patel DR, Kanungo S. Common metabolic disorder (inborn errors of

metabolism) concerns in primary care practice. Ann Transl Med 2018; 6(24): 469.
[http://dx.doi.org/10.21037/atm.2018.12.34] [PMID: 30740400]

[112] Castellazzi L, Mantero M, Esposito S. Update on the management of pediatric acute osteomyelitis and septic arthritis. Int J Mol Sci 2016; 17(6): 855.
[http://dx.doi.org/10.3390/ijms17060855] [PMID: 27258258]

[113] Montgomery NI, Epps HR. Pediatric septic arthritis. Orthop Clin North Am 2017; 48(2): 209-16.
[http://dx.doi.org/10.1016/j.ocl.2016.12.008] [PMID: 28336043]

[114] Ravelli A, Schiappapietra B, Verazza S, Martini A. Juvenile idiopathic arthritis The Heart in Rheumatic, Autoimmune and Inflammatory Diseases. Elsevier 2017; pp. 167-87.
[http://dx.doi.org/10.1016/B978-0-12-803267-1.00007-7]

[115] Duckworth AD, Jenkins PJ, Aitken SA, Clement ND, Court-Brown CM, McQueen MM. Scaphoid fracture epidemiology. J Trauma Acute Care Surg 2012; 72(2): E41-5.
[http://dx.doi.org/10.1097/TA.0b013e31822458e8] [PMID: 22439232]

[116] Vitello S, Dvorkin R, Sattler S, Levy D, Ung L. Epidemiology of nursemaid's elbow. West J Emerg Med 2014; 15(4): 554-7.
[http://dx.doi.org/10.5811/westjem.2014.1.20813] [PMID: 25035767]

[117] Franklin CC, Weiss JM. The natural history of pediatric and adolescent shoulder dislocation. J Pediatr Orthop 2019; 39(6,) (Supplement 1 Suppl 1): S50-2.
[http://dx.doi.org/10.1097/BPO.0000000000001374] [PMID: 31169649]

[118] Casadei K, Kiel J. Proximal Humeral Epiphysiolysis (Little League Shoulder) StatPearls. StatPearls Publishing 2020. Internet

[119] Williams CM, James AM, Tran T. Metatarsus adductus: development of a non-surgical treatment pathway. J Paediatr Child Health 2013; 49(9): E428-33.
[http://dx.doi.org/10.1111/jpc.12219] [PMID: 23647850]

[120] Atik A, Ozyurek S. Flexible flatfoot. North Clin Istanb 2014; 1(1): 57-64.
[http://dx.doi.org/10.14744/nci.2014.29292] [PMID: 28058304]

[121] Wicart P. Cavus foot, from neonates to adolescents. Orthop Traumatol Surg Res 2012; 98(7): 813-28.
[http://dx.doi.org/10.1016/j.otsr.2012.09.003] [PMID: 23098772]

[122] Basit S, Khoshhal KI. Genetics of clubfoot; recent progress and future perspectives. Eur J Med Genet 2018; 61(2): 107-13.
[http://dx.doi.org/10.1016/j.ejmg.2017.09.006] [PMID: 28919208]

[123] Choi JY, Park HJ, Suh JS. Operative treatment for fourth curly toe deformity in adults. Foot Ankle Int 2015; 36(9): 1089-94.
[http://dx.doi.org/10.1177/1071100715579758] [PMID: 25857938]

[124] Ramponi DR, Baker C. Sever's Disease (Calcaneal Apophysitis). Adv Emerg Nurs J 2019; 41(1): 10-4.
[http://dx.doi.org/10.1097/TME.0000000000000219] [PMID: 30702528]

[125] Schuh AM, Whitlock KB, Klein EJ. Management of toddler's fractures in the pediatric emergency department. Pediatr Emerg Care 2016; 32(7): 452-4.
[http://dx.doi.org/10.1097/PEC.0000000000000497] [PMID: 26087443]

[126] Qin S, Zheng X, Jiao S, Wang Y, Zang J, Pan Q, *et al.* Genu Varum, Genu Valgum, and Osteoarthritis of Knee Lower Limb Deformities. Springer 2020; pp. 571-624.
[http://dx.doi.org/10.1007/978-981-13-9604-5_14]

[127] Accadbled F, May O, Thévenin-Lemoine C, de Gauzy JS. Slipped capital femoral epiphysis management and the arthroscope. J Child Orthop 2017; 11(2): 128-30.
[http://dx.doi.org/10.1302/1863-2548-11-160281] [PMID: 28529661]

[128] Foris LA, Varacallo M, Maddox JP. Baker Cyst 2019.

[129] Circi E, Atalay Y, Beyzadeoglu T. Treatment of Osgood-Schlatter disease: review of the literature. Musculoskelet Surg 2017; 101(3): 195-200.
[http://dx.doi.org/10.1007/s12306-017-0479-7] [PMID: 28593576]

[130] Rodriguez L. Anterior Knee Pain in Adolescents. Pediatric Orthopedics, An Issue of Physician Assistant Clinics. E-Book 2020; 5(4): 497.

[131] Yang S, Zusman N, Lieberman E, Goldstein RY. Developmental dysplasia of the hip. Pediatrics 2019; 143(1)e20181147
[http://dx.doi.org/10.1542/peds.2018-1147] [PMID: 30587534]

[132] Han J-T. Effect of Induced Leg Length Discrepancy on the Limitation of Stability and Static Postural Balance. PNF and Movement 2018; 16(2): 267-73.

[133] Lerch TD, Eichelberger P, Baur H, *et al.* Prevalence and diagnostic accuracy of in-toeing and out-toeing of the foot for patients with abnormal femoral torsion and femoroacetabular impingement: implications for hip arthroscopy and femoral derotation osteotomy. Bone Joint J 2019; 101-B(10): 1218-29.
[http://dx.doi.org/10.1302/0301-620X.101B10.BJJ-2019-0248.R1] [PMID: 31564157]

[134] Rampal V, Clément J-L, Solla F. Legg-Calvé-Perthes disease: classifications and prognostic factors. Clin Cases Miner Bone Metab 2017; 14(1): 74-82.
[http://dx.doi.org/10.11138/ccmbm/2017.14.1.074] [PMID: 28740529]

[135] Swarup I, Goodbody C, Goto R, Sankar WN, Fabricant PD. Risk factors for contralateral slipped capital femoral epiphysis: a meta-analysis of cohort and case-control studies. J Pediatr Orthop 2020; 40(6): e446-53.
[http://dx.doi.org/10.1097/BPO.0000000000001482] [PMID: 32501913]

[136] Huntley JS. Transient Synovitis The Pediatric and Adolescent Hip. Springer 2019; pp. 327-46.
[http://dx.doi.org/10.1007/978-3-030-12003-0_12]

[137] Pahys JM, Guille JT. What's new in congenital scoliosis? J Pediatr Orthop 2018; 38(3): e172-9.
[http://dx.doi.org/10.1097/BPO.0000000000000922] [PMID: 28009797]

[138] Sheehan DD, Grayhack J. Pediatric Scoliosis and Kyphosis: An Overview of Diagnosis, Management, and Surgical Treatment. Pediatr Ann 2017; 46(12): e472-80.
[http://dx.doi.org/10.3928/19382359-20171113-01] [PMID: 29227524]

[139] Tomczak KK, Rosman NP. Torticollis. J Child Neurol 2013; 28(3): 365-78.
[http://dx.doi.org/10.1177/0883073812469294] [PMID: 23271760]

[140] Ferri I, Ristori G, Lisi C, Galli L, Chiappini E. Characteristics, Management and Outcomes of Spondylodiscitis in Children: A Systematic Review. Antibiotics (Basel) 2020; 10(1): 30.
[http://dx.doi.org/10.3390/antibiotics10010030] [PMID: 33396379]

[141] Cepela DJ, Tartaglione JP, Dooley TP, Patel PN. Classifications In Brief: Salter-Harris Classification of Pediatric Physeal Fractures. Clin Orthop Relat Res 2016; 474(11): 2531-7.
[http://dx.doi.org/10.1007/s11999-016-4891-3] [PMID: 27206505]

[142] Noordin S, Allana S, Hilal K, *et al.* Osteoid osteoma: Contemporary management. Orthop Rev (Pavia) 2018; 10(3): 7496.
[http://dx.doi.org/10.4081/or.2018.7496] [PMID: 30370032]

[143] Tong K, Liu H, Wang X, *et al.* Osteochondroma: Review of 431 patients from one medical institution in South China. J Bone Oncol 2017; 8: 23-9.
[http://dx.doi.org/10.1016/j.jbo.2017.08.002] [PMID: 28932679]

[144] Nacev BA, Jones KB, Intlekofer AM, *et al.* The epigenomics of sarcoma. Nat Rev Cancer 2020; 20(10): 608-23.
[http://dx.doi.org/10.1038/s41568-020-0288-4] [PMID: 32782366]

[145] Ullah S, Bin Ayaz S, Zaheer Qureshi A, Samir Tantawy S, Fe Flandez M. Characteristics and

functional outcomes of pediatric stroke survivors at a rehabilitation unit in Saudi Arabia. J Clin Neurosci 2020; 81: 403-8.
[http://dx.doi.org/10.1016/j.jocn.2020.10.014] [PMID: 33222951]

[146] Stafstrom CE, Carmant L. Seizures and epilepsy: an overview for neuroscientists. Cold Spring Harb Perspect Med 2015; 5(6)a022426
[http://dx.doi.org/10.1101/cshperspect.a022426] [PMID: 26033084]

[147] Kelly M, Strelzik J, Langdon R, DiSabella M. Pediatric headache: overview. Curr Opin Pediatr 2018; 30(6): 748-54.
[http://dx.doi.org/10.1097/MOP.0000000000000688] [PMID: 30157045]

[148] Langdon R, DiSabella MT. Pediatric headache: an overview. Curr Probl Pediatr Adolesc Health Care 2017; 47(3): 44-65.
[http://dx.doi.org/10.1016/j.cppeds.2017.01.002] [PMID: 28366491]

[149] Pick AM, Sweet DC, Begley KJ. A review of pediatric bacterial meningitis. US Pharm 2016; 41(5): 41-5.

[150] Thompson C, Kneen R, Riordan A, Kelly D, Pollard AJ. Encephalitis in children. Arch Dis Child 2012; 97(2): 150-61.
[http://dx.doi.org/10.1136/archdischild-2011-300100] [PMID: 21715390]

[151] Absoud M, Greenberg BM, Lim M, Lotze T, Thomas T, Deiva K. Pediatric transverse myelitis. Neurology 2016; 87(9) (Suppl. 2): S46-52.
[http://dx.doi.org/10.1212/WNL.0000000000002820] [PMID: 27572861]

[152] Kolb SJ, Kissel JT. Spinal muscular atrophy. Neurol Clin 2015; 33(4): 831-46.
[http://dx.doi.org/10.1016/j.ncl.2015.07.004] [PMID: 26515624]

[153] Varkal MA, Uzunhan TA, Aydınlı N, Ekici B, Çalışkan M, Özmen M. Pediatric Guillain-Barré syndrome: Indicators for a severe course. Ann Indian Acad Neurol 2015; 18(1): 24-8.
[PMID: 25745306]

[154] Peragallo JH, Ed. Pediatric myasthenia gravis Seminars in Pediatric Neurology. Elsevier 2017.

[155] Rosenberg AS, Puig M, Nagaraju K, Hoffman EP, Villalta SA, Rao VA, *et al.* Immune-mediated pathology in Duchenne muscular dystrophy. Science translational medicine 2015; 7(299) 299rv4-rv4.
[http://dx.doi.org/10.1126/scitranslmed.aaa7322]

[156] Phillips PH, Sheldon CA. Pediatric pseudotumor cerebri syndrome. J Neuroophthalmol 2017; 37 (Suppl. 1): S33-40.
[http://dx.doi.org/10.1097/WNO.0000000000000548] [PMID: 28806347]

[157] Copp AJ, Adzick NS, Chitty LS, Fletcher JM, Holmbeck GN, Shaw GM. Spina bifida. Nat Rev Dis Primers 2015; 1(1): 15007.
[http://dx.doi.org/10.1038/nrdp.2015.7] [PMID: 27189655]

[158] Dubourg C, Bendavid C, Pasquier L, Henry C, Odent S, David V. Holoprosencephaly. Orphanet J Rare Dis 2007; 2(1): 8.
[http://dx.doi.org/10.1186/1750-1172-2-8] [PMID: 17274816]

[159] Kahle KT, Kulkarni AV, Limbrick DD Jr, Warf BC. Hydrocephalus in children. Lancet 2016; 387(10020): 788-99.
[http://dx.doi.org/10.1016/S0140-6736(15)60694-8] [PMID: 26256071]

[160] Park JR, Eggert A, Caron H. Neuroblastoma: biology, prognosis, and treatment. Pediatr Clin North Am 2008; 55(1): 97-120, x.
[http://dx.doi.org/10.1016/j.pcl.2007.10.014] [PMID: 18242317]

[161] Shatat IF, Brady TM. Editorial: Pediatric Hypertension: Update. Front Pediatr 2018; 6: 209.
[http://dx.doi.org/10.3389/fped.2018.00209] [PMID: 30109219]

[162] Cleto-Yamane TL, Gomes CLR, Suassuna JHR, Nogueira PK. Acute Kidney Injury Epidemiology in

pediatrics. J Bras Nefrol 2019; 41(2): 275-83.
[http://dx.doi.org/10.1590/2175-8239-jbn-2018-0127] [PMID: 30465591]

[163]   Kaspar CD, Bholah R, Bunchman TE. A review of pediatric chronic kidney disease. Blood Purif 2016; 41(1-3): 211-7.
[http://dx.doi.org/10.1159/000441737] [PMID: 26766175]

[164]   Teitelbaum I, Kooienga L. Nephrotic syndrome versus nephritic syndrome CURRENT Diagnosis and Treatment: Nephrology and Hypertension New York. NY: McGraw-Hill 2009; pp. 211-6.

[165]   Rodriguez-Iturbe B, Haas M. Post-streptococcal glomerulonephritis Streptococcus pyogenes: Basic Biology to Clinical Manifestations. University of Oklahoma Health Sciences Center 2016. Internet

[166]   Talarico V, Aloe M, Monzani A, Miniero R, Bona G. Hemolytic uremic syndrome in children. Minerva Pediatr 2016; 68(6): 441-55.
[PMID: 27768015]

[167]   Arlen AM, Cooper CS. Controversies in the management of vesicoureteral reflux. Curr Urol Rep 2015; 16(9): 64.
[http://dx.doi.org/10.1007/s11934-015-0538-2] [PMID: 26199037]

[168]   Miah T, Kamat D. Pediatric nephrolithiasis: a review. Pediatr Ann 2017; 46(6): e242-4.
[http://dx.doi.org/10.3928/19382359-20170517-02] [PMID: 28599030]

[169]   Aldrink JH, Heaton TE, Dasgupta R, *et al.* Update on Wilms tumor. J Pediatr Surg 2019; 54(3): 390-7.
[http://dx.doi.org/10.1016/j.jpedsurg.2018.09.005] [PMID: 30270120]

[170]   Holland AJ, Nassar N, Schneuer FJ. Undescended testes: an update. Curr Opin Pediatr 2016; 28(3): 388-94.
[http://dx.doi.org/10.1097/MOP.0000000000000335] [PMID: 27138807]

[171]   Jacobsen FM, Rudlang TM, Fode M, *et al.* The impact of testicular torsion on testicular function. World J Mens Health 2020; 38(3): 298-307.
[http://dx.doi.org/10.5534/wjmh.190037] [PMID: 31081295]

[172]   McConaghy JR, Panchal B. Epididymitis: An Overview. Am Fam Physician 2016; 94(9): 723-6.
[PMID: 27929243]

[173]   Bingham G, Rentea RM. Posterior Urethral Valve. StatPearls 2020. [Internet]

[174]   Montag S, Palmer LS. Abnormalities of penile curvature: chordee and penile torsion. ScientificWorldJournal 2011; 11: 1470-8.
[http://dx.doi.org/10.1100/tsw.2011.136] [PMID: 21805016]

[175]   Raveenthiran V. Paraphimosis Normal and Abnormal Prepuce. Springer 2020; pp. 181-94.
[http://dx.doi.org/10.1007/978-3-030-37621-5_19]

[176]   Shono T. Phimosis Operative General Surgery in Neonates and Infants. Springer 2016; pp. 343-6.

[177]   Snodgrass WT. Hypospadias Pediatric Urology. Springer 2011; pp. 177-90.
[http://dx.doi.org/10.1007/978-1-60327-420-3_9]

[178]   Eyk NV, Allen L, Giesbrecht E, *et al.* Pediatric vulvovaginal disorders: a diagnostic approach and review of the literature. J Obstet Gynaecol Can 2009; 31(9): 850-62.
[http://dx.doi.org/10.1016/S1701-2163(16)34304-3] [PMID: 19941710]

[179]   McGonagle D, Aziz A, Dickie LJ, McDermott MF. An integrated classification of pediatric inflammatory diseases, based on the concepts of autoinflammation and the immunological disease continuum. Pediatr Res 2009; 65(5 Pt 2): 38R-45R.
[http://dx.doi.org/10.1203/PDR.0b013e31819dbd0a] [PMID: 19190531]

[180]   Genuneit J, Seibold AM, Apfelbacher CJ, *et al.* Overview of systematic reviews in allergy epidemiology. Allergy 2017; 72(6): 849-56.
[http://dx.doi.org/10.1111/all.13123] [PMID: 28052339]

[181] Modell V, Orange JS, Quinn J, Modell F. Global report on primary immunodeficiencies: 2018 update from the Jeffrey Modell Centers Network on disease classification, regional trends, treatment modalities, and physician reported outcomes. Immunol Res 2018; 66(3): 367-80.
[http://dx.doi.org/10.1007/s12026-018-8996-5] [PMID: 29744770]

[182] Bousfiha A, Jeddane L, Picard C, *et al.* Human inborn errors of immunity: 2019 update of the IUIS phenotypical classification. J Clin Immunol 2020; 40(1): 66-81.
[http://dx.doi.org/10.1007/s10875-020-00758-x] [PMID: 32048120]

CHAPTER 2

Updates on Pediatric Rheumatologic Diseases

Anju Gupta[1,*]

[1] *Department of Pediatrics, Postgraduate Institute of Medical Education and Research, Chandigarh, India*

Abstract: Rheumatological disorders pose a challenge to clinicians because of multisystemic involvement, relapsing-remitting course, and nonspecific clinical features, which can mimic infections, malignancies, and even genetic disorders. Common symptoms at presentation are joint pain, fever, weight loss, malaise, muscle weakness, rash, and ulcers. While diseases, such as juvenile idiopathic arthritis, juvenile dermatomyositis, and IgA vasculitis, are relatively easy to diagnose because of typical clinical manifestations, others such as systemic lupus erythematosus, scleroderma, and various vasculitides are much more challenging. No laboratory investigation is diagnostic of a particular rheumatological disorder. Investigations, such as antinuclear antibodies and antineutrophilic cytoplasmic antibodies, are associated with a high false-positive rate and should be used judiciously. Most diseases except for Kawasaki disease and IgA vasculitis are chronic and require long-term immunosuppression for control of disease activity. Long-term prognosis has improved over the past few decades due to better immunosuppressive regimens and better monitoring. With an improvement in mortality rates, many children are living into adulthood and facing issues with persistent disease activity and morbidity related to therapeutic regimens. Future research should focus on finding better therapeutic protocols, which should result in further improvements in survival while simultaneously reducing drug toxicity. There is also an urgent need to define better monitoring tools for most rheumatological conditions.

Keywords: ANCA associated vasculitis, Antiphospholipid syndrome, IgA vasculitis, Juvenile dermatomyositis, Juvenile idiopathic arthritis, Juvenile systemic sclerosis, Kawasaki disease, Localized scleroderma, Macrophage activation syndrome, Neonatal lupus, Polyarteritis nodosa, Rheumatological disorders, Systemic lupus erythematosus, Takayasu arteritis, Uveitis, Vasculitis.

RHEUMATOLOGICAL DISEASES IN CHILDREN

Rheumatological diseases pose a real challenge to physicians because of multiple reasons. Signs and symptoms may either be non-specific like fever, weight loss,

* **Corresponding author Anju Gupta:** Department of Pediatrics, Advanced Pediatrics Centre, Postgraduate Institute of Medical Education and Research, Chandigarh, India; Tel: +91-7087008315; Fax: 91-172-2745078; E-mail: anjupgi@gmail.com

Nima Rezaei and Noosha Samieefar (Eds.)

malaise, rash, and joint pains or may point to any organ system in the body. For this reason, these patients may present to any subspecialty of pediatrics. The differential diagnosis in such settings is wide, ranging from infections, inflammatory conditions, malignancies, and sometimes even genetic disorders.

Common manifestations with which patients are brought to pediatric rheumatological services are joint pain, fever, weight loss, malaise, muscle weakness, rash, and ulcers. This chapter will discuss the differential diagnosis of common rheumatological symptoms before discussing specific rheumatological conditions and their management.

When to Suspect Rheumatologic Disorders

Approach to a Child with Joint Pains

Joint pain is the most common symptom of children presenting to pediatric rheumatology services. Physicians need to be able to answer the following three questions after history and physical examination in children presenting with body pains:

1. Whether the pain is articular or not?
2. If articular,
   a. Is the pain inflammatory or non-inflammatory?
3. In case of inflammatory articular pain
   a. Is the involvement acute or chronic?
   b. The pattern of joint involvement: Number of joints involved, symmetry of involvement, peripheral *vs.* axial involvement, small *vs.* large joint involvement, fixed *vs.* migratory *vs.* additive involvement.
   c. Presence or absence of extra-articular features.

These three questions help in the further differential diagnosis. Pediatric gait, arms, legs, and spine (pGALS) test is a useful screening tool for musculoskeletal examination [1]. Though it is not specific to joint disease, it has been shown to improve musculoskeletal examination skills. Detection of any abnormality in pGALS should be followed by a detailed and focused examination of joints and supporting structures.

Whether the Pain is Articular or Not?

Articular pain tends to occur across joint lines, whereas the location of non-articular pain may vary. Articular pain is usually deep, diffuse, occurs along all planes of movement, and occurs on both passive and active movements (Table 1). Such pain suggests pathology in the synovium, cartilage, and joint capsule.

Table 1. Differences between articular and periarticular pain.

Clinical Feature	Articular Pain	Periarticular Pain
Anatomic structure	Synovium, cartilage, capsule	Tendon, bursa, ligament, muscle, bone
Location of pain	Diffuse, deep	Focal "pin-point"
Pain on movement	Active/passive, in all planes	Active, in a few planes
Swelling	Common	Uncommon; focal if present

On the other hand, periarticular pain is more focal, rather pinpoint, and occurs in few planes. Periarticular pain gets exacerbated with active movements. Such pain is seen due to pathology in tendons, bursa, ligaments, muscles, or bone. Common etiologies are enthesitis, fractures, and osteomyelitis in the metaphyseal region.

Is the Pain Inflammatory or Non-inflammatory?

Inflammatory pain is associated with early morning stiffness and gelling. Early morning stiffness refers to pain and difficulty in moving the joints in the morning on waking up, and it usually tends to last for half an hour or more. Gelling is similar to early morning stiffness but tends to happen after prolonged rest in the daytime. Joint swelling (Fig. **1**) is also indicative of joint inflammation. Redness over the joint is rarely seen except in septic arthritis and reactive arthritis. Warmth and limitation of movement of joints also point to inflammatory causes (Table **2**).

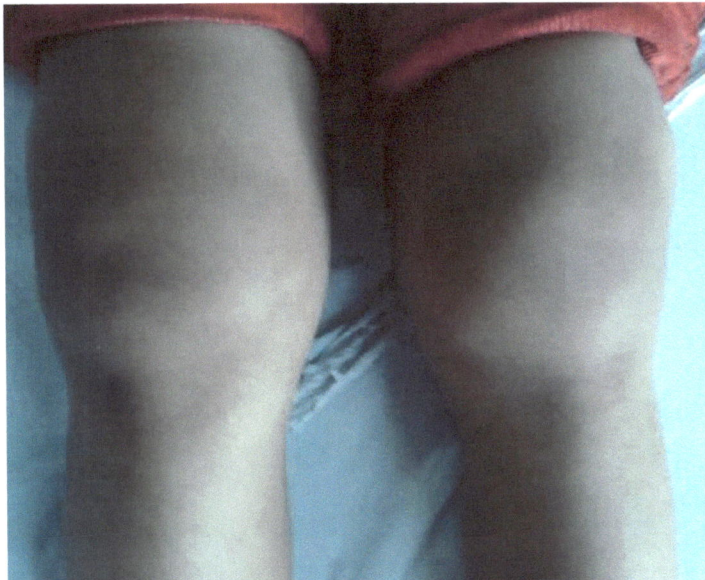

Fig. (1). Joint swelling in both knees suggestive of arthritis.

Table 2. Differences between inflammatory and noninflammatory articular pain.

Clinical Feature	Inflammatory Articular Pain	Noninflammatory Articular Pain
Pain	Morning	Evening
Swelling	Soft tissue	Bony
Redness	Occasional	Absent
Warmth	Sometimes	Absent
Stiffness	Prominent	Usually absent
Limitation of joint movements	Frequent	Absent
Systemic features	Sometimes	Absent
Erythrocyte sedimentation rate (ESR), C-reactive protein (CRP)	Usually elevated	Not elevated

Pains occurring predominantly at night are more typical of malignancies like acute leukemia or neuroblastoma. In such a setting, pain is not restricted to the joint line. Other red flag signs for malignancy are inability to bear weight, severe pain needing intravenous analgesics, and symptoms disproportionately more than signs.

Noninflammatory articular pain is typical in hereditary arthropathies, intraarticular arteriovenous malformations, hypermobility, and certain orthopedic conditions such as Perthes disease or avascular necrosis of the femoral head and slipped upper femoral epiphysis. Children with hereditary coagulopathy may show features of inflammation like warmth, swelling, and limitation of movements in a joint with acute hemarthrosis.

Is the Involvement Acute or Chronic?

The duration of articular involvement helps to narrow down the diagnosis. Whereas septic arthritis presents over hours to days, disease duration is longer over days to weeks in viral and post-viral etiologies, rheumatic fever, and reactive arthritis. A cut-off of 6 weeks differentiates between acute and chronic arthritis. Though this cut-off is arbitrary, it helps the clinician rule out etiologies like viral arthritis, acute rheumatic fever, septic arthritis, transient synovitis, *etc.*, from the differential diagnosis of a child presenting with chronic arthritis. Disease duration of more than 6 weeks is seen in juvenile idiopathic arthritis (JIA) and as the joint manifestation of other autoimmune diseases like systemic lupus erythematosus (SLE), juvenile dermatomyositis (JDM), and various vasculitides. Autoinflammatory syndromes can present with both acute recurrent arthritis and chronic arthritis. Tuberculosis and human immunodeficiency virus (HIV) infection can present with chronic arthritis.

Pattern of Joint Involvement

Certain features like the number of joints involved, symmetry of involvement, peripheral or axial skeleton involvement, and small or large joint involvement are useful in the differential diagnosis of arthritis. The pattern of involvement, whether fixed, migratory, or additive, also helps in the differential diagnosis. Whereas infections like tuberculosis typically involve a single joint, many joints may be involved in HIV infection. Most patients with infective endocarditis typically have only arthralgia; however, arthritis can be seen. Poststreptococcal arthritis can affect both large and small joints as well as the axial skeleton. Reactive arthritis causes asymmetric involvement of large joints of lower limbs. JIA can involve any number of joints. Systemic vasculitides and connective tissue disorders can present with either arthralgia or arthritis involving any number of joints. Painless contractures of limbs suggest etiology other than JIA and could be a pointer to skeletal dysplasia, Farber's disease, and mucopolysaccharidosis. Features of inflammation are absent in these conditions. Associated short stature, coarse facies, and developmental delay or regression may be present.

Extra-articular Involvement

Extra-articular involvement in a child with chronic arthritis usually suggests a possibility beyond JIA except when involvement occurs in the form of uveitis in JIA and macrophage activation syndrome (MAS) and amyloidosis in systemic JIA [2, 3].

What is Arthritis

The term "arthritis" means inflammation of joints [2]. Clinically it is defined as a swollen joint or presence of at least two of the following features: limited range of motion, redness, and warmth over the joint. Arthritis of deep joints like the hip, shoulder, spine, and sacroiliac joint may not show obvious joint swelling. Before giving a label of chronic arthritis, it is important to be sure that it is chronic and there is arthritis, meaning thereby that swelling is not arising from juxta-articular structures.

Arthritis could be monoarticular (involving single joint), oligoarticular (2-4 joints), and polyarticular (5 or more joints). Differential diagnosis of chronic arthritis is wide and is depicted in Table **3**. A good history and focused examination help in a majority of cases.

Table 3. Causes of chronic arthritis.

Cause	Examples
Related to Infection	Reactive arthritis, Tuberculosis, HIV, Poststreptococcal arthritis, Infective endocarditis
Malignancy	Leukemia, Neuroblastoma
Inflammation	JIA, Inflammatory bowel disease, Connective tissue diseases, Systemic vasculitides, Systemic autoinflammatory syndromes
Hemarthrosis	Coagulopathy, Synovial hemangioma
Mechanical (Arthritis mimics)	Trauma, Hypermobility syndrome
Hereditary (Arthritis mimics)	Genetic arthropathies, Skeletal dysplasia, Farber's disease, Mucopolysaccharidoses

Conditions Mimicking Chronic Arthritis

- Genetic arthropathies: These are hereditary conditions that are often misdiagnosed as JIA. Typically pain occurs only at extreme movements because of contractures. There are no features of inflammation on examination or in investigations. Typical examples are Progressive Pseudo rheumatoid Arthropathy of childhood (PPAC), epiphyseal dysplasias, and Camptodactyly-arthropathy-coxa vara-pericarditis (CACP) syndrome.
- The intra-articular arteriovenous malformation can present with joint swelling; however, there are no features of inflammation.
- Target joint of coagulation disorders like hemophilia can present with a swollen joint with restricted movements. Recurrent episodes of acute pain and swelling in one joint and a history of bleeds at other sites may give a diagnosis. The history of trauma may, however, not be obvious.

Approach to a Child with a Multisystem Disorder

Systemic lupus erythematosus (SLE) is a multisystemic disease and can present with manifestations related to any organ system [4]. Rash, oral ulcers, and joint pains are typical early clinical manifestations. Arthritis of both small and large joints can occur and is usually non-deforming.

Juvenile Dermatomyositis (JDM) is a multisystem disease [5]. Most children present with typical skin and muscle manifestations. Arthralgia and arthritis can both occur in JDM.

Scleroderma is associated with the tightening of skin to underlying tissues [6]. Early symptoms and signs may be very subtle, leading to a frequent delay in diagnosis.

Approach to a Child with Suspected Vasculitis

Vasculitis refers to inflammation of the vessel wall [7]. Nonspecific manifestations are fever, fatigue, malaise, weight loss, anorexia, and features of inflammation on investigations (leucocytosis, thrombocytosis, and elevated ESR/CRP). Specific manifestations vary with the size of the involved vessel (Table **4**) and the organ system in which vessel involvement occurs (Table **5**). For classification, vessels are broadly classified into three major types [8]:

Table 4. Clinical features of vasculitis depending on the type of vessel involved.

Type of Vessel Involved	Prototype	Common Features
Large vessel vasculitis	Takayasu arteritis	Absent pulses, claudication, congestive cardiac failure, cardiomyopathy, differential hypertension, stroke, syncope
Medium vessel vasculitis	Kawasaki disease (KD) Polyarteritis nodosa (PAN)	Cutaneous ulcers, livedo reticularis, tender nodules, hypertension, abdominal angina, orchitis, gangrene, mononeuritis multiplex
Small vessel vasculitis	IgA vasculitis (IgAV) Antineutrophilic cytoplasmic antibody (ANCA) associated vasculitis (AAV)	Purpura, glomerulonephritis, diffuse alveolar hemorrhage, abdominal angina

Table 5. Clinical features of vasculitis depending on the organ system involved.

Organ System	Manifestations
Skin and mucosa	Purpura, nodules, cutaneous ulcers, livedo reticularis, gangrene, panniculitis, oral and nasal ulcers
Gastrointestinal	Abdominal angina, hematochezia, malaena, intussusception
Genitourinary	Hypertension, hematuria, proteinuria, epididymo-orchitis
Neurological	Stroke, mononeuritis multiplex, focal neurological deficits
Cardiac	Myocarditis, valvular incompetence, myocardial ischemia, congestive cardiac failure, pulmonary artery hypertension
Ear, nose, and throat	Nasal ulceration, chronic ear discharge, subglottic stenosis, depressed nasal bridge
Eyes	Uveitis, scleritis/episcleritis, exudates/periphlebitis on fundus examination

1. Large-sized arteries are the aorta and its main branches.
2. The arterioles, venules, and capillaries form the small-sized blood vessels.
3. All other arteries between large-sized arteries and small-sized vessels are classified as medium-sized blood vessels.

In nutshell, rheumatological disorders can present with wide-ranging clinical manifestations and can present to many pediatric subspecialists. They can also present in an intensive care setting with multisystemic manifestations.

Investigations in Rheumatology

In pediatric rheumatology, physicians use many investigations that are also used in other subspecialties. Besides, we use certain investigations which are used exclusively in this field. These investigations can help confirm the diagnosis but should not be used to search for a rheumatologic diagnosis.

Hemogram

Anemia in rheumatologic conditions is multifactorial and can occur due to anemia of chronic disease, nutritional causes due to poor appetite and gastrointestinal losses due to nonsteroidal anti-inflammatory drugs (NSAID), and steroid therapy. Autoimmune hemolysis is seen in conditions like SLE, where direct Coomb's test may be positive. Rarely, bone marrow suppression may also be seen in SLE.

Leucocyte counts can be increased or decreased in rheumatologic conditions. Autoinflammatory conditions like systemic JIA (sJIA) are associated with leucocytosis and thrombocytosis unless there is associated MAS [3]. Leucocytosis, if present, is mild in polyarthritis and oligoarthritis. Leucopenia and especially lymphopenia is an important marker of disease activity in SLE [9]. Thrombocytopenia can be seen in SLE. Most vasculitides have thrombocytosis or normal platelet count [8]. Thrombocytopenia excludes the possibility of chronic vasculitides.

ESR measures the rate of sedimentation of RBC in anticoagulated blood and correlates with serum fibrinogen levels. It is raised in most rheumatologic conditions except conditions like MAS, where it is low because of falling serum fibrinogen [10]. High ESR is nonspecific and can be seen in many infectious and malignant conditions and should not be considered synonymous with a rheumatologic condition. The trend in ESR values over days is more helpful, especially in MAS, where falling ESR is an early diagnostic marker, much before the onset of clinical manifestations.

Liver Function Test

Liver function tests include aspartate aminotransferase (AST), alanine amino-transferase (ALT), alkaline phosphatase, serum proteins, and serum albumin. AST and ALT elevations are seen in liver involvement. Disproportionate elevation in AST compared to ALT is seen in a setting of hemolysis or inflammatory myopathy. Serum protein and globulins can be raised in rheumatologic conditions because of inflammation. Serum albumin may be low because of inflammation, malnutrition, or because of renal loss due to glomerular involvement.

Coagulogram

In a child with SLE, elevated activated partial thromboplastin time (aPTT) and normal prothrombin time (PT) give a clue to the presence of antiphospholipid (aPL) antibodies [11]. Both PT and aPTT are increased in hepatic involvement and MAS. In MAS, fibrinogen levels are low and D-dimer can be raised [12].

C-reactive Protein (CRP)

CRP levels rise many folds within hours of tissue injury or inflammation and fall back quickly once the stimulus subsides. The magnitude of CRP rise correlates with the severity of inflammation. Further, the CRP level is not affected by the number and morphology of red blood cells and serum immunoglobulin concentration. CRP levels are raised in infections, most rheumatological conditions, and malignancies. The only exception is SLE, where CRP levels are low during flares [4]. However, children with SLE, who has arthritis, serositis, or infection can have raised CRP. In most settings, ESR and CRP go hand in hand except MAS, which is characterized by very impressive elevations of CRP with falling ESR [13]. Since this investigation is very sensitive to underlying stimuli, it can be used to follow-up rheumatologic conditions.

Renal Function Tests

Renal function tests include blood urea, serum creatinine, and urine examination. A good urine examination is a must in rheumatology as the kidney is frequently involved in rheumatological conditions. The presence of proteinuria and microscopic hematuria can predict glomerular or microvascular involvement which is seen in SLE [14] and many vasculitides [7]. Renal function can be gauged by seeing blood urea and creatinine levels.

Lipid Profile

Fasting hypertriglyceridemia can be seen in many inflammatory conditions including MAS [15].

Serum Ferritin

Elevated serum ferritin levels are common in inflammation. In a child with sJIA, serum ferritin levels above 684 ng/ml are used as a mandatory criterion to classify

MAS [15]. It is common to have far more impressive elevations of ferritin levels in MAS.

Radiology

The main use of radiology in JIA lies in ruling out genetic arthropathies (Fig. **2**) and skeletal dysplasia. Changes like periarticular osteopenia, erosions, and change in joint space occur late during the course of JIA and hence are not routinely recommended in this condition. Radiographs are sometimes ordered before surgery in children with JIA and significant deformities. Ultrasound examination is commonly used when the clinical examination is suspicious of arthritis. It is also used while giving intraarticular injections, especially in deep-seated joints. Magnetic resonance imaging (MRI) is useful in the evaluation of sacroiliac joints in patients with enthesitis-related arthritis (ERA) [16]. It is useful in children with "single joint" involvement to exclude differentials like tuberculosis and intraarticular arteriovenous malformations. Chest radiographs may be useful in systemic rheumatological conditions. They may show features of diffuse alveolar hemorrhage in AAV [17] or SLE [18]. Features of interstitial lung disease (ILD) and pulmonary infarcts may be seen in systemic sclerosis [19] and antiphospholipid syndrome (APS), respectively.

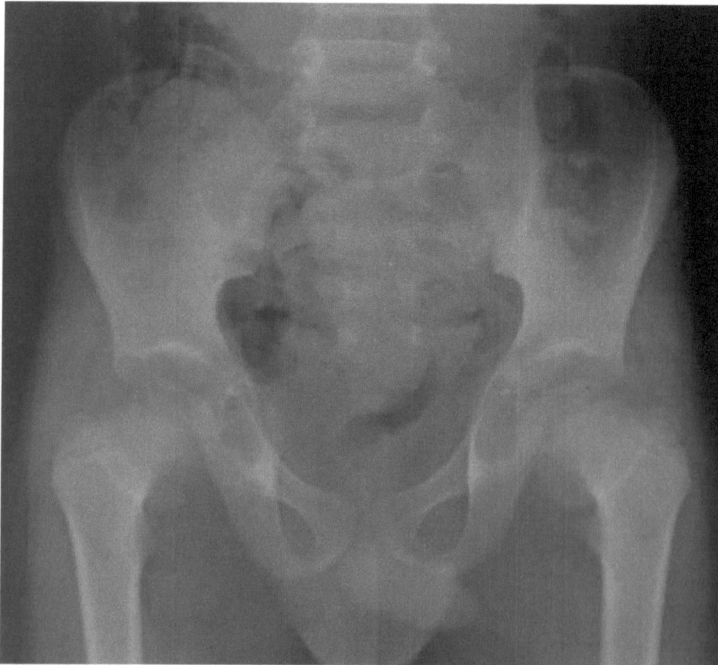

Fig. (2). X-ray of pelvis showing acetabular cysts in a child with Camptodactyly-arthropathy-coxa vara - pericarditis (CACP) syndrome.

MRI is useful in the evaluation of inflammatory myopathies [20]. Conventional or digital subtraction angiography is used to assist in the diagnosis of large (Takayasu arteritis) or medium vessel (PAN, KD) vasculitides [7]. Small vessel vasculitides cannot be diagnosed based on angiography and require tissue diagnosis. Echocardiography is useful in many rheumatologic conditions. It may pick up pericardial, myocardial, or endocardial involvement in diseases like SLE. It is useful to pick up coronary artery involvement in KD [21]. Besides characteristic coronary artery involvement, features of pericardial effusion, myocarditis, or valvular involvement can also be seen in the acute phase of KD [21]. The evolution of coronary abnormalities like ectasia or aneurysmal dilatation in the subacute phase is considered diagnostic of KD, even when all the typical clinical features are not present.

Complement

High C3 levels can be seen in many inflammatory conditions. Low C3 and C4 levels are common in SLE with nephritis because of complement consumption [14]. It is worth mentioning that all children with SLE do not have low complement levels [22].

Autoantibodies

Rheumatoid Factor (RF)

This test detects IgM antibodies directed against antigenic determinants on the Fc portion of IgG using the latex agglutination test. RF can be positive in many acute and chronic inflammatory conditions. In JIA, RF is used as a prognostic marker in polyarthritis [2].

Antinuclear Antibody (ANA)

ANA are autoantibodies directed against nuclear, nucleolar, or perinuclear antigens and are seen in many autoimmune diseases [23]. In an appropriate clinical setting, persistent positivity of ANA in high titers suggests autoimmunity. Positive ANA testing is included in the classification criteria for SLE, mixed connective tissue disease (MCTD), and Sjögren syndrome. Up to 20% of healthy children can have positive ANA. Therefore, the results of ANA testing must be interpreted while keeping clinical features in mind.

ANA can be detected by ELISA and indirect immunofluorescence (IIF). ELISA is commonly used in routine laboratory practice but tends to produce more false-positive and true weak-positive results. The recommended method to detect ANA is IIF using HEp-2 cell line [23]. Both strength and pattern of staining are important. The pattern of staining reflects the specific nuclear antigens to which the ANA is binding. The use of ANA pattern to diagnose specific autoimmune disorders has low sensitivity and specificity. Hence, if ANA is positive in an appropriate setting, one should try to confirm it with antibodies to specific nuclear antigens.

Anti-histone and anti-dsDNA antibodies typically produce homogenous patterns of ANA. Anti-dsDNA antibodies can also cause a peripheral or rim pattern on IIF (Fig. **3**) [24]. The speckled pattern can be seen with antibodies like anti-Sm (anti-Smith), anti-SSA, and anti-SSB antibodies. The nucleolar pattern is related to anti-Scl70 antibodies in systemic sclerosis, and the centromere pattern is seen with antibodies to the kinetochore in the CREST (Calcinosis, Raynaud phenomenon, Esophageal disease, Sclerodactyly, Telangiectasia) syndrome. ANA is frequently positive in oligoarthritis [2] and does not predict the development of SLE. ANA positivity in oligoarthritis is associated with a high risk of chronic uveitis [25].

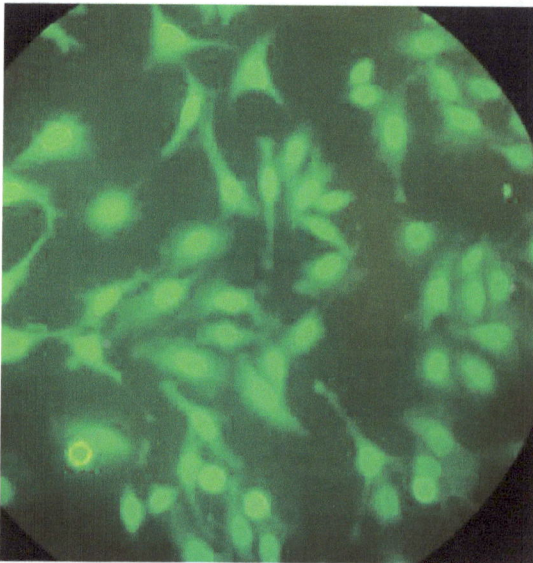

Fig. (3). Homogenous pattern with rim enhancement of ANA on IIF[16].

Anti-dsDNA antibody, though not sensitive, is moderately specific for SLE [24]. Anti-dsDNA levels have been found to correlate with disease activity and can be used to monitor the disease. Coming to specific antibodies, anti-SSA and anti-SSB antibodies are found in SLE and Sjögren syndrome. Mothers with these antibodies are at risk of having babies with congenital heart block, a manifestation of neonatal lupus [24]. Anti-RNP antibody is classical of MCTD. Anti-Scl-70 antibody is found in scleroderma and at low frequency in the CREST syndrome. Anti-Sm antibody is said to be a highly specific marker for SLE, though it occurs in a small minority [22]. Anti-histone antibodies are seen in drug-induced lupus [24].

ANCA (Anti-neutrophil Cytoplasmic Antibody)

There are different kinds of ANCA. ANCA with cytoplasmic staining (cANCA) and ANCA with perinuclear staining (pANCA) are most important [26]. Granulomatosis with polyangiitis (GPA) is associated with cANCA, which is mainly directed against proteinase 3 (PR3), while pANCA is associated with microscopic polyangiitis (MPA) and is mainly directed against myeloperoxidase. ANCA tests use either IIF or ELISA technique. IIF tests are more sensitive but less specific than ELISA and are operator dependent.

Antiphospholipid Antibodies

Anticardiolipin (aCL), anti-beta 2 glycoprotein 1 (aβ_2GP1) and lupus anticoagulant (LA) are common aPL antibodies in clinical use [27]. The persistent presence of one or more of these antibodies in association with thrombosis confirms the diagnosis of APS in children [11]. APS can be seen in association with rheumatologic conditions like SLE [28].

Tissue Diagnosis

Biopsies of various tissues are useful in rheumatologic diagnosis. Renal biopsy is useful in a child presenting with nephrosis or rapidly progressive glomerulonephritis, which are the common renal manifestations of rheumatologic conditions. Histopathology, along with immunofluorescence, helps in distinguishing SLE from a vasculitic group of disorders [14, 17]. Muscle biopsy is occasionally used in inflammatory myopathies when typical skin manifestations are not present [29]. Tissue biopsies from the skin, kidney, lung, muscle, *etc.,* are useful in the diagnosis of specific vasculitis. Skin biopsy in IgA vasculitis shows leukocytoclastic vasculitis with IgA deposition on immunofluorescence [30].

SPECIFIC RHEUMATOLOGICAL CONDITIONS

JUVENILE IDIOPATHIC ARTHRITIS

Juvenile idiopathic arthritis (JIA) is the commonest rheumatological disease in children, with a prevalence of 1 in 1000 children [31]. It is described from all over the world.

ILAR Classification

International League of Associations for Rheumatology (ILAR) classification has tried to classify JIA based on the number of joints involved, course of the disease, and extraarticular complications [31]. The seven groups are:

1. Oligoarthritis
2. Rheumatoid factor (RF) positive polyarthritis
3. Rheumatoid factor negative polyarthritis
4. Enthesitis related arthritis (ERA)
5. Juvenile psoriatic arthritis (JPsA)
6. Systemic JIA (sJIA)
7. Undifferentiated arthritis

There are some controversies regarding this classification. Instead of the number of joints, it is now clear that ANA positivity defines course and prognosis better. ILAR classification may undergo changes in years to come.

Oligoarthritis

Oligoarthritis typically involves less than five joints in the first six months of onset. This subtype is the commonest in the West, contributing to as many as 60-70% of children with JIA [2]. The peak age at onset is 1-3 years with a distinct female preponderance. Typically there is asymmetrical involvement of large joints of lower limbs, usually knee or ankle. Small joints are rarely involved, and if involved, one needs to ask for a family history of psoriasis. Swelling is usually disproportionate to pain. These children may limp early in the morning due to morning stiffness. Monoarthritis can be a diagnostic challenge since infectious etiologies like tuberculosis become important differential diagnoses. The presence of chronic anterior uveitis, ANA positivity, and sometimes, clinical response to NSAID or intraarticular steroids help in ruling out tubercular arthritis.

Laboratory investigations do not show any increase in inflammatory parameters. Nearly two-thirds of these children may show ANA positivity. Chronic anterior uveitis is the most common extra-articular manifestation in this subtype [25]. Commonly these children are not able to communicate any visual problems, even though the eye disease may be significantly advanced. Hence, these children must be screened for uveitis at the time of diagnosis and periodically thereafter. ANA positivity predicts a higher chance of chronic anterior uveitis.

Management requires the use of NSAIDs and steroids (intraarticular or oral) depending on severity. Some children need disease-modifying antirheumatic drugs (DMARDs) like methotrexate. DMARDs are required in children who develop uveitis, extended oligoarthritis or fail repeated intraarticular steroids [32]. Biologicals are rarely needed for joint disease in these children but may be required in children with refractory uveitis [32].

Besides uveitis, common articular complications are contractures, limb length discrepancy, and asymmetry in bone growth due to joint inflammation. Most children continue to have oligoarthritis and are labeled as "persistent oligoarthritis". Some children with oligoarthritis in the first six months of disease onset progress to involve more joints later in the course and are labeled as "extended oligoarthritis". These children are treated with polyarthritis.

Polyarthritis

Arthritis of more than 4 joints in the first six months of disease onset is labeled polyarthritis [2]. Polyarthritis is itself a heterogeneous type and includes two main subtypes:

1. Rheumatoid factor negative polyarthritis: This subtype has two peaks of onset: 2-4 years and 6-12 years. Small joint involvement does occur but is not too symmetrical. Temporomandibular joint involvement is common and can lead to micrognathia, retrognathia and malocclusion. Cervical spine involvement can also occur and lead to restricted neck movements. These children can have ANA positivity and risk developing chronic anterior uveitis like the children with oligoarthritis.
2. Rheumatoid factor positive polyarthritis: This subtype behaves like adult rheumatoid arthritis. It is typically seen in older adolescent girls who present symmetrical involvement of metacarpophalangeal and proximal interphalangeal joints. Other joints like wrists, elbows, knees, and ankles are commonly involved. Distal interphalangeal joints are spared. These children may also have subcutaneous nodules, which may resolve spontaneously. By definition, RF is positive. This needs to be reconfirmed three months later since the RF can be false-positive after many infectious illnesses [33]. This subtype is least likely to be in remission without therapy and is likely to continue into adulthood. These children carry the risk of significant deformities if not treated appropriately in time. Limb length discrepancy, retrognathia, and micrognathia are not common since onset is later in life when growth is nearly complete.

Risk factors for poor prognosis in polyarthritis include positive RF, positive anti-cyclic citrullinated peptide (anti-CCP) antibody, and joint damage [34].

For management, DMARDs have to be initiated early. Methotrexate is recommended over other drugs like leflunomide and sulfasalazine because of its safety and vast experience. Intraarticular steroids are used as adjuncts. Bridge steroids can be used for moderate and high disease activity. Biologic agents can be used upfront in children who have involvement of high-risk joints like cervical spine, wrist, or hip. They are also to be used in case of persistent moderate/high disease activity, despite the use of methotrexate for 3 months. NSAIDs are not appropriate as monotherapy for chronic persistent synovitis. There is no role of chronic low dose steroids [34].

Enthesitis Related Arthritis (ERA)

ERA describes a heterogeneous group of children who have enthesitis with or without arthritis, juvenile ankylosing spondylitis, and arthritis in children with inflammatory bowel disease [16]. The peak age at onset is 12 years though it can occur any time after 6 years of age. There is a male preponderance, with 60% of children being boys. Diagnosis requires the presence of arthritis and enthesitis [31]. If either of these features is not present, then two of the following features should be present for diagnosis:

1. Sacroiliac joint tenderness or inflammatory back pain
2. Positive HLA B27
3. The onset of arthritis in a male after 6 years of age
4. Family history of HLA B27 associated disease

Usually, there is asymmetrical involvement of large joints of lower limbs. Knees, ankles, hips, and midfoot joints are the typical joints involved. The axial disease may not be present at onset. Symptomatic sacroiliitis develops in 15% and 53% of patients within 2 and 4 years of disease onset, respectively [16]. History of inflammatory back pain or examination for tenderness over sacroiliac joints is not sensitive to pick up sacroiliitis. Sacroiliitis is a poor prognostic sign in ERA and may progress to juvenile ankylosing spondylitis. It does not respond to NSAIDs and DMARDs.

Enthesitis is inflammation of entheses, sites where the tendon, ligament, or joint capsule is attached to bone [35]. In ERA, enthesitis is a typical clinical feature and commonly involves tibial tuberosity, plantar fascial insertion at calcaneum, and Achilles tendon insertion at calcaneum. It is also seen in psoriatic arthritis and adult spondyloarthropathies. Enthesitis may not parallel arthritis activity and can significantly affect the activities of daily living. It also may not respond well to therapy.

These children are prone to develop uveitis. Unlike uveitis of oligoarthritis, uveitis in ERA is acute and is associated with redness, pain, and photophobia [25]. It is recurrent and commonly affects one eye only. Though the risk of complications is lower in this type of uveitis, severe inflammation in the acute stage and recurrent inflammation can cause complications.

There is no diagnostic test for ERA. Nearly one-half of these children are positive for HLA B27, but HLA B27 is not specific for ERA [16]. It can also be seen in arthropathy related to inflammatory bowel disease and reactive arthritis. These children are typically negative for ANA and RF.

Treatment includes NSAIDs, bridge steroids (oral or intraarticular), and anti-TNF agents [34]. Anti TNF agents have been shown to prevent the progression of axial skeleton involvement. Methotrexate may be useful in patients with concomitant peripheral arthritis but has no role in enthesitis and sacroiliitis. It has also been used as an adjunct to prevent antibody formation against anti-TNF agents. Physiotherapy is recommended.

Juvenile Psoriatic Arthritis

JIA patients are classified as juvenile psoriatic arthritis (JPsA) if they have a psoriatic rash or have at least two of the following minor criteria: first-degree relative with psoriasis, nail pitting, or onycholysis and dactylitis [31].

Age at onset is bimodal [36]. The first peak is seen at 2-4 years of age, and there is a distinct female preponderance. These children behave like those with oligoarthritis and may have ANA positivity as well as chronic uveitis. Nail pitting, dactylitis (Fig. **4**) and distal interphalangeal joint involvement are important differences in these children compared to oligoarthritis. Older children with JPsA behave more like spondyloarthropathy [37, 38].

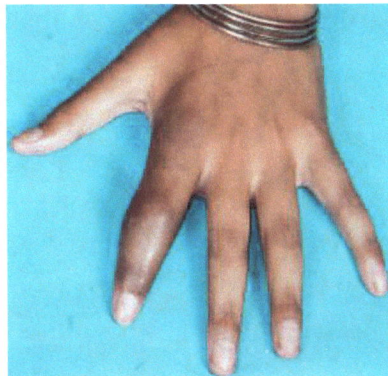

Fig. (4). Dactylitis in a child with JPsA.

Undifferentiated Arthritis

ILAR classifies all patients with JIA who do not fulfil criteria for any category or fulfil criteria for more than two categories as undifferentiated arthritis [31].

Systemic JIA

Systemic JIA (sJIA) was first described by Dr. Frederick Still in 1897 and is called "Still's disease". It is a systemic inflammatory condition. ILAR defines sJIA as the presence of arthritis with or preceded by a fever of at least 2 weeks duration for at least 3 consecutive days plus one of the following:-

- Evanescent non-fixed rash
- Generalized lymphadenopathy
- Hepatomegaly or splenomegaly
- Serositis

Diagnosis of sJIA also requires exclusion of the following conditions:

- Psoriasis or history of psoriasis in patient or first-degree relatives
- Arthritis in HLA B27 positive males beginning after the age of 6 years
- Presence of ankylosing spondylitis, enthesitis-related arthritis, sacroiliitis with inflammatory bowel disease, Reiter's syndrome, acute anterior uveitis in the patient, or history of any such disorder in first-degree relatives
- Presence of IgM RF on at least 2 occasions at least 3 months apart.

Epidemiology

sJIA can occur at any age throughout childhood and there is no sexual predilection. The incidence described in Western literature is roughly 0.4-0.9/100,000 per year [3].

Pathophysiology

The main abnormality seems to be cytokine dysregulation. Levels of proinflammatory cytokines are significantly elevated, and levels of anti-inflammatory cytokines are decreased. The IL-1β elevation is associated with fever, anorexia, and joint destruction. Serum levels of IL-6 parallel fever and acute phase reactants. IL-6 elevation is also associated with joint destruction. This condition is associated with a lack of specific antibodies and definite HLA locus.

Clinical Features

The most common presentation in sJIA is with the fever of unknown origin. Fever is classically high grade and intermittent with 1-2 spikes per day, often appearing at the same time each day. Typically the child looks sick when he is febrile but looks well in between the fever spikes. The fever may be accompanied by a transient faint pink rash noticed on face/inner arms, chest/back, and inner thighs. The rash is usually asymptomatic but sometimes can be itchy. The rash can be induced with minor trauma or a warm shower (Koebner phenomenon). Hepatosplenomegaly, generalized lymphadenopathy, and pleural and/or pericardial effusions can be seen.

Arthritis, if present at the onset, aids in diagnosis but can appear after years into illness. This can make diagnosis difficult, especially early on in the course of the illness. It usually affects large peripheral joints like wrists, shoulders, elbows, hips, knees, and ankles. Ankylosis of the cervical spine and wrist are common complications in inadequately treated patients.

Investigations

Laboratory features of inflammation such as neutrophilic leucocytosis, thrombocytosis, anemia of inflammation, hypoalbuminemia, very high ESR and CRP, and high serum fibrinogen are frequent [3]. When children present with febrile illness of a few weeks' duration, differential diagnoses are many and include infections, malignancy, and autoimmune diseases. These systemic diseases must be ruled out before making a diagnosis of sJIA. Bone marrow aspiration is routine in many centres to rule out malignancy before starting steroids.

Treatment

Treatment is aimed at the suppression of active features. While systemic features are dominant at the onset, the disease can evolve into persistent systemic disease with arthritis, persistent systemic disease with little or no arthritis, or persistent arthritis alone.

According to the American College of Rheumatology (ACR) guidelines, sJIA patients are classified according to the clinical severity of disease and prognostic features [39].

sJIA with Active Systemic Features (and Without Active Arthritis)

Features of Poor Prognosis

Six-month duration of significant active systemic disease, defined by fever, elevated inflammatory markers, or requirement for treatment with systemic glucocorticoids.

Disease Activity Levels

Active fever AND global physician assessment of overall disease activity 7 of 10.

Active fever AND systemic features of high disease activity (*e.g.* significant serositis) that result in global physician assessment of overall disease activity of >7/10.

Treatment

NSAIDs are first-line drugs in children with active systemic features. If there is a good response, NSAIDs are continued. If the response is inadequate or features that suggest high disease activity at onset, systemic corticosteroids are initiated. Good response in disease activity warrants a gradual tapering of corticosteroids with a plan to stop steroids by the end of 6 months.

Methotrexate can be added at a dose of 15-20 mg/m^2 for these children if they also have active arthritis. Intra-articular steroids can be used as an adjunct for arthritis.

Biologicals are recommended from the outset in patients with both high disease activity and poor prognostic features at the onset. Either IL-1 inhibitor (anakinra) or IL-6 inhibitor (tocilizumab) can be used. Anakinra is started at 2 mg/kg/day as a subcutaneous injection and continued for several months, maximum up to 4 mg/kg/day. It is highly effective in patients who present with MAS.

Tocilizumab is a humanized monoclonal antibody against IL6 receptor. It is given as an intravenous infusion at an 8 mg/kg dose in patients above 30 kg and 12 mg/kg in those under 30 kg every 2-4 weeks. It blunts CRP response and may make it difficult to recognize infection and MAS in these children. It is well-tolerated and is not associated with a significant risk of serious infections.

Thalidomide and calcineurin inhibitors have been used in sJIA to reduce systemic inflammation, particularly in settings where access to biologicals is impossible [3]. In MAS, cyclosporine A is used as second-line therapy after systemic steroids. Thalidomide has been shown to reduce systemic inflammation and thus acts as a steroid-sparing agent. However, it can be associated with side effects such as sedation and irreversible peripheral neuropathy.

sJIA with Active Arthritis (without Active Systemic Features)

Features of poor prognosis (must satisfy 1)

- Arthritis of the hip
- Radiographic damage (erosions or joint space narrowing by radiograph)

Disease activity levels

- Low disease activity (must satisfy all)
  - 4 or fewer active joints
  - Erythrocyte sedimentation rate or C-reactive protein level normal
  - Physician global assessment of overall disease activity 4 of 10
  - Patient/parent global assessment of overall well-being 2 of 10
- Moderate disease activity (does not satisfy criteria for low or high activity)
  - 1 or more features greater than low disease activity level AND fewer than 3 features of high disease activity
- High disease activity (must satisfy at least 3)
  - 8 or more active joints
  - Erythrocyte sedimentation rate or C-reactive protein level greater than the twice upper limit of normal
  - Physician global assessment of overall disease activity 7 of 10
  - Patient/parent global assessment of overall well-being of > 5/10

Treatment

NSAIDs, intra-articular steroids, and early methotrexate or leflunomide are the recommended options [39]. Systemic steroids can be used as a bridge for initial 2-3 months until the effect of methotrexate takes over.

Hydroxychloroquine and sulfasalazine do not have much additional benefit. If adding leflunomide or methotrexate does not work or is not tolerated, the next option is to consider biological therapy, usually with anakinra, tocilizumab, or abatacept.

For systemic arthritis with active systemic features or active arthritis, systemic steroids should not be used as monotherapy for more than 1 month. Similarly, NSAID monotherapy is not recommended for more than 1 month if the disease continues to be active [39].

Outcome

The course of sJIA is unpredictable. Some children tend to have a monocyclic course. In others, it can evolve into illness with predominant systemic features or predominant arthritis, or both. Common complications seen in sJIA are MAS [40], amyloidosis [41], growth failure, chronic anemia, and deformities. While MAS is a complication that can be seen even at the onset of disease, secondary amyloidosis is a late complication in children with inadequate control of inflammation. Proteinuria is one of the early clinical features of amyloidosis. Later renal dysfunction can set in. The diagnosis of amyloidosis can be confirmed by histopathology from the rectum, skin fat pad, duodenum, or kidney. In literature, renal biopsies have been associated with torrential bleeds and hence generally avoided [41]. With the availability of more effective therapies, the risk of amyloidosis has reduced significantly. In the West, amyloidosis is rarely described now. Good control of underlying inflammation helps in controlling amyloidosis.

Growth failure and chronic anemia are seen in patients who are inadequately controlled. Persistent inflammation, reduced appetite, and use of steroids contribute to growth failure. Significant deformities of major joints like hips, shoulders, wrists, cervical spine, and temporomandibular joints are common in children with prolonged arthritis.

SYSTEMIC LUPUS ERYTHEMATOUS (SLE)

SLE is a prototype multisystem autoimmune disorder with remitting-relapsing course and a potential to affect almost every organ of the body [4]. About 10-20% of all SLE patients have onset before the age of 18 years. Out of all childhood SLE patients, 60% have the disease onset after 10 years [4]. Only 5% of all childhood SLE have the disease onset before the age of 5 years and these children are likely to have a strong genetic predisposition. In adults, SLE in adolescence has a gender predilection towards females (male to female ratio 1:9). However, in prepubertal patients, gender predilection is less prominent (male to female 1:3-5) [4]. In general, childhood SLE is phenotypically similar to adult SLE but is associated with more severe disease and more organ damage [42].

Clinical Features

As SLE can affect any organ of the body, it can have a myriad of clinical manifestations. Organ-systems commonly affected at presentation include mucocutaneous, renal, and hematological [4].

Mucocutaneous involvement: The most characteristic manifestation is acute erythematous 'malar' or 'butterfly' rash (Fig. **5**) [43]. This rash is photosensitive and typically spares the nasolabial folds. Chronic elevated 'discoid' rash, commonly involving face and ears, is another specific clinical finding of SLE. Children can have many other types of rash, including vasculitic rash, chill-blain-like lesions, targetoid lesions, amongst others. Alopecia is also a common clinical feature and may present as a receding hairline or focally sparse hair. Painless oral ulcers affecting the palate (Fig. **6**) and nasal cavity are common. They typically occur in crops and heal without scarring.

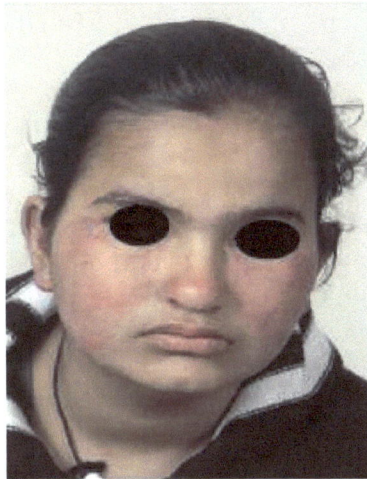

Fig. (5). Malar rash in a child with SLE.

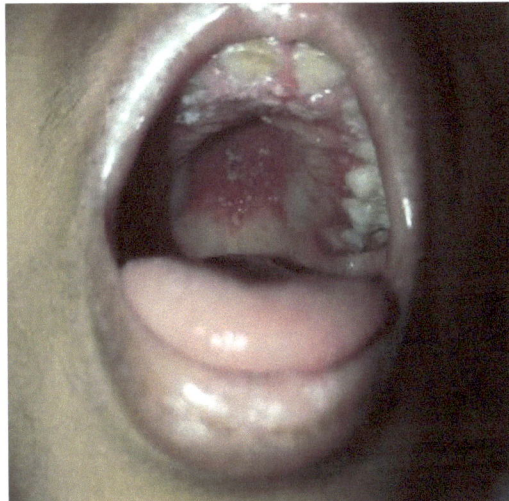

Fig. (6). Ulcer on hard palate in a child with SLE.

Renal involvement: Renal manifestations are more florid and frequent in childhood SLE as compared to adults. Common presentations include nephritic syndrome or nephrotic-nephritic pictures. However, renal involvement may be elusive, manifesting only as hypertension or abnormalities in urine microscopies such as hematuria, proteinuria, and urinary casts. Renal manifestations most commonly occur in the first year of presentation and need to be actively looked for. Renal involvement in SLE is classified into stages I-VI based on the renal pathology according to the International Society of Nephrology/Renal Pathology Society revised classification [44]. This classification takes into account both disease activity and chronicity. In general, proliferative lesions are more amenable to immunosuppressive therapy and should be treated aggressively to reduce the risk of developing end-stage renal disease.

Hematological involvement: Anemia of chronic disease is very common. Hemolytic anemia is another common manifestation and is associated with positive direct Coomb's test. Thrombocytopenia may be symptomatic as petechiae or mucosal bleeds and usually occurs due to immune destruction. Sometimes, it can be a manifestation of underlying APS. Leucopenia is common. Lymphopenia correlates with disease activity [45].

Musculoskeletal involvement: Arthralgia, non-erosive polyarthritis, myalgia, and myositis are described.

Serositis: Serositis is a common clinical feature and may present as asymptomatic effusions. Pericarditis and pleuritis (Fig. **7**) are common. Pericarditis requires the presence of two or more than two features in the form of pericardial pain, pericardial rub, typical features on electrocardiogram, and pericardial effusion [22].

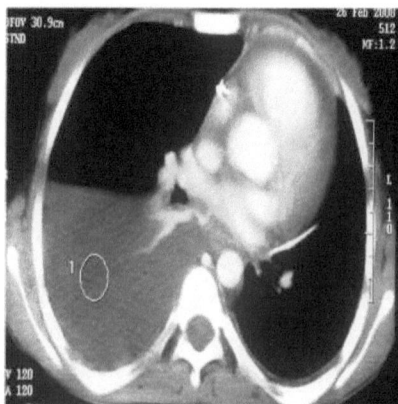

Fig. (7). CT scan showing pleural effusion in SLE

Central nervous system (CNS) involvement: CNS involvement is less common in children than adults but is a significant concern throughout the illness. SLE can have a myriad of clinical features, including headache, seizures, focal neurological defects, and psychiatric manifestations.

SLE can result in the involvement of the heart (lupus carditis), blood vessels (lupus vasculitis), gastrointestinal tract (lupus enteritis), pancreas, liver, gonads, amongst others. Recurrent infections, due to both immunosuppressive medications and genetic predisposition, are also common in pediatric SLE. Systemic features such as fever, fatigue, and generalized lymphadenopathy are common.

In general, renal, neuropsychiatric, and hematological involvement is more common in childhood SLE. In neuropsychiatric involvement, seizures, psychosis, chorea, and encephalopathy are more common in childhood SLE, and cranial neuropathies are less common. There is less gender bias towards females, especially in prepubertal children. The disease severity is greater, and organ damage occurs more frequently because of the accrual of damage occurring over time. Raynaud phenomenon, pleuritis, and sicca features are less common in children compared to adults.

Genetic Forms of SLE

Lastly, monogenic forms of SLE are increasingly being recognized [46]. C1q deficiency is the most common genetic cause of SLE in children. Specific clinical scenarios where such genetic forms need to be considered include early age at presentation (<6 years), poor response to treatment, male gender, the predominance of CNS involvement, normal complements despite active disease, speckled pattern of ANA positivity with anti-dsDNA negativity and family history of SLE or consanguinity.

Investigations

Hemogram may show anemia, reticulocytosis (hemolysis), leukopenia, lymphopenia, and thrombocytopenia. Direct Coomb's test may be positive even in the absence of laboratory evidence of hemolysis. ESR is often elevated in the active disease; however, CRP is normal as a result of impaired IL-6 signaling in SLE. CRP may be elevated in concomitant infection, arthritis or serositis.

Biochemistry may show elevated transaminases and/or lactate dehydrogenase as a result of hemolysis. Hypoalbuminemia may occur due to chronic inflammation or renal losses. Hyperglobulinemia may be due to chronic inflammation, resulting in a reversal of the albumin/globulin ratio. Urine microscopy can reveal crenated/dysmorphic red blood cells reflective of glomerulonephritis, often called 'active' sediment. Proteinuria is often an accompaniment. Analysis of complement (C3, C4) may show decreased levels in active disease due to excessive consumption; however, this is not universal.

Autoantibody testing shows ANA positivity in almost all the patients. Negative ANA has a high negative predictive value in ruling out SLE. ANA positivity can be seen in up to 10-20% of normal subjects, and hence, it has a low positive predictive value [24]. Homogenous ANA pattern with rim enhancement in HEp-2 cell-based kits on IIF is called the 'lupus' pattern (Fig. **3**) and specifically points towards SLE. The pathognomonic autoantibody for diagnosis is anti-dsDNA which has a specificity of >95% for SLE. However, it may be negative in as many as 60% of patients with SLE. Other autoantibodies that can be positive in patients with lupus include aPL and other less relevant antibodies like anti-C1q, anti-prothrombin, *etc.*

Kidney biopsy is essential for the proper management of significant SLE nephritis [14]. As the kidney damage is typically immune-mediated, glomeruli show concomitant deposition of complement, various immunoglobulin subtypes, and free light chains called the 'full-house' pattern. This pattern on immunochemistry is so specific that it may obviate the need to fulfill the clinical criteria for the diagnosis of SLE. The biopsy may also show evidence of antiphospholipid nephropathy, which may not respond well to immunosuppressive therapy.

Diagnosis

Various criteria have been proposed for the classification of SLE, notably ACR 1997 criteria [47], SLE International Collaborating Clinics (SLICC) criteria [10], and the most recent European League against Rheumatism (EULAR)/ACR classification criteria. EULAR/ACR classification criteria have been divided the criteria into two broad categories: clinical and immunological [22, 43]. A positive ANA titre by HEp2 on IIF ≥ 1:80 is mandatory for diagnosis. Clinical criteria are divided into seven categories namely systemic, hematological, central nervous system, mucocutaneous, serositis, joint, and renal manifestations. Immunological criteria include aPL antibodies, complement levels, anti-dsDNA, and anti-Smith antibodies. Each criterion has been given relative weightage. A total of ≥ 10 points in addition to 1 clinical criterion helps in classification as SLE.

Treatment

Treatment of SLE requires the use of immunosuppression to control disease activity. The choice of immunosuppression depends on the severity of the disease and the organs involved at presentation. Minor organ lupus, which includes mucocutaneous and joint involvement, is usually treated with low-dose steroids in addition to supportive therapy.

Major organ lupus includes the involvement of any major organ and can be organ or life-threatening. Here treatment is divided into two phases: induction phase to induce remission with aggressive immunosuppression and maintenance phase to maintain the patient in remission with less aggressive immunosuppression. Induction is achieved with steroid pulses followed by oral steroids and the use of agents such as cyclophosphamide or mycophenolate mofetil. The usual aim is to achieve remission quickly and no later than six months. Different doses and routes of administration have been used for both steroids and cyclophosphamide [45]. In general, children require more dose of steroids for control of disease compared to adults.

Once remission is achieved, the maintenance phase requires the use of lower doses of mycophenolate mofetil or azathioprine. There is no consensus on the duration of maintenance treatment, especially in patients with severe manifestations at the onset. Most physicians will continue maintenance therapy for 3-5 years if the patient is doing well.

Hydroxychloroquine (HCQ) has been shown to reduce the number of flares and increase long-term survival [45]. It is also shown to provide some protection against thrombosis. All children with SLE should be on HCQ. It is given at a dose of 4-5 mg/kg/day at bedtime. Hyperpigmentation and retinal toxicity are common long-term complications. All children on this drug should be evaluated for retinal toxicity yearly. The retinal toxicity is irreversible, and risk depends on cumulative dose [45].

Photoprotection is an important management strategy as exposure to ultraviolet radiation is associated with a higher risk of flares [4]. All patients should be advised to wear clothes that cover the body as much as possible, wear a hat, and use an umbrella. A sunscreen with a sun protection factor ≥30 is recommended and it needs to be applied at least 3-4 times during the day. An adequate amount of sunscreen is also critical as sun protection is directly proportional to the thickness of the sunscreen applied over the skin. As a rule of thumb, 5 ml each is applied on the face, throat and neck, hands and feet.

Monitoring

All patients are evaluated for clinical manifestations, blood pressure, and urine microscopy and spot urine protein estimation at each visit. Complement levels and anti-dsDNA titers are useful markers of disease activity and may show a rise before a clinical flare.

Outcome

Improvements in management protocols have led to significant improvement in mortality rates in childhood SLE [45, 48]. Infections, disease activity in the form of severe lupus nephritis, and barriers to treatment have been important causes of mortality [48]. With improvement in survival, these children live longer and are at risk of more organ damage related to disease activity and treatment. Damage is most often seen in musculoskeletal, cardiovascular, and central nervous systems.

Conclusion

SLE is an autoimmune disease with the potential to involve any organ system. No investigation is diagnostic. Treatment protocols include steroids, HCQ, sun protection and steroid-sparing immunosuppressive agents. Mortality has reduced significantly with the use of better immunosuppression. Infections, disease activity, and barriers to treatment are responsible for higher mortality in developing countries. Future efforts should focus on reducing mortality and decreasing damage to provide a good quality of life.

Neonatal Lupus

Newborns born to mothers with anti-SSA and/or anti-SSB antibodies are prone to develop this condition. Mothers may themselves be either asymptomatic or may have SLE or Sjögren syndrome [49]. This condition occurs due to the transplacental passage of these antibodies. Mothers with anti-SSA and/or anti-SSB antibodies carry a 2% risk of having a baby with neonatal lupus. However, this risk increases tenfold in mothers who have a previously affected baby [49].

Since this condition occurs due to transplacental passage of antibodies, which disappear within a few months after birth, most of the clinical manifestations of neonatal lupus are transient except for atrioventricular (AV) block.

Typical organ systems involved in neonatal lupus are skin, hematological, hepatic and cardiac. There are no skin manifestations at birth, and the rash appears or gets exacerbated within 48 hours of sunlight exposure. The head and neck are most commonly involved, followed by the trunk and extremities. The rash is seen as macular erythema, papular lesions, or plaque-like lesions with central clearing and regular borders. Some of these lesions may become coalescent. The rash disappears within 7 months in 80% of patients and, at maximum, can persist till 12 months. In 20% of patients, the rash may leave behind telangiectasia, atrophy, and hyperpigmentation [49].

Hematological involvement is transient and seen as anemia, thrombocytopenia, and leucopenia. In case of severe cytopenias, a newborn would need steroids and/or IVIg in addition to blood component therapy to tide over the crisis. Liver involvement can manifest as transaminitis, cholestasis and hepatomegaly. Like skin manifestations, hematological and hepatic manifestations are transient and usually recover within 4 months.

Most worrisome and persistent complication of neonatal lupus is congenital AV block. This occurs between 18-26 weeks of gestation and is usually complete AV block [50]. In utero, it can be seen as fetal bradycardia with normal atrial rate and low ventricular rate. If the ventricular rate becomes significantly low, it can cause cardiomegaly and hydrops fetalis. After birth, a significantly low ventricular rate may manifest with pallor and congestive heart failure. Some of the severely affected newborns may develop cardiomyopathy.

All newborns should avoid sun exposure. Breastfeeding is not contraindicated and should be encouraged. In newborns with severe cytopenias, blood component therapy with steroids and/or IVIg may be required. A pacemaker is required for most children with congenital complete AV block. The timing of pacemaker insertion may vary depending on symptoms and ventricular rate.

All mothers at risk of having a baby with neonatal lupus should be counseled. Serial echocardiography is required starting from 16th week of gestation till 26th week of gestation. If there is no evidence of AV block by 26 weeks of gestation, then it is unlikely that the baby will have serious cardiac manifestations. However, such newborns can develop other manifestations of neonatal lupus after birth. If AV block is detected *in utero,* it can progress from first degree to complete heart block within a few weeks. Administration of betamethasone or IVIg to the mother is not useful to prevent progression of AV block [50]. HCQ is advised for all mothers at risk of having babies with neonatal lupus.

JUVENILE SCLERODERMA

Juvenile scleroderma is the third most common childhood rheumatological disease after JIA and SLE. It has two major subtypes: Juvenile localized scleroderma (JLS) and Juvenile systemic sclerosis (JSSc) [6]. JLS is more common in children compared to JSSc [6].

Juvenile Localized Scleroderma (JLS)

JLS is a group of disorders characterized by the involvement of skin and subdermal tissues [51]. Internal organ involvement is not very frequent, unlike JSSc. It can occur at any age and the mean age at onset was reported as 7.3 years

[6]. Based on the type of skin lesions, JLS is classified into five major types:

Linear Scleroderma

Linear scleroderma is the most common subtype of JLS. It is characterized by linear indurated streaks involving the dermis and subcutaneous tissues (Fig. **8**). Sometimes, these streaks can extend to the underlying bone. It is most commonly seen in limbs and the trunk. Linear scleroderma of the face is known as "en coup de saber" because the lesion resembles depression caused by a sword wound [6]. Parry Romberg syndrome is characterized by unaffected skin and loss of underlying tissues on one side of the face that may involve the dermis, subcutaneous tissue, muscle, and bone [52].

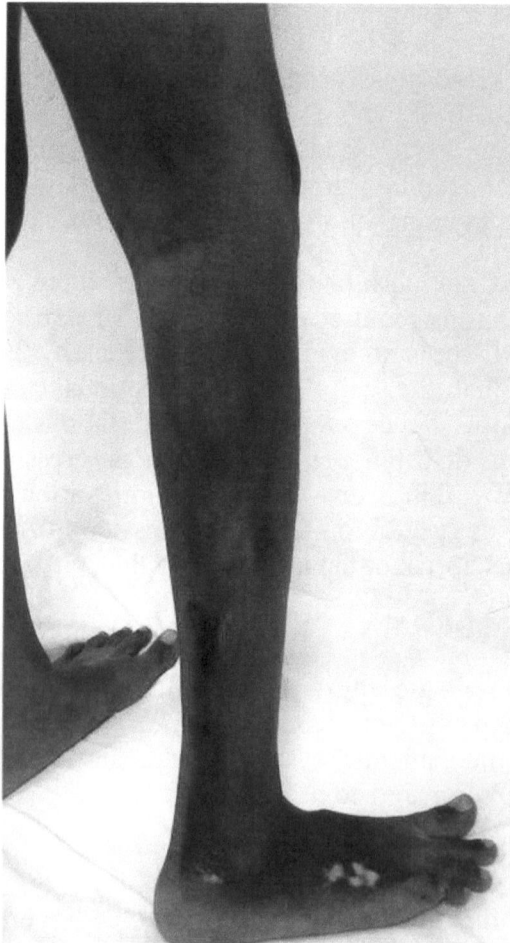

Fig. (8). Linear scleroderma of lower limb[17].

Circumscribed Morphea

This variant is characterized by oval or round areas of skin induration with altered pigmentation surrounded by a violaceous erythematous halo (Fig. **9**). The lesions can be single or multiple. When such lesions involve subcutaneous tissue or deeper areas like fascia and muscle, it is called deep circumscribed morphea. Rarely, the primary site of involvement is in the subcutaneous tissue without the involvement of the skin. This variant is seen more often on the trunk.

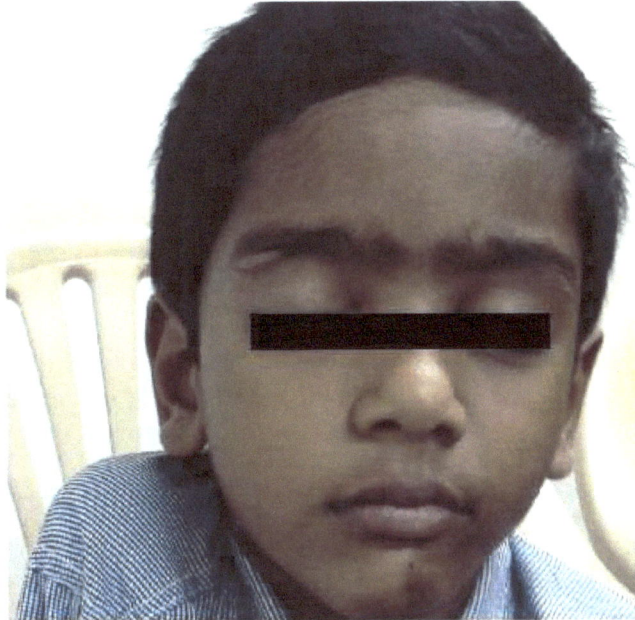

Fig. (9). Localized scleroderma of left side of face[19].

Generalized Morphea

Generalized morphea is diagnosed when more than four circumscribed morphea lesions, each larger than 3 cm, become confluent and involve two of seven anatomical sites [6]. The circumscribed morphea lesions can be superficial or deep.

Pansclerotic Morphea

Pansclerotic morphea is diagnosed when there is circumferential involvement of limbs affecting the skin, subcutaneous tissue, muscle and bone. Auto-amputation can occur due to fibrotic strictures and occlusion of vascular supply. The lesion may involve trunk, face, and scalp but typically has no internal organ involvement. Fingertips and toes are spared, differentiating it from JSSc.

Mixed Subtype

A mixed subtype is diagnosed when more than one type of JLS lesion is seen in a single patient.

Extracutaneous Manifestations

Extracutaneous manifestations are seen in 20% of patients with JLS [19]. Arthritis is most commonly described in patients with linear scleroderma. Linear scleroderma of the face may be associated with neurological features such as seizures, headaches, and learning disabilities. MRI may show white matter changes, calcifications, and vascular malformations [6]. JLS patients also have a higher association with many autoimmune diseases like type I diabetes mellitus, Hashimoto's thyroiditis.

Investigations

The diagnosis of JLS is clinical. Routine blood tests such as hemogram, blood chemistry, and urine analysis are normal. Biopsy from skin lesion shows an initial marked inflammatory reaction, followed by matrix deposition, fibrosis, and ultimately atrophy. ANA may be positive. Anti-histone antibodies may be positive especially in generalized and linear scleroderma.

Treatment

Treatment decisions in JLS depend on the subtype of JLS and disease activity. Circumscribed LS is associated with cosmetic concerns and can be treated with topical treatments like corticosteroids, imiquimod and phototherapy. Other forms of JLS need systemic therapy. The early inflammatory phase is associated with progression to multiple or extensive lesions, then stabilization, and finally improvement with softening of the skin and increased pigmentation around the lesions. The active inflammatory phase may last for years leaving behind significant disability by the time lesion becomes inactive. Hence all active JLS lesions except circumscribed JLS need to be treated with early aggressive systemic therapy.

Systemic therapy is usually initiated with weekly oral or subcutaneous methotrexate therapy along with a bridge course of oral corticosteroids. If effective, methotrexate is continued for a minimum of 2 years as a shorter duration of methotrexate has been associated with higher relapse rates. Refractory disease may need the addition of mycophenolate mofetil or biological disease modifiers.

Outcome

Even though JLS is not associated with significant internal organ involvement, it is associated with significant morbidity. Limb growth and development can be affected. Linear scleroderma of the face is associated with cosmetic issues.

Juvenile Systemic Sclerosis (JSSc)

JSSc is a multisystemic autoimmune disease characterized by vasculopathy and organ fibrosis [53]. It accounts for 3% of all SSc patients. Overlap syndrome contributes to a significant proportion of JSSc patients, unlike in adults [54]. Even though it is rare in children, the morbidity associated with this condition outweighs morbidity associated with any other rheumatological condition.

Clinical Features

Early features of SSc are extremely insidious, and progression is gradual over months and years. This is why most patients are picked up late during the course of the disease with well-established internal organ involvement [53].

Dermatologic involvement manifests as swollen fingers and toes in the early phase. This is followed by the gradual tightening of the skin of fingers. Skin changes lead to a typical waxy texture with the skin getting adhered to underlying tissues leading to "sclerodactyly" (Fig. 10) and "typical expressionless pinched face" (Fig. 11) Vascular involvement manifests as Raynaud phenomenon, digital pitting (Fig. 12), ulcers (Fig. 13), and gangrene. Subcutaneous calcifications can be seen in 20% of patients; most commonly over elbows, metacarpophalangeal joints and knees.

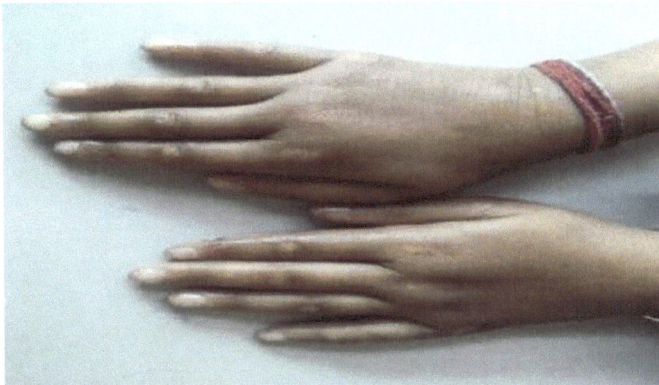

Fig. (10). Thin tapering fingers suggestive of sclerodactyly.

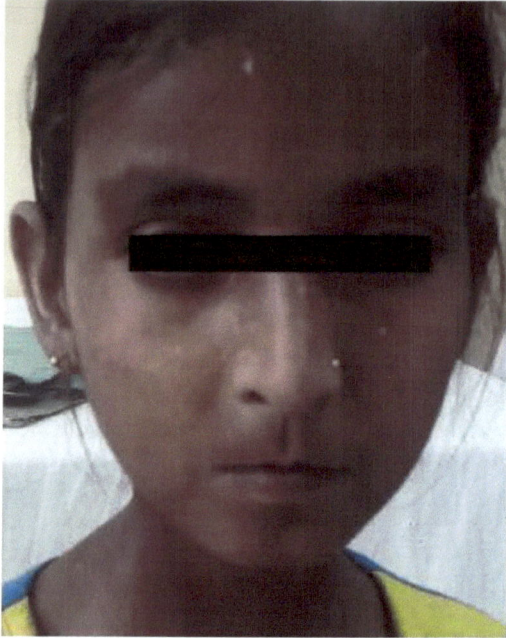

Fig. (11). Thin pinched face in a child with JSSc.

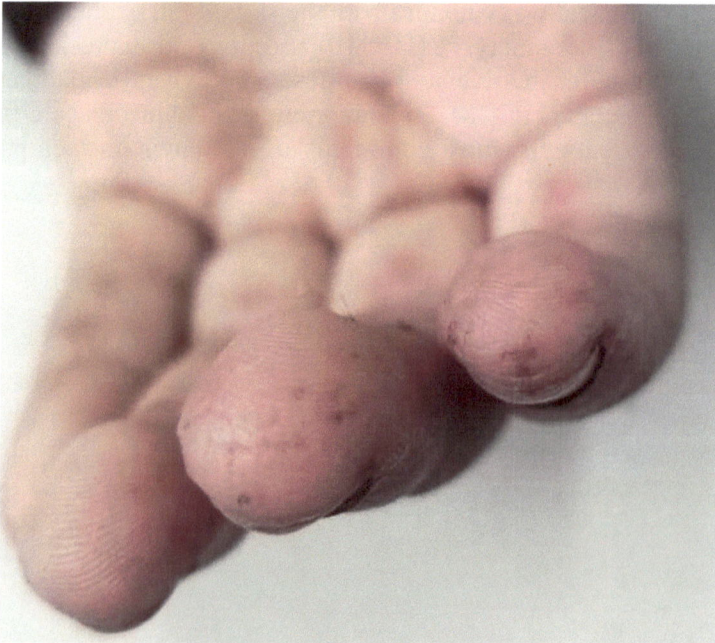

Fig. (12). Digital pitting in a child with JSSc.

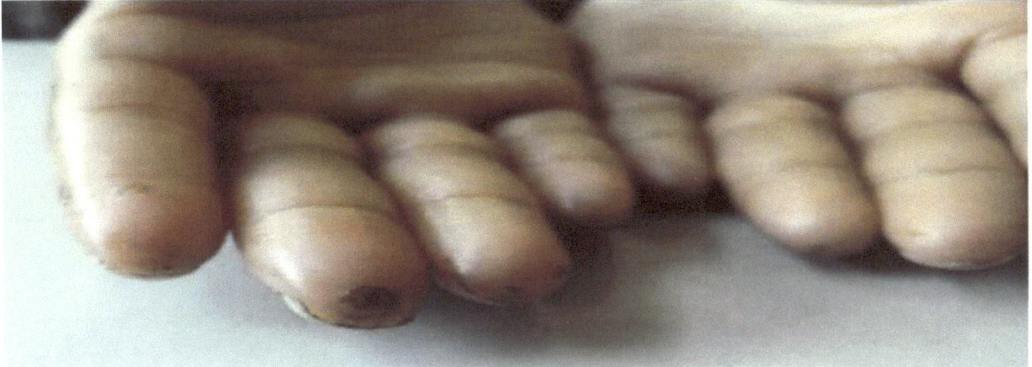

Fig. (13). Digital ulcers in a child with JSSc.

Besides skin and vascular changes, extracutaneous features are common in JSSc:

Musculoskeletal: Arthralgia, arthritis, muscle weakness, contractures

Gastrointestinal: Gastritis, dysphagia, gastroesophageal dysmotility, malabsorptive diarrhea

Cardiopulmonary: Dry hacking cough, breathlessness on exertion, pulmonary fibrosis, pulmonary artery hypertension, cardiac fibrosis leading to conduction defects, arrhythmia, ventricular dysfunction

Renal: Proteinuria, reduced renal function, renal crisis (acute onset of severe hypertension and renal failure)

In comparison to adults, children show less frequent involvement of internal organs at onset [19]. Pulmonary fibrosis (Fig. **14**), renal crisis, and gastroesophageal dysmotility are seen less frequently in children compared to adults, whereas arthritis and muscle involvement are more common in children [6]. Multiorgan involvement is common. Most commonly involved organ systems are skin, vascular, musculoskeletal, gastrointestinal and pulmonary systems [53].

Diagnosis

The diagnosis of JSSc is clinical. Pediatric Rheumatology European Society (PReS)/ACR/EULAR provisional classification criteria for JSSc require the mandatory presence of sclerosis/induration of the skin proximal to metacarpophalangeal or metatarsophalangeal joints in a child aged less than 16 years of age along with at least 2 of the 20 minor criteria [55]. The classification criteria are depicted in Table **6**.

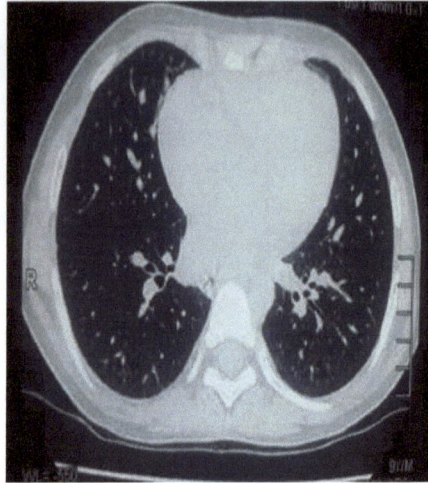

Fig. (14). CT images showing evidence of interstitial lung disease in JSSc.

Table 6. PReS/ACR/EULAR provisional classification criteria for JSSc [55].

Major Criteria	Sclerosis/Induration of the Skin Proximal to Metacarpophalangeal or Metatarsophalangeal Joints	
Minor Criteria	Skin	Sclerodactyly
	Vascular	Raynaud phenomenon Digital tip ulcers Nailfold capillary abnormalities
	Gastrointestinal	Dysphagia Gastroesophageal reflux
	Renal	Renal crisis New-onset arterial hypertension
	Cardiac	Arrhythmia Heart failure
	Respiratory	Pulmonary fibrosis Low diffusing capacity of the lung for carbon monoxide Pulmonary hypertension
	Musculoskeletal	Tendon friction rubs Arthritis Myositis
	Neurological	Neuropathy Carpal tunnel syndrome
	Serology	ANA SSc selective autoantibodies (anticentromere, anti-topoisomerase I, anti-fibrillarin, anti-PM-Scl, anti-fibrillin or anti-RNA polymerase I or III)

Investigations

ANA is positive in high titers in a large majority of patients and the typical pattern is speckled and nucleolar. Antitopoisomerase I (anti-Scl-70) antibodies are present in 28-34% of patients with JSSc. Anti centromere antibody positivity has been described less frequently in JSSc [53]. Anti-PM-Scl and anti-U1RNP antibodies correlate with features of scleroderma in overlap syndromes. RF and aCL antibodies are present in about 15% of children with SSc. Nailfold capillaroscopy is helpful in showing features of vasculopathy as thin capillary loops, markedly reduced capillary density, and less florid tortuosity of capillary loops ('scleroderma' pattern).

Treatment

Treatment of JSSc is especially challenging. Immunosuppression with methotrexate, cyclophosphamide, or mycophenolate mofetil is central in the overall management of JSSc. Steroids have been used in JSSc with no significant association with renal crisis [53]. Table 7 depicts other therapeutic agents which can be used in other manifestations of the disease.

Table 7. Common therapeutic agents for clinical manifestations of JSSc.

Clinical Manifestation	Drugs
Pulmonary arterial hypertension	Endothelin receptor antagonists Phosphodiesterase inhibitors Intravenous prostanoids
Pulmonary fibrosis	Cyclophosphamide Steroids
Hypertensive crises	Angiotensin converting enzyme (ACE) inhibitors Prostacyclin
Digital vasculopathy	Vasodilators Prostacyclin Endothelin receptor antagonists Phosphodiesterase inhibitors

Outcome

JSSc is associated with lower mortality due to a lower frequency of major internal organ involvement compared to SSc in adults. Literature from Europe has reported survival rates of 89%, 87%, and 82% at 5, 10, and 20 years, respectively [56]. Death is usually related to the involvement of cardiac, renal, and pulmonary systems [54]. Morbidity is a major issue in this disease, with most patients reporting poor quality of life scores and poor functional status in multiple organ systems.

JUVENILE DERMATOMYOSITIS (JDM)

JDM is an inflammatory disorder characterized by skin and muscle involvement [5]. It is the most common idiopathic inflammatory myositis (IIM) in children. It predominantly affects children in the latter part of the first decade of life, and there is no overwhelming gender predilection.

Clinical Features

Skin involvement in JDM is characteristic and may offer spot diagnosis to clinicians [5]. Gottron papules (Fig. **15**) are erythematous or pale atrophic skin lesions predominantly located over the dorsal surface of the metacarpophalangeal and interphalangeal joints of the hand [57]. These lesions can sometimes be present on the volar surface of these joints and are termed as 'inverse' Gottron papules. Besides, these lesions may be present over other bony prominences such as elbows or malleoli (Gottron sign) [57]. Heliotrope (Fig. **16**) is a violaceous rash (after the violet-colored flower heliotrope) over the eyelids and adjoining periorbital skin. Sometimes mild periorbital edema may accompany. A diffuse photosensitive erythematous macular rash (Fig. **17**) may be seen over the face, neck, and upper trunk.

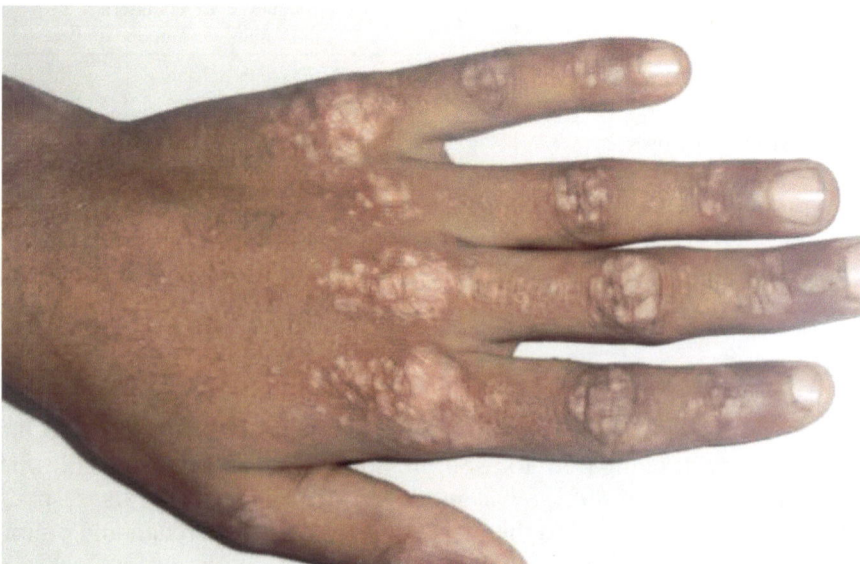

Fig. (15). Gottron papules in a child with JDM.

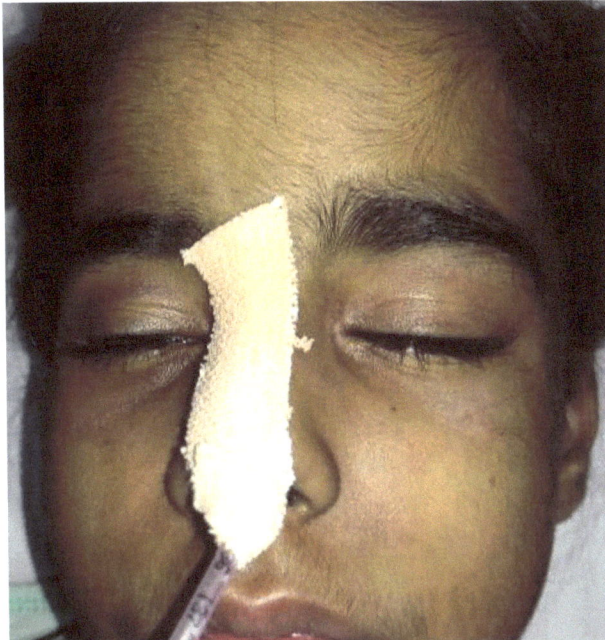

Fig. (16). Heliotrope in a child with JDM.

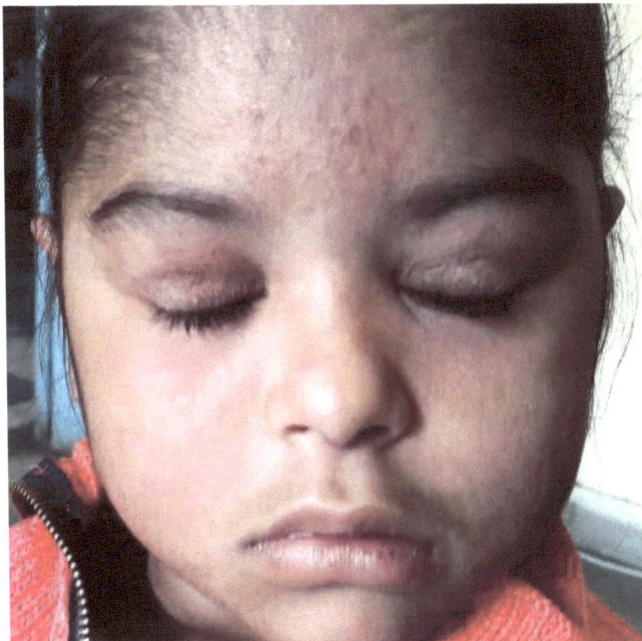

Fig. (17). Diffuse erythema over face in a child with JDM.

In contrast to lupus, the facial rash does not spare the nasolabial folds; however, there may be perioral sparing. In the neck and upper dorsal trunk, photosensitive rash gives rise to a 'shawl' sign resembling a shawl placed around and over the shoulders. Anteriorly, this erythematous rash may give rise to a 'V' sign resembling the V-shaped neck of the upper garments. Additionally, the skin of the nail folds may have visible telangiectatic capillary loops, and that over the tip and pulp of fingers may have scars reminiscent of vasculopathic lesions (Fig. **18**). More commonly, the capillary anomalies of the nail folds are better visualized by a capillaroscope (Fig. **19**) In a subset of patients, there may be diffuse hyperkeratotic thickening of the palms called 'mechanic hands'. The skin lesions in JDM, especially Gottron papules and heliotrope, are virtually pathognomonic of the disease and may help in the clinical diagnosis even when muscle weakness is not prominent. Children presenting with muscle weakness and the above-mentioned skin findings virtually have no differential diagnosis.

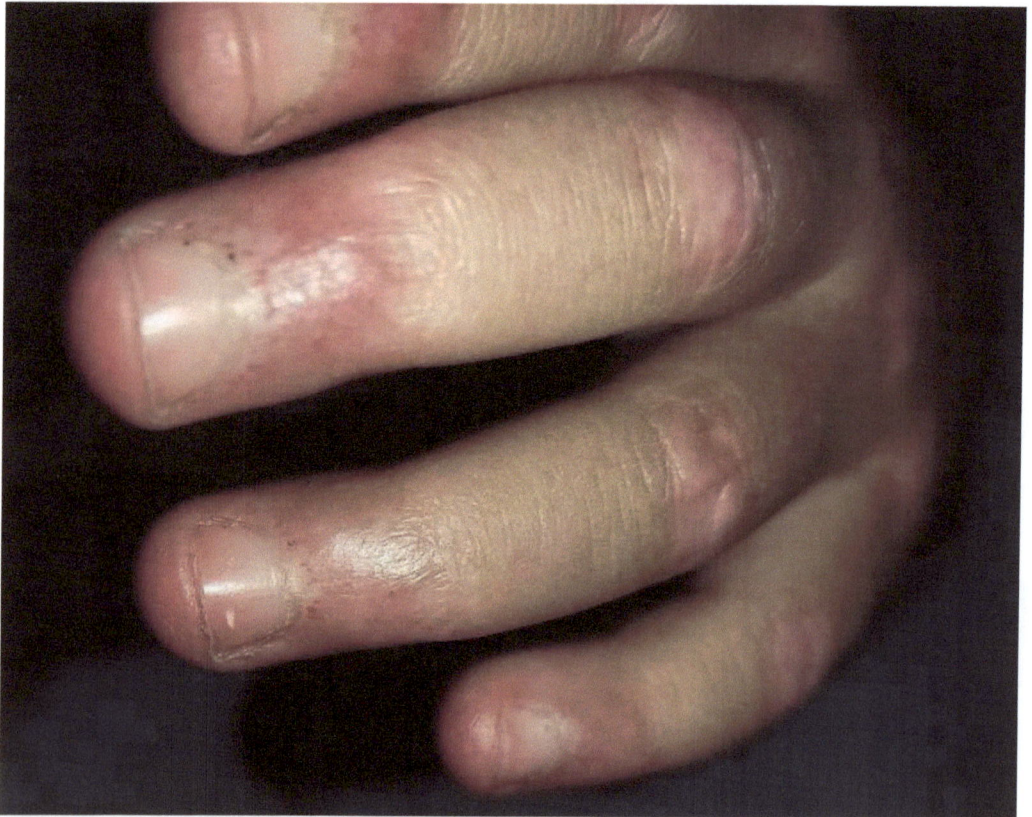

Fig. (18). Nail changes in a child with JDM.

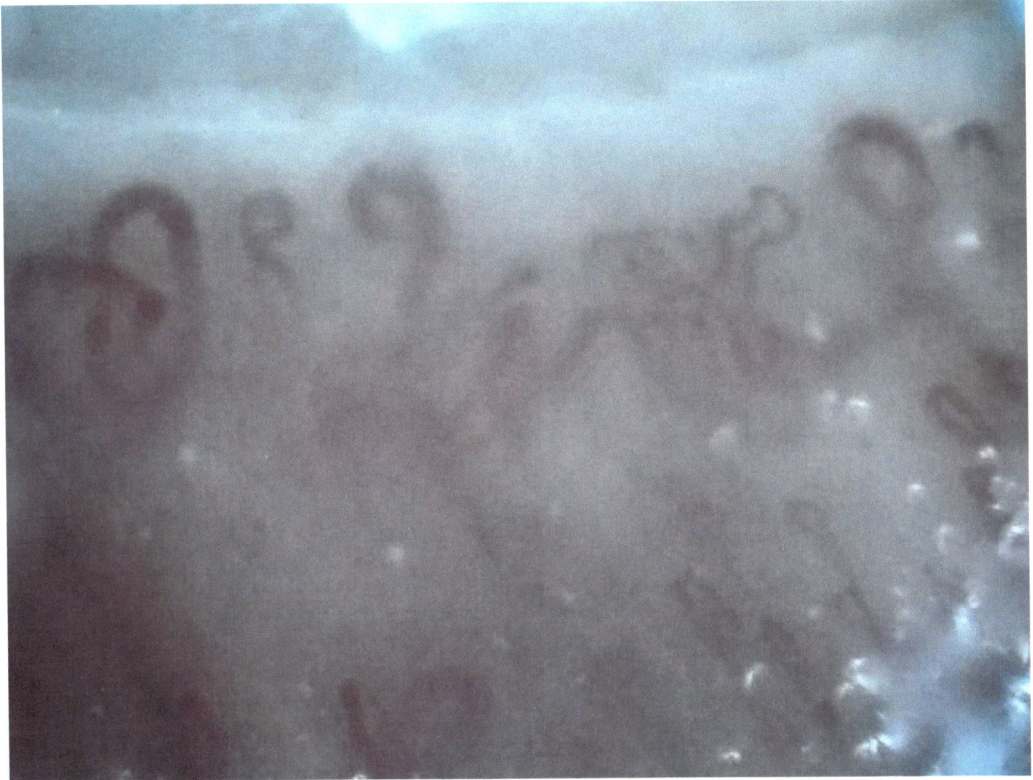

Fig. (19). Nailfold capillaroscopy in a child with JDM.

The muscle involvement in JDM is characterized by weakness of the proximal musculature and progresses to involve axial musculature, pharyngeal musculature, and diaphragm. Common symptoms include difficulty in squatting, getting-up, climbing stairs, and manipulating objects overhead. Pharyngeal muscle weakness is manifested as a change in voice, nasal twang, difficulty in swallowing, choking, and nasal regurgitation of feeds. Aspiration may result, which may often prove fatal. Diaphragmatic muscle involvement may lead to respiratory failure and death. Often children complain of easy fatigability, exercise intolerance, or inability to keep up with peers during play before manifesting with florid muscle weakness.

Besides the clinical manifestations mentioned above, other clinical features reflecting the underlying vasculopathy include gastrointestinal bleeding, which may be massive and life-threatening, and central nervous system vasculopathy. These manifestations are usually seen at the initial presentation or during relapses.

Investigations

Amongst the baseline laboratory investigations, complete blood count may show anemia of chronic disease, high-normal platelet count suggestive of inflammation and elevated ESR. Biochemistry often shows elevated alanine and aspartate aminotransferases. Muscle enzymes such as creatinine phosphokinase, aldolase, and lactate dehydrogenase may be elevated. However, muscle enzymes correlate poorly with disease activity [57]. Other modalities to document muscle involvement include electromyography (EMG), muscle biopsy, and fat-suppressed T2-weighted magnetic resonance imaging (MRI) of muscles. EMG shows increased insertional activity, fibrillation, decreased amplitude of muscle action potential, and polyphasic potentials. Muscle biopsy shows characteristic perifascicular atrophy with perivascular mononuclear cell infiltrate. Since both EMG and muscle biopsy are invasive and difficult to do in children, they are now reserved for children where the diagnosis of JDM is in doubt. Fat suppressed T2-weighted MRI of muscles is a useful noninvasive modality for documenting muscle inflammation and has replaced invasive investigations in patients with typical clinical manifestations.

Autoantibody testing shows ANA positivity in 80% of patients [20]. Extensive research over the last two decades has shown several auto-antibodies to be positive in patients with JDM. These autoantibodies have been broadly classified into two categories: myositis-specific autoantibodies (MSAs) and myositis-associated autoantibodies (MAAs) [20]. Examples of MSAs include anti-melanoma differentiating antigen-5 (anti-MDA5), anti-nuclear matrix protein-2 (anti-NXP2), anti-transcriptional intermediary factor 1 (anti-TIF-1), anti-histidy--tRNA synthetase (anti-Jo-1), anti-alanyl-tRNA synthetase (anti-PL-12), and other anti-tRNA synthetase autoantibodies. Examples of MAAs include anti-U1 small ribonucleoprotein (anti-U1-RNP), anti-Ro, anti-polymyositis scleroderma antibody (anti-PM-Scl), and anti-Ku. Although studies in adults have shown a strong phenotypic correlation with a specific autoantibody positivity, the correlation in the pediatric population is less stringent and less studied. Important correlations include anti-NXP2 with calcinosis and persistent disease activity, anti-MDA5 with skin ulcerations, milder muscle disease and ILD, anti-TIF-1 with bad cutaneous involvement and lipodystrophy, and anti-synthetase antibodies with arthritis, mechanic's hands, Raynaud phenomenon, and ILD (anti-synthetase syndrome).

Nail-fold capillaroscopy is a useful modality to visualize vasculopathy in JDM. The principle of this technique is that the capillaries in the nail folds run parallel to the skin surface and hence can be visualized throughout their course. This is in contrast to the capillary loops at other places in the skin, where they run perpendicular to the skin surface. Findings include dilated tortuous loops, hemorrhages, and capillary loss. Excessive tortuosity may resemble a tree-like pattern called 'arborized' capillary loops. This pattern (myositis pattern) differs from the pattern seen in JSSc.

Diagnosis

The diagnosis of JDM has traditionally been based on the Bohan and Peter criteria published way back in 1975 [58]. The diagnosis requires the presence of one of the two characteristic skin manifestations (Gottron papules or heliotrope rash), in addition to three of four features suggestive of muscle involvement (proximal muscle weakness on clinical examination, elevated muscle enzymes, suggestive EMG findings, and suggestive muscle biopsy findings). However, EMG is technically challenging in children, and muscle biopsy has largely been supplanted by MRI. In the revised diagnostic criteria, MRI findings have been added as one diagnostic criterion. Therefore, JDM can be diagnosed in children without the need for EMG or muscle biopsy. However, muscle biopsy may still be required in doubtful cases and in cases where skin manifestations are not present.

EULAR/ACR classification criteria for adult and juvenile IIM have been developed [59]. According to these criteria, the probability of having IIM is calculated based on a scoring system that includes both clinical and laboratory features. Muscle biopsy is not a must for this scoring system. An online calculator is available for calculating the probability of having IIM. In a patient who is classified as definite IIM, diagnosis of JDM requires age at onset of < 18 years, and presence of any one skin manifestation (heliotrope, Gottron papule, or Gottron sign).

Complications

The two most important complications of JDM include calcinosis and lipodystrophy/lipoatrophy. Calcinosis (Figs. **20** and **21**) develops during the disease course and is seldom present at disease onset. Risk factors for calcinosis include long duration of disease, suboptimal therapy at disease presentation, and positivity for anti-NXP2 and anti-PM-Scl antibodies. Similar to calcinosis, lipoatrophy/dystrophy develops late during the disease course. It is often associated with features suggestive of metabolic syndrome: acanthosis nigricans (insulin resistance), dyslipidemia, hypertension, steatohepatitis, and hyperandro-genism. Early aggressive therapy of JDM decreases the risk of lipodystrophy and calcinosis. Other complications include vasculopathic skin ulcers, ILD and cardiac involvement.

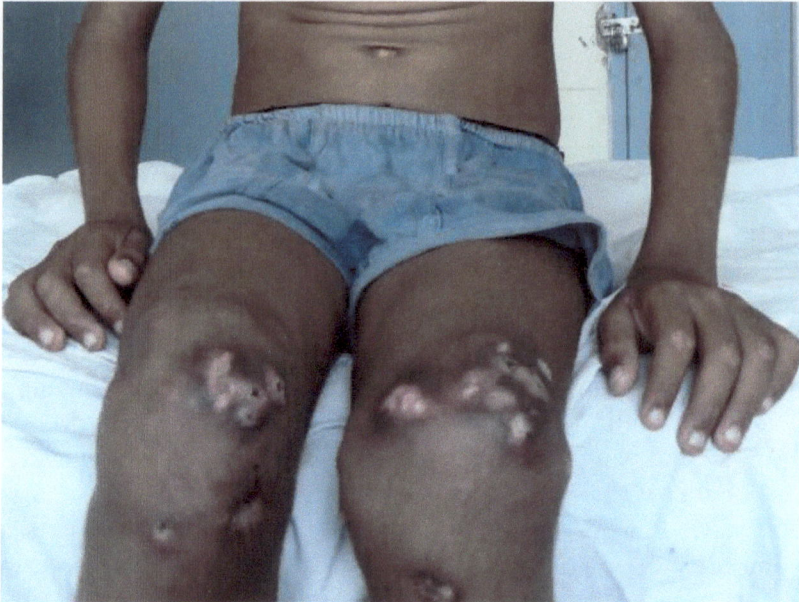

Fig. (20). Calcinosis over knees in a patient with JDM.

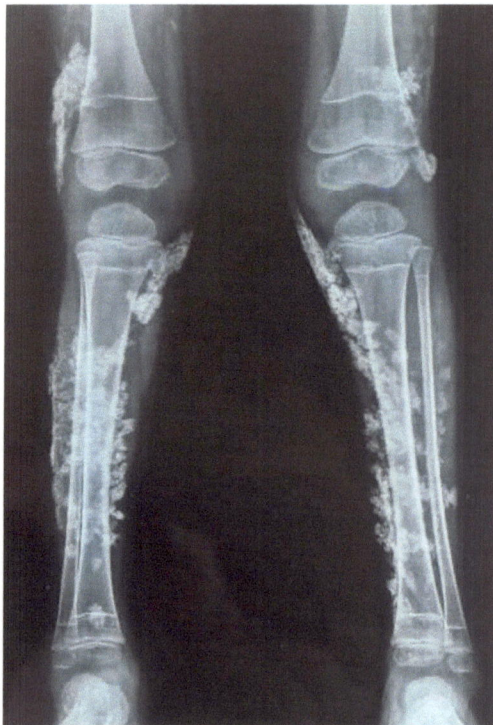

Fig. (21). X-ray showing extensive calcinosis in a child with JDM.

Treatment

Treatment aims to control the disease activity, prevent organ damage, and improve quality of life.

Control of disease activity is achieved by immunosuppressive therapy. Steroids and parenteral methotrexate are the most common immunosuppressants used in the management of JDM [5]. There is no consensus on the route of steroids for patients presenting with mild to moderate JDM. However, in severe cases, it is recommended that steroids be given as pulse therapy intravenously. This is especially important in patients with significant edema where gut absorption of medications may be compromised. There is no consensus on the duration of steroids. Steroids are gradually weaned off as patients show clinical improvement. Commonly employed doses for methotrexate are 15-20 mg/m^2 given subcutaneously every week. Methotrexate is recommended for all children with mild to moderate weakness. Children on methotrexate therapy require frequent monitoring with complete blood count and liver transaminase measurement. There is no consensus on when to stop therapy. If the patient has been off steroids and doing well on methotrexate alone for 1 year, one may consider withdrawing methotrexate.

Inadequate response to therapy warrants intensification of treatment within first 12 weeks. This is required to preserve muscle mass and strength and reduce the risk of chronic complications. There is no fixed protocol for intensification and various agents like intravenous immunoglobulin (IVIg), mycophenolate mofetil, cyclosporine, cyclophosphamide, and biological agents such as rituximab, infliximab and adalimumab have been used. IVIg has been used as an adjunct in children with moderate JDM and those with persistent skin disease [29]. No specific regimen has been recommended in the literature for IVIg. Cyclosporine is effective in children with JDM. However, because of the adverse side-effect profile, it can be reserved as an alternative in children who are either intolerant or have contraindications to methotrexate.

High-risk patients such as those with a severe disability defined as the inability to get out of bed, aspiration, dysphagia, gastrointestinal vasculitis, cardiac involvement, skin ulcerations, and onset in infancy need more intense immunosuppression at the onset itself [5]. Intravenous cyclophosphamide pulse therapy is reserved for such patients. Cyclophosphamide is given as 500 mg/m^2 as a single intravenous monthly dose for six months, followed by the addition of parenteral methotrexate or oral mycophenolate mofetil.

HCQ is a useful and common adjunct in the treatment protocol of children with JDM; especially in those with significant skin disease. Sun protection with sunscreen and physical barriers should be advised to all patients.

Supportive care is equally important, especially in the acute phase. Pharyngeal involvement needs to be checked in all patients and a nasogastric tube should be placed for feeding in all children with pharyngeal weakness. Frequent oropharyngeal suction may be required in these children. Daily respiratory muscle assessment is vital during acute phase.

Physiotherapy and occupational therapy have been used to improve the range of motion at various joints, muscle strength, and physical function. Frequent position changes may be required in children unable to change their position on their own to prevent bedsores.

Monitoring

Assessment of disease activity is clinical. Muscle disease is monitored by utilizing the childhood myositis assessment scale or manual muscle testing scales. Skin assessment is done by using cutaneous assessment tools and nail fold capillaroscopy. Swallowing dysfunction should be assessed on every follow-up visit. Persistent or worsening skin rash reflects systemic disease activity, which requires hiking up of the immunosuppression. Muscle enzymes are not used routinely to monitor disease activity due to their poor correlation. Screening for ILD may be prudent in a subset of patients with JDM with anti-synthetase antibodies.

Outcome

Before the steroid era, the outcome was often stated in the form of "one-third" formula, with one-third succumbing to the illness, one-third having a spontaneous remission, and one-third having a persistent disease. Modern-day treatment has reduced mortality to around 1%, with sustained remission in more than three-fourths of the children [29]. One-half of all children with JDM are able to stop immunosuppression within 2-3 years of disease onset. However, 40-50% of children may continue to require immunosuppressive therapy because of persistent disease activity or relapsing disease. With the increasing life span of these children, the focus has shifted to reducing long-term morbidities such as calcinosis and lipodystrophy.

VASCULITIS IN CHILDREN

Vasculitis means inflammation of blood vessels. There can be many causes of vasculitis in children. Secondary causes like infections, autoimmune diseases, and malignancy predominate [8]. Primary causes are less common in children compared to secondary causes. Out of all primary systemic vasculitides, IgA vasculitis (IgAV, Henoch-Schönlein purpura) and KD are common in childhood.

Similarly, vasculitides can also be classified based on the course of the disease. A chronic course is typical of Takayasu arteritis and PAN [60]. Acute course is typical with KD and IgAV. Acute inflammation of vessel wall can cause occlusion or weakening of vessel wall causing aneurysms and rupture [7]. Chronic inflammation in the vessel wall can also lead to fibrosis and consequent stenosis. Occlusion and stenosis of vessels can cause ischemic injury to the organs [8].

Pathophysiologically, vasculitis can be divided into large vessel, medium vessel and small vessel vasculitis based on the size of involved vessels. Clinical manifestations vary according to the type of involved vessel and involved organ systems (Table **8**).

Table 8. Features of vasculitides based on the type of vessel involved.

	Large Vessel Vasculitis	**Medium Vessel Vasculitis**	**Small Vessel Vasculitis**
Type of vessels involved	Aorta and its immediate branches	All other vessels except mentioned under large and small-vessel vasculitis	Arterioles, capillaries, venules
Clinical features	• Pulse discrepancy • Differential hypertension • Bruits • Features of ischemia in limbs esp on exertion	• Syndromic features of KD • Systemic involvement of PAN due to microaneurysms and stenosis of blood vessels (lungs are usually spared)	• Palpable purpura • Renal involvement (Glomerulonephritis) • GI involvement • Arthritis • Lung involvement (pulmonary capillaritis)
Diagnostic modalities	Imaging of vessels (Angiography)	Imaging of vessels (Angiography, Echocardiography), biopsy	Biopsy, ANCA
Examples	Takayasu arteritis	KD, PAN	IgAV, AAV

Whereas small vessel vasculitis can be easily diagnosed by demonstration of inflammation in the vessel wall in a biopsy from the involved organ system, the same may not be feasible in larger vessels because of the risk of rupture. Hence vascular imaging to show inflammation in the vessel wall, and its after-effects like stenosis and aneurysms plays a major role in the diagnosis of large and medium vessel vasculitides.

IgA Vasculitis (IgAV)

Previously known as Henoch-Schönlein purpura (HSP), it is the commonest primary vasculitis of children with an annual incidence of 3-27 per 1,00,000 children [61, 62]. Though it can be seen at any age, peak age at onset is 4-6 years and 90% of childhood-onset IgAV occur in children less than 10 years of age [30]. There is a slight male predominance, unlike many other autoimmune diseases.

Pathophysiology

Exact pathophysiology of this disease remains unknown. It is hypothesized that elevated abnormal IgA leads to the formation of circulating immune complexes, which in turn cause complement activation and cytokine release [30]. Infectious triggers like viral and bacterial infections have been implicated and can explain seasonal predilection seen in this disease [63, 64]. Genetic factors include many protective and susceptibility risk factors [30].

Clinical Features

Previously well child usually presents with acute onset of skin rash, which is typically symmetrical, palpable purpuric rash predominant in lower limbs and buttocks (Figs. **22** and **23**). The skin rash may also extend to the upper limbs and trunk. Rarely, this rash may become more confluent and show a bullous appearance. Sometimes, a preceding transient urticarial rash is seen. In addition to skin rash, a classic triad of musculoskeletal, gastrointestinal, and renal involvement is seen.

Musculoskeletal involvement: Transient arthralgia or arthritis is described in as many as 70-90% of patients. Arthritis involves a few joints of the lower limbs [30]; however, upper limb joints may also be involved. Sometimes, the skin overlying a particular joint may be involved due to rash and may mimic arthritis.

Gastrointestinal involvement: Gastrointestinal involvement is the major cause of acute morbidity associated with this disease. Colicky abdominal pain after feeds is typical of bowel angina and is present in 70% of children. Gastritis, duodenitis, gastrointestinal mucosal ulcerations, and purpura are common features. Significant gastrointestinal bleeding can present as malena or hematemesis. Intussusception, either ileoileal or ileocolic, can be a presenting feature. Hence, an ultrasound should be done to rule out an intussusception in any child with IgAV and severe abdominal pain [65].

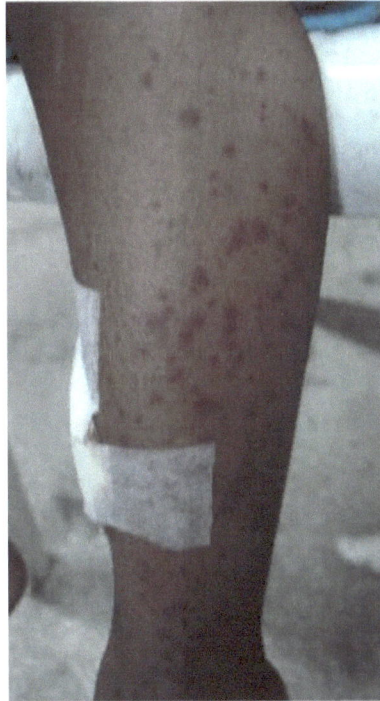

Fig. (22). Palpable purpura in lower limbs in IgAV.

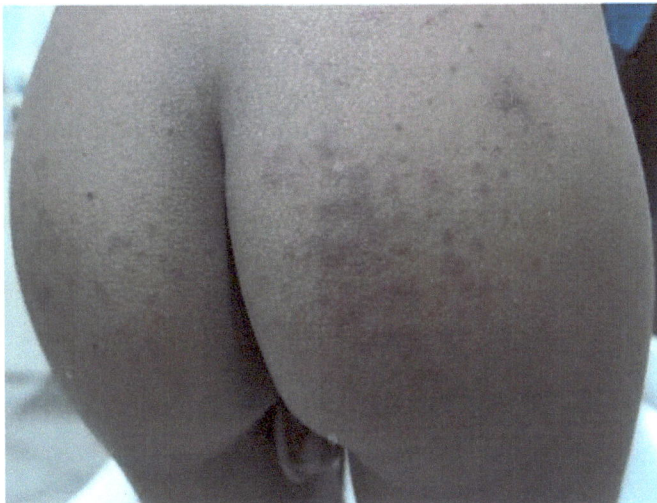

Fig. (23). Palpable purpura in gluteal region in a child with IgAV.

Renal involvement: Renal involvement is the major cause of chronic morbidity and mortality in IgAV. It is seen in 40-50% patients and can vary from mild manifestations like microscopic hematuria and mild proteinuria to severe rapidly progressive glomerulonephritis [30]. It is seen within the first 6-12 months after the acute disease. Hence, all children with IgAV should be monitored for the development of nephritis by periodic urine examinations by microscopy and urine protein to creatinine ratio, blood pressure measurements, and assessment of glomerular filtration rate for at least 1 year after the acute illness.

Long-term risk of developing end-stage renal disease is low (~1.6%) for children who have mild renal involvement presenting as microscopic hematuria with or without mild to moderate proteinuria. This risk is higher (~20%) for children who present with nephritis or nephrotic syndrome.

Mild IgAV nephritis (normal GFR and mild or moderate proteinuria) does not warrant kidney biopsy, and if kidney biopsy is done, it usually correlates with the International Study of Kidney Disease in Children histological Class I (minimal changes) or Class II (mesangial changes only). The presence of severe persistent proteinuria and/or impaired GFR correlates with a higher histological class [65]. Table **9** depicts the classification of IgAV nephritis based on kidney biopsy and laboratory features.

Table 9. Classification of IgAV nephritis[2].

Severity of IgAV Nephritis	Definition
Mild	Normal GFR and mild or moderate proteinuria
Moderate	<50% crescents on renal biopsy and impaired GFR or severe persistent proteinuria
Severe	>50% crescents on renal biopsy and impaired GFR or severe persistent proteinuria
Persistent proteinuria	Spot urine protein: urine creatinine (UP:UC) ratio >250 mg/mmol or 2.2 mg/mg for 4 weeks UP:UC ratio >100 mg/mmol or 0.88 mg/mg for 3 months UP:UC ratio >50 mg/mmol or 0.44 mg/mg for 6 months

Other organs: Testicular inflammation is another important emergency, sometimes mimicking testicular torsion. It is important to differentiate the two since orchitis responds briskly to steroids, whereas testicular torsion requires urgent surgery. Uncommonly, nervous system involvement may also be seen during the acute phase.

Investigations

Skin Biopsy

Skin biopsy is not routinely required for typical clinical presentations of IgAV. For atypical presentations, skin biopsy with immunofluorescence should be done from the most recent skin lesions. Evidence of leukocytoclastic vasculitis with IgA deposition is typical, but the absence of IgA from the lesions does not exclude the diagnosis of IgAV.

Indications of Kidney Biopsy

Renal biopsy is indicated in a child with IgAV [65] if the patient has:

- Severe proteinuria (>250 mg/mmol or >2.2 mg/mg) for at least 4 weeks
- Persistent moderate (100-250 mg/mmol or 0.88-2.2 mg/mg) proteinuria
- Impaired glomerular filtration rate (GFR)
- Acute kidney injury with worsening renal function as a part of rapidly progressive glomerulonephritis

Diagnosis

There is no single diagnostic test, and diagnosis relies on clinical and laboratory findings (Table **10**). The ACR criteria (1990) were found to have 87% sensitivity and specificity to distinguish from other forms of vasculitides [66]. EULAR/Pediatric Rheumatology International Trials Organization (PRINTO)/ Pediatric Rheumatology European Society (PReS) endorsed criteria (2008) rely on clinical features and have been found to have 100% sensitivity and 87% specificity to distinguish from other forms of vasculitides [67]. Skin biopsy is not mandatory to make a diagnosis; however, it should be done in case of atypical rashes like diffuse or very extensive rash [64]. It should be remembered that classification criteria should not be used for diagnostic purposes.

Treatment

Typically IgAV is an acute self-limiting illness; hence treatment is primarily supportive. The only exception is renal inflammation which has the potential to cause scarring and end-stage renal disease.

Analgesia: Adequate analgesia is required for IgAV associated arthritis and gastrointestinal manifestations. Single Hub and Access point for Paediatric Rheumatology in Europe (SHARE) guidelines recommend the use of NSAIDs or paracetamol for relief of joint pain. The presence of microscopic hematuria does not contraindicate the use of NSAIDs.

Table 10. Classification criteria of IgA vasculitis.

ACR Criteria (1990) [66][3]	EULAR/PRINTO/PReS Endorsed Criteria (2008) [67][4]
At least 2 out of the 4 following criteria Palpable purpura Age of onset ≤ 20 years Acute abdominal pain Skin biopsy showing granulocytes in small arterioles or venules	Mandatory criterion • Purpura or petechiae with lower limb predominance At least 1 out of 4 • Acute onset diffuse abdominal colicky pain (may include intussusception and gastrointestinal bleeding) • Histology showing leukocytoclastic vasculitis or proliferative glomerulonephritis with predominant IgA deposition. • Acute onset arthralgia or arthritis • Either proteinuria or hematuria

Corticosteroids: Corticosteroids are indicated for orchitis, cerebral vasculitis, pulmonary hemorrhage, and other severe organ- or life-threatening vasculitic manifestations. Corticosteroids may also be considered in children with severe abdominal pain and/or rectal bleeding. Oral prednisolone is started at 1-2 mg/kg/day for 1-2 weeks, followed by weaning over the next 2-3 weeks. Pulse methylprednisolone may be used in children with severe vasculitic manifestations. Corticosteroid use early in the disease course does not reduce the risk of development of IgAV nephritis.

Treatment of IgAV Nephritis

SHARE guidelines recommend using ACE inhibitors or angiotensin receptor blockers in all patients of IgAV nephritis with persistent proteinuria to prevent secondary glomerular injury.

Children with macroscopic hematuria with normal renal functions and no proteinuria or non-persistent proteinuria do not need renal biopsy but require periodic follow-up for progression [65]. On the other hand, children with persistent/severe proteinuria or impaired renal function need a kidney biopsy. Corticosteroids should be used in patients with moderate to severe IgAV nephritis. Azathioprine or mycophenolate mofetil may be used as first or second-line treatment in moderate nephritis. Intravenous cyclophosphamide along with pulse methylprednisolone is used to induce remission in severe nephritis, whereas for maintenance, azathioprine or mycophenolate mofetil may be used.

ANCA Associated Vasculitis (AAV)

AAV is a group of pauci-immune necrotizing vasculitides of small to medium-sized blood vessels [8]. This group includes three primary systemic vasculitides with multisystem involvement:

1. Granulomatosis with polyangiitis (GPA), formerly called Wegener's granulomatosis
2. Microscopic polyangiitis (MPA)
3. Eosinophilic granulomatosis with polyangiitis (EGPA), formerly called Churg Strauss syndrome

Besides these, renal limited ANCA vasculitis is also included in this group. This group is characterized by severe clinical manifestations, frequent relapses, and high morbidity and mortality. Detection of ANCA to proteinase-3 (PR3) or myeloperoxidase (MPO) is the cornerstone of diagnosis.

Epidemiology

GPA is more common than EGPA and MPA in childhood [68]. The typical age at onset is adolescence and there is a female preponderance.

Clinical Features

Clinical features of GPA, MPA, and EGPA are depicted in Table **11**. Children with EGPA have a prolonged history of atopy, symptoms related to ears and sinuses, and severe steroid-dependent asthma for years before the diagnosis of vasculitis [69, 70].

Table 11. Clinical features of AAV.

	GPA	MPA	EGPA
Pathology	Granulomatous inflammation of medium and small arteries	Nongranulomatous inflammation of small vessels	Granulomatous inflammation of medium-sized arteries and small vessels
Upper respiratory tract	Common Epistaxis, sinusitis, otitis media, nasal septal perforation, saddle nose deformity, subglottic stenosis	Rare	Common Sinusitis, nasal polyps, allergic rhinitis, otitis media

(Table 11) cont.....

	GPA	MPA	EGPA
Lower respiratory tract	Common Nodules (Fig. **24**), cavities, fixed infiltrates, pulmonary hemorrhage	Common Diffuse alveolar hemorrhage (Fig. **25**)	Common Severe asthma, Nonfixed pulmonary infiltrates
Kidney	Common Pauci-immune necrotizing glomerulonephritis	Common Pauci-immune necrotizing glomerulonephritis	Rare
Less common manifestations	• Ocular: scleritis, conjunctivitis, ocular pseudotumor • Mucocutaneous: oral and genital ulcers, skin rash • Musculoskeletal: arthritis, arthralgia, muscular pain • Gastrointestinal	• Peripheral neuropathy • Ocular: Episcleritis, conjunctivitis • Mucocutaneous: oral and genital ulcers, skin rash • Musculoskeletal: arthritis, arthralgia, muscular pain	• Systemic symptoms: fatigue, weight loss, fever • Skin: nodules, papules, palpable purpura • Cardiac: pericarditis, heart failure, hypertension, arrhythmia • Gastrointestinal: Abdominal pain, colitis • Musculoskeletal: arthritis, arthralgia, muscular pain • Neurological: mononeuritis, polyneuropathy, central nervous system involvement

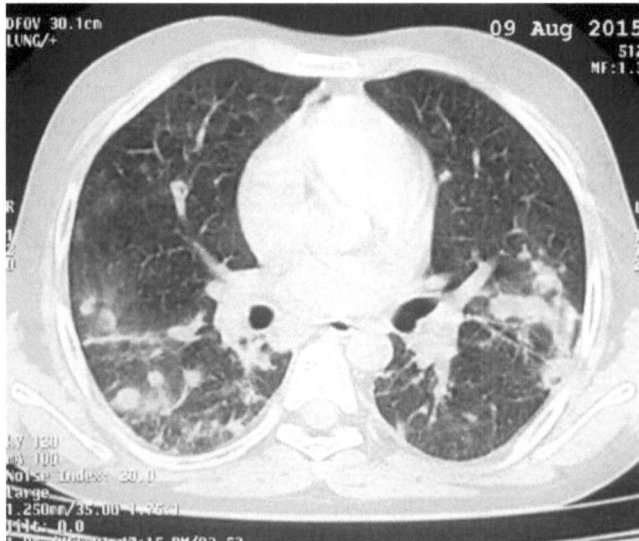

Fig. (24). CT images showing pulmonary nodules in a child with GPA.

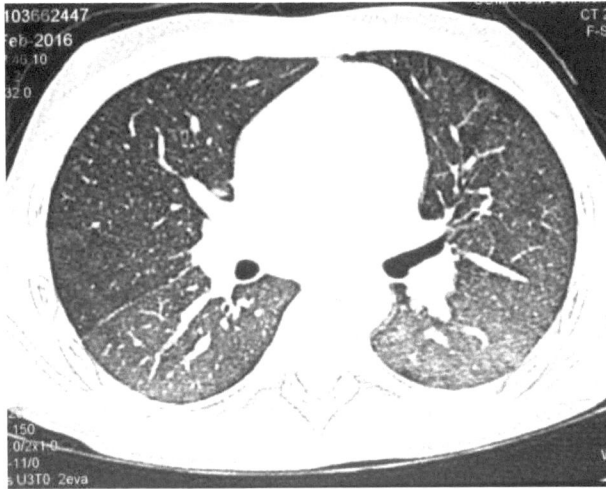

Fig. (25). CT images in a child with diffuse alveolar hemorrhage.

Diagnosis

Diagnosis is based on histopathologic demonstration of vascular involvement. Even though children may present with diffuse alveolar hemorrhage secondary to pulmonary capillaritis, lung biopsy is difficult in hypoxic children. Biopsies from the kidney, skin, upper respiratory tract, or orbital pseudotumor are used more often for diagnosis.

Most patients show positivity for ANCA. In GPA, majority of patients show positivity for c-ANCA with antigen specificity for PR3. On the other hand, in MPA, p-ANCA may be positive with antigen specificity for MPO. In EGPA, ANCA positivity is seen in only 30-40% of patients and it is usually seen against MPO. Peripheral blood eosinophilia and tissue eosinophilia are commonly seen in EGPA. Type of ANCA is useful to predict prognosis. PR3-ANCA positivity has been associated with a higher risk of disease relapse and death.

Treatment

Owing to the rarity of the disease and paucity of randomized control trials in children, most treatment protocols have been adapted from adult literature. Therapy consists of remission induction and maintenance. In life- or organ-threatening AAV, induction of remission is achieved by pulse corticosteroids with cyclophosphamide or rituximab. Maintenance of remission can be achieved by low dose steroids along with the drugs like methotrexate, azathioprine, rituximab, or mycophenolate mofetil. Therapy should be continued for a minimum duration of 24 months after achieving sustained remission [68]. Plasmapheresis has been used in acute settings of severe alveolar hemorrhage or rapidly progressive glomerulonephritis not responding appropriately to induction therapy.

Outcome

AAV are severe life- or organ-threatening pauci-immune vasculitides with high relapse rates and morbidity. Early diagnosis and initiation of appropriate therapy are the cornerstone to a favorable outcome. Morbidity is usually attributed to complications like end-stage renal disease, saddle nose deformity, chronic sinusitis, or side effects of therapy like infertility and avascular necrosis.

Kawasaki Disease

KD is an acute medium vessel systemic vasculitis of unknown etiology [21]. It was first described by Dr. Tomisaku Kawasaki in 1967 from Japan. Since then, it has been described from all continents of the world and has become a leading cause of acquired heart disease in children in developed nations.

Epidemiology

The highest incidence rates are described from Japan, Korea, and Taiwan. Annual incidence rates in Japan and US have been described as 308/1,00,000 [71] and 19/1,00,000 [72] children less than 5 years of age, respectively. Incidence is intermediate in Asians living in US. Risk in siblings is estimated at 2.1%, which is ten times the risk in the general population in Japan [21]. Recurrence risk is estimated at 3%, with maximum risk in the first 2 years after the disease [73]. Maximum incidence is seen in children between 6-11 months. Nearly 80% of children are less than 5 years at diagnosis [21]. A distinct seasonal predilection has been seen. In US, most cases occur in winters and early spring. Similar seasonality has been observed in other countries in the Northern hemisphere except for those lying in the tropics.

Etiology

The etiology of KD remains unknown even though 50 years have passed since its first description. Factors like the seasonality of cases, nationwide epidemics, and self-limiting nature of the disease point to an infectious cause. On the other hand, high incidence rates in Japan, intermediate rates in Japanese children staying in US, and relatively lower rates in US point to genetic factors. High concordance rates in siblings further support the genetic predisposition. The most accepted theory is that infection caused by a widely distributed agent evokes an abnormal immunologic response in genetically susceptible persons. However, no causative agent has been identified consistently.

Pathogenesis

KD is a generalized systemic vasculitis that affects medium-sized arteries throughout the body. Both innate and adaptive immune systems are involved [21]. In the first two weeks (acute phase), neutrophilic infiltration is seen in the vessel wall. After a few weeks, a phase of subacute or chronic vasculitis with predominant lymphocytic infiltration sets in. The resultant inflammation causes the destruction of luminal endothelial cells, elastic lamina, and smooth muscle of media, further leading to loss of structural integrity, arterial wall dilation, and aneurysm formation [74]. Irregular blood flow in aneurysms leads to further endothelial damage and thrombi formation. Tendency to form thrombi is further increased by the prothrombotic state induced by active inflammation. Finally, this phase is replaced by luminal myofibroblastic proliferation, leading to luminal narrowing and may cause myocardial ischemia.

Arterial remodeling in aneurysms can cause regression, occlusion, stenosis, and further extension of an aneurysm. Regression and occlusion occur due to luminal myofibroblastic proliferation and layered thrombi formation within aneurysms. Calcification is common in aneurysms with layered thrombi and usually occurs after 5 years of diagnosis.

Stenosis is progressive over the years and is commonly seen proximal and distal to aneurysms. Further extension of coronary aneurysms can be seen in up to 3% coronary artery lesions over 10 years. Virtually all mortality and morbidity in patients with KD are attributed to giant aneurysms.

It is hypothesized that coronary artery lesions of KD may predispose to premature atherosclerosis. Intimal thickening and endothelial dysfunction are seen in both KD and atherosclerosis. Vascular lesions of KD are considered distinct and different from atherosclerotic lesions. However, there is evidence of persistent endothelial dysfunction, increased reactive oxygen radicals, dyslipidemia, and decreased vascular elasticity in KD. All these risk factors may increase the risk of atherosclerosis.

Clinical Features

The acute febrile phase is characterized by fever and mucocutaneous inflammation. Fever is high spiking and intermittent and usually does not respond well to antipyretics. Mucocutaneous inflammation manifests as nonpurulent bilateral conjunctivitis (Fig. **26**), oral mucosa and lip changes (Figs. **27** and **28**) and nonspecific, diffuse maculopapular eruption. Erythema of palms and soles and firm induration of dorsum of hands and feet (Fig. **29**) are common. Periungual desquamation of fingers and toes (Figs. **30** and **31**) is not seen in the acute phase.

Perianal desquamation (Fig. **32**) is also described and occurs a few days earlier than periungual desquamation. Clinical features related to mucocutaneous inflammation are evanescent and may be altogether absent in infants.

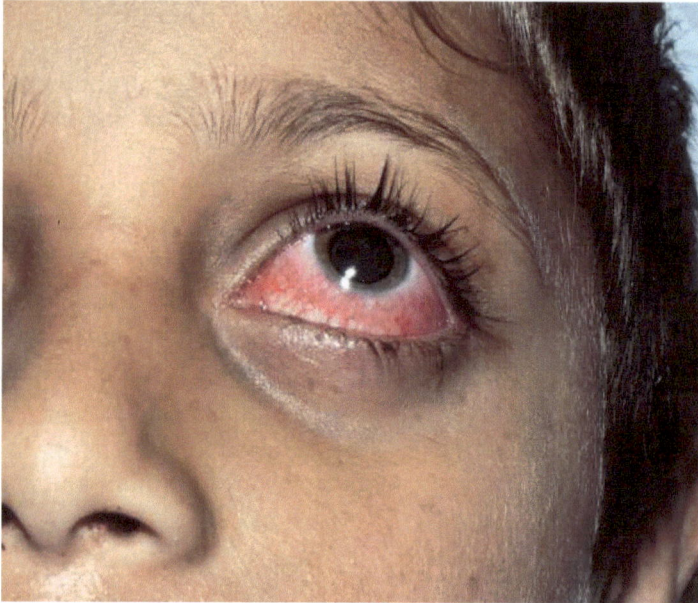

Fig. (26). Nonpurulent conjunctivitis in a child with KD.

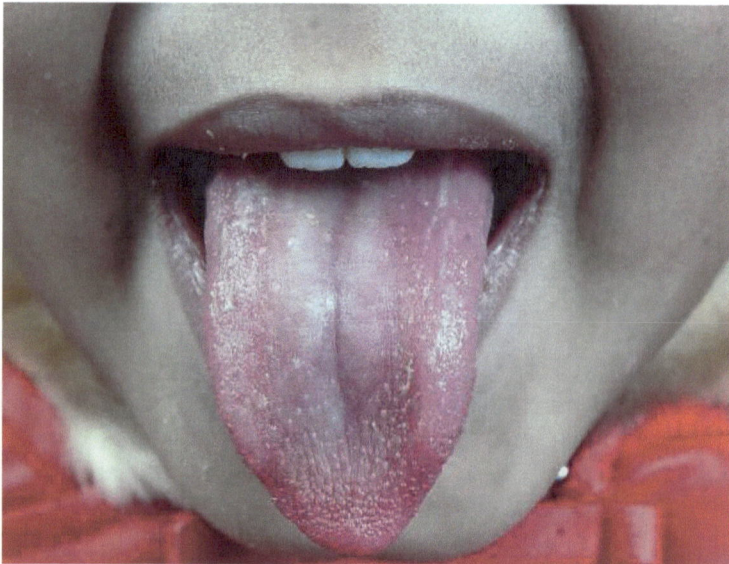

Fig. (27). Strawberry tongue in KD.

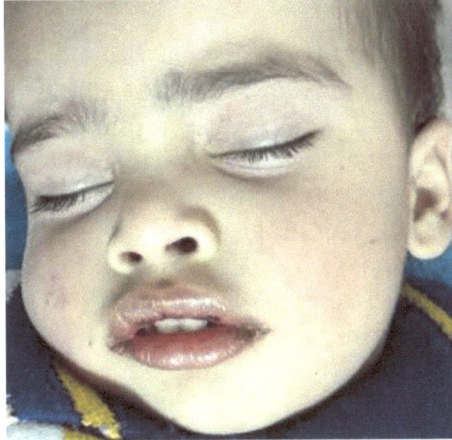

Fig. (28). Lip changes in KD.

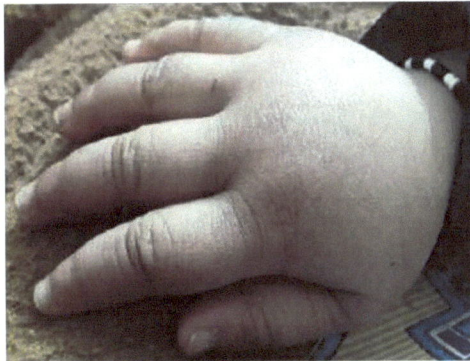

Fig. (29). Induration of dorsum of hand in acute KD.

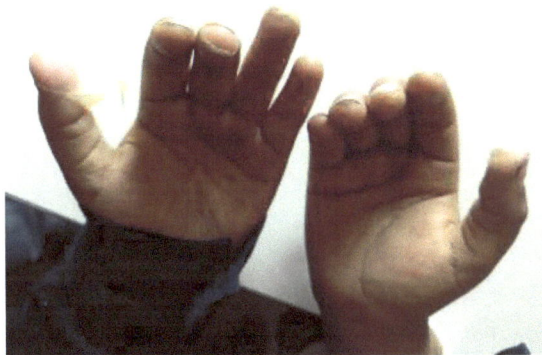

Fig. (30). Early periungual desquamation in KD.

Unilateral cervical adenopathy may be seen. Most children, especially infants, have an extreme degree of persistent irritability due to aseptic meningitis. It is important to think of KD in all infants with prolonged unexplained fever, marked irritability, and increased acute phase reactants, even in the absence of any other typical features. Polyarthritis of small joints, arthralgia, and gastrointestinal manifestations like diarrhea, vomiting, and abdominal pain are other important manifestations in the acute phase. Evidence of gall bladder hydrops may be seen due to acalculous cholecystitis. In countries where BCG vaccine is administered, BCG site reactivation is seen frequently, especially in younger children. Urethritis is frequent and is seen as sterile pyuria on urine microscopy. Cardiac involvement can be seen as myocarditis, pericarditis, shock, and valvular regurgitation by echocardiography in the acute phase. Coronary artery dilatation is unusual in the first week of illness.

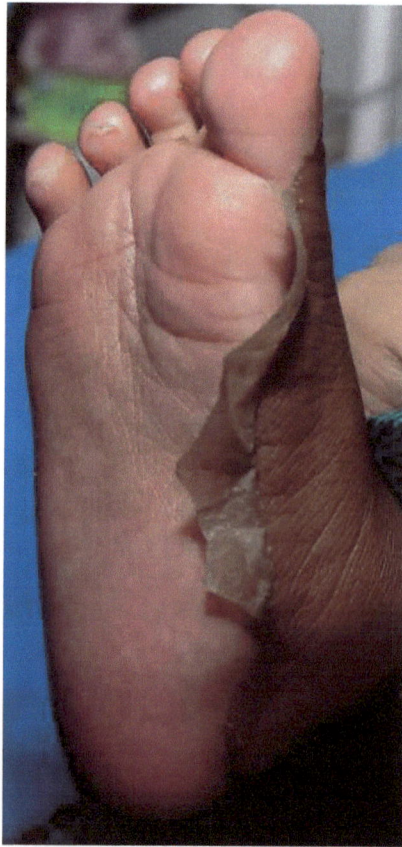

Fig. (31). Extensive desquamation in soles in KD.

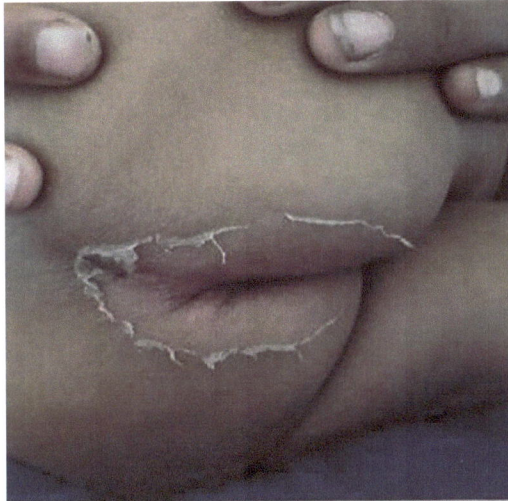

Fig. (32). Perianal desquamation in KD.

When fever and other signs start to disappear, the subacute phase begins. During this phase, the child is at greatest risk for death because of coronary vasculitis and a high risk of thrombosis due to markedly elevated platelet count and hypercoagulable state. In this phase, certain characteristic features like periungual peeling and thrombocytosis are seen.

The convalescent phase begins at around 4-6 weeks when all signs of illness have disappeared, and it continues until acute phase reactants have returned to normal. Beau lines may appear on nails and depict temporary growth arrest during the acute phase (Fig. **33**). This is a nonspecific finding of the disease. Arthritis involving large joints may be seen during this phase.

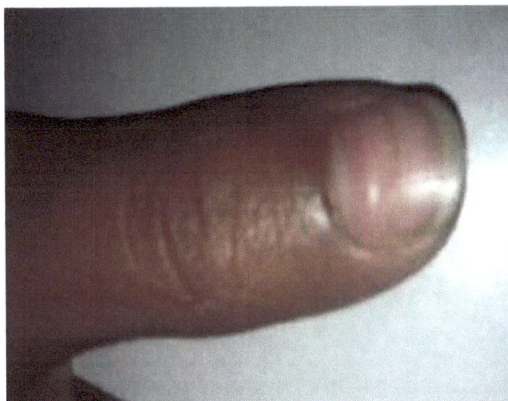

Fig. (33). Beau lines in KD.

The chronic phase encompasses the long-term management of children in whom coronary artery abnormalities develop during the acute phase.

Investigations

No single laboratory investigation is diagnostic of KD. The role of investigations in KD is to rule out the differential diagnosis, to show inflammation and to pick up coronary involvement.

Inflammation is depicted by anemia, leucocytosis, raised ESR and CRP, sterile pyuria and hypoalbuminemia in the acute phase. Sterile pyuria occurs due to urethritis and urine collected directly from the urinary bladder will not show pyuria. Acalculous cholecystitis leads to ultrasonographic evidence of gall bladder hydrops. Other less common laboratory findings include mild to moderate elevation in serum transaminases, hyponatremia and hypoalbuminemia. Thrombocytosis is seen in the second and third weeks of illness and can support the clinical diagnosis. Thrombocytopenia can occur in acute phase due to consumptive coagulopathy and is associated with elevated D-dimer.

A normal echocardiographic examination does not rule out KD. In the first week of illness, most children have no evidence of coronary dilatation. Rather one is more likely to see evidence of small pericardial effusion, mitral valvulitis, and myocardial dysfunction. Early coronary involvement within the first 10 days predicts the development of coronary artery aneurysms (Fig. **34**) during the next few days. Internal dimensions of coronary segments are measured and normalized based on body surface area and expressed as "z scores" [73]. The severity of dilatation is classified in Table **12**.

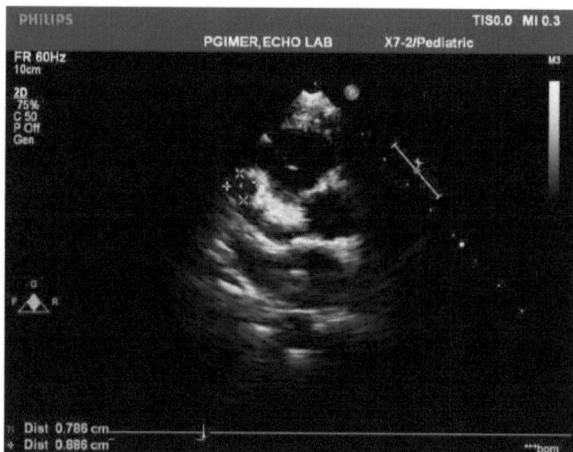

Fig. (34). Echocardiography showing coronary aneurysm in KD.

Table 12. American Heart Association (AHA) Classification of coronary artery lesions in KD [73]⁵.

Z Score of Internal Dimensions of Coronary Segments	Category
< 2	Normal
2 to <2.5	Transient dilatation
≥ 2.5 to <5	Small aneurysm
≥5 to <10	Medium aneurysm
≥10	Giant aneurysm

The coronary artery lesions are classified as follows:

• Ectasia: Dilatation of an artery without a segmental aneurysm.
• Saccular aneurysm: When axial and lateral diameters of an aneurysm are nearly equal.
• Fusiform aneurysm: Symmetrical dilatation of an artery with gradual proximal and distal tapering.

It is important to note that transient dilatation of coronary arteries can occur in many febrile illnesses. Echocardiographic examinations at diagnosis, after 1-2 weeks and after 4-6 weeks, suffice for most children with KD who respond briskly to standard therapy. Resolution at 6-8 weeks is most likely in patients with coronary dilatation with z scores of 2 to <2.5.

However, in children who have high-risk factors or show coronary z scores of > 2 at first examination need more frequent echocardiographic examinations until dimensions of aneurysms stabilize [21]. CT or conventional angiography may help in better delineation of giant aneurysms and complications like stenosis or calcification.

Diagnosis

There is no diagnostic test for KD. Diagnosis is essentially clinical. Classic KD is diagnosed according to criteria given by AHA (Table **13**) [74].

Table 13. Diagnosis of Classic KD [74]⁶.

o Fever for at least 5 days
o Presence of at least four out of five principal clinical features
o Bilateral bulbar conjunctival injection without exudates
o Rash: maculopapular, diffuse erythroderma or erythema multiforme like rash
o Erythema and cracking of lips, strawberry tongue and/or erythema of the oral and pharyngeal mucosa
o Erythema and edema of hands and feet in the acute phase and/or periungual desquamation in the subacute phase
o Cervical lymphadenopathy (≥ 1.5 cm, usually unilateral)

These criteria are neither 100% sensitive nor 100% specific. It has been shown that as high as 27% of patients may not be treated if these criteria are used strictly for diagnosis.

Incomplete KD

Incomplete KD is suspected when a patient has a fever for at least 5 days with no other explanation but has fewer than four of the clinical criteria required for the diagnosis of classic KD (Table **13**). It is more common in infants. About 10% of all KD patients fall into this group [75]. Laboratory findings are similar to those of KD. Delayed diagnosis is frequent because of the incomplete clinical picture, and hence, the risk of coronary artery aneurysms is high.

AHA recommends that all such children should be screened with ESR and CRP [73]. If CRP is $\geq$ 3 mg/dl and/or ESR $\geq$ 40 mm per hour, one needs to look at other laboratory findings and echocardiography. The laboratory features include anemia for age, leucocytosis (TLC>$15*10^9$/L), thrombocytosis after day 7 of fever, low serum albumin, high serum alanine transaminase, and high leucocyte count in urine. If more than three of these laboratory findings are present, the the patient should be labeled "incomplete KD" and treated. Similarly, if echocardiography shows any of the three following features, the child should be labeled as "incomplete KD" and treated.

- Z score of left anterior descending coronary artery or right coronary artery $\geq$2.5
- Coronary artery aneurysm
- $\geq$3 suggestive features
    - Decreased left ventricular function
    - Mitral regurgitation
    - Pericardial effusion
    - Z scores in the left anterior descending coronary artery or right coronary artery of 2 to < 2.5

Differential Diagnosis

Differential diagnoses include viral infections, such as measles, scarlet fever, toxic shock syndrome, drug hypersensitivity reactions, Stevens-Johnson syndrome, rickettsial infection, and sJIA [73]. Certain clinical and laboratory features should alert one to the possibility of alternate diagnosis:

- Generalized lymphadenopathy
- Purulent conjunctivitis
- Vesicular rash

- Discrete ulcers in the mouth
- Tonsillar exudates
- Low total leukocyte count
- Lymphocyte predominance

Treatment

The aim of treatment in the acute phase is to reduce inflammation as early as possible and reduce the risk of thrombosis in developing aneurysms.

Intravenous immunoglobulin (IVIg): IVIg was initially used in KD without any evidence. Now it has been proven beyond doubt that timely initiation of IVIg reduces the incidence of coronary artery aneurysms from 25% to about 4%. With timely IVIg, transient coronary dilation, coronary artery aneurysms and giant aneurysms are seen in 20%, 5%, and 1% patients, respectively. Single IVIg infusion at a dose of 2 g/kg over 10-12 hours is recommended. This is preferred over splitting the dose over 2-5 days, as lower peak serum IgG levels have been associated with a longer duration of fever, longer duration to normalize inflammatory parameters, and higher risk of coronary artery aneurysms. In most children, this treatment alone leads to rapid clinical improvement. The mechanism of action of IVIg is not clearly defined and many mechanisms have been implicated. Though children with KD should receive IVIg within the first 10 days of therapy for maximum efficacy, AHA recommends that all children who present after day 10 of illness receive this treatment if they have persistent fever, features of ongoing inflammation, or have developed coronary artery aneurysms [73]. AHA recommends against use of IVIg in children with KD after 10 days if they are clinically well and have normal laboratory investigations and echocardiography study. IVIg administration is associated with an increase in ESR. Hence, ESR should not be used to monitor inflammation in patients after administration of IVIg.

Aspirin: Aspirin was initially used at a dose of 80-100 mg/kg/day in 3-4 divided doses. In Japan and Europe, a lower dose at 30-50 mg/kg/day is being used because of gastrointestinal side effects due to higher doses. There is no data to suggest higher efficacy with either dose. It also does not seem to have any effect on the development of coronary artery lesions. The dose is further reduced to antiplatelet doses (3-5 mg/kg/day) once the child remains afebrile for 48-72 hours. Duration of aspirin depends on coronary artery involvement. It is recommended that aspirin should be stopped if there is no evidence of coronary involvement on echocardiography at 6-8 weeks of disease.

Anticoagulation: Children who develop giant aneurysms are at the highest risk of developing thrombosis, and this risk is maximum in the first three months of illness. Unfractionated heparin or low molecular weight heparin is preferred in the acute phase. Later on, the patients can be switched over to oral anticoagulants.

Steroids: Early literature on the role of steroids in KD was controversial. Later with the proven efficacy of IVIg, steroids were not used much in the treatment. A recent meta-analysis published by *Chen et al* have shown that a combination of corticosteroids along with IVIg is associated with a significant reduction in coronary artery aneurysms as compared to IVIg alone [72]. It seems to be a promising adjunct for children at high risk of developing coronary artery aneurysms. Many centers in Europe now use steroids along with IVIg as the first-line therapy for high-risk patients with KD. AHA recommends a longer course of corticosteroids with tapering over 2–3 weeks for the treatment of high-risk patients with acute KD along with standard IVIg and aspirin. It recommends against using single-dose pulse methylprednisolone along with IVIg as a routine primary therapy for patients with KD [73].

Other options: Monoclonal antibodies directed against TNF-α, such as infliximab, have been used in patients with IVIg resistance and as an intensification of initial therapy for high-risk children.

IVIg Resistance

IVIg resistance is defined as persistent or recurrent fever after $\geq$ 36 hours after completion of the initial IVIg infusion. This is seen in about 10-20% children with KD. Multiple risk factors such as age less than 1 year, male sex, initial thrombocytopenia, low albumin, and high liver enzymes have been shown to predict IVIg resistance. These children are at higher risk of developing coronary artery lesions and need additional anti-inflammatory treatment and frequent echocardiography studies till the stabilization of coronary dimensions. Many agents have been used as anti-inflammatory agents in this group of patients but none of them are as beneficial as IVIg therapy for initial treatment of KD. The second dose of IVIg, steroids and infliximab have been used in literature. Alternative treatments with cyclosporine, anakinra, cyclophosphamide, and plasmapheresis have been tried in a few cases. There is no consensus on which agent to use. There is also a need to intensify primary therapy in patients at high risk of coronary artery lesions rather than using additional therapy once IVIg resistance is documented.

Long-term Management

Long-term management of KD patients depends on the severity of coronary involvement. All children who have had KD, should be assessed and counseled about known cardiovascular risk factors. Periodic cardiac evaluation is needed for all patients who develop coronary artery aneurysms. The frequency of assessment depends both on the maximum diameter of the lesion and the degree of regression. Table **14** depicts long-term management according to the maximum z scores observed in the patient.

Table 14. Long-term management of KD [73].

Z Scores	Long-term Management
< 2	Antiplatelet agents for 4-6 weeks
2 to < 2.5	Antiplatelet agents until regression documented
≥ 2.5 to < 5	Low dose aspirin Lifelong surveillance Serial echocardiography and electrocardiography Assessment for inducible myocardial ischemia Statins ±
≥ 5 to <10	Long term antiplatelet agents (double agent used may be considered) Lifelong surveillance Serial echocardiography and electrocardiography Assessment for inducible myocardial ischemia Statins ±
≥ 10	Low molecular weight heparin or Vitamin K antagonists + aspirin Beta-blockers ± Statins ± Serial echocardiography and electrocardiography Assessment for inducible myocardial ischemia Angiography

Conclusion

KD is an important cause of acquired heart disease in children in developed countries. Coronary artery aneurysms are described in up to 25% of untreated children. Timely treatment with IVIg and aspirin is the gold standard and has been proven to decrease the risk of coronary artery aneurysms to less than 5%. There is a growing consensus on the intensification of initial therapy for children at high risk of developing coronary artery aneurysms. There is no consensus on second-line treatment for IVIg resistant cases. Long-term management varies with the severity of coronary artery aneurysms.

Polyarteritis Nodosa

PAN is a rare necrotizing medium vessel vasculitis with the usual involvement of visceral, renal, and soft tissue vessels. It spares lungs, unlike AAV. Association with infections is described, most commonly with Hepatitis B virus (HBV), though most cases are idiopathic. The genetic association has been seen with loss of function mutations in the gene encoding for adenosine deaminase 2 (ADA2) [76].

Clinical Features

Constitutional features like fever, malaise, weight loss, arthralgia, and myalgia are common. Almost all organ systems can be involved, with common features being mononeuritis multiplex, skin nodules, necrotic ulcers, livedo reticularis, abdominal pain, lower gastrointestinal bleeding, and testicular pain or swelling. Renal involvement is seen as impaired glomerular filtration rate, hypertension, hematuria and proteinuria. Limb claudication and gangrene can also be seen.

Since it is a medium vessel vasculitis, glomerulonephritis and pulmonary capillaritis, which are typical features of AAV, do not occur in PAN. Organ-specific manifestations occur due to microaneurysm formation with arterial occlusions leading to ischemia.

Investigations

No investigations are specific to PAN. Laboratory investigations like increased ESR, increased CRP, thrombocytosis, and anemia are suggestive of inflammation. ANCAs are typically negative.

A tissue biopsy can show evidence of necrotizing vasculitis in medium and small-sized arteries [76]. Vascular lesions are typically segmental and occur at branching sites. Demonstration of different stages of inflammation in the vessel wall is typical of PAN. Biopsies from symptomatic sites are likely to give a higher yield. Renal biopsy should be avoided because of the risk of rupture of aneurysms. Skin, muscle, and sural nerve biopsies can be used as they are less invasive and fraught with less danger. In the absence of a histopathologic diagnosis, vascular imaging can be used for diagnosis. Typical findings on imaging are the demonstration of microaneurysms and stenotic lesions in visceral arteries [60]. Renal infarcts may also be seen but are not diagnostic of PAN [76].

Treatment

Owing to rarity of disease, no evidence-based guidelines exist for management of childhood PAN. Therapy is based on the use of corticosteroids and immunosuppressive agents. Steroids are the mainstay of therapy. Patients with mild PAN are treated with oral steroids, which are gradually tapered once remission is achieved. Methotrexate or azathioprine may be added in children with mild PAN when one is not able to taper steroids or there are unacceptable side-effects related to steroids. In patients with renal insufficiency, gastrointestinal or cardiac involvement, aggressive immunosuppression should be used from the beginning. Monthly pulse cyclophosphamide therapy for 6-9 months is preferred along with pulse steroids for induction. This is followed by maintenance therapy with azathioprine or mycophenolate mofetil. There is no consensus on the duration of therapy.

Surgery may be required in the acute stage for gastrointestinal perforation or bleeding in internal organs. HBV-related PAN requires seroconversion of HBV status to maintain long-term remission.

Takayasu Arteritis

Takayasu arteritis is a chronic granulomatous large vessel vasculitis of the aorta and its major branches [77]. It is a panarteritis involving all the three layers of the vessel wall producing a typical pathology characterized by stenosis, occlusions, aneurysms, and rarely rupture. Clinical features are ascribed to inflammation and distal ischemia.

Epidemiology

For the initial 40 years after its first description, this disease was described only from Japan [77]. However, now this disease has been described from all over the world. The usual age at onset is 10-40 years, with 20-30% cases occurring in childhood. Females are 2-4 times more likely to be affected [78].

Pathology

Pathologically, the disease can be seen in acute florid inflammatory or healed fibrotic phases [79]. In the acute phase, initial involvement occurs in vasa vasorum in the adventitia. There is infiltration by lymphocytes and occasional giant cells in media followed by neovascularization and intimal thickening. In the chronic phase, there is fibrosis with the destruction of elastic tissue. The lumen is narrowed in a patchy distribution, often affecting multiple areas. Aneurysms occur due to significant inflammation occurring over a short period of time, which does not give enough time for fibrosis to set in. Aneurysms are uncommon in children.

Clinical Features

Clinical features depend on the site of vascular involvement and organs supplied by that vessel.

Involvement of arch of aorta with origins of major vessels from it results in impalpable or weak vessels in upper limbs and neck, upper limb claudication, syncope, or stroke. Such children may have evidence of ischemic retinopathy due to the involvement of the carotid trunk.

The involvement of thoracoabdominal aorta distal to the origin of upper limb vessels results in weak lower limb vessels and hypertension in the upper limbs. Such children may show evidence of hypertensive retinopathy. They may also have cardiac involvement in the form of congestive heart failure due to myocardial inflammation or due to outflow obstruction. Reduced renal flow due to renal artery involvement or suprarenal aortic involvement is responsible for hypertension. Hypertension is usually severe and may or may not be associated with differential pulses depending on the site involved. Advanced stenosis in bilateral renal arteries could lead to renal dysfunction.

Claudication is not a common symptom in childhood, probably because of the inability to express this symptom. Bruits are common at the site of arterial involvement because of irregular flow across a stenotic lesion. Though mesenteric circulation is usually affected in Type 3 and 4 disease, mesenteric ischemia is distinctly uncommon because of extensive collaterals. Impalpable pulses, especially in vessels like brachial, carotid or femoral arteries, indicate proximal obstruction, which is an important sign of the disease. Carotidodynia (tenderness on palpating carotid arteries) is uncommon.

Prepulseless disease (before the onset of stenosis) presents with nonspecific features like fever, malaise, night sweats, anorexia, and weight loss. In this stage, no specific clinical features exist, and hence diagnosis is rarely made. Some authors have used positron emission tomography (PET) scan in this stage to make a diagnosis, however, this modality is not well standardized for diagnosis.

Types

Table **15** gives the angiographic classification of Takayasu arteritis.

Table 15. Angiographic classification of Takayasu arteritis, Takayasu conference 1994 [80][7,8].

Type	Arterial Territory Involved
Type I	Branches from the aortic arch
Type IIa	Ascending aorta, aortic arch and its branches
Type IIb	Ascending aorta, aortic arch and its branches, descending thoracic aorta
Type III	Thoracic descending aorta, abdominal aorta, and/or renal arteries
Type IV	Abdominal aorta and/or renal arteries
Type V	Combined features of types IIb and IV

There are regional differences in type of the disease. In Japan, Type 1 and 2a are the most common variants, and hence the typical clinical features of absent pulses in upper limb (pulseless disease) and features of CNS ischemia. Eye examination may show features of ischemic retinopathy and retinal microaneurysms. Upper limbs will not have hypertension.

In India, Type 3 and 4 are the common variants, thus explaining an entirely different clinical presentation [80]. These types are not associated with "pulselessness" in upper limbs and CNS and eye ischemia features. Instead, lower limb pulses would be feeble with significant hypertension in the upper limbs. Cardiac decompensation is more frequent, and CNS involvement occurs due to severe hypertension. The eye may show features of hypertensive retinopathy.

Diagnosis

Takayasu arteritis is the prototype large vessel vasculitis in children. Vascular imaging by angiography is the gold standard for diagnosis. Ultrasound with a doppler can be used to look for kidney size and evidence of arterial stenosis. Echocardiography is used to look for cardiac dysfunction. Unilateral renal artery stenosis may present with a discrepancy in renal size, whereas bilateral stenosis may not show the discrepancy. Doppler of renal and carotid arteries is useful in picking up stenosis.

Most errors are committed at the stage of history and examination. In all children presenting with congestive heart failure, visual complaints, stroke, seizures and syncope, it is necessary to look for pulses in all four limbs as well as carotids and take blood pressure. If the child is hypertensive, one must take blood pressure in all four limbs. This basic examination is enough to make one think of this disease in most settings.

Once this disease is suspected, the gold standard for diagnosis is angiography. The vascular imaging can show occlusion, stenosis (usually proximal and ostial), dilatation, and aneurysms (Fig. **35**). Usually, there is contiguous involvement of arteries; however, skip lesions may be seen. Status of the vessel wall is not seen by conventional angiography and is better seen with CT or MR angiography.

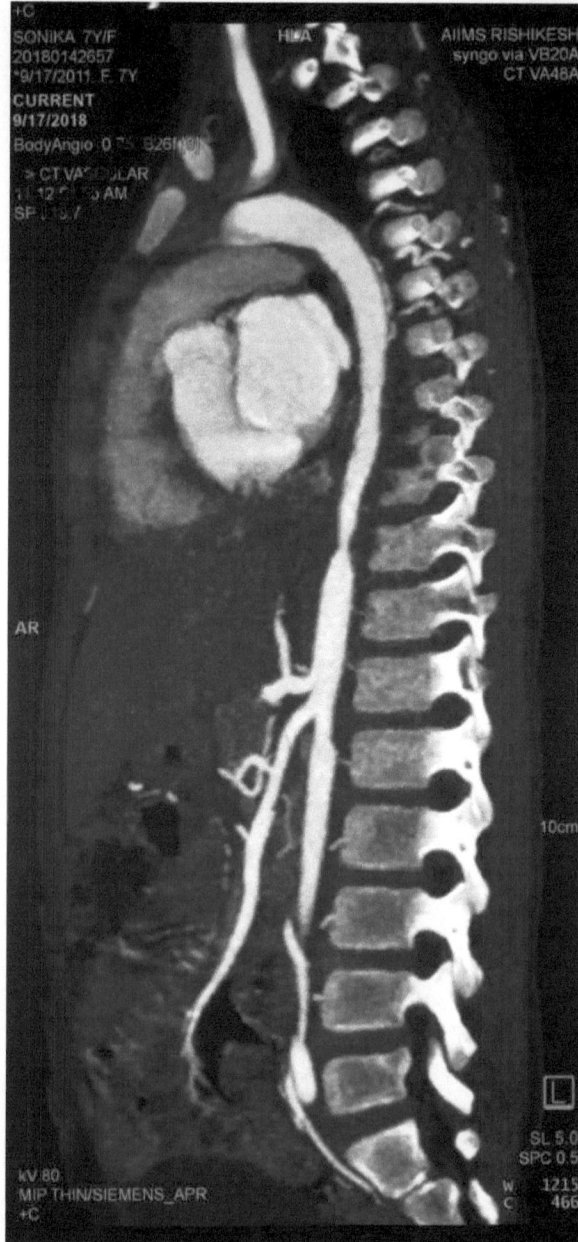

Fig. (35). Angiography study showing stenosis of thoracoabdominal aorta in Takayasu arteritis.

PET scan has been used to detect inflammation in the arterial wall. It is based on the principle of excessive glucose metabolism by inflammatory cells. However, it is expensive and is associated with a significant radiation dose. This investigation has still not become the gold standard for diagnosis.

Tables **16** and **17** depict ACR criteria [81] and EULAR/PReS classification criteria for Takayasu arteritis [82].

Table 16. 1990 ACR criteria for the classification of Takayasu arteritis [81][9].

A Diagnosis of Takayasu Arteritis Requires that at least 3 of the 6 Criteria are Met.
Age at disease onset <40 years Claudication of extremities Decreased brachial artery pulse Systolic blood pressure difference >10 mm Hg between arms Bruit over subclavian arteries or aorta Arteriogram abnormality (narrowing or occlusion of the entire aorta, its primary branches or large arteries in the proximal upper or lower extremities, not caused by arteriosclerosis, fibromuscular dysplasia or similar causes; changes usually focal or segmental)

Table 17. EULAR/PReS classification criteria for Takayasu arteritis [82][10].

Angiographic abnormalities plus the Presence of **at least one** of the features
Decreased peripheral artery pulse(s) or claudication of extremities Blood pressure difference >10 mmHg Bruits over the aorta or its major branches Hypertension (related to childhood normative data)

Differential Diagnosis

Coarctation of the aorta is a common differential diagnosis of Type 3 and 4 Takayasu arteritis and usually presents with hypertension in upper limbs, decreased pulses in lower limbs, and radio-femoral delay. Hypertension is chronic and hence associated with left ventricular hypertrophy. Collaterals are more common because of the long duration of illness. Echocardiography and doppler help in diagnosis. Angiography shows a discrete lesion in the aorta in juxtaductal region and post-stenotic dilatation.

Infectious aortitis can occur due to tuberculosis and syphilis. Syphilitic aortitis has not been described in children. Tubercular aortitis presents more often with aneurysms rather than stenosis.

IgG4 related aortitis has been described recently in adults. It is arteritis involving both media and adventitia and may be associated with systemic features. Again, aneurysms are more common. It is a predominantly pathologic diagnosis.

Treatment

Management aims at suppressing vessel wall inflammation and relieving distal ischemia.

Steroids are the mainstay to suppress inflammation and can be given intravenously as a pulse dose or orally. Most patients would need additional immunosuppression, and various drugs like methotrexate, azathioprine, and mycophenolate have been used. There is hardly any literature to support the use of one drug over another. Parenteral methotrexate is used as the first line drug because of large experience, low cost, and relatively few side-effects. Clinical effect requires 8-12 weeks of weekly subcutaneous doses, and meanwhile, steroids are tapered to a low single daily dose. Mycophenolate mofetil has been used at some centers as first-line drug along with steroids.

In patients with severe manifestations such as Takayasu retinopathy, secondary hypertension, aortic regurgitation, or aneurysm formation, some authors recommend using more aggressive immunosuppression. This can be achieved by pulse cyclophosphamide or by using biologic disease modifiers such as tocilizumab. Duration of immunosuppression is variable, usually for a few years. As vessel wall histopathology is not feasible and good serological biomarkers are not available, it is difficult to pinpoint when to stop immunosuppression. Most centers will continue it for 2-3 years if there have been no relapses of the disease.

Relief of distal ischemia is achieved by percutaneous or surgical procedures. This is usually required in children with carotid, thoracic/abdominal aorta, or renal artery involvement. Percutaneous procedures have been proven safe with similar recurrence rates as surgical procedures [83]. Percutaneous procedures are preferred for short-segment, critical arterial stenosis. Long-segment stenosis with extensive periarterial fibrosis or occlusion may require surgical bypass; however, this also carries the risk of anastomotic aneurysm and graft failure. As a general rule, if the condition of the patient permits, these procedures are avoided during the acute inflammatory phase because of the high risk of dissection, anastomotic aneurysms, and leaks [76].

Supportive therapy is required for the control of hypertension and congestive heart failure. Renovascular hypertension is severe and needs multiple antihypertensive agents. Angiotensin-converting enzyme inhibitors are very effective in this form of hypertension, but that control occurs at the cost of reducing blood flow further to the compromised kidney. In patients with bilateral renal artery stenosis or significant suprarenal aortic stenosis, this can lead to frank renal failure. Aggressive control of hypertension is also not warranted as this leads to compromised blood flow distal to the area of stenosis. In patients with carotid stenosis, this can manifest as worsening sensorium and stroke.

Antiplatelet agents are given as a routine to reduce the risk of thrombosis. Role of antitubercular therapy is controversial.

Monitoring

All children should be monitored for disease activity and adverse drug effects. Symptoms of worsening ischemia, physical examination for new signs like the absence of pulse, bruit, or blood pressure difference, and inflammatory parameters like ESR and CRP are not sensitive in picking up disease activity. Repeated angiography to look for involvement of new vessels or worsening of stenosis in a previously involved vessel is associated with a high radiation risk. MR angiography and PET scans may be useful.

Outcome

It is a chronic disease with a relapsing course. In fact, it is very difficult to define remission because of the paucity of serological biomarkers. A monophasic course is seen in about 20% of patients. Adult survival rates of 94-97% at 10-15 years have been achieved with immunosuppression and revascularization procedures [78]. Higher mortality is seen in children because of cardiac involvement due to both hypertension and cardiomyopathy.

Hypertension and myocardial inflammation is common. Nervous system ischemia can cause seizures, syncope, and stroke. Claudication is not a common complaint in children. Diagnosis is not difficult once suspected. Vascular imaging is the gold standard for diagnosis. Management is aimed at suppressing vessel wall inflammation and relieving distal ischemia. Inflammation is controlled by steroids and other steroid-sparing immunosuppressants. Relief of distal ischemia is achieved by percutaneous or surgical procedures, usually done once inflammation subsides.

ANTIPHOSPHOLIPID SYNDROME (APS)

APS is an acquired multisystem autoimmune disorder associated with an increased risk of thrombosis [11] and accounts for 20% of young patients with stroke or venous thromboembolism. Prevalence and incidence rates are reported to be 40-50 per lakh population and 5 per lakh population per year, respectively [84]. Children with APS differ from adults in having lower female preponderance.

It is characterized by a combination of clinical features (thrombosis and/or recurrent pregnancy loss) and laboratory tests showing persistent positivity for one or more of the following aPL antibodies: anticardiolipin (aCL), anti-beta 2 glycoprotein 1 ($a\beta_2GP1$) or lupus anticoagulant (LA) [27]. The thrombosis may be the arterial or venous, or small vessel but should not be due to a vasculitic disorder.

This syndrome is associated with two anomalous laboratory tests: aCL antibodies giving false-positive syphilis test and LA phenomenon. LA can prolong *in vitro* phospholipid-dependent clotting assays. Because this prolongation of clotting time occurs due to the presence of an inhibitor (antibody), it gets corrected by adding excess phospholipid reagent [85].

APS can be of two types: primary APS (when no underlying cause is found) and secondary APS (when an underlying autoimmune disease, usually SLE, is responsible for APS) [11]. It has been observed that a proportion of SLE patients may initially present like primary APS and go on to develop SLE on follow-up [27]. Primary APS accounts for 38-50% of all childhood APS.

APS has been described in all age groups; however, it is described less often in children, likely due to the rarity of defining clinical criteria, namely thrombosis and/or recurrent pregnancy loss in children. An additional life-threatening emergency called catastrophic APS (CAPS) is described, though rare in children [86].

Pathogenesis

The pathogenesis of APS is not clear [27]. aPL antibodies are directed against several plasma proteins and proteins expressed on endothelium and platelets. These antibodies have been shown to induce a procoagulant state by their actions on endothelial cells, platelets, and monocytes [87]. Production of aPL antibodies can be triggered by infections, vaccination, and dietary intake of β_2GPI.

However, aPL antibodies alone are not enough for the production of clinical manifestations. A second hit in the form of infections, vaccination, surgery, autoimmune disease, or malignancy is required for clinical manifestations to develop. More than 50% of adult patients with thrombosis attributable to aPL have been observed to have at least one non-aPL thrombotic risk factor such as inherited thrombophilia or acquired conditions like malignancy, central venous catheter.

Because transient production of aPL antibodies is common in response to multiple triggers, classification criteria for APS require the persistent presence of these antibodies over a minimum duration of 12 weeks. It is important to recognize that not every positive aPL profile is clinically significant. Risk categorization depends on the type and titers of aPL antibodies, presence of additional risk factors, and a "second hit" [27]. Table **18** depicts the risk categorization of aPL profile.

Table 18. Risk categorization of aPL profile[11].

Risk Category	Criteria
High-risk profile	Positive LA with or without Moderate to high titers of aCL/aβ2GP1 IgG/M
Moderate risk profile	Negative LA + Moderate to high titers of aCL/aβ2GP1 IgG/M
Low-risk profile	Negative LA + Low titers of aCL/aβ2GP1 IgG/M

In a healthy population, high risk aPL profile is very rare [27], whereas in SLE, 20-30% of patients have been reported to have persistent moderate to high risk aPL profile.

Inflammation, thrombosis, and vasculopathy have been implicated in the causation of clinical manifestations [27, 88]. These vascular lesions have been shown to be resistant to anticoagulation [88] and may respond to the mammalian target of rapamycin (mTOR) inhibitors like sirolimus.

LA has been shown to be most predictive of clinical manifestations [11]. LA is strictly *in vitro* phenomenon and is not associated with the bleeding tendency in vivo. It is important that a test for LA is performed before the patient is started on anticoagulation. LA can be false negative in acute thrombotic events and in certain inflammatory conditions. Neonatal APS has been described in newborns born to mothers with aPL positivity. However, de novo production of aPL has also been implicated in neonatal APS.

Clinical Features

Children with aPL positivity can be classified into four broad categories

1. No clinical manifestations
2. With nonthrombotic manifestations
3. With thrombosis
4. CAPS

Clinical manifestations of APS have been classified into thrombotic and non thrombotic manifestations. Thrombosis may involve veins, arteries, or microvasculature; however venous thrombosis is most common and can present as deep venous thrombosis. Arterial thrombosis presents commonly as stroke. Microcirculation can be involved, commonly presenting as peripheral gangrene (Fig. **36**). Embolism from the deep venous system as well as from the heart can occur. In the heart, both valvular thickening as well as sterile endocarditis has been described. In Ped-APS registry, 60% of patients had venous thrombosis [11].

Arterial and microvasculature thrombosis was seen in 32% and 6% of patients, respectively.

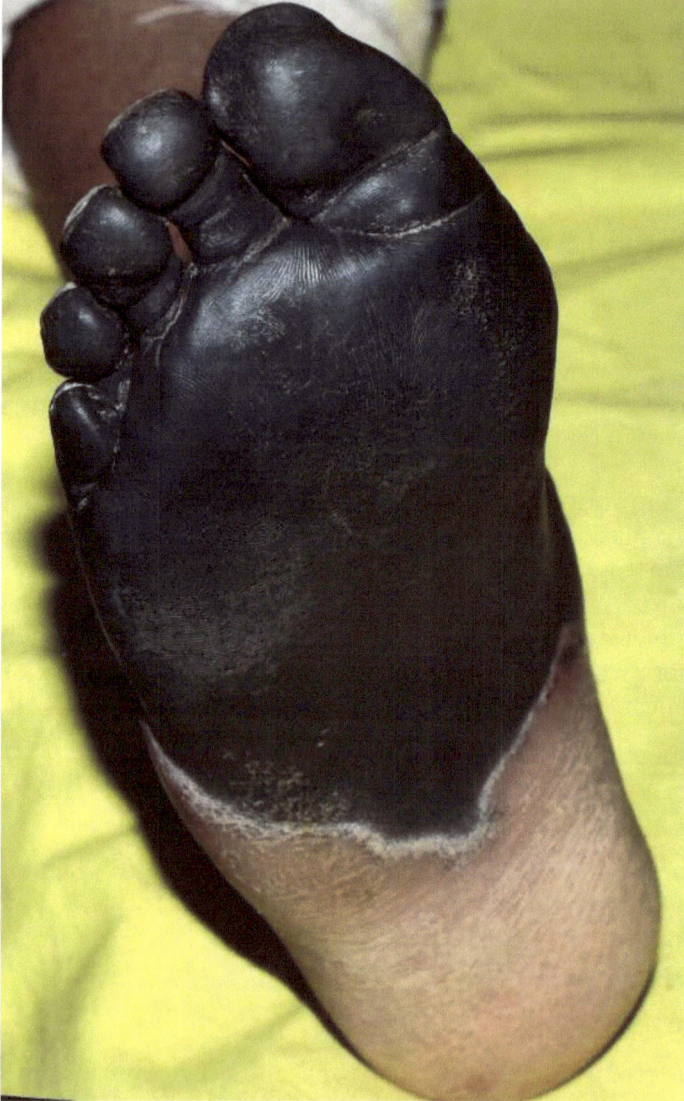

Fig. (36). Peripheral gangrene in a child with APS.

APS is an important cause of acquired thrombophilia. Like other genetic prothrombotic factors, it does not have an "all or none" association with thrombosis. The risk of thrombosis is modified by many factors like aPL profile and persistence, associated autoimmune conditions, and presence of other prothrombotic risk factors. Whereas LA has been found to have the strongest correlate with thrombosis out of the three prototype antibodies, an association of antiβ2GP1 and aCL with thrombosis is far weaker and less well understood. For thrombosis, anti-β_2GP1 IgG antibodies are more sensitive and specific than IgA, and IgM and aCL antibodies are most sensitive but least specific. Triple antibody positivity confers the highest risk of thrombosis.

Associated autoimmune conditions like SLE and prothrombotic risk factors like hypercholesterolemia, smoking, and hypertension increase the risk of thrombosis. In SLE patients, LA and isolated aCL positivity at medium to high titers have been found to increase the risk of thrombosis.

Nonthrombotic manifestations involve the nervous system (seizures, headache, chorea, demyelinating disease), hematological system (thrombocytopenia, hemolytic anemia), kidneys (aPL nephropathy), heart (cardiac valve disease) and lungs (pulmonary artery hypertension, diffuse alveolar hemorrhage). Thrombosis in microcirculation, complement activation, release of various cytokines, and direct neurotoxicity have been implicated in some of the neurological features. Livedo reticularis has been described as one of the important skin manifestations.

CATASTROPHIC APS (CAPS)

CAPS is a syndrome associated with acute onset of multiple small vessel occlusions resulting in multiorgan failure. It is associated with high mortality. Extensive microthrombosis and systemic inflammatory response syndrome are important pathophysiologic mechanisms [89].

Diagnosis requires at least 3 organ systems to be clinically involved over a short time along with laboratory evidence of small vessel occlusion and aPL antibodies [90]. Large vessel thrombosis may occur but is not included for diagnosis. Common organ systems involved are the kidney, liver, central nervous system, heart, lung, and skin. In the International CAPS registry, the profile of 45 children with CAPS has been reported [86]. Infection was the commonest trigger in 60% of children. More than two-thirds of these children had primary APS. About one-half of these children had peripheral vessel thrombosis. Among laboratory features, thrombocytopenia is frequent [89]. Evidence of microangiopathic hemolytic anemia may be present.

Diagnosis

There are no validated diagnostic criteria for the diagnosis of pediatric APS. Updated Sapporo criteria may be adapted for children by removing the pregnancy morbidity criterion [84].

Treatment

Aim of treatment of APS includes:

- Treatment of clinical manifestations
  - Thromboembolic manifestations
  - Nonthrombotic manifestations
- Prevention of thrombotic manifestations
  - Secondary prevention
  - Primary prevention
- Elimination of aPL antibodies and targeting other pathophysiologic pathways

Treatment of Clinical Manifestations

Thrombotic manifestations need anticoagulation. In the acute stage, the preferred anticoagulant is heparin. Heparin has been shown to have an inhibitory effect on complement activation in addition to its thrombolytic and fibrinolytic effects. Anticoagulation is not useful for nonthrombotic manifestations of APS, aPL nephropathy, and microthrombosis.

Since systemic inflammatory response syndrome is an important component of CAPS, various strategies have been used to reduce inflammation to reduce mortality. Steroids, plasma exchange, and intravenous immunoglobulins have been used most frequently [89]. Some patients may need cyclophosphamide and biological disease modifiers. Appropriate management of treatable triggers is important [86].

Immune therapy to reduce or eliminate aPL has been shown to have only transient effects; hence, it is not used to treat or prevent thrombosis in APS [84]. Recent literature stresses the paradigm shift from thrombosis prevention to the prevention of autoimmune damage and vascular proliferation. Sirolimus is useful in reducing vascular proliferation in kidneys in APS patients [88].

Prevention of Thrombotic Manifestations

Secondary Prevention

Secondary prevention is directed at preventing recurrence of thrombosis in patients with APS. Strict control of associated prothrombotic risk factors like hypertension, hypercholesterolemia and smoking should be achieved irrespective of the previous thrombosis.

For venous thrombosis, vitamin K antagonists are preferred for secondary prevention with an aim to maintain an international normalized ratio (INR) between 2.0 and 3.0. For arterial thrombosis, low dose aspirin is added to this regimen or anticoagulation is aimed at maintaining INR > 3.0, however, this increases the risk of bleeding significantly.

Duration of prophylaxis depends on site of thromboembolism, aPL profile, and whether venous thromboembolism was provoked or not. Pulmonary thromboembolism, high-risk aPL profile, and presence of autoimmune conditions or associated prothrombotic condition warrant lifelong treatment. Duration can be shortened in case of single antibody positivity and a provoked thromboembolism.

Primary Prevention

For patients who have persistent aPL positivity without an underlying autoimmune disease and no episode of thrombosis, the role of prophylactic aspirin is controversial since the risk of thrombosis is estimated at 1% per year. Strict control of additional risk factors and anticoagulation during high-risk situations like surgery and prolonged immobilization are advised.

For patients who have persistent moderate to high-risk aPL profile without thrombosis but with an underlying autoimmune condition like SLE, the risk of thrombosis is estimated at 3-4% every year [87]. In such cases, aspirin may be used for the prevention of thrombosis. HCQ is protective for both arterial and venous thrombosis in adult SLE patients.

Conclusion

APS is a fascinating disease that confers a high risk of thrombosis. Many nonthrombotic clinical manifestations have been described, though they are not a part of diagnostic criteria. Laboratory diagnosis requires persistent positivity for aPL antibodies. Clinical events correlate most strongly with LA and with aCL and anti-β_2GP1 IgG in moderate to high titers. Lifelong thromboprophylaxis with oral vitamin K antagonists is recommended for all APS patients with high-risk aPL profiles or SLE. The presence of SLE in a patient with persistent aPL positivity increases the risk of thrombosis. In the absence of thrombosis, all high-risk patients should be on low-dose aspirin. The addition of HCQ is beneficial in SLE patients with aPL positivity.

UVEITIS

Inflammation of the uvea, which is the middle layer of the eye, is called uveitis. Onset in childhood accounts for 5-10% of all cases of uveitis [25]. Anatomically, it can involve anterior (iris and ciliary body), intermediate (vitreous) or posterior (choroid and usually retina) compartments. When all the three compartments are involved, it is termed "panuveitis". Anterior uveitis is the commonest type in children [91]. Chronic uveitis is usually bilateral and is more common in children compared to acute or acute recurrent uveitis.

Uveitis is a syndromic diagnosis and can occur secondary to infections or autoimmune causes. Acute uveitis is seen in viral infections such as *Herpes simplex* virus (HSV), and *Varicella zoster* virus (VZV). *Cytomegalovirus* can cause posterior uveitis in immunocompromised children. Tuberculosis can cause uveitis by the immune phenomenon. Parasitic infections like cysticercus, *Toxocara,* and *Toxoplasma* cause posterior uveitis.

JIA is the commonest known autoimmune cause of uveitis in children. About 10-20% of children with JIA develop uveitis during the disease [77]. Oligoarthritis and RF negative polyarthritis carry the highest risk of developing chronic anterior uveitis [32]. ERA is associated with acute recurrent uveitis. There is no significant risk of uveitis in children with sJIA. JIA-associated uveitis typically presents after the onset of arthritis; however, in 3-7% of cases, uveitis can precede arthritis manifestations [91]. Three-fourth of children with uveitis in JIA have bilateral involvement.

Other less common autoimmune causes of uveitis include reactive arthritis, Blau syndrome, KD, Behçet's disease, and tubulointerstitial nephritis-uveitis (TINU) syndrome. More often, no obvious systemic cause can be identified, leading to "idiopathic uveitis" diagnosis.

Clinical Features

Clinical features of uveitis depend on the anatomic localization. Pain, redness, and decreased vision are presenting features of anterior uveitis. JIA associated uveitis is typically silent with no obvious manifestations; probably due to the very young age of children. Visual impairment is common and can occur due to significant inflammation in anterior or posterior chambers or due to complications such as cataracts, glaucoma, and macular edema.

Role of Ophthalmologist

In any child with uveitis, an ophthalmologist should look for disease activity and complications. Cells and flare are examined by slit-lamp examination and graded according to Standardization of Uveitis Nomenclature (SUN) criteria (Table **19**) [92]. Optical coherence tomography can identify cystoid macular edema at an early stage.

Table 19. Standardization of Uveitis Nomenclature (SUN) criteria for uveitis activity[12].

Grading Scheme for Anterior Chamber Cells	
Grade	**Cells in field[13]**
0	< 1
0.5 +	1-5
1 +	6-15
2 +	16-25
3 +	26-50
4 +	> 50
Grading Scheme for Anterior Chamber Flare	
Grade	Description
0	None
1 +	Faint
2 +	Moderate (iris and lens details clear)
3 +	Marked (iris and lens details hazy)
4 +	Intense (fibrin or plastic aqueous)
Activity of Uveitis Terminology	
Term	**Definition**
Inactive	Grade 0 cells in anterior chamber
Worsening activity	Two-step increase in level of inflammation (*e.g.* anterior chamber cells, vitreous haze) or increase from grade 3+ to grade 4+
Improved activity	Two-step decrease in level of inflammation (*e.g.* anterior chamber cells, vitreous haze) or decrease to grade 0
Remission	Inactive disease for ≥ 3 months after discontinuing all treatments for eye disease

Role of Pediatrician

Pediatrician's role lies in the evaluation of a systemic cause for uveitis. Good history and examination are required to look for any systemic cause. In the absence of any such clue, it is highly unlikely that investigations would be useful in identifying a secondary cause. Arthritis may point towards JIA or Blau syndrome. In Blau syndrome, maculopapular skin rash and deforming arthritis with synovial proliferation are seen. Tubulointerstitial nephritis and deafness are seen in TINU syndrome. Lung involvement and mediastinal node enlargement are seen in sarcoidosis.

Investigations

The role of laboratory investigations lies in confirming an underlying cause and monitoring for drug toxicity. In a child with oligoarthritis or polyarthritis, ANA predicts the risk of uveitis in JIA [91]. Blau syndrome requires a genetic diagnosis. Work up for tuberculosis is required in developing countries where tuberculosis is prevalent. Chest radiograph and tuberculin test are routinely done in all children with uveitis. These tests also help to rule out latent tuberculosis infection as tuberculosis may flare up while these patients are on immuno-suppression for uveitis. The polymerase chain reaction from aqueous/vitreous humor may help in confirming the diagnosis of tubercular uveitis, but the yield of this investigation is very low due to immune mediated injury.

Hemogram, liver and renal function tests, and serology for hepatitis B surface antigen (HBsAg) are required before initiating patients on immunosuppression.

Treatment

Treatment of uveitis depends on underlying cause. Infectious causes require specific therapy. In autoimmune causes, aim should be to achieve a quick and sustained suppression of inflammation by using immunosuppression. This helps in reducing the risk of complications.

Immunosuppression can be achieved by using steroids either topically or systemically. Topical steroid drops are useful only in anterior uveitis. In severe cases, additional systemic steroids may be required to control inflammation. Topical steroids should not be used as monotherapy in the presence of continued activity after 12 weeks. Overdependence on topical steroids is associated with significant side-effects, namely cataract, glaucoma, and systemic steroid toxicity. Systemic steroids are needed in complications like cystoid macular edema, where vision can be lost over hours to days if not treated. In addition, topical mydriatics help in reducing the risk of synechiae formation.

Methotrexate is first line therapy for most children with uveitis. It is administered once a week by either oral or subcutaneous route. It is started at 10-15 mg/m^2/dose and is increased gradually to 25-30 mg/m^2/dose depending on response and tolerance. The onset of action is slow and takes 8-12 weeks. During this time, steroids may be required to suppress inflammation. Methotrexate is a relatively safe drug and requires periodic monitoring for hepatic and hematological toxicity. Nausea and vomiting are more common and may be distressing enough to lead to drug withdrawal. Nearly three-fourths of children show a response to methotrexate. It can be gradually tapered and stopped if the disease has been inactive for 12-24 months after withdrawal of steroids. While tapering, the patient should be evaluated periodically for disease activity.

If methotrexate is not tolerated or contraindicated, other immunosuppressive agents such as azathioprine, mycophenolate mofetil, and calcineurin inhibitors can be used upfront. Experience with most of these drugs is not as vast as with methotrexate. Nonresponse to methotrexate after 12 weeks is another indication to intensify immunosuppression with any of these drugs. Biological disease modifiers are, no doubt, effective but extremely expensive [25]. Anti-TNF agents like infliximab and adalimumab have been shown to be effective [25, 91], whereas etanercept has been shown to worsen uveitis in a few studies.

Complications like cataract, band-shaped keratopathy (if affecting vision due to central cornea affection), glaucoma, *etc.* may require surgery. Surgery should be avoided during active inflammation as disturbing inflamed tissue can cause more tissue injury. Ideally, surgery should be done if the eye has been inactive for at least 3 months.

Monitoring

All children with uveitis should be evaluated by ophthalmologists frequently till they achieve remission and less frequently thereafter. Visual acuity can be affected both due to activity and structural complications. Slit-lamp examination should be done to look for cells and flare. The presence of cells in aqueous and vitreous humor depicts activity whereas flare can be seen with both activity and structural damage to the eye. Cells and flare are graded according to SUN classification [79] as it helps in better monitoring and resultant therapeutic decisions. The presence or worsening of structural complications should be looked for. Intraocular pressure (IOP) of > 21 mmHg is defined as intraocular hypertension. Intraocular hypertension, along with pathologic cupping of the optic disc or visual field defects, is defined as glaucoma. IOP of < 6 mmHg is defined as ocular hypotony and signals the development of phthisis.

Outcome

Posterior synechiae formation is a common complication of anterior uveitis and can lead to irregular pupil. Band-shaped keratopathy involving the central cornea can cause visual impairment. Cataracts can develop secondary to both uveitis and steroids. Ocular hypertension can occur due to increased secretion and decreased drainage of aqueous humor and due to steroids. Cystoid macular edema is an acute sight-threatening complication. Early diagnosis and immediate steroid therapy can save vision in such a condition. Phthisis is a delayed complication with a poor prognosis.

Conclusion

Uveitis is a syndromic diagnosis. Many infections and autoimmune diseases can have uveitis as either their sole presentation or one of the systemic manifestations. JIA is the commonest known cause of chronic anterior uveitis. Posterior uveitis occurs commonly due to infections, whereas no cause is identifiable for intermediate uveitis. Every child with uveitis should have a periodic evaluation for disease activity, structural complications, and visual acuity. A pediatrician is required to identify the systemic disease and manage immunosuppression. Overreliance on topical steroids can be harmful leading to complications such as cataract, glaucoma, and systemic steroid toxicity. Systemic immunosuppression in the form of subcutaneous methotrexate is safe and effective with periodic monitoring of potential side effects. Biological disease modifiers (anti-TNF agents like infliximab and adalimumab) are effective but extremely expensive. Early diagnosis and appropriate therapy help in reducing complications and improving visual outcomes.

RHEUMATOLOGICAL EMERGENCIES

Many emergencies are seen in pediatric rheumatology practice. Hence, these children can present to intensivists also. If the emergency presentation is the first presentation of the disease, it can be a real diagnostic challenge. Table **20** enumerates common emergencies seen in pediatric rheumatology.

Table 20. Common emergencies seen in pediatric rheumatological disorders.

Disease	Common Rheumatological Emergencies
JIA	MAS in sJIA
SLE	Organ dysfunction of major organs, thrombosis, MAS, infections
JDM	Severe weakness, aspiration pneumonia, gastrointestinal vasculitis
CAPS	Multiorgan dysfunction due to microvascular thrombosis
Vasculitis	Pulmonary renal syndrome, severe hypertension, peripheral gangrene, ischemia of major organs

MACROPHAGE ACTIVATION SYNDROME (MAS)

MAS is a severe hyperinflammatory reaction characterized by cytokine storm and excessive activation and expansion of T lymphocytes and macrophages, showing hemophagocytic activity [10]. This term is used interchangeably with secondary hemophagocytic lymphohistiocytosis (HLH) [10]. It is a result of an exuberant immune response to a variety of triggers [12].

HLH can be idiopathic or can occur secondary to a systemic illness like infection, autoimmune and autoinflammatory diseases, or malignancy. In rheumatology practice, MAS is commonly seen in a setting of sJIA. It can also be seen in SLE, KD, and periodic fever syndromes [10].

In idiopathic HLH, genetic defects in cytolytic pathways lead to decreased apoptosis of virus-infected cells by cytolytic cells such as CD8 positive T lymphocytes and Natural Killer (NK) cells [93]. The end result is the expansion of CD8 positive T-lymphocytes and macrophages and excessive production of many cytokines. This process itself is enough to produce a hyperinflammatory state labeled as HLH.

In secondary HLH, partial genetic defects and triggers like infections, inflammation, or malignancy play an additive role. It has been observed that children with MAS who have partial genetic defects in ≥ 1 primary HLH related genes have more recurrences of MAS.

sJIA is a condition associated with activation of innate immune system. Decreased NK cell activity has been reported in patients with sJIA and MAS; however, it may improve on control of disease activity of sJIA. Activated macrophages seem to be responsible for high serum ferritin seen in this condition. Overt MAS is seen in 10% of patients with sJIA but subclinical or mild MAS is more common in 30-40% of patients with sJIA. MAS can be the first presentation of sJIA. Usage of biologics has reduced the incidence of MAS [12]. It is unlikely that biologics increase the risk of MAS as an increased dose of the same biologic helps to control it. However, the use of some biologics like tocilizumab makes it difficult to recognize MAS.

Clinical Features

Clinical manifestations of MAS and HLH are strikingly similar. Children present with acute onset fever, which is high grade and sustained, unlike quotidian fever of sJIA. Fever may not be very impressive in patients on biologics. These children may also have lymphadenopathy and hepatosplenomegaly. Bleeding tendency occurs due to consumptive coagulopathy. Central nervous system involvement may vary from mild irritability to seizures and coma. Congestive heart failure, renal failure, and lung involvement can occur in a small proportion of children.

Multiorgan failure is the commonest cause of mortality. Paradoxical improvement in clinical features of underlying inflammatory diseases like arthritis in patients with sJIA is common [13]. Patients of sJIA on biologics like tocilizumab can have masking of symptoms, especially fever. Such patients also tend to have lower CRP and ferritin levels [94].

Investigations

Investigations may show cytopenias, liver dysfunction, and coagulopathy. High serum ferritin is considered an important marker of the disease. Usually, serum ferritin levels are more than 10,000 μg/L. In the absence of renal failure, such elevations of serum ferritin have been found to be very specific for MAS. Serum ferritin can, however, be less than 1000 μg/L in the presence of MAS [12]. Inflammatory markers like CRP are high, but erythrocyte sedimentation rate (ESR) is paradoxically low due to low fibrinogen. Both increased fibrinogen consumption and hepatic dysfunction contribute to low fibrinogen. Lactate dehydrogenase and serum triglycerides are elevated.

Diagnosis

Prompt diagnosis is essential for a good outcome in MAS. Clinical and laboratory features are relatively nonspecific and can mimic infections. Table **21** depicts the diagnostic criteria of HLH [95]. When these criteria are used for the diagnosis of MAS, certain difficulties are encountered. Molecular diagnosis is a time-consuming investigation, and results are not available immediately for the management decision. Moreover, all children with MAS do not have genetic defects. Hemophagocytosis is seen in only 50-60% of patients with MAS. NK cell activity and sCD25 are not available in routine laboratories. Since sJIA is an inflammatory condition, it is associated with neutrophilia, thrombocytosis, elevated fibrinogen, and elevated serum ferritin. Serum ferritin > 500 μg/L is so commonly seen in sJIA itself. When MAS sets in a patient with sJIA, it takes time for neutrophils, platelets and fibrinogen to fall to such low levels as depicted in HLH 2004 criteria. This occurs too late in the clinical course and can account for high mortality. For all these reasons, HLH2004 criteria are not good for the diagnosis of MAS in sJIA. In fact, these criteria were met in only 38% of episodes in patients with sJIA [40]. For this reason, 2016 MAS classification criteria are being used (Table **22**) [15].

Table 21. Diagnostic criteria of HLH 2004 [95][14].

The diagnosis of HLH can be established if one of either 1 or 2 below is fulfilled.
1. A molecular diagnosis consistent with HLH.
2. Diagnostic criteria for HLH fulfilled (5 out of the 8 criteria below)
Initial diagnostic criteria (to be evaluated in all patients with HLH).
o Clinical criteria
▪ Fever
▪ Splenomegaly

(Table 21) cont.....

o <u>Laboratory criteria</u> • Cytopenias (affecting ≥ 2 of 3 lineages in the peripheral blood) • Hemoglobin (<90 g/L), Platelets (<100 x 10⁹/L), Neutrophils (<1.0 x 10⁹/L) (In infants <4 weeks: Hemoglobin <100 g/L) • Hypertriglyceridemia and/or hypofibrinogenemia (fasting triglycerides ≥3.0 mmol/L (i e ≥265 mg/dL), fibrinogen ≤1.5 g/L) o <u>Histopathologic criteria</u> • Hemophagocytosis in bone marrow or spleen or lymph nodes. No evidence of malignancy 3. New diagnostic criteria a. Low or absent NK-cell activity (according to local laboratory reference) b. Ferritin ≥500 µg/L c. Soluble CD25 (*i.e.* soluble IL-2 receptor) ≥2400 U/ml

Table 22. 2016 MAS classification criteria [15][15].

A febrile patient with known or suspected sJIA is classified as having MAS if the following criteria are met: Serum ferritin ≥ 684 µg/L with any two of the following: Platelet count ≤ 181*10⁹ /L SGOT > 48 IU/L Triglycerides > 1.56 g/L Fibrinogen ≤ 3.6 g/L

Children with SLE, who develop MAS, have no difference in clinical features compared to other children with SLE. They, however, have a higher chance of developing cytopenias and carry higher mortality.

Treatment

MAS is associated with high mortality if not recognized in time [10, 94]. A high degree of clinical suspicion coupled with prompt immunosuppressive therapy is a key to a good outcome. Therapy of MAS has evolved with time. Initially, the HLH2004 protocol, which uses dexamethasone, cyclosporine, and high dose etoposide, was used as a bridge to bone marrow transplant. This is a must for primary HLH but was considered to be too toxic for MAS.

Most rheumatologists rely on high-dose steroids as pulse methylprednisolone for first-line therapy [96]. Dexamethasone may be preferred in children with CNS involvement because of better CNS penetration. For steroid-refractory disease or sicker children, cyclosporin, plasmapheresis, biologics, and IVIg are used in addition to pulse steroids. IVIg should not be used as the only therapy in children with MAS. Antithymocyte globulin has been used in refractory cases. Among biologics, anakinra, canakinumab, and tocilizumab have been used most frequently in MAS [94].

Conclusion

MAS is associated with high mortality. It is important to recognize it early and treat it aggressively. In rheumatological conditions, especially sJIA, it may be difficult to recognize MAS because of persistent inflammation due to sJIA itself. Serial monitoring of laboratory and clinical features helps in early diagnosis. Abnormalities in laboratory investigations usually precede clinical features. High dose pulse steroids as pulse methylprednisolone are the first-line therapy.

NOTES

[1] Zulian F, Woo P, Athreya BH, Laxer RM, Medsger TA, Lehman TJA, *et al*. The Pediatric Rheumatology European Society/American College of Rheumatology/ European League against Rheumatism provisional classification criteria for juvenile systemic sclerosis. Arthritis Rheum. 2007 Mar 15;57(2):203–12.

[2] Ozen S, Marks SD, Brogan P, Groot N, de Graeff N, Avcin T, *et al*. European consensus-based recommendations for diagnosis and treatment of immunoglobulin A vasculitis—the SHARE initiative. Rheumatology. 2019 Sep 1;58(9):1607–16.

[3] Mills JA, Michel BA, Bloch DA, Calabrese LH, Hunder GG, Arend WP, *et al*. The American College of Rheumatology 1990 criteria for the classification of henoch-schönlein purpura. Arthritis Rheum. 2010 Aug 17;33(8):1114–21

[4] Ozen S, Pistorio A, Iusan SM, Bakkaloglu A, Herlin T, Brik R, *et al*. EULAR/PRINTO/PRES criteria for Henoch-Schonlein purpura, childhood polyarteritis nodosa, childhood Wegener granulomatosis and childhood Takayasu arteritis: Ankara 2008. Part II: Final classification criteria. Ann Rheum Dis. 2010 May 1;69(5):798–806.

[5] McCrindle BW, Rowley AH, Newburger JW, Burns JC, Bolger AF, Gewitz M, *et al*. Diagnosis, Treatment, and Long-Term Management of Kawasaki Disease: A Scientific Statement for Health Professionals From the American Heart Association. Circulation [Internet]. 2017 Apr 25 [cited 2020 May 21];135(17). Available from: https://www.ahajournals.org/doi/10.1161/CIR.0000000000000484

[6] McCrindle BW, Rowley AH, Newburger JW, Burns JC, Bolger AF, Gewitz M, *et al*. Diagnosis, Treatment, and Long-Term Management of Kawasaki Disease: A

Scientific Statement for Health Professionals From the American Heart Association. Circulation [Internet]. 2017 Apr 25 [cited 2020 May 21];135(17). Available from: https://www.ahajournals.org/doi/10.1161/CIR.0000000000000484

[7] Adapted from Moriwaki R, Noda M, Yajima M, Sharma BK, Numano F. Clinical Manifestations of Takayasu Arteritis in India and Japan— New Classification of Angiographic Findings. Angiology. 1997 May;48(5):369–79.

[8] According to this classification system, involvement of the coronary or pulmonary arteries should be designated as C (+) or P (+), respectively.

[9] Arend WP, Michel BA, Bloch DA, Hunder GG, Calabrese LH, Edworthy SM, *et al.* The American College of Rheumatology 1990 criteria for the classification of Takayasu arteritis. Arthritis Rheum. 1990 Aug;33(8):1129–34.

[10] Ozen S. EULAR/PReS endorsed consensus criteria for the classification of childhood vasculitides. Ann Rheum Dis. 2005 Nov 3;65(7):936–41.

[11] Adapted from Garcia D, Erkan D. Diagnosis and Management of the Antiphospholipid Syndrome. *N Engl J Med.* 2018;378(21):2010-2021. doi:10.1056/NEJMra1705454

[12] Adapted from Jabs DA, Nussenblatt RB, Rosenbaum JT; Standardization of Uveitis Nomenclature (SUN) Working Group. Standardization of uveitis nomenclature for reporting clinical data. Results of the First International Workshop. Am J Ophthalmol. 2005;140:509-516.

[13] Field size is a 1 mm by 1 mm slit beam.

[14] Adapted from Henter JI, Horne A, Aricó M, *et al.* HLH-2004: Diagnostic and therapeutic guidelines for hemophagocytic lymphohistiocytosis. *Pediatr Blood Cancer.* 2007;48(2):124-131. doi:10.1002/pbc.21039

[15] Adapted from Ravelli A, Minoia F, Davì S, Horne A, Bovis F, Pistorio A, *et al.* 2016 Classification Criteria for Macrophage Activation Syndrome Complicating Systemic Juvenile Idiopathic Arthritis: A European League Against

Rheumatism/American College of Rheumatology/Paediatric Rheumatology International Trials Organisation Collaborative Initiative: EULAR/ACR CLASSIFICATION CRITERIA FOR MAS. Arthritis Rheumatol. 2016 Mar;68(3):566–76.

[16] Courtesy: Dr Aaqib Banday, Postgraduate Institute of Medical Education and Research (PGIMER), Chandigarh

[17] Courtesy: Dr Suma Balan, Amrita Institute of Medical Sciences (AIMS), Kochi

[18] Courtesy: Dr Suma Balan, Amrita Institute of Medical Sciences (AIMS), Kochi

CONSENT FOR PUBLICATION

Not applicable.

CONFLICT OF INTEREST

The author declares no conflict of interest, financial or otherwise.

ACKNOWLEDGEMENTS

The author thanks Dr. Dharmagat Bhattarai, Dr. Aaqib Banday and Dr. Murugan Sudhakar for the review of the manuscript and providing constructive criticism. The author is also grateful to Dr. Suma Balan, AIMS, Kochi, for providing clinical photographs of localized scleroderma.

REFERENCES

[1]   Foster HE, Jandial S. pGALS - paediatric Gait Arms Legs and Spine: a simple examination of the musculoskeletal system. Pediatr Rheumatol Online J 2013; 11(1): 44.
        [http://dx.doi.org/10.1186/1546-0096-11-44] [PMID: 24219838]

[2]   Crayne CB, Beukelman T. Juvenile Idiopathic Arthritis: Oligoarthritis and Polyarthritis. Pediatr Clin North Am 2018; 65(4): 657-74.
        [http://dx.doi.org/10.1016/j.pcl.2018.03.005] [PMID: 30031492]

[3]   Cimaz R. Systemic-onset juvenile idiopathic arthritis. Autoimmun Rev 2016; 15(9): 931-4.
        [http://dx.doi.org/10.1016/j.autrev.2016.07.004] [PMID: 27392503]

[4]   Aggarwal A, Srivastava P. Childhood onset systemic lupus erythematosus: how is it different from adult SLE? Int J Rheum Dis 2015; 18(2): 182-91.
        [http://dx.doi.org/10.1111/1756-185X.12419] [PMID: 24965742]

[5]   Bellutti Enders F, Bader-Meunier B, Baildam E, *et al.* Consensus-based recommendations for the management of juvenile dermatomyositis. Ann Rheum Dis 2017; 76(2): 329-40.
        [http://dx.doi.org/10.1136/annrheumdis-2016-209247] [PMID: 27515057]

[6]   Zulian F. Scleroderma in children. Best Pract Res Clin Rheumatol 2017; 31(4): 576-95.

[http://dx.doi.org/10.1016/j.berh.2018.02.004] [PMID: 29773274]

[7] Ozen S, Sag E. Childhood vasculitis. Rheumatology (Oxford) 2020; 59 (Suppl. 3): iii95-iii100.
[http://dx.doi.org/10.1093/rheumatology/kez599] [PMID: 32348513]

[8] Singh-Grewal D, Durkan AM. Pediatric Vasculitis. Indian J Pediatr 2016; 83(2): 156-62.
[http://dx.doi.org/10.1007/s12098-015-1876-2] [PMID: 26365154]

[9] Borgia RE, Silverman ED. Childhood-onset systemic lupus erythematosus: an update. Curr Opin Rheumatol 2015; 27(5): 483-92.
[http://dx.doi.org/10.1097/BOR.0000000000000208] [PMID: 26200474]

[10] Crayne C, Cron RQ. Pediatric macrophage activation syndrome, recognizing the tip of the Iceberg. Eur J Rheumatol 2019; 7: 1-8.
[PMID: 31804174]

[11] Aguiar CL, Soybilgic A, Avcin T, Myones BL. Pediatric antiphospholipid syndrome. Curr Rheumatol Rep 2015; 17(4): 27.
[http://dx.doi.org/10.1007/s11926-015-0504-5] [PMID: 25854492]

[12] Cron RQ, Davi S, Minoia F, Ravelli A. Clinical features and correct diagnosis of macrophage activation syndrome. Expert Rev Clin Immunol 2015; 11(9): 1043-53.
[http://dx.doi.org/10.1586/1744666X.2015.1058159] [PMID: 26082353]

[13] Ravelli A, Davì S, Minoia F, Martini A, Cron RQ. Macrophage Activation Syndrome. Hematol Oncol Clin North Am 2015; 29(5): 927-41.
[http://dx.doi.org/10.1016/j.hoc.2015.06.010] [PMID: 26461152]

[14] Wenderfer SE, Eldin KW. Lupus Nephritis. Pediatr Clin North Am 2019; 66(1): 87-99.
[http://dx.doi.org/10.1016/j.pcl.2018.08.007] [PMID: 30454753]

[15] Ravelli A, Minoia F, Davì S, *et al.* 2016 Classification Criteria for Macrophage Activation Syndrome Complicating Systemic Juvenile Idiopathic Arthritis: A European League Against Rheumatism/American College of Rheumatology/Paediatric Rheumatology International Trials Organisation Collaborative Initiative. Arthritis Rheumatol 2016; 68(3): 566-76.
[http://dx.doi.org/10.1002/art.39332] [PMID: 26314788]

[16] Weiss PF. Diagnosis and treatment of enthesitis-related arthritis. Adolesc Health Med Ther 2012; 2012(3): 67-74.
[http://dx.doi.org/10.2147/AHMT.S25872] [PMID: 23236258]

[17] Calatroni M, Oliva E, Gianfreda D, *et al.* ANCA-associated vasculitis in childhood: recent advances. Ital J Pediatr 2017; 43(1): 46.
[http://dx.doi.org/10.1186/s13052-017-0364-x] [PMID: 28476172]

[18] Levy DM, Kamphuis S. Systemic lupus erythematosus in children and adolescents. Pediatr Clin North Am 2012; 59(2): 345-64.
[http://dx.doi.org/10.1016/j.pcl.2012.03.007] [PMID: 22560574]

[19] Denton CP, Derrett-Smith EC. Juvenile-onset systemic sclerosis: children are not small adults. Rheumatology (Oxford) 2009; 48(2): 96-7.
[http://dx.doi.org/10.1093/rheumatology/ken418] [PMID: 19028745]

[20] Wu Q, Wedderburn LR, McCann LJ. Juvenile dermatomyositis: Latest advances. Best Pract Res Clin Rheumatol 2017; 31(4): 535-57.
[http://dx.doi.org/10.1016/j.berh.2017.12.003] [PMID: 29773272]

[21] Newburger JW, Takahashi M, Burns JC. Kawasaki Disease. J Am Coll Cardiol 2016; 67(14): 1738-49.
[http://dx.doi.org/10.1016/j.jacc.2015.12.073] [PMID: 27056781]

[22] Aringer M, Costenbader K, Daikh D, *et al.* 2019 European League Against Rheumatism/American College of Rheumatology Classification Criteria for Systemic Lupus Erythematosus. Arthritis Rheumatol 2019; 71(9): 1400-12.

[http://dx.doi.org/10.1002/art.40930] [PMID: 31385462]

[23] Satoh M, Vázquez-Del Mercado M, Chan EKL. Clinical interpretation of antinuclear antibody tests in systemic rheumatic diseases. Mod Rheumatol 2009; 19(3): 219-28.
[http://dx.doi.org/10.3109/s10165-009-0155-3] [PMID: 19277826]

[24] Kumar Y, Bhatia A, Minz RW. Antinuclear antibodies and their detection methods in diagnosis of connective tissue diseases: a journey revisited. Diagn Pathol 2009; 4(1): 1.
[http://dx.doi.org/10.1186/1746-1596-4-1] [PMID: 19121207]

[25] Clarke SLN, Sen ES, Ramanan AV. Juvenile idiopathic arthritis-associated uveitis. Pediatr Rheumatol Online J 2016; 14(1): 27.
[http://dx.doi.org/10.1186/s12969-016-0088-2] [PMID: 27121190]

[26] Bosch X, Guilabert A, Font J. Antineutrophil cytoplasmic antibodies. Lancet 2006; 368(9533): 404-18.
[http://dx.doi.org/10.1016/S0140-6736(06)69114-9] [PMID: 16876669]

[27] Garcia D, Erkan D. Diagnosis and Management of the Antiphospholipid Syndrome. 2018.
[http://dx.doi.org/10.1056/NEJMra1705454]

[28] Meroni PL, Tsokos GC. Editorial: Systemic Lupus Erythematosus and Antiphospholipid Syndrome. Front Immunol 2019; 10: 199.
[http://dx.doi.org/10.3389/fimmu.2019.00199] [PMID: 30858846]

[29] Huber AM. Update on the clinical management of juvenile dermatomyositis. Expert Rev Clin Immunol 2018; 14(12): 1021-8.
[http://dx.doi.org/10.1080/1744666X.2018.1535901] [PMID: 30308133]

[30] Oni L, Sampath S. Childhood IgA Vasculitis (Henoch Schonlein Purpura)-Advances and Knowledge Gaps. Front Pediatr 2019; 7: 257.
[http://dx.doi.org/10.3389/fped.2019.00257] [PMID: 31316952]

[31] Petty RE, Southwood TR, Manners P, *et al.* International League of Associations for Rheumatology classification of juvenile idiopathic arthritis: second revision, Edmonton, 2001. J Rheumatol 2004; 31(2): 390-2.
[PMID: 14760812]

[32] Davies R, Carrasco R, Foster HE, *et al.* Treatment prescribing patterns in patients with juvenile idiopathic arthritis (JIA): Analysis from the UK Childhood Arthritis Prospective Study (CAPS). Semin Arthritis Rheum 2016; 46(2): 190-5.
[http://dx.doi.org/10.1016/j.semarthrit.2016.06.001] [PMID: 27422803]

[33] Ingegnoli F, Castelli R, Gualtierotti R. Rheumatoid factors: clinical applications. Dis Markers 2013; 35(6): 727-34.
[http://dx.doi.org/10.1155/2013/726598] [PMID: 24324289]

[34] Ringold S, Angeles-Han ST, Beukelman T, *et al.* 2019 American College of Rheumatology/Arthritis Foundation Guideline for the Treatment of Juvenile Idiopathic Arthritis: Therapeutic Approaches for Non-Systemic Polyarthritis, Sacroiliitis, and Enthesitis. Arthritis Rheumatol 2019; 71(6): 846-63.
[http://dx.doi.org/10.1002/art.40884] [PMID: 31021537]

[35] Mistry RR, Patro P, Agarwal V, Misra DP. Enthesitis-related arthritis: current perspectives. Open Access Rheumatol 2019; 11: 19-31.
[http://dx.doi.org/10.2147/OARRR.S163677] [PMID: 30774484]

[36] Zisman D, Gladman DD, Stoll ML, *et al.* The Juvenile Psoriatic Arthritis Cohort in the CARRA Registry: Clinical Characteristics, Classification, and Outcomes. J Rheumatol 2017; 44(3): 342-51.
[http://dx.doi.org/10.3899/jrheum.160717] [PMID: 28148698]

[37] Ravelli A, Consolaro A, Schiappapietra B, Martini A. The conundrum of juvenile psoriatic arthritis. Clin Exp Rheumatol 2015; 33(5) (Suppl. 93): S40-3.
[PMID: 26470604]

[38] Butbul Aviel Y, Tyrrell P, Schneider R, *et al.* Juvenile Psoriatic Arthritis (JPsA): juvenile arthritis with psoriasis? Pediatr Rheumatol Online J 2013; 11(1): 11.
[http://dx.doi.org/10.1186/1546-0096-11-11] [PMID: 23497068]

[39] Ringold S, Weiss PF, Beukelman T, *et al.* 2013 Update of the 2011 American College of Rheumatology Recommendations for the Treatment of Juvenile Idiopathic Arthritis: Recommendations for the Medical Therapy of Children With Systemic Juvenile Idiopathic Arthritis and Tuberculosis Screening Among C: ACR 2013 Updated Recommendations for the Medical Treatment of JIA. Arthritis Rheum 2013; 65(10): 2499-512.
[http://dx.doi.org/10.1002/art.38092] [PMID: 24092554]

[40] Aytaç S, Batu ED, Ünal Ş, *et al.* Macrophage activation syndrome in children with systemic juvenile idiopathic arthritis and systemic lupus erythematosus. Rheumatol Int 2016; 36(10): 1421-9.
[http://dx.doi.org/10.1007/s00296-016-3545-9] [PMID: 27510530]

[41] Real de Asúa D, Costa R, Galván JM, Filigheddu MT, Trujillo D, Cadiñanos J. Systemic AA amyloidosis: epidemiology, diagnosis, and management. Clin Epidemiol 2014; 6: 369-77.
[http://dx.doi.org/10.2147/CLEP.S39981] [PMID: 25378951]

[42] Lo MS. Insights Gained From the Study of Pediatric Systemic Lupus Erythematosus. Front Immunol 2018; 9: 1278.
[http://dx.doi.org/10.3389/fimmu.2018.01278] [PMID: 29922296]

[43] Tedeschi SK, Johnson SR, Boumpas DT, *et al.* Multicriteria decision analysis process to develop new classification criteria for systemic lupus erythematosus. Ann Rheum Dis 2019; 78(5): 634-40.
[http://dx.doi.org/10.1136/annrheumdis-2018-214685] [PMID: 30692164]

[44] Bajema IM, Wilhelmus S, Alpers CE, *et al.* Revision of the International Society of Nephrology/Renal Pathology Society classification for lupus nephritis: clarification of definitions, and modified National Institutes of Health activity and chronicity indices. Kidney Int 2018; 93(4): 789-96.
[http://dx.doi.org/10.1016/j.kint.2017.11.023] [PMID: 29459092]

[45] Rodriguez-Smith J, Brunner HI. Update on the treatment and outcome of systemic lupus erythematous in children. Curr Opin Rheumatol 2019; 31(5): 464-70.
[http://dx.doi.org/10.1097/BOR.0000000000000621] [PMID: 31107290]

[46] Lo MS. Monogenic Lupus. Curr Rheumatol Rep 2016; 18(12): 71.
[http://dx.doi.org/10.1007/s11926-016-0621-9] [PMID: 27812953]

[47] Hochberg MC. Updating the American College of Rheumatology revised criteria for the classification of systemic lupus erythematosus. Arthritis Rheum 1997; 40(9): 1725-5.
[http://dx.doi.org/10.1002/art.1780400928] [PMID: 9324032]

[48] Tektonidou MG, Lewandowski LB, Hu J, Dasgupta A, Ward MM. Survival in adults and children with systemic lupus erythematosus: a systematic review and Bayesian meta-analysis of studies from 1950 to 2016. Ann Rheum Dis 2017; 76(12): 2009-16.
[http://dx.doi.org/10.1136/annrheumdis-2017-211663] [PMID: 28794077]

[49] Vanoni F, Lava SAG, Fossali EF, *et al.* Neonatal Systemic Lupus Erythematosus Syndrome: a Comprehensive Review. Clin Rev Allergy Immunol 2017; 53(3): 469-76.
[http://dx.doi.org/10.1007/s12016-017-8653-0] [PMID: 29116459]

[50] Izmirly P, Saxena A, Buyon JP. Progress in the pathogenesis and treatment of cardiac manifestations of neonatal lupus. Curr Opin Rheumatol 2017; 29(5): 467-72.
[http://dx.doi.org/10.1097/BOR.0000000000000414] [PMID: 28520682]

[51] Li SC. Scleroderma in Children and Adolescents: Localized Scleroderma and Systemic Sclerosis. Pediatr Clin North Am 2018; 65(4): 757-81.
[http://dx.doi.org/10.1016/j.pcl.2018.04.002] [PMID: 30031497]

[52] El-Kehdy J, Abbas O, Rubeiz N. A review of Parry-Romberg syndrome. J Am Acad Dermatol 2012; 67(4): 769-84.

[http://dx.doi.org/10.1016/j.jaad.2012.01.019] [PMID: 22405645]

[53]   Stevens BE, Torok KS, Li SC, *et al.* Clinical Characteristics and Factors Associated With Disability and Impaired Quality of Life in Children With Juvenile Systemic Sclerosis: Results From the Childhood Arthritis and Rheumatology Research Alliance Legacy Registry. Arthritis Care Res (Hoboken) 2018; 70(12): 1806-13.
[http://dx.doi.org/10.1002/acr.23547] [PMID: 29457372]

[54]   Stevens AM, Torok KS, Li SC, Taber SF, Lu TT, Zulian F. Immunopathogenesis of Juvenile Systemic Sclerosis. Front Immunol 2019; 10: 1352.
[http://dx.doi.org/10.3389/fimmu.2019.01352] [PMID: 31293569]

[55]   Zulian F, Woo P, Athreya BH, *et al.* The Pediatric Rheumatology European Society/American College of Rheumatology/European League against Rheumatism provisional classification criteria for juvenile systemic sclerosis. Arthritis Rheum 2007; 57(2): 203-12.
[http://dx.doi.org/10.1002/art.22551] [PMID: 17330294]

[56]   Martini G, Vittadello F, Kasapçopur O, *et al.* Factors affecting survival in juvenile systemic sclerosis. Rheumatology (Oxford) 2009; 48(2): 119-22.
[http://dx.doi.org/10.1093/rheumatology/ken388] [PMID: 18854345]

[57]   Findlay AR, Goyal NA, Mozaffar T. An overview of polymyositis and dermatomyositis. Muscle Nerve 2015; 51(5): 638-56.
[http://dx.doi.org/10.1002/mus.24566] [PMID: 25641317]

[58]   Bohan A, Peter JB. Polymyositis and dermatomyositis (first of two parts). N Engl J Med 1975; 292(7): 344-7.
[http://dx.doi.org/10.1056/NEJM197502132920706] [PMID: 1090839]

[59]   Bottai M, Tjärnlund A, Santoni G, *et al.* EULAR/ACR classification criteria for adult and juvenile idiopathic inflammatory myopathies and their major subgroups: a methodology report. RMD Open 2017; 3(2): e000507.
[http://dx.doi.org/10.1136/rmdopen-2017-000507] [PMID: 29177080]

[60]   Barut K, Şahin S, Adroviç A, Kasapçopur Ö. Diagnostic approach and current treatment options in childhood vasculitis. Turk Pediatri Ars 2015; 50(4): 194-205.
[http://dx.doi.org/10.5152/TurkPediatriArs.2015.2363] [PMID: 26884688]

[61]   Piram M, Maldini C, Biscardi S, *et al.* Incidence of IgA vasculitis in children estimated by four-source capture-recapture analysis: a population-based study. Rheumatology (Oxford) 2017; 56(8): 1358-66.
[http://dx.doi.org/10.1093/rheumatology/kex158] [PMID: 28444335]

[62]   Ruperto N, Ozen S, Pistorio A, *et al.* EULAR/PRINTO/PRES criteria for Henoch-Schönlein purpura, childhood polyarteritis nodosa, childhood Wegener granulomatosis and childhood Takayasu arteritis: Ankara 2008. Part I: Overall methodology and clinical characterisation. Ann Rheum Dis 2010; 69(5): 790-7.
[http://dx.doi.org/10.1136/ard.2009.116624] [PMID: 20388738]

[63]   Jauhola O, Ronkainen J, Koskimies O, *et al.* Clinical course of extrarenal symptoms in Henoch-Schonlein purpura: a 6-month prospective study. Arch Dis Child 2010; 95(11): 871-6.
[http://dx.doi.org/10.1136/adc.2009.167874] [PMID: 20371584]

[64]   Hwang HH, Lim IS, Choi B-S, Yi DY. Analysis of seasonal tendencies in pediatric Henoch-Schönlein purpura and comparison with outbreak of infectious diseases. Medicine (Baltimore) 2018; 97(36): e12217.
[http://dx.doi.org/10.1097/MD.0000000000012217] [PMID: 30200139]

[65]   Ozen S, Marks SD, Brogan P, *et al.* European consensus-based recommendations for diagnosis and treatment of immunoglobulin A vasculitis-the SHARE initiative. Rheumatology (Oxford) 2019; 58(9): 1607-16.
[http://dx.doi.org/10.1093/rheumatology/kez041] [PMID: 30879080]

[66] Mills JA, Michel BA, Bloch DA, *et al.* The American College of Rheumatology 1990 criteria for the classification of Henoch-Schönlein purpura. Arthritis Rheum 1990; 33(8): 1114-21.
[http://dx.doi.org/10.1002/art.1780330809] [PMID: 2202310]

[67] Ozen S, Pistorio A, Iusan SM, *et al.* EULAR/PRINTO/PRES criteria for Henoch-Schönlein purpura, childhood polyarteritis nodosa, childhood Wegener granulomatosis and childhood Takayasu arteritis: Ankara 2008. Part II: Final classification criteria. Ann Rheum Dis 2010; 69(5): 798-806.
[http://dx.doi.org/10.1136/ard.2009.116657] [PMID: 20413568]

[68] Jariwala MP, Laxer RM. Primary Vasculitis in Childhood: GPA and MPA in Childhood. Front Pediatr 2018; 6: 226.
[http://dx.doi.org/10.3389/fped.2018.00226] [PMID: 30167431]

[69] Fina A, Dubus J-C, Tran A, *et al.* Eosinophilic granulomatosis with polyangiitis in children: Data from the French RespiRare® cohort. Pediatr Pulmonol 2018; 53(12): 1640-50.
[http://dx.doi.org/10.1002/ppul.24089] [PMID: 29943913]

[70] Eleftheriou D, Gale H, Pilkington C, Fenton M, Sebire NJ, Brogan PA. Eosinophilic granulomatosis with polyangiitis in childhood: retrospective experience from a tertiary referral centre in the UK. Rheumatology (Oxford) 2016; 55(7): 1263-72.
[http://dx.doi.org/10.1093/rheumatology/kew029] [PMID: 27026726]

[71] Makino N, Nakamura Y, Yashiro M, *et al.* Epidemiological observations of Kawasaki disease in Japan, 2013-2014. Pediatr Int 2018; 60(6): 581-7.
[http://dx.doi.org/10.1111/ped.13544] [PMID: 29498791]

[72] Kim GB. Reality of Kawasaki disease epidemiology. Korean J Pediatr 2019; 62(8): 292-6.
[http://dx.doi.org/10.3345/kjp.2019.00157] [PMID: 31319643]

[73] McCrindle BW, Rowley AH, Newburger JW, *et al.* Diagnosis, Treatment, and Long-Term Management of Kawasaki Disease: A Scientific Statement for Health Professionals From the American Heart Association. Circulation 2017; 135(17): e927-99.
[http://dx.doi.org/10.1161/CIR.0000000000000484] [PMID: 28356445]

[74] Sundel RP. Kawasaki disease. Rheum Dis Clin North Am 2015; 41(1): 63-73, viii.
[http://dx.doi.org/10.1016/j.rdc.2014.09.010] [PMID: 25399940]

[75] Ramphul K, Mejias SG. Kawasaki disease: a comprehensive review. Arch Med Sci Atheroscler Dis 2018; 3(1): e41-5.
[http://dx.doi.org/10.5114/amsad.2018.74522] [PMID: 30775588]

[76] Forbess L, Bannykh S. Polyarteritis nodosa. Rheum Dis Clin North Am 2015; 41(1): 33-46, vii.
[http://dx.doi.org/10.1016/j.rdc.2014.09.005] [PMID: 25399938]

[77] Numano F. The story of Takayasu arteritis. Rheumatology (Oxford) 2002; 41(1): 103-6.
[http://dx.doi.org/10.1093/rheumatology/41.1.103] [PMID: 11792888]

[78] Johnston SL, Lock RJ, Gompels MM. Takayasu arteritis: a review. J Clin Pathol 2002; 55(7): 481-6.
[http://dx.doi.org/10.1136/jcp.55.7.481] [PMID: 12101189]

[79] Arnaud L, Haroche J, Mathian A, Gorochov G, Amoura Z. Pathogenesis of Takayasu's arteritis: a 2011 update. Autoimmun Rev 2011; 11(1): 61-7.
[http://dx.doi.org/10.1016/j.autrev.2011.08.001] [PMID: 21855656]

[80] Moriwaki R, Noda M, Yajima M, Sharma BK, Numano F. Clinical manifestations of Takayasu arteritis in India and Japan--new classification of angiographic findings. Angiology 1997; 48(5): 369-79.
[http://dx.doi.org/10.1177/000331979704800501] [PMID: 9158381]

[81] Arend WP, Michel BA, Bloch DA, *et al.* The American College of Rheumatology 1990 criteria for the classification of Takayasu arteritis. Arthritis Rheum 1990; 33(8): 1129-34.
[http://dx.doi.org/10.1002/art.1780330811] [PMID: 1975175]

[82]   Ozen S, Ruperto N, Dillon MJ, *et al.* EULAR/PReS endorsed consensus criteria for the classification of childhood vasculitides. Ann Rheum Dis 2006; 65(7): 936-41.
[http://dx.doi.org/10.1136/ard.2005.046300] [PMID: 16322081]

[83]   Sharma S, Gupta A. Visceral Artery Interventions in Takayasu's Arteritis. Semin Intervent Radiol 2009; 26(3): 233-44.
[http://dx.doi.org/10.1055/s-0029-1225668] [PMID: 21326568]

[84]   Cervera R. Antiphospholipid syndrome. Thromb Res 2017; 151 (Suppl. 1): S43-7.
[http://dx.doi.org/10.1016/S0049-3848(17)30066-X] [PMID: 28262233]

[85]   Graf J. Central Nervous System Manifestations of Antiphospholipid Syndrome. Rheum Dis Clin North Am 2017; 43(4): 547-60.
[http://dx.doi.org/10.1016/j.rdc.2017.06.004] [PMID: 29061241]

[86]   Go EJL, O'Neil KM. The catastrophic antiphospholipid syndrome in children. Curr Opin Rheumatol 2017; 29(5): 516-22.
[http://dx.doi.org/10.1097/BOR.0000000000000426] [PMID: 28632503]

[87]   Ruiz-Irastorza G, Crowther M, Branch W, Khamashta MA. Antiphospholipid syndrome. Lancet 2010; 376(9751): 1498-509.
[http://dx.doi.org/10.1016/S0140-6736(10)60709-X] [PMID: 20822807]

[88]   Siddique S, Risse J, Canaud G, Zuily S. Vascular Manifestations in Antiphospholipid Syndrome (APS): Is APS a Thrombophilia or a Vasculopathy? Curr Rheumatol Rep 2017; 19(10): 64.
[http://dx.doi.org/10.1007/s11926-017-0687-z] [PMID: 28871481]

[89]   Carmi O, Berla M, Shoenfeld Y, Levy Y. Diagnosis and management of catastrophic antiphospholipid syndrome. Expert Rev Hematol 2017; 10(4): 365-74.
[http://dx.doi.org/10.1080/17474086.2017.1300522] [PMID: 28277850]

[90]   Al-Haddad C, BouGhannam A, Abdul Fattah M, Tamim H, El Moussawi Z, Hamam RN. Patterns of uveitis in children according to age: comparison of visual outcomes and complications in a tertiary center. BMC Ophthalmol 2019; 19(1): 137.
[http://dx.doi.org/10.1186/s12886-019-1139-5] [PMID: 31248388]

[91]   Heiligenhaus A, Minden K, Föll D, Pleyer U. Uveitis in Juvenile Idiopathic Arthritis 2015.https://www.aerzteblatt.de/10.3238/arztebl.2015.0092
[http://dx.doi.org/10.3238/arztebl.2015.0092]

[92]   Jabs DA, Nussenblatt RB, Rosenbaum JT. Standardization of uveitis nomenclature for reporting clinical data. Results of the First International Workshop. Am J Ophthalmol 2005; 140(3): 509-16.
[http://dx.doi.org/10.1016/j.ajo.2005.03.057] [PMID: 16196117]

[93]   Grom AA, Horne A, De Benedetti F. Macrophage activation syndrome in the era of biologic therapy. Nat Rev Rheumatol 2016; 12(5): 259-68.
[http://dx.doi.org/10.1038/nrrheum.2015.179] [PMID: 27009539]

[94]   Yasin S, Schulert GS. Systemic juvenile idiopathic arthritis and macrophage activation syndrome: update on pathogenesis and treatment. Curr Opin Rheumatol 2018; 30(5): 514-20.
[http://dx.doi.org/10.1097/BOR.0000000000000526] [PMID: 29870499]

[95]   Henter J-I, Horne A, Aricó M, *et al.* HLH-2004: Diagnostic and therapeutic guidelines for hemophagocytic lymphohistiocytosis. Pediatr Blood Cancer 2007; 48(2): 124-31.
[http://dx.doi.org/10.1002/pbc.21039] [PMID: 16937360]

[96]   Lerkvaleekul B, Vilaiyuk S. Macrophage activation syndrome: early diagnosis is key. Open Access Rheumatol 2018; 10: 117-28.
[http://dx.doi.org/10.2147/OARRR.S151013] [PMID: 30214327]

CHAPTER 3

Updates on Common Oral Diseases in Children

Heliya Ziaei[1,2], **Shahrzad Banan**[3] and **Donya Alinejhad**[4,*]

[1] *Network of Immunity in Infection, Malignancy and Autoimmunity (NIIMA), Universal Scientific Education and Research Network (USERN), Tehran, Iran*

[2] *Maxillofacial Surgery & Implantology & Biomaterial Research foundation, Tehran, Iran*

[3] *School of Dentistry, Guilan University of Medical Sciences, Rasht, Iran*

[4] *Department of Pediatric Dentistry, School of Dentistry, Tehran University of Medical Sciences, Tehran, Iran*

Abstract: Oral and dental diseases are among the most common problems in children worldwide. If these problems remain untreated, they can have long-term effects on the orofacial system, chewing and speaking abilities, oral health-related quality of life, and overall health status. Dental caries, periodontitis and gingivitis, dental malocclusion, dental trauma, and some oral soft tissue lesions are among the most common oral disorders in children. Early diagnosis and management of these conditions by pediatric dentists and pediatricians necessitate being aware of the clinical manifestations of each disease at every age. Implementing preventive intervention, accurate diagnosis, proper treatment, and performing regular follow-ups are among the key factors for eliminating harmful long-life consequences of poor oral and dental health status in children and adolescents.

Keywords: Aphthous ulcer, Bruxism, Childhood caries, Children, Cyst, Dental caries, Eruption hematoma, Gingivitis, Hemangioma, Infection, Lip biting, Lymphangioma, Malocclusion, Oral habits, Periodontitis, Thumb sucking, Tongue, Tongue thrusting, Tooth, Trauma.

INTRODUCTION

Oral and dental diseases are among the most common problems in children worldwide. If these problems remain untreated, they can have long-term effects on the orofacial system, chewing and speaking abilities, oral health-related quality of life, and overall health status. Pediatric dentists and pediatricians should be aware of the signs and symptoms of these oral conditions for accurate diagnosis from the early steps and proper management to prevent further harmful consequences in the overall health status.

* **Corresponding author Donya Alinejhad:** Department of Pediatric Dentistry, School of Dentistry, Tehran University of Medical Sciences, Tehran, Iran; Tel: 00989153046375; E-mail: donya_alinejhad@yahoo.com

Nima Rezaei and Noosha Samieefar (Eds.)

DENTAL CARIES

Dental caries is the most common chronic infection among children worldwide; *Streptococcus mutans* bacteria are considered the main etiological factor for this common oral disease [1]. According to the World Health Organization (WHO), in 2020, more than 530 million children suffer from dental caries of deciduous teeth; also, permanent teeth dental caries are the most common health issue based on a global assessment of 354 diseases in 2017 [2]. The DMFT index indicates the number of permanent teeth decayed, missing, and filled teeth, which is used as a global index for evaluating dental caries conditions worldwide. Due to the fact that this major public health issue is completely preventable, public health policymakers paid significant attention to implementing strategies to prevent this disease from childhood [3].

Early Childhood Caries (ECC) is one of the major public health problems worldwide; its prevalence is 12-27% among 2 to 3-year-old children, and it reaches 48% in up to 6 years old children. ECC is defined as "the presence of one or more decayed (non-cavitated or cavitated lesions), missing (due to caries), or filled tooth surfaces in any primary tooth in a child under the age of six" [4, 5]. This early onset disease can have major long-term consequences during the lifetime, such as premature teeth loss, future orthodontic problems, speech difficulties, masticatory and chewing issues, higher risk of further carious lesions in permanent teeth, impact on the development and eruption of permanent dentition, and orofacial dysfunction [6]. Thus, it has become one of the priorities of planning preventive interventions among public health managers.

ECC has multifactorial etiology, such as socio-economic status, dietary factors, behavioral problems, and genetic factors [4]; however, inadequate dental plaque removal of the primary teeth in addition to a sugary diet leads to accelerating this process [7]. One of the most prevalent examples of a sugary diet is prolonged usage of baby bottles with sugary contents, especially during the sleep period [4]. Based on a systematic review and meta-analysis, ECC's most important risk factors in high-income families were frequent sweetened meals, improper oral health care, and visible plaque in the oral cavity [8].

However, ECC can involve all primary teeth; it usually involves maxillary incisors (compared to mandibular incisors), followed by molars and canines, consequently (Figs. **1**, **2A**, **2B** and **3**) [9]. One of the most significant character-istics of ECC is the rapid progression of initial white spot lesions in the gingival margin to cavitated lesions in the labial or lingual surfaces of the primary teeth, which is not common in the routine form of tooth decay at this age [4, 9].

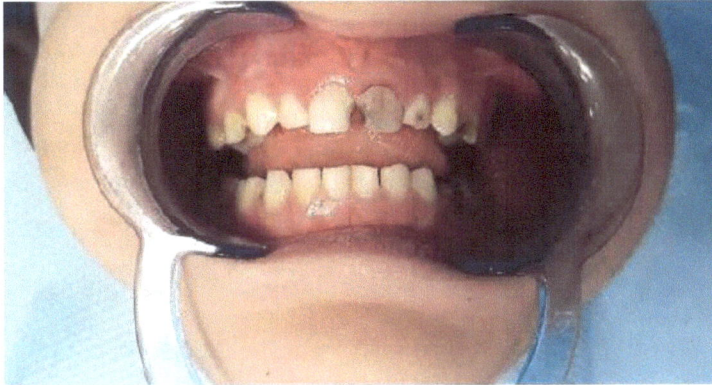

Fig. (1). ECC involving anterior maxillary incisors in a 5-years-old male child.

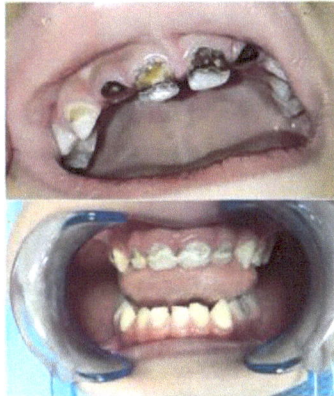

Fig. (2). A.ECC involving almost all primary teeth of 3-years-old children. The central and lateral primary incisors have severe tooth caries leading to complete disruption of the lateral crowns. **B.**ECC in the anterior maxillary incisors in a 4-years-old female patient.

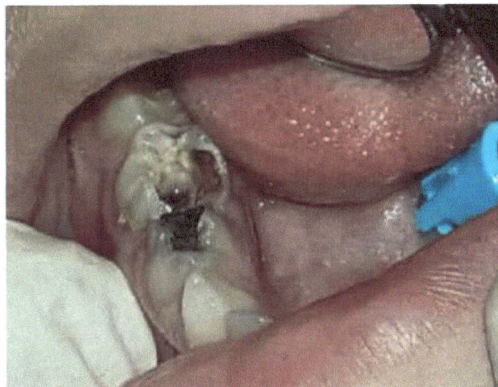

Fig. (3). Cavitated untreated tooth caries in the second primary molar of a 6-years-old child.

There are various proposed techniques to prevent ECC; first of all, regular oral health care management and plaque removal reduce the cariogenic bacterial load, leading to decelerating the caries progression. Second, reducing the frequency and amount of glucose-containing food for the children and changing dietary habits omit one of the main components of this vicious cycle. Also, applying topical fluoride on recently erupted teeth increases the resistance of primary teeth enamel to caries, which has to be done by dental professionals in the dental office [9].

PERIODONTITIS AND GINGIVITIS

Periodontal disease, including gingivitis and periodontitis, is another common oral disease with a high prevalence comparable to dental caries among children. Based on the American Academy of Pediatric Dentistry (AAPD) statement, "gingivitis is nearly universal in children and adolescents." Studies reveal that gingivitis involves half of four or five-year-old children. The frequency and severity of gingivitis are aggravated with age, with a peak in puberty [10, 11]. Although the prevalence and severity of gingival disease decrease after the adolescent period, it has an inclination regarding periodontitis during the lifetime [11]. Periodontitis is an inflammatory disease of supporting tissue of dental apparatus such as alveolar bone, periodontal ligaments, cementum, and gingiva, which can be destructive, leading to progressive clinical attachment loss (CAL) and bone loss [12]. Accumulation of dental plaque and bacteria in a deep periodontal pocket leads to the progression of the attachment apparatus destruction [13]; preventive protocols (plaque removal, regular follow-ups, antibacterial mouthwashes, *etc.*) would be very beneficial during the early phase of these conditions at an early age to stop this vicious cycle. Fig. (**4**) shows early onset gingivitis during infancy.

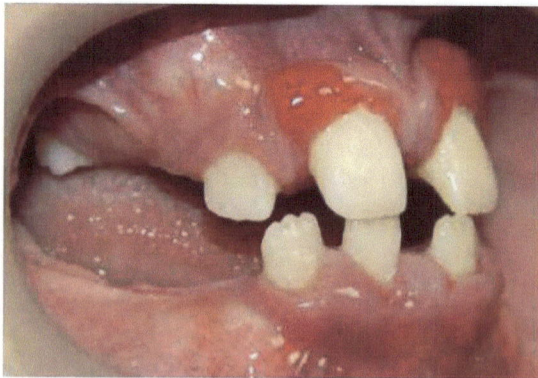

Fig. (4). Early onset gingivitis in a 9-years-old child.

It should be noted that the normal anatomy of children's gingiva and periodontium has a significant difference compared to adults. Table **1** [14, 15] indicated these differences for accurate diagnosis of gingivitis and periodontitis in children and preventing any misdiagnosis.

Table 1. Differences between normal gingival tissue and periodontium in children compared to adults.

Children	Adult
Lower width of the attached gingiva	higher width of the attached gingiva
Edematous, erythematous, and rounded gingival margin (especially during tooth eruption)	Normal gingival margin in colar pink color with no evidence of reddened or edematous area.
Greater probing depth	Normal probing depth
Lack of stippling	Normal stippling can be seen in a healthy gingiva

Fig. (**5**) [12, 14] and Fig. (**6**) [16, 17] specify the classification of gingivitis and periodontitis in children. In non-plaque induced gingivitis, plaque is not the main etiology of the inflammation; plaque removal and improving oral health status do not have a significant positive effect on reducing the inflammation.

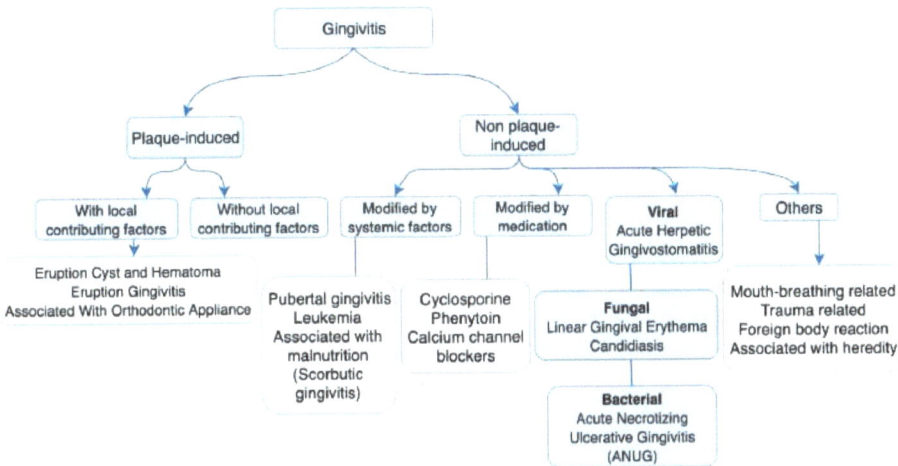

Fig. (5). Classification of gingivitis in children and adolescent.

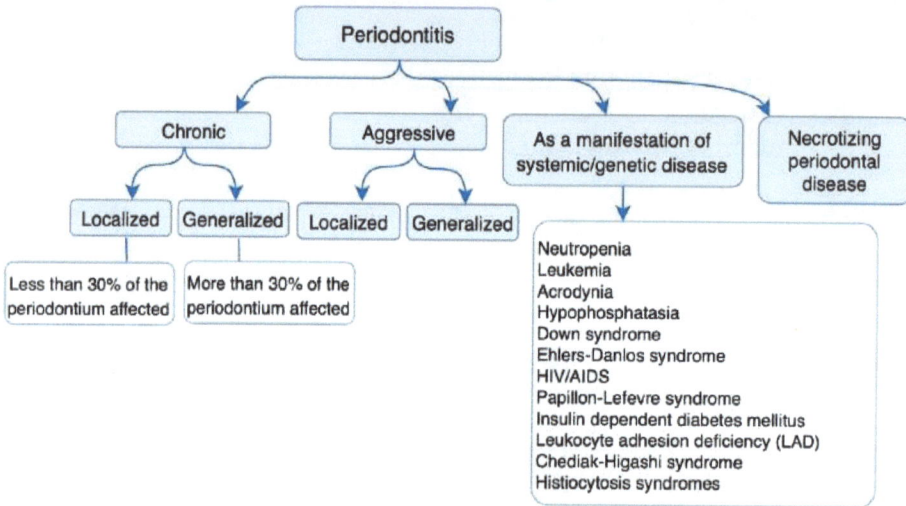

Fig. (6). Classification of periodontitis in children and adolescent.

Localized aggressive periodontitis is mostly seen in children and adolescents with severe bone loss, especially around permanent first molars and incisors, and with rapid progression. Antibiotics with root surgical debridement are one of the best management procedures for treating this periodontal condition. On the other hand, chronic periodontitis is more frequent in adults with a slower progression compared to the aggressive type; it is classified into mild, moderate, and severe forms [16, 17].

Necrotizing uncreative periodontitis usually is seen in children with underlying conditions such as systemic disease, compromised immunity, malnutrition, *etc.*; it is associated with severe gingival pain, ulceration, and necrosis [16].

Periodontal and gingival indexes such as bleeding on probing (BOP), probing depth, plaque, and calculus indexes should be recorded in the follow-up sessions to evaluate the progression/amelioration of these conditions [18].

MALOCCLUSION

Malocclusion is one of the most common dental problems in children and adolescents worldwide [19, 20]. Based on a systematic review and meta-analysis in 2020, the global prevalence of malocclusion was 56%; but a range of 20% to 100% is reported by different studies 19,21.

Various hereditary, environmental, or a combination of both factors are responsible for malocclusion in children; oral habits and dental diseases are among the principal etiological factors [21 - 24]. Table **2** indicates some major environmental and genetic factors causing malocclusion in children.

Malocclusion is known as an early onset problem that is preventable if it is diagnosed and treated properly from early childhood. In case of no treatment, it can result in significant problems such as facial disharmony, masticatory problems, oral and maxillofacial discrepancy, temporomandibular disorders, abnormal jaw interrelationships, and impact on the quality of life [25 - 27]. Management and treatment of oral dysfunctions, treating oral and dental problems affecting normal dentition, and maintaining normal tooth development and eruption in both deciduous and permanent dentition can effectively prevent malocclusion in children and adolescents [21].

Malocclusion can be classified as skeletal and dental; each of them can have multifactorial etiology. While the exact cause of each classification of malocclusion is unknown, genetic factors and congenital craniofacial disorders have a significant role in skeletal malocclusion [28].

Table **2.** Major environmental and genetic etiological factors causing malocclusion in children [22,23,29,30].

Environmental	Genetic
Oral habits Pacifier habit Lip habit Nail biting Airway obstruction Tongue thrusting Mouth breathing Finger sucking Unilateral mastication habit Bruxism	Size of the maxilla and mandible
Early childhood caries	Arch form
Pulpal and periapical lesions of primary teeth	Tooth size
Trauma of primary teeth	Tooth morphology
-	Congenital tooth missing (primary or permanent)

Oral Habits

The high prevalence of some deleterious oral habits in early childhood, which affects dental, skeletal, and craniofacial growth, emphasizes the importance of paying attention to early diagnosis of them at this age [31]. Consultation with an orthodontist and psychiatrist from early childhood may help in treating oral habits prior to entering the mixed and permanent dentition period to prevent further consequences.

In this section, a number of common oral habits that affect normal occlusion in children are discussed.

Finger (Thumb) Sucking

The position of fingers in the oral cavity while sucking causes loss of normal force balance in the oral cavity; it applies lingual pressure to the lower anterior teeth and labial pressure to the upper incisors [32]. In addition, the lower position of the tongue causes less lingual pressure on the posterior teeth and more buccal pressure from the cheek. This can result in constriction of the maxilla or V-shape arch form in severe cases [33]. Nonnutritive sucking behavior, especially in children more than two years old, causes more occlusion problems compared to children with no sucking behavior, such as protruded upper incisors, anterior open bite, excessive overjet, posterior crossbite, and maxillary arch constriction [33, 34]. The duration and frequency of the behavior have a direct relationship with the severity of malocclusion [35 - 37]. In general, dental effects of finger sucking are reversible, if it is inhibited before the permanent dentition period.

Lip Biting (Sucking)

This habit is usually found with or as a substitution for finger sucking. The position of the lower lip between the upper and lower incisors applies lingual force to the lower anterior incisors and labial force to the upper incisors, which increases the overjet, causes anterior open bite, and leads to deepening of the mento-labial sulcus [21, 38].

Nail-biting (Onychophagia)

This habit is common in children with a previous finger biting habit and usually is not seen in younger than three-year-old children [38, 39]. Biting the nails between the incisal edge of the maxillary and mandibular anterior teeth causes anterior teeth attrition and malalignment, small fractures of the incisal edge of these teeth, and protrusion of the upper maxillary incisors [39].

Pacifier Habits

Using pacifiers before three years of age may not have serious harmful effects on the dentition. But in children older than three years, especially those older than 5, it may cause severe oral consequences [32, 40]. Although the usage of both conventional and orthodontic pacifiers increased the occurrence of malocclusion, the usage of orthodontic pacifiers may have priorities based on recent researches, but further studies are needed to approve it [41, 42]. Based on an observational study in 3-5-year-old children who started using orthodontic pacifiers from the first three months of life, the risk of harmful oral habits or malocclusion in the primary dentition was not increased, despite long-term usage of them [43]; also, the risk of finger sucking is reduced in these children too. The most considerable clinical effects of pacifiers in the dental apparatus include narrow and deep palate, posterior crossbite, and anterior open bite [44, 45].

Among nutritive sucking behaviors, breastfeeding can reduce the risk of malocclusion in children compared to bottle feeding [46, 47]. The longer duration of breastfeeding has a positive relationship with the lower risk of malocclusion [22], but more well-designed studies with a high number of cases are needed to prove its positive effects.

Bruxism

Sleep bruxism is an unconscious condition with a wide range of 3.5 - 40.6% prevalence in children based on a systematic review study [48]. Children with long-term sleep bruxism are more prone to temporomandibular joint disorders; also, they represent clinical manifestations such as teeth erosion and consequent teeth hypersensitization, and hypertrophy of the masticatory muscles [45, 49].

Tongue Thrusting

Tongue thrust swallowing is a physiological characteristic during infancy, in which the tongue is positioned between upper and lower gum pads while swallowing. This type of swallowing is atypical in children older than four and can have oral and dental harmful effects [32]. The anterior and lateral pressure of the tongue to the teeth, instead of its pressure to the hard palate in normal swallowing, may result in an anterior open bite and proclination and spacing of the anterior teeth. Posterior crossbite and narrow hard palate due to the lower resting position of the tongue are other clinical features [22, 50].

Mouth Breathing

The etiology of mouth breathing in children can be related to habitual, anatomical (short lower lip), or obstructive reasons [51]. Allergic rhinitis and adenotonsillar hypertrophy are among the most important causes of obstructive mouth breathing [52, 53]. The open posture of the mouth, elongation of the vertical facial height, deep mental sulcus, convex facial pattern, lip incompetency, and lower position of the tongue are among common clinical features associated with mouth breathing

[53, 54]. Anterior open bite, proclination of the incisor teeth, and supra eruption of the lower anterior teeth are some dental alterations due to mouth breathing [51].

TRAUMA

Dental trauma is highly prevalent among children and adolescents worldwide; this emphasizes the importance of planning preventive interventions for reducing the occurrence of it in different age groups [55, 56]. Rapid diagnosis and management of a dental injury can be crucial to improve the prognosis and make it possible to save the injured teeth [57]. Falling and playing sports were the most common accidents that were associated with teeth injuries [56].

Traumatic dental injuries can be divided into trauma to dental tissue trauma (hard tissue), supporting dental tissue trauma, or both [58].

Based on a recent systematic review and meta-analysis, the most common dental trauma was enamel fracture, followed by dentin fracture, contusion, and fractures with pulp exposure, consequently, in children and adolescents [56]. Trauma to the primary and permanent dentition can be classified as it is mentioned in Table **3**.

Although the primary dentition is temporary and replaced by the permanent dentition in the oral cavity, paying attention to any trauma to these teeth is crucial. The first and foremost issue about trauma to the primary teeth is its harmful effects in odontogenesis of the permanent dentition; it can be explained by the close relationship of the primary teeth apices and permanent teeth buds (Figs. **7** & **8**) [59]. Even minor traumatic injuries to the primary dentition, especially during the first five years of life, have a harmful effect on the permanent tooth development; defects in enamel formation of the permanent teeth (hypoplasia or discoloration) are the most common type after trauma to the primary dentition [56, 59, 60]. It should be mentioned that reimplantation of the avulsed primary tooth is completely contraindicated, as a result of its probable trauma to the underlying permanent tooth [60]. But reimplantation of the avulsed permanent teeth is a treatment option following the standard instruction [61].

Table 3. Types of dental trauma to the primary and permanent dentition [57].

Classification	Types of Trauma	Description
Hard tissue injury	Infraction	Incomplete fracture of the enamel (Crack)
	Uncomplicated crown fracture	Fracture of enamel or dentin of the tooth without pulp exposure
	Complicated crown fracture	Fracture of enamel and dentin of the tooth with pulp exposure
	Crown and root fracture	Fracture of enamel, dentin, and cementum of the tooth with or without pulp exposure
	Root fracture	Fracture of dentin and cementum of the tooth with pulp exposure
Tooth supporting tissue injury	Concussion	No mobility or bleeding
	Subluxation	Bleeding from the marginal gingiva
	Lateral luxation	Lateral displacement of the tooth (It usually can be associated with alveolar trauma or fracture)
	Intrusion	Apical displacement of the tooth, with severe trauma to the periodontal ligament and usually associated with alveolar bone condensation or fracture.
	Extrusion	Axial displacement of the tooth from the socket (with loose attachment to the socket)
	Avulsion	Complete dislocation of the teeth out of the socket (Fig. **5**).

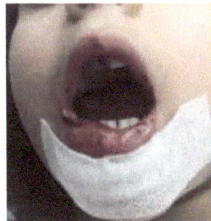

Fig. (7). A child with trauma (Avulsion of the right central and lateral maxillary incisors).

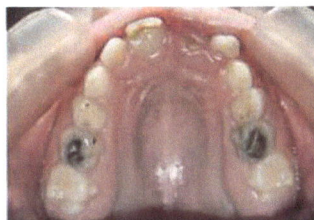

Fig. (8). Traumatic injury to the primary dentition caused impairment in the enamel formation in the permanent incisors.

The most common trauma to the tooth-supporting structures is intrusive luxation that is one of the most destructive traumas to the supporting bone and tissues [62].

If any traumatic injury is neglected, and a proper treatment plan is not considered for it, it can have a long-life consequence in oral health and quality of life of the children and adolescents [63]. Accordingly, regular follow-up sessions are mandatory for children with previous dental trauma to monitor the state of tooth vitality and prognosis.

ORAL SOFT TISSUE LESIONS

Eruption Hematoma and Cyst

Eruption cyst or hematoma is a benign pathologic condition overlying erupting primary or permanent teeth, shortly before emerging into the oral cavity [64, 65]. It is characterized by its translucent, dome-shaped, bluish swelling over the alveolar ridge 66. Fluid accumulation with or without blood in the follicular space of the erupting teeth causes this condition, so this lesion is fluctuant in palpation. This lesion is usually seen in 6-9-year-old children, during the early mixed dentition [65, 67]. The most common involved teeth are primary mandibular incisors and permanent mandibular molars [68]. Its size is variable and depends on the size and number of the affected teeth.

It is resolved spontaneously just after the appearance of the tooth crown in the oral cavity. But if it remains for a longer time, it may interfere with the tooth eruption, and surgical intervention is needed [66].

Erythema Migrans (Benign Migratory Glossitis or Geographic Tongue)

Erythema migrans is a chronic inflammatory condition of the tongue, that is mostly seen during childhood and early adolescence [69]. It typically involves the dorsum and, in some cases, ventrum of the tongue. It is characterized by multiple map-like irregular and well-demarcated areas on the tongue. These erythematous areas are formed because of atrophy of the filiform papillae, surrounded by elevated yellowish-white borders [69, 70]. The size, shape, and location of these zones change within days and weeks. It is usually asymptomatic, but it causes sore tongue in some cases; it is mostly seen in association with fissured tongue [70]. It should be noted that this condition is not related to erythema migrans of Lyme disease.

Aphthous Ulcer (Recurrent Aphthous Stomatitis)

It is a common idiopathic condition, characterized by recurrent painful ulcerative lesions in the oral mucosa, affecting children and adolescents more than adults [71, 72]. Buccal and labial mucosa are the most affected sites; it is mostly seen in non-keratinized oral mucosa [73]. The treatment protocols for the management of these lesions are long-term and complicated, interfering with daily activity and children's quality of life [71]. The erythematous shallow and round ulcers covered with fibrinous pseudo-membrane have a distinct margin. It is classified into three typical forms: minor, major, and herpetiform; the minor type is the most prevalent with ulcers with less than 1 cm in diameter [73, 74]. Major aphthous ulcers have lesions with more than 1 cm in diameter, remain longer in the oral cavity, and leave a scar after healing. Herpetiform type is rare and characterized by multiple small and deep ulcers, that can merge together and form larger lesions [73].

Traumatic Lesions

Morsicatio Buccarum

Oral frictional hyperkeratosis or Morsicatio buccarum is a benign white plaque or patch lesion in the buccal mucosa caused by chronic biting or chewing of the oral mucosa. It is usually seen along with the occlusal plane as irregular localized to diffuse rough white lesions that can be extended into the labial mucosa. This lesion should not be termed as leukoplakia, as it has an obvious etiological factor. This asymptomatic lesion is usually seen in the first decade of life. It usually needs no treatment, and the lesion regresses by the elimination of the harmful oral habit [75, 76].

Burns

Oropharyngeal burn injuries take place due to chemical, electrical, and thermal results. It is common in the first and second decades of life [76]. The most common causes of oral burn injuries are chemical burns, and overheated foods and drinks consequently [77, 78]. The most common sites of burn injuries are lips and tongue, following, palate, pharynx, and buccal mucosa [77]. Comprehensive treatment protocol with regular follow-up sessions is necessary for these children with a focus on pain relief and infection control [78]. A typical oral burn lesion is a white plaque which is not adherent to the underlying mucosa, along with erythematous erosion and ulcer [76].

TONGUE

Ankyloglossia

Ankyloglossia, also known as tongue-tie, is characterized by a short lingual frenum that extends from the tip of the tongue to the floor of the mouth and toward the lingual gingival tissue. It causes limitation of tongue movement and speech disorders (Fig. **9**). In infants, tongue-tie can lead to breastfeeding problems. The following techniques are indicated for treatment of children with ankyloglossia: Frenotomy, Frenectomy, and Lingual frenuloplasty [79].

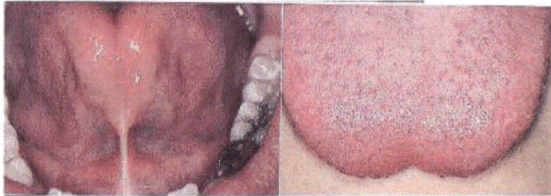

Fig. (9). Tongue-tie. A short lingual frenum that extends from the tip of the tongue to the floor of the mouth, limiting tongue movements.

Geographic Tongue

The geographic tongue, which is also known as benign migratory glossitis, is characterized by depapillated and erythematous patches with whitish borders that cause a map-like pattern on the dorsal and lateral surfaces of the tongue (Fig. **10**). The pattern of the lesions is not stable, and it is changeable. The etiology of the geographic tongue is unknown. However, it can be associated with some predisposing factors such as stress, Vitamin B deficiency, hereditary factors, allergy, and immunological factors. Geographic tongue is usually discovered as an accidental finding during routine oral examination by dentists. Most of the time, the geographic tongue is asymptomatic and does not require any treatment [80, 81].

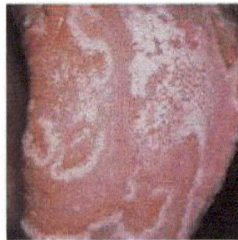

Fig. (10). Benign migratory glossitis. The depapillated and erythematous patches with whitish borders can be seen on the dorsal and lateral surfaces of the tongue.

Fissured Tongue

Fissured tongue is characterized by fissures or grooves with variable depth along with the dorsal or lateral surfaces of the tongue. The etiology of the fissured tongue is unknown 80. Fissured tongue can be related to some diseases such as psoriasis, Down's syndrome, hypothyroidism, and diabetes. It is usually asymptomatic and symmetrical, and no treatment is necessary (Fig. **11**) [79].

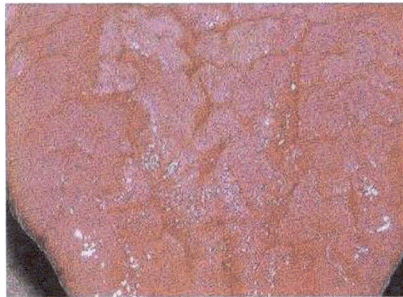

Fig. (11). Fissured tongue. The fissures or grooves along with the dorsal or lateral surfaces of the tongue with variable depth.

Coated Tongue (Hairy Tongue)

Coated tongue is a benign condition on the dorsal surface of the tongue. It is characterized by a whitish substance that may become yellowish-brown or black by foods and drugs. It is caused by hyperkeratinization and lengthening of the papillae and comprises of food residue, bacteria, blood metabolites, saliva, and desquamated epithelial cells among the papillae (Fig. **12**) [82]. The contributing factors on the coated tongue are oral hygiene, diet, age, oral breathing, drugs, systemic diseases, fever, stress, immunological factors, and an abnormality in salivary flow [83]. Drinking more water and good oral hygiene such as brushing the tongue can improve this condition [79].

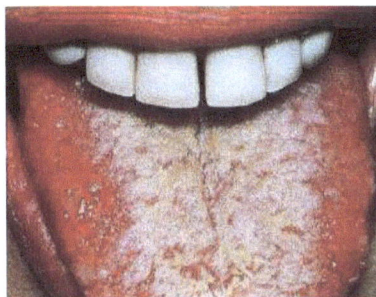

Fig. (12). Coated tongue.

Bifid Tongue

Bifid tongue is a rare congenital condition that occurs during the fetal period. Bifid tongue is characterized by a groove running along the tip of the tongue [84]. It has been presented with some other orofacial anomalies and syndromes, and it is not common solely. Bifid tongue causes speech disorders and swallowing problems, so immediate treatment is significant [85].

INFECTIONS

Primary Herpetic Gingivostomatitis

Primary herpetic gingivostomatitis is the most common clinical manifestation of primary Herpes simplex virus infection and is caused in 90% of cases by HSV-1 [86]. It is usually transmitted by direct contact. The onset of primary herpes gingivostomatitis is abrupt, and it occurs with fever, anterior cervical lymphadenopathy, malaise, vomiting, anorexia, languor, and painful oral lesions [87]. Originally oral lesions are characterized by multiple pinpoint vesicles. These vesicles burst and produce small ulcers with a yellow membrane [88]. The oral lesions may be found on any area of the oral mucosa concluding the tongue, lips, buccal mucosa, and the hard and soft palate [89, 67]. The predisposing factors may be stress, systemic disease, and trauma [87]. The presence of the satellite vesicles around the perioral site is common. If the child puts her finger into the mouse, the herpes virus might be transmitted to any part of the body by touching them. In this case, the mild conditions improve between 7 to 14 days [67]. Primary herpetic gingivostomatitis is mainly self-limited and can be managed by drinking enough water. It is suggested that acyclovir cream is effective, too [87].

Oropharyngeal Candidiasis

Oropharyngeal candidiasis is a prevalent infection that is caused by Candida Albicans [90]. It is highly associated with immunodeficiency. Other predisposing factors are prolonged usage of broad-spectrum antibiotics, reduced saliva, corticosteroid therapy, diabetes mellitus, extreme malnutrition in children, and HIV [91, 92].

Pseudomembranous and Erythematous candidiasis are the most frequent forms of candidiasis in children [93]. Pseudomembranous candidiasis is characterized by creamy-white curded plaques, similar to cottage cheese or curdled milk on the tongue, oral mucosa, oropharynx, mucobuccal folds, and palate. These plaques can be wiped out with dry gauze, leaving an erythematous area [67, 92, 93].

Erythematous candidiasis is more frequent than Pseudomembranous candidiasis. It is characterized by red macules, a burning sensation, and disappearing the filiform papilla. The commonly involved areas are buccal mucosa, the dorsal surface of the tongue, and the hard palate's posterior region [67]. Oropharyngeal candidiasis can cause many problems such as pain, burning tongue, and eating difficulties; it can also affect taste and speech [94].

Secondary Herpetic Ulcer

Reactivation of the herpes simplex virus causes Recurrent Herpetic Infection [95]. The stimulating factors may be emotional stress, menstruation, fever, prolonged exposure to sunlight, and trauma [67, 96]. This condition is also known as Herpes Labialis, cold sore, or fever blister [67]. Vermillion rim and perioral skin are the most prevalent area of relapse [97].

The most affected intraoral areas are the hard palate, dorsal surface of the tongue, and attached gingiva [93]. Prodromal symptoms containing burning, pain, scratching, and tingling appear 24 hours before the herpetic lesions [67, 95]. The lesion is characterized by numerous small papules that develop into a fluid-filled pustule [98]. The pustules burst, and then the crusts are recognized within two days [67]. The healing process takes place within 6 to 10 days [93]. When the finger is affected by a Herpes infection, it is called Herpetic Whitlow. This condition may be caused by thumb sucking or nail biting in a child with orofacial herpes infection [98].

Angular Cheilitis

Angular cheilitis, which is also known as perleche, is an inflammatory condition that appears at one or both corners of the mouth [99, 100]. It is characterized by red and crusty fissuring and ulcers in the commissure region 101,102. Candida Albicans is the most common etiology of angular cheilitis [99]. Some predisposing factors may be iron deficiency, contact allergy, orthodontic treatment, and nutritional deficiencies [99, 100, 102]. It is also associated with Down syndrome [103]. Regularly thumb sucking and licking lips may cause angular cheilitis [104].

Hand-Foot-Mouth Disease

Hand-foot-mouth disease is a viral infection that usually affects children less than ten years old. It is mainly caused by Coxsackievirus A16 and Enterovirus A17 [105].

This contagious disease usually presents a mild self-limited illness and starts with a low-grade fever, malaise, loss of appetite, weakness, sore throat, and vesicles in the mouth. Vesicular rush is found on the hands, feet, tongue, or buttocks [106].

One or two days after the fever begins, the child gets painful mouth sores. These ulcers are usually found on the tongue, buccal mucosa, and palate. Currently, there is no approved vaccination for hand-foot-mouth disease. One of the protective factors for hand-foot-mouth disease is washing hands [107]. Most of the patients get well over a few weeks with complications; however, some serious complications such as persistent stomatitis, aseptic meningitis, encephalitis, Guillain-Barre syndrome, acute flaccid paralysis may occur in a limited number of cases [105, 108].

Periapical Primary Teeth Lesions

Periapical Abscess

Periapical abscess manifests as the collection of bacteria and their productions at the apex of the tooth, which produces pus [109]. A periapical abscess is followed by dental caries, trauma, and unsuccessful root canal therapy [110, 111]. It is characterized by pain, swelling of soft tissue and sensitivity to percussion (Fig. 13) [93]. Systemic appearances may be fever, lymphadenopathy, and trismus [112]. The affected tooth does not react to vitality tests [67]. Treatment includes incision and drainage, root canal therapy or extraction, but the most significant step of the treatment is eliminating the origin of the infection [79, 93].

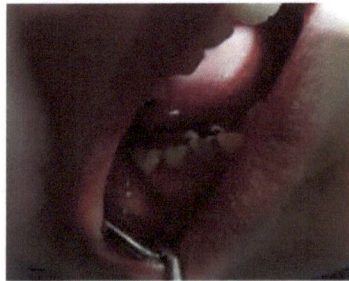

Fig. (13). Periapical abscess of the first and second primary molars of the mandible.

Cellulitis

Cellulitis is an acute and diffuse infection of soft tissue originating from a necrosis tooth and can affect the fascial planes [79, 67, 113]. It manifests as noticeable facial swelling and edema. Redness, warmth, and firmness are the features of swelling [79, 93]. It is more commonly observed in younger children and can be life-threatening. Multiple complications of cellulitis can be observed, such as Ludwig Angina, Cavernous sinus thrombosis, brain abscess, and airway obstruction [114].

When diffuse cellulitis affects the submandibular, sublingual, and submental spaces, it is called Ludwig Angina [79]. The etiology of Ludwig Angina is the infection of mandibular teeth, especially the molars [115]. In this condition, the elevated tongue and the swelling of the floor of the mouth lead to airway obstruction, and it causes dysphagia. Untreated cellulitis in maxillary teeth can affect the eyes and lead to brain abscess and cavernous sinus thrombosis [79].

CONGENITAL DISEASES

Abnormal Tooth Development

Hyperdontia

Hyperdontia is a tooth developmental abnormality and is characterized by any number of extra teeth. The most common supernumerary tooth is called mesiodens, and it is located in the palatal midline between two maxillary central incisors [116]. Hyperdontia is more common in permanent teeth, and the most common site of an extra tooth is located in the maxillary arch (Fig. **14**) [93, 117]. Based on the location, the supernumerary tooth is classified into three groups, including mesiodens, distomolar, and paramolar. Distomolar is referred to as extra fourth molar, and paramolar is referred to as a posterior supernumerary tooth located buccally or lingually to a molar [67]. Hyperdontia is associated with multiple syndromes and abnormalities such as Cleidocranial dysplasia, Gardner's syndrome (Fig. **15**), Incontinentia pigmenti, Ehler-Danlos syndrome, cleft lip/palate [116 - 118]. Some of the dental complications associated with supernumerary teeth are malocclusion, diastema, crowding, eruption failure, delayed tooth eruption, crown resorption, tooth displacement, and cystic lesions [93, 119].

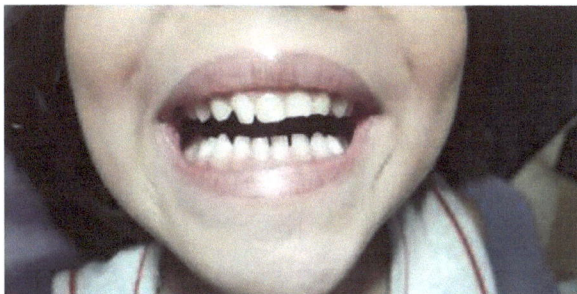

Fig. (14). Hyperdontia in primary dentition.

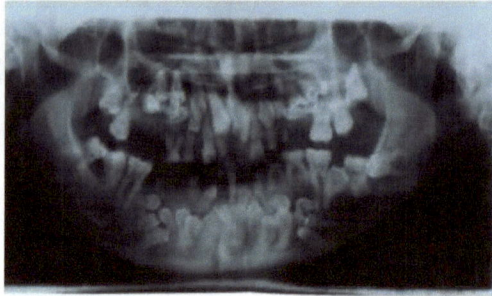

Fig. (15). Gardner's syndrome.

Hypodontia

Hypodontia is referred to congenitally missing teeth other than the third molar [120]. The most frequently missing teeth are permanent second lower premolars, upper lateral incisors, and upper second premolars [121]. When there are six or more absent teeth, it is called oligodontia (Fig. **16A**). ANADONTIA refers to completely absent dentitions [120]. Missing permanent teeth is more common than deciduous teeth (Fig. **16A, C**). This condition is usually non-syndromic, but it can be associated with some syndromes and abnormalities such as Ectodermal dysplasia, Down syndrome, and cleft lip with or without cleft palate [122].

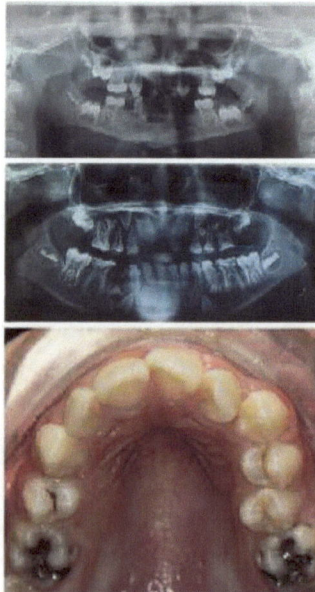

Fig. (16). A) Oligodontia. **B)** Hypodontia. **C)** Missing of left upper second premolar.

Taurodontism

Taurodontism is a morpho-anatomical anomaly, and it is characterized by an elongated pulp chamber, shortening of the roots, and apical shift of bifurcation [123]. It can be seen in both permanent and primary teeth, but more frequently in permanent teeth. The most commonly affected teeth are permanent molars [124].

Dens Invaginatus

Dens invaginatus, which is also known as dens in dente, is a developmental malformation of the tooth and occurs due to the invagination of the enamel into the dental structure [125]. The permanent maxillary laterals are the most prevalently affected teeth. These teeth are presented by a deep groove on the lingual surface of the tooth. This unusual anatomy may enhance the risk of caries, and pulpal and periapical infections [126].

Dens Evaginatus

Dens evaginatus is a developmental dental anomaly characterized by an extra cusp or tubercle containing enamel, dentin, and pulp [127]. The cusp-like prominence is located on the occlusal surface of mandibular premolars and in the cingulum of anterior teeth (Fig. **17**). Due to malocclusion and occlusal force, the tubercle may be fractured, and it is followed by pulp exposure, pulpitis, loss of vitality, and abscess [128].

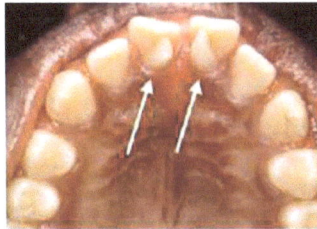

Fig. (17). Dens evaginatus in the cingulum of anterior maxillary incisors.

Amelogenesis Imperfecta

Amelogenesis imperfecta is an inherited developmental disorder with a heterogeneous etiology that affects the enamel [129]. Both dentitions are affected by this condition. Amelogenesis imperfecta has been categorized into four types such as hypoplastic, hypomaturation, hypocalcified, and hypoplastic-hypomaturation. Hypoplastic type is characterized by a lack of enamel quantity, reduced thickness of enamel, and rough and pitted surface [129, 130]. The hypomaturation type presents normal thickness, but mottled opaque in appearance and reduced hardness. In the affected teeth, variable degrees of discoloration and enamel cracking can be observed [129, 131]. The hypocalcified type of Amelogenesis imperfecta is characterized by poorly calcifications of enamel, yellowish-brown discoloration, rapid destruction of the tooth, and opaque appearance [130, 132]. The last type is associated with Taurodontism and is characterized by thin pitted yellow-brown enamel [131] (Fig. **18**).

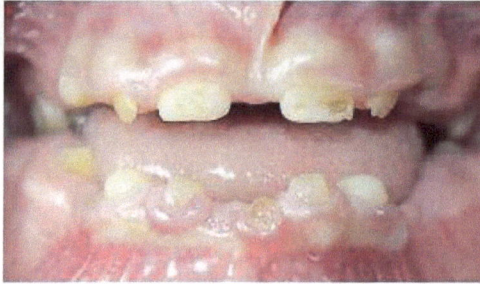

Fig. (18). Amelogenesis imperfecta.

HEMANGIOMA AND LYMPHANGIOMA

Hemangioma, which is also known as infantile hemangioma, is the most common benign vascular tumor of endothelial origin in childhood. It usually occurs in the head and neck region of the children. The most common locations of oral soft tissue hemangiomas are tongue, lips, and buccal mucosa [79]; it presents as single or multiple lesions with variable diameters [133]. Based on depth, it is divided into three groups, including superficial plaque-type, deeper plaque-type, and mixed type [134]. The superficial lesions are bright red, and the deep ones tend to be bluish hue plaque [135]. Based on the extent of involvement, it is classified into three groups, including localized, segmental, and multifocal. Perioral involvement may have some complications such as feeding problems, ulceration, and cosmetic deformations [134]. Most of the hemangioma lesions do not need any treatment, and the treatment of the other ones depends on size, type, location, and complications [135].

Lymphangioma is an uncommon benign congenital tumor of the lymphatic system. The most common site of lymphangioma is the head and neck. Congenital lymphangioma is mainly presented at birth, and 90% of the lesions appear within two years of life [79]. The clinical features are based on the depth of the lesions. The superficial ones have a pebbly surface that looks like a cluster of translucent vesicles and may have the same color as the adjacent mucosa, and they give a frog-egg or tapioca pudding appearance. The deeper lesions are characterized by soft and ill-defined masses [67]. Oral lymphangioma mostly occurs on the anterior two-third part of the dorsal surface of the tongue, lips, and buccal mucosa [67, 136]. Tongue involvement usually causes macroglossia. Head and neck lymphangioma may have some complications such as malocclusion, dysphagia, speech disorders, mastication problems, and respiratory problems [93, 137].

GINGIVAL

Cyst of Newborn

Epstein Pearls

Epstein pearls are frequently detected in newborn infants. They are characterized by small white-yellowish nodules in the mid palatal raphe or beside the junction of the hard and soft palate. They are caused by entrapped keratin during the development of the palate. These keratin-filled cysts are harmless and benign, and they will disappear on their own. No treatment is required, and dentists should comfort parents [138].

Bohn Nodule

Bohn nodule is described as a mucous gland and keratin-filled cyst that occurs along buccal and lingual surfaces of the alveolar ridge and far from the midline of the palate. These small multiple white grayish cysts are self-limited, and they apparently resolve on their own, and no treatment is needed [138, 139].

Gingival Cyst of the Newborn (Dental Lamina Cyst)

Gingival cyst of newborns, known as dental lamina cyst, is a very prevalent lesion in newborns, and it is rarely observed after three months of birth [140]. These cysts present as multiple or solitary, white to small yellowish nodules on the alveolar ridge. These nodules are not usually larger than 2-3 millimeters. These keratin-filled cysts are originated from the rest of the dental lamina. These cysts can be classified into two groups. The ones that are located in midline raphe are named palatal cysts, while those that appear on the crest of alveolar ridges are called alveolar cysts. They are self-limited, and no treatment is needed [139, 141].

CONCLUSION

Oral and dental diseases are among the most common problems in children worldwide. Dental caries, periodontitis and gingivitis, dental malocclusion, dental trauma, and some oral soft tissue lesions are among the most common oral disorders in children. Early diagnosis and management of these conditions by pediatric dentists and pediatricians necessitate being aware of the clinical manifestations of each disease at every age. Implementing preventive intervention, accurate diagnosis, proper treatment, and performing regular follow-ups are among the key factors for eliminating harmful long-life consequences of poor oral and dental health status in children and adolescents.

CONSENT FOR PUBLICATION

Not applicable.

CONFLICT OF INTEREST

The authors declare no conflict of interest, financial or otherwise.

ACKNOWLEDGEMENT

Declared none.

REFERENCES

[1]   Aas JA, Griffen AL, Dardis SR, *et al.* Bacteria of dental caries in primary and permanent teeth in children and young adults. J Clin Microbiol 2008; 46(4): 1407-17.
        [http://dx.doi.org/10.1128/JCM.01410-07] [PMID: 18216213]

[2]   James SL, Abate D, Abate KH, *et al.* Global, regional, and national incidence, prevalence, and years lived with disability for 354 diseases and injuries for 195 countries and territories, 1990-2017: a systematic analysis for the Global Burden of Disease Study 2017. Lancet 2018; 392(10159): 1789-858.
        [http://dx.doi.org/10.1016/S0140-6736(18)32279-7] [PMID: 30496104]

[3]   Bourgeois DM, Llodra JC. Global burden of dental condition among children in nine countries participating in an international oral health promotion programme, 2012-2013. Int Dent J 2014; 64 (Suppl. 2): 27-34.
        [http://dx.doi.org/10.1111/idj.12129] [PMID: 25209648]

[4]   Colak H, Dülgergil CT, Dalli M, Hamidi MM. Early childhood caries update: A review of causes, diagnoses, and treatments. J Nat Sci Biol Med 2013; 4(1): 29-38.
        [http://dx.doi.org/10.4103/0976-9668.107257] [PMID: 23633832]

[5]   Drury TF, Horowitz AM, Ismail AI, Maertens MP, Rozier RG, Selwitz RH. Diagnosing and reporting early childhood caries for research purposes. A report of a workshop sponsored by the National Institute of Dental and Craniofacial Research, the Health Resources and Services Administration, and the Health Care Financing Administration. J Public Health Dent 1999; 59(3): 192-7.
        [http://dx.doi.org/10.1111/j.1752-7325.1999.tb03268.x] [PMID: 10649591]

[6]   Collado V, Pichot H, Delfosse C, Eschevins C, Nicolas E, Hennequin M. Impact of early childhood caries and its treatment under general anesthesia on orofacial function and quality of life : A prospective comparative study. Med Oral Patol Oral Cir Bucal 2017; 22(3): e333-41.
        [http://dx.doi.org/10.4317/medoral.21611] [PMID: 28390125]

[7]   Meyer F, Enax J. Early Childhood Caries: Epidemiology, Aetiology, and Prevention. Int J Dent 2018; 2018: 1415873.
        [http://dx.doi.org/10.1155/2018/1415873] [PMID: 29951094]

[8]   Kirthiga M, Murugan M, Saikia A, Kirubakaran R. Risk Factors for Early Childhood Caries: A Systematic Review and Meta-Analysis of Case Control and Cohort Studies. Pediatr Dent 2019; 41(2): 95-112.
        [PMID: 30992106]

[9]   Seow WK. Early Childhood Caries. Pediatr Clin North Am 2018; 65(5): 941-54.

[http://dx.doi.org/10.1016/j.pcl.2018.05.004] [PMID: 30213355]

[10]   Classification of Periodontal Diseases in Infants. Children, Adolescents, and Individuals with Special Health Care Needs 2019.

[11]   Bimstein E, Huja PE, Ebersole JL. The potential lifespan impact of gingivitis and periodontitis in children. J Clin Pediatr Dent 2013; 38(2): 95-9.
[http://dx.doi.org/10.17796/jcpd.38.2.j525742137780336] [PMID: 24683769]

[12]   Al-Ghutaimel H, Riba H, Al-Kahtani S, Al-Duhaimi S. Common periodontal diseases of children and adolescents. Int J Dent 2014; 2014: 850674.
[http://dx.doi.org/10.1155/2014/850674] [PMID: 25053946]

[13]   Rosier BT, De Jager M, Zaura E, Krom BP. Historical and contemporary hypotheses on the development of oral diseases: are we there yet? Front Cell Infect Microbiol 2014; 4: 92.
[http://dx.doi.org/10.3389/fcimb.2014.00092] [PMID: 25077073]

[14]   Pari A, Ilango P, Subbareddy V, Katamreddy V, Parthasarthy H. Gingival diseases in childhood - a review. J Clin Diagn Res 2014; 8(10): ZE01-4.
[PMID: 25478471]

[15]   Bhatia G, Kumar A, Khatri M, Bansal M, Saxena S. Assessment of the width of attached gingiva using different methods in various age groups: A clinical study. J Indian Soc Periodontol 2015; 19(2): 199-202.
[http://dx.doi.org/10.4103/0972-124X.152106] [PMID: 26015672]

[16]   Chauhan V, Chauhan R, Devkar N, Vibhute A, More S. Gingival and Periodontal Diseases in Children and Adolescents. J Dent Allied Sci 2012; 1(1): 26.
[http://dx.doi.org/10.4103/2277-4696.159114]

[17]   Oh T-J, Eber R, Wang H-L. Periodontal diseases in the child and adolescent. J Clin Periodontol 2002; 29(5): 400-10.
[http://dx.doi.org/10.1034/j.1600-051X.2002.290504.x] [PMID: 12060422]

[18]   Clerehugh V, Tugnait A. Diagnosis and management of periodontal diseases in children and adolescents. Periodontol 2000 2001; 26(1): 146-68.
[http://dx.doi.org/10.1034/j.1600-0757.2001.2260108.x] [PMID: 11452903]

[19]   Lombardo G, Vena F, Negri P, et al. Worldwide prevalence of malocclusion in the different stages of dentition: A systematic review and meta-analysis. Eur J Paediatr Dent 2020; 21(2): 115-22.
[PMID: 32567942]

[20]   CARVALHO CAP de, SALES-PERES A, Magalhães BASTOS JR de, Carvalho SALES-PERES SH de: Epidemiology of malocclusion in children and adolescents: a critic review. RGO -. Rev Gaucha Odontol 2014; 62: 253.

[21]   Zou J, Meng M, Law CS, Rao Y, Zhou X. Common dental diseases in children and malocclusion. Int J Oral Sci 2018; 10(1): 7.
[http://dx.doi.org/10.1038/s41368-018-0012-3] [PMID: 29540669]

[22]   D'Onofrio L. Oral dysfunction as a cause of malocclusion. Orthod Craniofac Res 2019; 22(S1) (Suppl. 1): 43-8.
[http://dx.doi.org/10.1111/ocr.12277] [PMID: 31074141]

[23]   Nayak T, Sahoo S, Nanda S, Pattanaik S, Mohammad N, Panigrahi P. The Basic Genetics of Malocclusion. Indian J Public Health Res Dev 2018; 9(12): 2507.
[http://dx.doi.org/10.5958/0976-5506.2018.02146.0]

[24]   Rodrigues JA, Azevedo CB, Chami VO, Solano MP, Lenzi TL. Sleep bruxism and oral health-related quality of life in children: A systematic review. Int J Paediatr Dent 2020; 30(2): 136-43.
[http://dx.doi.org/10.1111/ipd.12586] [PMID: 31630473]

[25]   Shroff B. Malocclusion as a Cause for Temporomandibular Disorders and Orthodontics as a

Treatment. Oral Maxillofac Surg Clin North Am 2018; 30(3): 299-302.
[http://dx.doi.org/10.1016/j.coms.2018.04.006] [PMID: 29866453]

[26]   English JD, Buschang PH, Throckmorton GS. Does malocclusion affect masticatory performance? Angle Orthod 2002; 72(1): 21-7.
[PMID: 11843269]

[27]   Saccomanno S, Antonini G, D'Alatri L, D'Angelantonio M, Fiorita A, Deli R. Causal relationship between malocclusion and oral muscles dysfunction: a model of approach. Eur J Paediatr Dent 2012; 13(4): 321-3.
[PMID: 23270292]

[28]   Joshi N, Hamdan AM, Fakhouri WD. Skeletal malocclusion: a developmental disorder with a life-long morbidity. J Clin Med Res 2014; 6(6): 399-408.
[http://dx.doi.org/10.14740/jocmr1905w] [PMID: 25247012]

[29]   Dimberg L, Arnrup K, Bondemark L. The impact of malocclusion on the quality of life among children and adolescents: A systematic review of quantitative studies. Eur J Orthod 2014; 37.
[PMID: 25214504]

[30]   Doğramacı EJ, Rossi-Fedele G, Dreyer CW. Malocclusions in young children: Does breast-feeding really reduce the risk? A systematic review and meta-analysis. J Am Dent Assoc 2017; 148(8): 566-574.e6.
[http://dx.doi.org/10.1016/j.adaj.2017.05.018] [PMID: 28754184]

[31]   Jan H, Abuhamda ISB, Assiri A, *et al.* Meta-Analysis of Prevalence of Bad Oral Habits and Relationship with Prevalence of Malocclusion. 2017.

[32]   Gartika M. The effect of oral habits in the oral cavity of children and its treatment. Padjadjaran J Dent 2008; 20(2)
[http://dx.doi.org/10.24198/pjd.vol20no2.14142]

[33]   7:J/ NAR: Prevalence of Thumb Sucking Habit and its Relation to Malocclusion in Preschool Children. In: 2009.

[34]   Singh SP, Utreja A, Chawla HS. Distribution of malocclusion types among thumb suckers seeking orthodontic treatment. J Indian Soc Pedod Prev Dent 2008; 26 (Suppl. 3): S114-7.
[PMID: 19127028]

[35]   Haryett RD, Hansen FC, Davidson PO, Sandilands ML. Chronic thumb-sucking: the psychologic effects and the relative effectiveness of various methods of treatment. Am J Orthod 1967; 53(8): 569-85.
[http://dx.doi.org/10.1016/0002-9416(67)90069-3] [PMID: 4951439]

[36]   Tanaka O, Oliveira W, Galarza M, Aoki V, Bertaiolli B. Breaking the Thumb Sucking Habit: When Compliance Is Essential. Case Rep Dent 2016; 2016: 6010615.
[http://dx.doi.org/10.1155/2016/6010615] [PMID: 26904311]

[37]   Khayami S, Bennani F, Farella M. Fingers in mouths: from cause to management. N Z Dent J 2013; 109(2): 49-50, 52-54.
[PMID: 23767167]

[38]   Joelijanto R. Oral Habits That Cause Malocclusion Problems. Insisiva Dent J 2012; 1

[39]   Sachan A, Chaturvedi TP. Onychophagia (Nail biting), anxiety, and malocclusion. Indian J Dent Res 2012; 23(5): 680-2.
[http://dx.doi.org/10.4103/0970-9290.107399] [PMID: 23422619]

[40]   Castilho SD, Rocha MA. Pacifier habit: history and multidisciplinary view. J Pediatr (Rio J) 2009; 85(6): 480-9.
[PMID: 20016867]

[41]   Lima AA dos SJ, Alves CM, Ribeiro CC, *et al.* Effects of conventional and orthodontic pacifiers on

the dental occlusion of children aged 24-36 months old. Int J Paediatr Dent 2017; 27(2): 108-19.
[http://dx.doi.org/10.1111/ipd.12227] [PMID: 26856705]

[42] Medeiros R, Ximenes M, Massignan C, *et al.* Malocclusion prevention through the usage of an orthodontic pacifier compared to a conventional pacifier: a systematic review. Eur Arch Paediatr Dent 2018; 19(5): 287-95.
[http://dx.doi.org/10.1007/s40368-018-0359-3] [PMID: 30054865]

[43] Caruso S, Nota A, Darvizeh A, Severino M, Gatto R, Tecco S. Poor oral habits and malocclusions after usage of orthodontic pacifiers: an observational study on 3-5 years old children. BMC Pediatr 2019; 19(1): 294.
[http://dx.doi.org/10.1186/s12887-019-1668-3] [PMID: 31438904]

[44] Franco Varas V, Gorritxo Gil B. [Pacifier sucking habit and associated dental changes. Importance of early diagnosis]. An Pediatr (Barc) 2012; 77(6): 374-80.
[http://dx.doi.org/10.1016/j.anpedi.2012.02.020] [PMID: 22608913]

[45] Shahraki N, Yassaei S. GoldaniMoghadam M: Abnormal oral habits: A review. J Dent Oral Hyg 2012; 4: 12.

[46] Thomaz E, Alves C, Silva L, Ribeiro C. Seabra Soares de Britto e Alves M, Hilgert J, Wendland E: Breastfeeding Versus Bottle Feeding on Malocclusion in Children: A Meta-Analysis Study. J Hum Lact 2018; 34: 089033441875568.
[http://dx.doi.org/10.1177/0890334418755689]

[47] Peres KG, Cascaes AM, Nascimento GG, Victora CG. Effect of breastfeeding on malocclusions: a systematic review and meta-analysis. Acta Paediatr 2015; 104(467): 54-61.
[http://dx.doi.org/10.1111/apa.13103] [PMID: 26140303]

[48] Manfredini D, Restrepo C, Diaz-Serrano K, Winocur E, Lobbezoo F. Prevalence of sleep bruxism in children: a systematic review of the literature. J Oral Rehabil 2013; 40(8): 631-42.
[http://dx.doi.org/10.1111/joor.12069] [PMID: 23700983]

[49] de Oliveira Reis L, Ribeiro RA, Martins CC, Devito KL. Association between bruxism and temporomandibular disorders in children: A systematic review and meta-analysis. Int J Paediatr Dent 2019; 29(5): 585-95.
[http://dx.doi.org/10.1111/ipd.12496] [PMID: 30888712]

[50] Gowri sankar S, Chetan kumar: Tongue Thrust Habit - A Review. Ann Essences Dent, 2009.

[51] Singh S, Awasthi N, Gupta T. Mouth Breathing-Its Consequences, Diagnosis & Treatment. Acta Sci Dent Scienecs 2020; 4(5): 32-41.
[http://dx.doi.org/10.31080/ASDS.2020.04.0831]

[52] Grippaudo C, Paolantonio EG, Antonini G, *et al.* Association between oral habits, mouth breathing and malocclusion. Acta Otorhinolaryngol Ital organo Uff della Soc Ital di Otorinolaringol e Chir Cerv-facc 2016; 36: 386.

[53] Martins D, Lima L, Sales V, *et al.* The Mouth Breathing Syndrome: prevalence, causes, consequences and treatments. A Literature Review. J Surg Clin Res 2014; 5(1): 47.
[http://dx.doi.org/10.20398/jscr.v5i1.5560]

[54] Basheer B, Hegde KS, Bhat SS, Umar D, Baroudi K. Influence of mouth breathing on the dentofacial growth of children: a cephalometric study. J Int oral Heal JIOH 2014; 6: 50,

[55] Petti S, Glendor U, Andersson L. World traumatic dental injury prevalence and incidence, a meta-analysis-One billion living people have had traumatic dental injuries. Dent Traumatol 2018; 34(2): 71-86.
[http://dx.doi.org/10.1111/edt.12389] [PMID: 29455471]

[56] Azami-Aghdash S, Ebadifard Azar F, Pournaghi Azar F, *et al.* Prevalence, etiology, and types of dental trauma in children and adolescents: systematic review and meta-analysis. Med J Islam Repub Iran 2015; 29(4): 234.

[PMID: 26793672]

[57]   Tewari N, Bansal K, Mathur VP. Dental Trauma in Children: A Quick Overview on Management. Indian J Pediatr 2019; 86(11): 1043-7.
[http://dx.doi.org/10.1007/s12098-019-02984-7] [PMID: 31197645]

[58]   Andrade M, Americano G, Cruz L, Marsillac M, Campos V: Types of traumatic dental injuries to the primary dentition and the surface against which they occurred. RGO -. Rev Gaucha Odontol 2019; •••: 67.

[59]   Lenzi MM, da Silva Fidalgo TK, Luiz RR, Maia LC. Trauma in primary teeth and its effect on the development of permanent successors: a controlled study. Acta Odontol Scand 2019; 77(1): 76-81.
[http://dx.doi.org/10.1080/00016357.2018.1508741] [PMID: 30345854]

[60]   Flores MT, Onetto JE. How does orofacial trauma in children affect the developing dentition? Long-term treatment and associated complications. Dent Traumatol 2019; 35(6): 312-23.
[http://dx.doi.org/10.1111/edt.12496] [PMID: 31152620]

[61]   Müller DD, Bissinger R, Reymus M, Bücher K, Hickel R, Kühnisch J. Survival and complication analyses of avulsed and replanted permanent teeth. Sci Rep 2020; 10(1): 2841.
[http://dx.doi.org/10.1038/s41598-020-59843-1] [PMID: 32071357]

[62]   ANDRADE MRTC, AMERICANO GCA, CRUZ LR, MARSILLAC M de WS DE, CAMPOS V: Types of traumatic dental injuries to the primary dentition and the surface against which they occurred. RGO -. Rev Gaucha Odontol 2019; •••: 67.

[63]   Zaror C, Martínez-Zapata MJ, Abarca J, *et al.* Impact of traumatic dental injuries on quality of life in preschoolers and schoolchildren: A systematic review and meta-analysis. Community Dent Oral Epidemiol 2018; 46(1): 88-101.
[http://dx.doi.org/10.1111/cdoe.12333] [PMID: 28940434]

[64]   Şen-Tunç E, Açikel H, Sönmez IS, Bayrak Ş, Tüloğlu N. Eruption cysts: A series of 66 cases with clinical features. Med Oral Patol Oral Cir Bucal 2017; 22(2): e228-32.
[http://dx.doi.org/10.4317/medoral.21499] [PMID: 28160586]

[65]   Dhawan P, Kochhar GK, Chachra S, Advani S. Eruption cysts: A series of two cases. Dent Res J (Isfahan) 2012; 9(5): 647-50.
[http://dx.doi.org/10.4103/1735-3327.104889] [PMID: 23559935]

[66]   de Oliveira AJ, Silveira ML, Duarte DA, Diniz MB. Eruption Cyst in the Neonate. Int J Clin Pediatr Dent 2018; 11(1): 58-60.
[http://dx.doi.org/10.5005/jp-journals-10005-1485] [PMID: 29805237]

[67]   Neville B, Damm DD, Allen C, Chi A. Oral and Maxillofacial Pathology. 4th ed., 2015.

[68]   Bodner L, Goldstein J, Sarnat H. Eruption cysts: a clinical report of 24 new cases. J Clin Pediatr Dent 2004; 28(2): 183-6.
[http://dx.doi.org/10.17796/jcpd.28.2.038m4861g8547456] [PMID: 14969381]

[69]   McNamara KK, Kalmar JR. Erythematous and Vascular Oral Mucosal Lesions: A Clinicopathologic Review of Red Entities. Head Neck Pathol 2019; 13(1): 4-15.
[http://dx.doi.org/10.1007/s12105-019-01002-8] [PMID: 30693460]

[70]   Scully C. Erythema migrans.In: Scully C, ed Oral and Maxillofacial Medicine (Third Edition) Third Edit Churchill Livingstone. 2013; pp. 268-70.
[http://dx.doi.org/10.1016/B978-0-7020-4948-4.00041-6]

[71]   Edgar NR, Saleh D, Miller RA. Recurrent Aphthous Stomatitis: A Review. J Clin Aesthet Dermatol 2017; 10(3): 26-36.
[PMID: 28360966]

[72]   Challacombe SJ, Alsahaf S, Tappuni A. Recurrent Aphthous Stomatitis: Towards Evidence-Based Treatment? Curr Oral Health Rep 2015; 2(3): 158-67.

[http://dx.doi.org/10.1007/s40496-015-0054-y]

[73]   Akintoye SO, Greenberg MS. Recurrent aphthous stomatitis. Dent Clin North Am 2014; 58(2): 281-97.
        [http://dx.doi.org/10.1016/j.cden.2013.12.002] [PMID: 24655523]

[74]   Montgomery-Cranny JA, Wallace A, Rogers HJ, Hughes SC, Hegarty AM, Zaitoun H. Management of Recurrent Aphthous Stomatitis in Children. Dent Update 2015; 42(6): 564-566, 569-572.
        [http://dx.doi.org/10.12968/denu.2015.42.6.564] [PMID: 26506812]

[75]   Müller S. Frictional Keratosis, Contact Keratosis and Smokeless Tobacco Keratosis: Features of Reactive White Lesions of the Oral Mucosa. Head Neck Pathol 2019; 13(1): 16-24.
        [http://dx.doi.org/10.1007/s12105-018-0986-3] [PMID: 30671762]

[76]   CASAMASSIMO PS, MCTIGUE DJ, FIELDS HW, NOWAK AJ:. Pediatric Dentistry, Infancy through adolescence 2013.

[77]   Cowan D, Ho B, Sykes KJ, Wei JL. Pediatric oral burns: a ten-year review of patient characteristics, etiologies and treatment outcomes. Int J Pediatr Otorhinolaryngol 2013; 77(8): 1325-8.
        [http://dx.doi.org/10.1016/j.ijporl.2013.05.026] [PMID: 23786788]

[78]   Kang S, Kufta K, Sollecito TP, Panchal N. A treatment algorithm for the management of intraoral burns: A narrative review. Burns 2018; 44(5): 1065-76.
        [http://dx.doi.org/10.1016/j.burns.2017.09.006] [PMID: 29032979]

[79]   McDonald JS. Tumors of the Oral Soft Tissues and Cysts and Tumors of Bone.McDonald and Avery's Dentistry for the Child and Adolescent. 10th ed. St. Louis: Mosby 2016; pp. 603-26.
        [http://dx.doi.org/10.1016/B978-0-323-28745-6.00028-4]

[80]   Dafar A, Çevik-Aras H, Robledo-Sierra J, Mattsson U, Jontell M. Factors associated with geographic tongue and fissured tongue. Acta Odontol Scand 2016; 74(3): 210-6.
        [http://dx.doi.org/10.3109/00016357.2015.1087046] [PMID: 26381370]

[81]   Najafi S, Gholizadeh N, Akhavan Rezayat E, Kharrazifard MJ. Treatment of Symptomatic Geographic Tongue with Triamcinolone Acetonide Alone and in Combination with Retinoic Acid: A Randomized Clinical Trial. J Dent (Tehran) 2016; 13(1): 23-8.
        [PMID: 27536325]

[82]   Funahara M, Yanamoto S, Soutome S, Hayashida S, Umeda M. Clinical observation of tongue coating of perioperative patients: factors related to the number of bacteria on the tongue before and after surgery. BMC Oral Health 2018; 18(1): 223.
        [http://dx.doi.org/10.1186/s12903-018-0689-x] [PMID: 30572861]

[83]   Seerangaiyan K, Jüch F, Winkel EG. Tongue coating: its characteristics and role in intra-oral halitosis and general health-a review. J Breath Res 2018; 12(3): 034001.
        [http://dx.doi.org/10.1088/1752-7163/aaa3a1] [PMID: 29269592]

[84]   Surej KL, Kurien NM, Sivan MP. Isolated congenital bifid tongue. Natl J Maxillofac Surg 2010; 1(2): 187-9.
        [http://dx.doi.org/10.4103/0975-5950.79228] [PMID: 22442597]

[85]   Lee JY, Mohd Zainal H, Mat Zain MA. Bin: Bifid Tongue and Cleft Palate With and Without a Tessier 30 Facial Cleft: Cases of Rare Congenital Anomalies and a Review of Management and Literature. Cleft palate-craniofacial J Off Publ Am Cleft Palate-Craniofacial Assoc 2019; 56:1243

[86]   Goldman RD. Acyclovir for herpetic gingivostomatitis in children. Can Fam Physician 2016; 62(5): 403-4.
        [PMID: 27255621]

[87]   Aslanova M, Ali R, Zito PM. Herpetic Gingivostomatitis. 2020.

[88]   Kolokotronis A, Doumas S. Herpes simplex virus infection, with particular reference to the progression and complications of primary herpetic gingivostomatitis. Clin Microbiol Infect 2006;

12(3): 202-11.
[http://dx.doi.org/10.1111/j.1469-0691.2005.01336.x] [PMID: 16451405]

[89] Arduino PG, Porter SR. Herpes Simplex Virus Type 1 infection: overview on relevant clinico-pathological features. J Oral Pathol Med 2008; 37(2): 107-21.
[http://dx.doi.org/10.1111/j.1600-0714.2007.00586.x] [PMID: 18197856]

[90] Quindós G, Gil-Alonso S, Marcos-Arias C, *et al.* Therapeutic tools for oral candidiasis: Current and new antifungal drugs. Med Oral Patol Oral Cir Bucal 2019; 24(2): e172-80.
[http://dx.doi.org/10.4317/medoral.22978] [PMID: 30818309]

[91] Coronado-Castellote L, Jiménez-Soriano Y. Clinical and microbiological diagnosis of oral candidiasis. J Clin Exp Dent 2013; 5(5): e279-86.
[http://dx.doi.org/10.4317/jced.51242] [PMID: 24455095]

[92] Patil S, Rao RS, Majumdar B, Anil S. Clinical Appearance of Oral Candida Infection and Therapeutic Strategies. Front Microbiol 2015; 6: 1391.
[http://dx.doi.org/10.3389/fmicb.2015.01391] [PMID: 26733948]

[93] Nowak AJ, Mabry TR, Wells MH, Christensen JR, Townsend JA. Pediatric dentistry-e-book: Infancy through adolescence., 2019.

[94] Pankhurst CL. Candidiasis (oropharyngeal). Clin Evid 2013; 2013: 1304.
[PMID: 24209593]

[95] Saleh D, Yarrarapu SNS, Sharma S. 2020.

[96] Shulman JD. Recurrent herpes labialis in US children and youth. Community Dent Oral Epidemiol 2004; 32(6): 402-9.
[http://dx.doi.org/10.1111/j.1600-0528.2004.00157.x] [PMID: 15541155]

[97] Chi C-C. Herpes labialis. BMJ Clin Evid 2015 2015.

[98] Wald A, Corey L. Persistence in the population: epidemiology, transmission.Cambridge 2007.
[http://dx.doi.org/10.1017/CBO9780511545313.037]

[99] Gossman W, Gharbi A, Hafsi W. Cheilitis. Treasure Island, FL: StatPearls Publishing 2019.

[100] Cross D, Eide ML, Kotinas A. The clinical features of angular cheilitis occurring during orthodontic treatment: a multi-centre observational study. J Orthod 2010; 37(2): 80-6.
[http://dx.doi.org/10.1179/14653121042930] [PMID: 20567030]

[101] Cabras M, Gambino A, Broccoletti R, Lodi G, Arduino PG. Treatment of angular cheilitis: A narrative review and authors' clinical experience. Oral Dis 2019.
[PMID: 31464357]

[102] Oza N, Doshi JJ. Angular cheilitis: A clinical and microbial study. Indian J Dent Res Off Publ Indian Soc Dent Res 2017; 28(6): 661-5.
[http://dx.doi.org/10.4103/ijdr.IJDR_668_16] [PMID: 29256466]

[103] Al-Maweri SA, Tarakji B, Al-Sufyani GA, Al-Shamiri HM, Gazal G. Lip and oral lesions in children with Down syndrome. A controlled study. J Clin Exp Dent 2015; 7(2): e284-8.
[http://dx.doi.org/10.4317/jced.52283] [PMID: 26155347]

[104] Sharon V, Fazel N. Oral candidiasis and angular cheilitis. Dermatol Ther 2010; 23(3): 230-42.
[http://dx.doi.org/10.1111/j.1529-8019.2010.01320.x] [PMID: 20597942]

[105] Guerra AM, Waseem M. Hand foot and mouth disease 2017.

[106] Kua JA, Pang J. The epidemiological risk factors of hand, foot, mouth disease among children in Singapore: A retrospective case-control study. PLoS One 2020; 15(8): e0236711.
[http://dx.doi.org/10.1371/journal.pone.0236711] [PMID: 32780749]

[107] Nassef C, Ziemer C, Morrell DS. Hand-foot-and-mouth disease: a new look at a classic viral rash. Curr Opin Pediatr 2015; 27(4): 486-91.

[http://dx.doi.org/10.1097/MOP.0000000000000246] [PMID: 26087425]

[108] Cai K, Wang Y, Guo Z, *et al.* Clinical characteristics and managements of severe hand, foot and mouth disease caused by enterovirus A71 and coxsackievirus A16 in Shanghai, China. BMC Infect Dis 2019; 19(1): 285.
[http://dx.doi.org/10.1186/s12879-019-3878-6] [PMID: 30917800]

[109] Zhang W, Chen Y, Shi Q, Hou B, Yang Q. Identification of bacteria associated with periapical abscesses of primary teeth by sequence analysis of 16S rDNA clone libraries. Microb Pathog 2020; 141: 103954.
[http://dx.doi.org/10.1016/j.micpath.2019.103954] [PMID: 31891793]

[110] Erazo D, Whetstone DR. Dental Infections. StatPearls 2020. [Internet]

[111] Shweta , Prakash SK. Dental abscess: A microbiological review. Dent Res J (Isfahan) 2013; 10(5): 585-91.
[PMID: 24348613]

[112] Siqueira JFJ Jr, Rôças IN. Microbiology and treatment of acute apical abscesses. Clin Microbiol Rev 2013; 26(2): 255-73.
[http://dx.doi.org/10.1128/CMR.00082-12] [PMID: 23554416]

[113] Ritwik P, Fallahi S, Yu Q. Management of facial cellulitis of odontogenic origin in a paediatric hospital. Int J Paediatr Dent 2020; 30(4): 483-8.
[http://dx.doi.org/10.1111/ipd.12613] [PMID: 31894605]

[114] Bali RK, Sharma P, Gaba S, Kaur A, Ghanghas P. A review of complications of odontogenic infections. Natl J Maxillofac Surg 2015; 6(2): 136-43.
[http://dx.doi.org/10.4103/0975-5950.183867] [PMID: 27390486]

[115] An J, Madeo J, Singhal M. Ludwig Angina. Treasure Island, FL: StatPearls Publishing 2019.

[116] Subasioglu A, Savas S, Kucukyilmaz E, Kesim S, Yagci A, Dundar M. Genetic background of supernumerary teeth. Eur J Dent 2015; 9(1): 153-8.
[http://dx.doi.org/10.4103/1305-7456.149670] [PMID: 25713500]

[117] Alhashimi N, Al Jawad FHA, Al Sheeb M, Al Emadi B, Al-Abdulla J, Al Yafei H. The prevalence and distribution of nonsyndromic hyperdontia in a group of Qatari orthodontic and pediatric patients. Eur J Dent 2016; 10(3): 392-6.
[http://dx.doi.org/10.4103/1305-7456.184162] [PMID: 27403060]

[118] Bello S, Olatunbosun W, Adeoye J, Adebayo A, Ikimi N. Prevalence and presentation of hyperdontia in a non-syndromic, mixed Nigerian population. J Clin Exp Dent 2019; 11(10): e930-6.
[http://dx.doi.org/10.4317/jced.55767] [PMID: 31636863]

[119] Amini F, Rakhshan V, Jamalzadeh S. Prevalence and Pattern of Accessory Teeth (Hyperdontia) in Permanent Dentition of Iranian Orthodontic Patients. Iran J Public Health 2013; 42(11): 1259-65.
[PMID: 26171338]

[120] Al Jawad FHA, Al Yafei H, Al Sheeb M, Al Emadi B, Al Hashimi N. Hypodontia prevalence and distribution pattern in a group of Qatari orthodontic and pediatric patients: A retrospective study. Eur J Dent 2015; 9(2): 267-71.
[http://dx.doi.org/10.4103/1305-7456.156850] [PMID: 26038662]

[121] Williams MA, Letra A. The Changing Landscape in the Genetic Etiology of Human Tooth Agenesis. Genes (Basel) 2018; 9(5): 9.
[http://dx.doi.org/10.3390/genes9050255] [PMID: 29772684]

[122] Al-Ani AH, Antoun JS, Thomson WM, Merriman TR, Farella M. Hypodontia: An Update on Its Etiology, Classification, and Clinical Management. BioMed Res Int 2017; 2017: 9378325.
[http://dx.doi.org/10.1155/2017/9378325] [PMID: 28401166]

[123] Dineshshankar J, Sivakumar M, Balasubramanium AM, Kesavan G, Karthikeyan M, Prasad VS.

Taurodontism. J Pharm Bioallied Sci 2014; 6(5) (Suppl. 1): S13-5.
[http://dx.doi.org/10.4103/0975-7406.137252] [PMID: 25210354]

[124] Jafarzadeh H, Azarpazhooh A, Mayhall JT. Taurodontism: a review of the condition and endodontic treatment challenges. Int Endod J 2008; 41(5): 375-88.
[http://dx.doi.org/10.1111/j.1365-2591.2008.01388.x] [PMID: 18363703]

[125] Gallacher A, Ali R, Bhakta S. Dens invaginatus: diagnosis and management strategies. Br Dent J 2016; 221(7): 383-7.
[http://dx.doi.org/10.1038/sj.bdj.2016.724] [PMID: 27713460]

[126] Zhu J, Wang X, Fang Y, Von den Hoff JW, Meng L. An update on the diagnosis and treatment of dens invaginatus. Aust Dent J 2017; 62(3): 261-75.
[http://dx.doi.org/10.1111/adj.12513] [PMID: 28306163]

[127] Levitan ME, Himel VT. Dens evaginatus: literature review, pathophysiology, and comprehensive treatment regimen. J Endod 2006; 32(1): 1-9.
[http://dx.doi.org/10.1016/j.joen.2005.10.009] [PMID: 16410059]

[128] Chen J-W, Huang GT-J, Bakland LK. Dens evaginatus: Current treatment options. J Am Dent Assoc 2020; 151(5): 358-67.
[http://dx.doi.org/10.1016/j.adaj.2020.01.015] [PMID: 32209245]

[129] Ohrvik H, Hjortsjo C. Retrospective study of patients with amelogenesis imperfecta treated with different bonded restoration techniques. Clin Exp Dent Res 2019; 6

[130] Gadhia K, McDonald S, Arkutu N, Malik K. Amelogenesis imperfecta: an introduction. Br Dent J 2012; 212(8): 377-9.
[http://dx.doi.org/10.1038/sj.bdj.2012.314] [PMID: 22538897]

[131] Sabandal MMI, Schäfer E. Amelogenesis imperfecta: review of diagnostic findings and treatment concepts. Odontology 2016; 104(3): 245-56.
[http://dx.doi.org/10.1007/s10266-016-0266-1] [PMID: 27550338]

[132] Shivhare P, Shankarnarayan L, Gupta A, Sushma P. Amelogenesis Imperfecta: A Review. J Adv Oral Res 2016; 7(1): 1-6.
[http://dx.doi.org/10.1177/2229411220160101]

[133] Smith CJF, Friedlander SF, Guma M, Kavanaugh A, Chambers CD. Infantile Hemangiomas: An Updated Review on Risk Factors, Pathogenesis, and Treatment. Birth Defects Res 2017; 109(11): 809-15.
[http://dx.doi.org/10.1002/bdr2.1023] [PMID: 28402073]

[134] Abraham A, Job AM, Roga G. Approach to Infantile Hemangiomas. Indian J Dermatol 2016; 61(2): 181-6.
[http://dx.doi.org/10.4103/0019-5154.177755] [PMID: 27057018]

[135] George A, Mani V, Noufal A. Update on the classification of hemangioma. J Oral Maxillofac Pathol 2014; 18(4) (Suppl. 1): S117-20.
[http://dx.doi.org/10.4103/0973-029X.141321] [PMID: 25364160]

[136] Kolay SK, Parwani R, Wanjari S, Singhal P. Oral lymphangiomas - clinical and histopathological relations: An immunohistochemically analyzed case series of varied clinical presentations. J Oral Maxillofac Pathol 2018; 22(4) (Suppl. 1): S108-11.
[http://dx.doi.org/10.4103/jomfp.JOMFP_157_17] [PMID: 29491618]

[137] Nelson BL, Bischoff EL, Nathan A, Ma L. Lymphangioma of the Dorsal Tongue. Head Neck Pathol 2020; 14(2): 512-5.
[http://dx.doi.org/10.1007/s12105-019-01108-z] [PMID: 31823215]

[138] Ortiz LED, de , Mendez MD. Epstein Pearls 2018.

[139] Patil S, Rao RS, Majumdar B, Jafer M, Maralingannavar M, Sukumaran A. Oral Lesions in Neonates.

Int J Clin Pediatr Dent 2016; 9(2): 131-8.
[http://dx.doi.org/10.5005/jp-journals-10005-1349] [PMID: 27365934]

[140] Donley CL, Nelson LP. Comparison of palatal and alveolar cysts of the newborn in premature and full-term infants. Pediatr Dent 2000; 22(4): 321-4.
[PMID: 10969441]

[141] Moda A. Gingival Cyst of Newborn. Int J Clin Pediatr Dent 2011; 4(1): 83-4.
[http://dx.doi.org/10.5005/jp-journals-10005-1087] [PMID: 27616865]

CHAPTER 4

Updates on Pediatric Metabolic Syndrome

Caroline Brand[1], **Cézane P. Reuter**[1] and **Roya Kelishadi**[2,3,*]

[1] *Graduate Program in Health Promotion - University of Santa Cruz do Sul, Santa Cruz do Sul, Rio Grande do Sul, Brazil*

[2] *Child Growth and Development Research Center, Research Institute for Primordial Prevention of Non-Communicable Disease, Isfahan University of Medical Sciences, Isfahan, Iran*

[3] *USERN Office, Research Institute for Primordial Prevention of Non-Communicable Disease, Isfahan University of Medical Sciences, Isfahan, Iran*

Abstract: Metabolic Syndrome (MetS) is considered as the presence of clustering metabolic risk factors. It is rapidly increasing in children and adolescents, notably in low- and middle-income countries. It results from a complex interaction of lifestyle, environmental, and genetic factors. Although its universal definition needs to be determined in the pediatric age group, the main components are obesity, dyslipidemia in terms of elevated triglycerides, and elevated blood pressure. Respectively, fatness and fitness have a direct and inverse association with the development of MetS. Various metabolic responses that are involved in the adipose tissue promote a link between obesity, insulin resistance, inflammation, and future atherogenesis. Management of pediatric MetS would need multidisciplinary interventions, including a multicomponent approach, consisting of healthy eating, reducing screen time, increasing physical activity, as well as providing appropriate duration and quality of sleep. Limiting the exposure of pregnant mothers as well as children and adolescents with endocrine disrupting chemicals is beneficial for preventing the development of MetS. Lifestyle modification and family-centered interventions are the first-line approaches in the treatment of MetS, and the use of medication should be considered only for those who fail to reach healthy weight after lifestyle intervention and for those with underlying disease and complications. Prevention and early management of pediatric MetS are of main strategies for primordial/primary prevention of non communicable diseases.

Keywords: Children and adolescents, Environment, Epigenetics, Lifestyle, Metabolic syndrome, Prevention.

* **Corresponding author Roya Kelishadi:** Child Growth and Development Research Center, Research Institute for Primordial Prevention of Non-Communicable Disease, Isfahan University of Medical Sciences, Isfahan, Iran and USERN Office, Research Institute for Primordial Prevention of Non- Communicable Disease, Isfahan University of Medical Sciences, Isfahan, Iran; Tel: +983136691216, 37923321; E-mail: kelishadi@med.mui.ac.ir

INTRODUCTION

Metabolic Syndrome (MetS) is characterized as clustering of cardiometabolic risk factors. Although there is no uniform agreement regarding the diagnostic criteria for MetS among children and adolescents, most of the available definitions agree that hypertension, glucose intolerance, central obesity, and dyslipidemia should be included as the main components [1, 2]. In this context, obesity plays a central role, as it represents the main risk for developing metabolic alterations [3].

The prevalence of MetS has increased in the paediatric population in recent years as a result of improper lifestyle habits along with the development of early risk factors [4, 5]. Healthy behaviors, such as regular physical activity practice, healthy diet, adequate sleep patterns, as well as an active routine must be incorporated at an early age, once they are closely related to the development of metabolic complications [6, 7]. In addition, prenatal and postnatal environmental factors, including birth weight, obesity during pregnancy, gestational diabetes, as well as breastfeeding duration, have been considered relevant aspects for the onset of obesity and MetS [8 - 10].

Pediatric MetS is a predictor of this condition in adulthood [11], highlighting the need for the early management of this disease. As the first-line approach, the treatment includes interventions to promote adequate nutrition and physical activity practice, in which multicomponent interventions are the most effective [12, 13]. If this strategy does not result in beneficial effects, pharmacological treatment can be incorporated [14].

Therefore, MetS is a complex disorder that develops at an early age, necessitating the implementation of public health policies to prevent and treat it.Taking these aspects into consideration, this chapter aims to approach the factors associated with MetS development, prevention, and treatment in the pediatric age group.

DEFINITION AND PREVALENCE

MetS is recognized as an important health risk in children and adolescents [15]. It is characterized by a clustering of metabolic abnormalities that result in increased risk for the development of chronic diseases, mainly cardiovascular disease and type II diabetes [16]. In the pediatric age group, studies are proposing a set of different criteria to define MetS, and although there is no consensus among them, the diagnosis criteria agree that some essential components are present, such as glucose intolerance, central obesity, hypertension, and dyslipidemia [1, 17, 18].

In the absence of definitive definitions, adult criteria have been adapted to be applied in the field of pediatrics, and one of the most commonly used is the one proposed by the International Diabetes Federation (IDF) [1]. According to this group, the parameter required for the MetS diagnosis is the presence of three or more of the following criteria: waist circumference $\geq 90^{th}$ percentile, systolic blood pressure ≥ 130 mmHg; diastolic blood pressure ≥ 85 mmHg; triglycerides ≥ 1.69 mmol/L; high-density lipoprotein cholesterol (HDL-C) ≤ 1.03 mmol/L; fasting glucose ≥ 5.55 mmol/L. Another widely used definition is the one adapted from the Adult Treatment Panel III (ATP III) [2], in which MetS is defined by the presence of three or more of the following components: waist circumference $\geq 90^{th}$ percentile for age and gender; elevated systolic and/or diastolic blood pressure $\geq 90^{th}$ percentile for age, sex, and height; triglycerides ≥ 1.24 mmol/L; HDL ≤ 1.03 mmol/L; impaired fasting glucose ≥ 5.6 mmol/L. Although these definitions included the same components, they considered different cut-points for elevated blood pressure and hypertriglyceridemia. Also, the IDF criteria are suitable only for children 10 years or older, while the ATP III can be used for children below the age of 10 years.

There are important limitations attributed to these traditional criteria. Using a binary classification, it is only possible to determine the presence or the absence of the risk factor, which can lead to a lack of durability in the classification, mainly considering the individuals near the limit of individual cut-offs. The instability in the categorical diagnosis of MetS has been shown in studies developed with children and adolescents [19, 20]. Another limitation concerns the disregard of the influence of sex and ethnicity [21].

To overcome these barriers, it has been suggested that the components of MetS should be considered as continuous variables [22, 23]. Thus, several studies have proposed a continuous score to represent the clustering of MetS components, which is justified by the notion that this approach could be less error susceptible compared to the dichotomic one [24]. Additionally, it would provide full information on the health status and is more reliable in predicting young adult cardiovascular risk from childhood [25].

In addition to the traditional elements, some researchers have proposed that other components should be included in MetS diagnosis. According to Andersen *et al.* (2015), the inclusion of cardiorespiratory fitness and leptin could improve the diagnostic criteria. Furthermore, the consideration of non-alcoholic fatty liver disease, hyperuricemia, leptin/adiponectin ratio, and sleep disturbances have also been argued once are related to risks for metabolic impairment [15, 26].

The lack of a universal definition and the different characteristics between populations result in the varying MetS prevalence. A study developed with Chinese schoolchildren compared two definitions and showed that the prevalence of MetS for children older than ten years was 14.3% in the obese group and 3.7% in the overweight group according to the IDF definition. According to the modified ATP-III definition, the prevalence of MetS was 32.3% in obese and 8.4% in overweight children. Considering both definitions, central obesity was the most common component of MetS [26].

In a general sample of Canadian children and adolescents, the prevalence of MetS was 2.1%, although 37.7% presented at least one risk factor, and the most prevalent was abdominal obesity (21.6%) (this study considered the IDF definition) [27]. In the USA, considering the ATP II definition, this prevalence was higher. 4.2% of adolescents were affected and 28.7% of overweight adolescents were presented with the syndrome [28]. Around 18% of Brazilian adolescents with overweight and obesity were diagnosed with MetS [29].

Although there is high heterogeneity in the prevalence among studies, it is established that overweight and obese children are more affected by the syndrome, placing obesity as a central element for the development of MetS.

RISK FACTORS FOR METS: THE CENTRAL ROLE OF OBESITY

Obesity plays a crucial role in the development of MetS, especially because it is associated with endothelial dysfunction directly (production of pro-inflammatory adipokines and high levels of free fatty acids) and indirectly (mechanisms involved in insulin resistance) [30].

Thus, the different criteria for the diagnosis of MetS include obesity, using body mass index (BMI) or waist circumference (WC) to classify this condition [31]. However, most criteria consider WC for diagnosing MetS, and only the IDF criterion (2007) [1] considers central obesity as a mandatory component. In fact, obesity has been identified to play acentral role in the grouping of metabolic risk factors [26, 32], suggesting that this is the initial change in the etiological cascade that culminates in MetS [33].

Therefore, considering obesity as one of the central roles in the development of MetS, it is necessary to further investigate the metabolic mechanisms involved in adipose tissue, especially white adipose tissue, which is not only energy storage but also an important endocrine organ. In this sense, it is important to identify the mechanisms involved in white adipose tissue for a better understanding of aspects related to obesity and metabolic changes [34].

Fig. (1) illustrates a summary of the main metabolic responses resulting from increased body adiposity. It is observed that elevated BMI promotes increased secretion of several proteins (leptin and resistin, for instance) by adipocytes, in addition to pro-inflammatory cytokines (tumor necrosis factor-alpha (TNF-α) and interleukins). There is also an important immune response, with the action of macrophages and lymphocytes [35]. Thus, these metabolic responses involved in adipose tissue would promote a link between obesity, insulin resistance, inflammation, and atherogenesis [36].

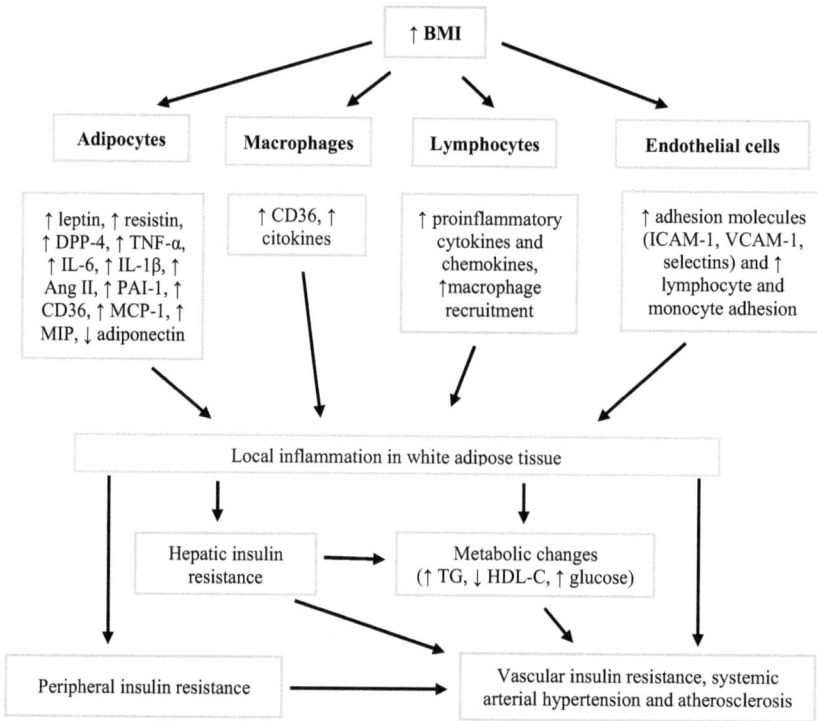

Fig. (1). Adapted from Gómez-Hernández *et al* . (2016).
BMI: body mass index; DPP-4: dipeptidyl peptidase-4; TNF-α: tumor necrosis factor- α; IL: interleukin; Ang: angiotensin; PAI-1: plasminogen activator inhibitor-1; CD36: differentiation cluster (glycoprotein IV); MCP-1: monocyte chemoattractant protein 1; MIP: macrophage inflammatory protein; ICAM-1: intercellular adhesion molecule 1; VCAM-1: vascular cell adhesion molecule 1; TG: triglycerides; HDL-c: high density lipoprotein cholesterol
Role of increased body mass index over white adipose tissue and metabolic responses.

On the other hand, the immune response induced by obesity is complex and involves not only the adipose tissue but also multiple organs, which increases the difficulty in understanding the precise mechanisms of MetS development. Therefore, knowing that various systems and organs are affected by obesity, prevention, control, and treatment strategies for this condition are important in maintaining metabolic health [37].

THE INFLUENCE OF LIFESTYLE AND EARLY RISK FACTORS

Lifestyle factors, including physical activity practice, healthy eating, limiting screen time, and healthy sleep habits, are considered primary goals for the prevention and treatment of MetS [4].Fig. (2) presents a summary of these items. Scientific recommendations emphasize that it is essential to increase physical activity and decrease total calorie intake in obese children and adolescents [38]. The World Health Organization suggests that to achieve benefits for health, children and adolescents should perform a minimum of 60 minutes of moderate to vigorous physical activity every day, along with activities that maintain or improve endurance and muscular strength at least three times a week [39].

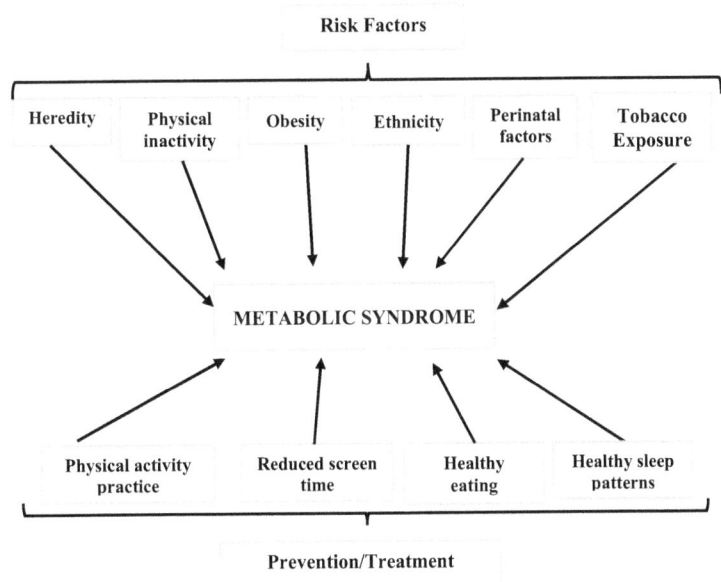

Fig. (2). Variables related to prevention/treatment and risk factors of metabolic syndrome.

Studies have investigated the association between MetS or its components with physical activity and physical fitness in children and adolescents. The literature suggests an inverse association between moderate to vigorous physical activity with a clustered metabolic syndrome risk factors, being that physical fitness (cardiorespiratory and muscular fitness) intervene in this relationship [40]. Moreover, the composition of different daily behaviors, such as sedentary time, light, moderate, and vigorous physical activity, was associated with different cardiometabolic biomarkers, including HDL-C, diastolic blood pressure, and waist circumference in American children and adolescents [6]. Nevertheless, approximately 80% of the pediatric population does not comply with the physical activity recommendation [41], leading to a worrying scenario.

Sleep patterns have been recognized as risk factors for MetS [42]. The National Sleep Foundation indicates that sufficient sleep is considered for children who sleep 9 to 11h and 8 to 10h for adolescents [43]. Following this guideline, a study developed with children and adolescents from Bogotá (Colombia), found that recommended sleep duration was associated with decreased fasting glucose levels, while poor sleep quality was related to lower HDL-C and higher triglyceride levels [7]. In agreement Cruz *et al.*, (2018) showed a worse cardiometabolic profile in children who sleep less than 9 hours 15 minutes.

Other lifestyle behaviors, such as active commuting, screen time and eating habits, have been shown to play a role in MetS. Cycling to school was associated with a lower incidence of MetS than passive transport, which was observed mainly in girls [44]. Additionally, Brazilian adolescents who spent ≥6 h/day in front of screens had an increased risk for MetS; however, this association was observed only for the ones who reported consumption of snacks in front of screens, indicating that both behaviors should be avoided to prevent metabolic complications [45].

In addition to the determining role of lifestyle, prenatal and postnatal environmental factors have been considered relevant aspects for developing obesity and Mets [46]. These aspects are related to the concept of developmental origins of health and disease, also known as fetal programming, which refers to the long-term control of tissue physiology and homeostasis, that is affected by the environment before birth or in the first years of life [47]. Such adaptive responses may lead to several diseases in adult life [10]. With the increasing prevalence of obesity and MetS among children and adolescents in the last years, the interest among the perinatal factors that are associated has increased, including birth weight, obesity during pregnancy, gestational diabetes, and breastfeeding duration [5, 8, 48].

Low birth weight is a relevant condition for health in pediatrics and adulthood. It is usually associated with high-calorie diets, which leading to adipose tissue deposition in the abdominal region and obesity, promoting the development of

MetS [49]. A study carried out with overweight/obese children and adolescents indicated that low birth weight and high-calorie diets were related to a higher probability of MetS [5]. Otherwise, high birth weight is also related to metabolic complications, as higher levels of glucose, triglycerides and abdominal obesity, as well as low concentrations of HDL-C in adolescents [46].

A recent systematic review investigated the association between being breastfed and the development of MetS in children and adolescents. Of 11 studies included, 7 found a protective association between breastfeeding and MetS and 4 found no association [9]. The role of breastfeeding duration was investigated in another study and data indicated an inverse associated with hypertriglyceridemia, low HDL-C and MetS [46].

The influence of maternal obesity, in both pre-pregnancy and during pregnancy, has also been addressed. It seems that children and adolescents whose mothers were overweight or obese during pregnancy were more susceptible to MetS development [50]. Furthermore, it is suggested that maternal pre-delivery BMI of 27.16 kg/m^2 could be the cut-off for predicting offspring overweight/obesity at the age of 2 years. Thus, for the mothers with a BMI lower of the cut-off, the chance of their children 's not presenting overweight/obesity will be approximately 95% [8]. Pre-pregnancy overweight/obesity also represents a risk factor for offspring insulin resistance, excess adiposity, and cardiometabolic disease risk [51].

Gestational diabetes mellitus is defined as a glucose tolerance disorder developed during pregnancy, leading to raised feto-maternal morbidity and complications in mother and child [52]. One of these complications is MetS, which seems to manifest in children and adolescent offsprings of a mother with gestational diabetes [48, 53].

Taken together, this evidence highlights the need to consider MetS as a complex disorder related to many lifestyle aspects of children and adolescents, as well as perinatal factors. There is a need for multicomponent intervention, promoting physical activity practice, decreasing sedentary behavior, and encouraging healthy eating. Beyond that, normal weight status and healthy nutrition before and during pregnancy should be kept to prevent health issues in the pediatric population.

MANAGEMENT OF PEDIATRIC METS

The treatment of MetS, as well as its single components, includes non-pharmacological and pharmacological management. The non-pharmacological treatment consists of lifestyle modifications, which include healthy eating, regular physical activity practice, avoiding sedentary behavior, and adopting healthy sleep habits. This should be the first-line approach and then, if necessary, include pharmacological therapy [14].

Regular physical activity is an important strategy in treating obesity-related complications, including MetS. The magnitude of benefits may vary according to the characteristics of the exercise, including type, intensity, and duration. To achieve improvements on anthropometric and body composition indicators, such as BMI and fat mass, as well as cardiometabolic parameters (triglycerides, insulin, and glucose), it has been suggested that the physical exercise intervention be developed from four to twelve weeks, three times a week, with 60 minutes duration, each session [54]. Also, activities of moderate to vigorous intensity must be performed as they are inversely associated with the risk score of Mets in adolescents [55].

There are different guidelines concerning the recommendations of physical activity for health, but all of them place a strong emphasis on moderate to vigorous physical activity. The American Academy of Pediatrics and the World Health Organization recommend a minimum of 60 minutesof moderate to vigorous physical activity every day, incorporating vigorous physical activity at least three times a week [39, 56]. The Endocrine Society clinical guideline is more conservative, indicating that a minimum of 20 minutes of moderate to vigorous physical activity, along with a reduction of inactivity and a calorie-controlled diet, would positively affect metabolic health [57]. Concerning nutrition guidelines, the main approach for dietary changes in the pediatric population is increasing vegetable and fruit consumption and reducing sugar intake and saturated food, as suggested by the World Health Organization [58].

Therefore, adopting regular physical activity and healthy eating habits are essential for the treatment of MetS. Furthermore, the prevention and treatment of obesity and metabolic disorders is complex and requires a multicomponent approach, involving the family and working on social and individual aspects [12, 59]. In this context, the role of parents is crucial since it allows actions on multiple factors that affect health, encouraging, for example, the consumption of fruits and vegetables and limiting the consumption of sweets and processed foods, imposing rules that reduce the screen time and providing support for physical activity practice [60].

A systematic review of randomized clinical trials indicated that multidisciplinary interventions, including a combination of physical exercise and dietary interventions, indicated important changes in body composition in patients with metabolic syndrome [13]. Also, a multicomponent approach, consisting of exercise sessions, nutritional education sessions, and parental support, effectively decreased metabolic parameters in overweight/obese children [61].

There is a common agreement that lifestyle intervention is the first-line approach in the treatment of MetS in children and adolescents, and medication should be used only for those who failed to reach healthy weight after the lifestyle intervention and those with underlying diseases and those with complications. Thus, the treatment of pediatric MetS is composed of the management of disease-specific components, which includes pharmacologic treatment and bariatric surgery in the case of severe obesity [14, 62].

It is noteworthy to mention that exposure to environmental pollutants, mainly endocrine disruptor chemicals, is considered an underlying factor for developing insulin resistance, obesity, and MetS [63 - 65]. These associations might explain, at least in part, the reason for the development of MetS and its components in normal-weight individuals.

A multicomponent intervention, including physical activity, nutrition, and parental involvement, along with a multidisciplinary team composed of pediatricians, nutritionists and mental health practitioners, seem to achieve better results in the treatment of pediatric MetS.

CONCLUSION

Pediatric MetS, although well described in the literature, still does not have a universal definition. Knowing that several metabolic conditions are already present at this stage of life, a better discussion about this topic is necessary, from diagnosis to prevention, control and treatment strategies, to avoid possible health problems, either early or adult life. The establishment of healthy lifestyle habits, as well as early diagnosis and control of the MetS risk factors, are essential for the prevention and management of this complex disorder, and in turn, for primordial prevention of non-communicable diseases.

CONSENT FOR PUBLICATION

Not Applicable.

CONFLICT OF INTEREST

The authors declare no conflict of interest, financial or otherwise.

ACKNOWLEDGEMENT

Declared none.

REFERENCES

[1]   Zimmet P, Alberti KG, Kaufman F, *et al.* The metabolic syndrome in children and adolescents - an IDF consensus report. Pediatr Diabetes 2007; 8(5): 299-306.
[http://dx.doi.org/10.1111/j.1399-5448.2007.00271.x] [PMID: 17850473]

[2]   Executive Summary of The Third Report of The National Cholesterol Education Program (NCEP) Expert Panel on Detection, Evaluation, And Treatment of High Blood Cholesterol In Adults (Adult Treatment Panel III). JAMA 2001; 285(19): 2486-97.
[http://dx.doi.org/10.1001/jama.285.19.2486] [PMID: 11368702]

[3]   Ortega FB, Lavie CJ, Blair SN. Obesity and cardiovascular disease. Circ Res 2016; 118(11): 1752-70.
[http://dx.doi.org/10.1161/CIRCRESAHA.115.306883] [PMID: 27230640]

[4]   Wang LX, Gurka MJ, Deboer MD. Metabolic syndrome severity and lifestyle factors among adolescents. Minerva Pediatr 2018; 70(5): 467-75.
[http://dx.doi.org/10.23736/S0026-4946.18.05290-8] [PMID: 29968453]

[5]   Velazquez-Bautista M, López-Sandoval JJ, González-Hita M, Vázquez-Valls E, Cabrera-Valencia IZ, Torres-Mendoza BM. Association of metabolic syndrome with low birth weight, intake of high-calorie diets and acanthosis nigricans in children and adolescents with overweight and obesity. Endocrinol Diabetes Nutr 2017; 64(1): 11-7.
[http://dx.doi.org/10.1016/j.endinu.2016.09.004] [PMID: 28440765]

[6]   Carson V, Tremblay MS, Chaput JP, McGregor D, Chastin S. Compositional analyses of the associations between sedentary time, different intensities of physical activity, and cardiometabolic biomarkers among children and youth from the United States. PLoS One 2019; 14(7): e0220009.
[http://dx.doi.org/10.1371/journal.pone.0220009] [PMID: 31329609]

[7]   Pulido-Arjona L, Correa-Bautista JE, Agostinis-Sobrinho C, *et al.* Role of sleep duration and sleep-related problems in the metabolic syndrome among children and adolescents. Ital J Pediatr 2018; 44(1): 9.
[http://dx.doi.org/10.1186/s13052-018-0451-7] [PMID: 29334985]

[8]   Liu HK, Wu CY, Yang YN, *et al.* Association between maternal pre-delivery body mass index and offspring overweight/obesity at 1 and 2 years of age among residents of a suburb in Taiwan. PeerJ 2019; 7(2): e6473.
[http://dx.doi.org/10.7717/peerj.6473] [PMID: 30828490]

[9]   Wisnieski L, Kerver J, Holzman C, Todem D, Margerison-Zilko C. Breastfeeding and Risk of Metabolic Syndrome in Children and Adolescents: A Systematic Review. J Hum Lact 2018; 34(3): 515-25.
[http://dx.doi.org/10.1177/0890334417737038] [PMID: 29100483]

[10]   de Gusmão Correia ML, Volpato AM, Águila MB, Mandarim-de-Lacerda CA. Developmental origins of health and disease: experimental and human evidence of fetal programming for metabolic syndrome. J Hum Hypertens 2012; 26(7): 405-19.
[http://dx.doi.org/10.1038/jhh.2011.61] [PMID: 21697895]

[11]   Morrison JA, Friedman LA, Wang P, Glueck CJ. Metabolic syndrome in childhood predicts adult metabolic syndrome and type 2 diabetes mellitus 25 to 30 years later. J Pediatr 2008; 152(2): 201-6.
[http://dx.doi.org/10.1016/j.jpeds.2007.09.010] [PMID: 18206689]

[12]   Elvsaas IKØ, Giske L, Fure B, Juvet LK. Multicomponent Lifestyle Interventions for Treating Overweight and Obesity in Children and Adolescents: A Systematic Review and Meta-Analyses. J Obes 2017; 2017: 5021902.
[http://dx.doi.org/10.1155/2017/5021902] [PMID: 29391949]

[13]   Albert Pérez E, Mateu Olivares V, Martínez-Espinosa RM, Molina Vila MD, Reig García-Galbis M. New insights about how to make an intervention in children and adolescents with metabolic syndrome: Diet, exercise *vs.* changes in body composition. A systematic review of RCT. Nutrients 2018; 10(7): 878.

[http://dx.doi.org/10.3390/nu10070878] [PMID: 29986479]

[14] Fornari E, Maffeis C. Treatment of Metabolic Syndrome in Children. Front Endocrinol (Lausanne) 2019; 10: 702.
[http://dx.doi.org/10.3389/fendo.2019.00702] [PMID: 31681173]

[15] Bussler S, Penke M, Flemming G, *et al.* Novel Insights in the Metabolic Syndrome in Childhood and Adolescence. Horm Res Paediatr 2017; 88(3-4): 181-93.
[http://dx.doi.org/10.1159/000479510] [PMID: 28848168]

[16] DeBoer MD, Betancourt TS. Assessing and Managing the Metabolic Syndrome in Children and Adolescents. Nutrients 2019; 11(8): 673-80.
[http://dx.doi.org/10.3390/nu11081788] [PMID: 31382417]

[17] de Ferranti SD, Gauvreau K, Ludwig DS, Neufeld EJ, Newburger JW, Rifai N. Prevalence of the metabolic syndrome in American adolescents: findings from the Third National Health and Nutrition Examination Survey. Circulation 2004; 110(16): 2494-7.
[http://dx.doi.org/10.1161/01.CIR.0000145117.40114.C7] [PMID: 15477412]

[18] Weiss R, Dziura J, Burgert TS, *et al.* Obesity and the metabolic syndrome in children and adolescents. N Engl J Med 2004; 350(23): 2362-74.
[http://dx.doi.org/10.1056/NEJMoa031049] [PMID: 15175438]

[19] Goodman E, Daniels SR, Meigs JB, Dolan LM. Instability in the diagnosis of metabolic syndrome in adolescents. Circulation 2007; 115(17): 2316-22.
[http://dx.doi.org/10.1161/CIRCULATIONAHA.106.669994] [PMID: 17420347]

[20] Gustafson JK, Yanoff LB, Easter BD, *et al.* The stability of metabolic syndrome in children and adolescents. J Clin Endocrinol Metab 2009; 94(12): 4828-34.
[http://dx.doi.org/10.1210/jc.2008-2665] [PMID: 19837941]

[21] Deboer MD. Underdiagnosis of Metabolic Syndrome in Non-Hispanic Black Adolescents: A Call for Ethnic-Specific Criteria. Curr Cardiovasc Risk Rep 2010; 4(4): 302-10.
[http://dx.doi.org/10.1007/s12170-010-0104-x] [PMID: 21379366]

[22] Eisenmann JC. On the use of a continuous metabolic syndrome score in pediatric research. Cardiovasc Diabetol 2008; 7(17): 17.
[http://dx.doi.org/10.1186/1475-2840-7-17] [PMID: 18534019]

[23] Andersen LB, Lauersen JB, Brønd JC, Anderssen SA, Sardinha LB, Steene-Johannessen J, *et al.* A new approach to define and diagnose cardiometabolic disorder in children. J Diabetes Res 2015; (Cvd):

[24] Magge SN, Goodman E, Armstrong SC, *et al.* The Metabolic Syndrome in Children and Adolescents: Shifting the Focus to Cardiometabolic Risk Factor Clustering. Pediatrics 2017; 140(2): e20171603.
[http://dx.doi.org/10.1542/peds.2017-1603] [PMID: 28739653]

[25] Kelly AS, Steinberger J, Jacobs DR Jr, Hong CP, Moran A, Sinaiko AR. Predicting cardiovascular risk in young adulthood from the metabolic syndrome, its component risk factors, and a cluster score in childhood. Int J Pediatr Obes 2011; 6(2-2): e283-9.
[http://dx.doi.org/10.3109/17477166.2010.528765] [PMID: 21070100]

[26] Wang Q, Yin J, Xu L, *et al.* Prevalence of metabolic syndrome in a cohort of Chinese schoolchildren: comparison of two definitions and assessment of adipokines as components by factor analysis. BMC Public Health 2013; 13(1): 249.
[http://dx.doi.org/10.1186/1471-2458-13-249] [PMID: 23514611]

[27] MacPherson M, de Groh M, Loukine L, Prud'homme D, Dubois L. Prevalence of metabolic syndrome and its risk factors in Canadian children and adolescents: Canadian Health Measures Survey Cycle 1 (2007-2009) and Cycle 2 (2009-2011). Health Promot Chronic Dis Prev Can 2016; 36(2): 32-40.
[http://dx.doi.org/10.24095/hpcdp.36.2.03] [PMID: 26878492]

[28] Cook S, Weitzman M, Auinger P, Nguyen M, Dietz WH. Prevalence of a metabolic syndrome

phenotype in adolescents: findings from the third National Health and Nutrition Examination Survey, 1988-1994. Arch Pediatr Adolesc Med 2003; 157(8): 821-7.
[http://dx.doi.org/10.1001/archpedi.157.8.821] [PMID: 12912790]

[29]   Rizzo ACB, Goldberg TBL, Silva CC, Kurokawa CS, Nunes HRC, Corrente JE. Metabolic syndrome risk factors in overweight, obese, and extremely obese Brazilian adolescents. Nutr J 2013; 12(19): 19.
[http://dx.doi.org/10.1186/1475-2891-12-19] [PMID: 23363783]

[30]   Prieto D, Contreras C, Sánchez A. Endothelial dysfunction, obesity and insulin resistance. Curr Vasc Pharmacol 2014; 12(3): 412-26.
[http://dx.doi.org/10.2174/15701611112666140423221008] [PMID: 24846231]

[31]   Brambilla P, Lissau I, Flodmark CE, *et al.* Metabolic risk-factor clustering estimation in children: to draw a line across pediatric metabolic syndrome. Int J Obes 2007; 31(4): 591-600.
[http://dx.doi.org/10.1038/sj.ijo.0803581] [PMID: 17384660]

[32]   Wang D, Wang CL. [Orthogonal factor analysis of metabolic syndrome components in children and adolescents in the Xiaoshan District of Hangzhou, China]. Zhongguo Dang Dai Er Ke Za Zhi 2014; 16(6): 634-7.
[PMID: 24927442]

[33]   Alberti KGMM, Zimmet P, Shaw J. The metabolic syndrome--a new worldwide definition. Lancet 2005; 366(9491): 1059-62.
[http://dx.doi.org/10.1016/S0140-6736(05)67402-8] [PMID: 16182882]

[34]   Luo L, Liu M. Adipose tissue in control of metabolism. J Endocrinol 2016; 231(3): R77-99.
[http://dx.doi.org/10.1530/JOE-16-0211] [PMID: 27935822]

[35]   Gómez-Hernández A, Beneit N, Díaz-Castroverde S, Escribano Ó. Differential Role of Adipose Tissues in Obesity and Related Metabolic and Vascular Complications. Int J Endocrinol 2016; 2016: 1216783.
[http://dx.doi.org/10.1155/2016/1216783] [PMID: 27766104]

[36]   Zafar U, Khaliq S, Ahmad HU, Manzoor S, Lone KP. Metabolic syndrome: an update on diagnostic criteria, pathogenesis, and genetic links. Hormones (Athens) 2018; 17(3): 299-313.
[http://dx.doi.org/10.1007/s42000-018-0051-3] [PMID: 30171523]

[37]   Saltiel AR, Olefsky JM. Inflammatory linking obesity and metabolic disease and metabolic disease. J Clin Invest 2017; 127(1): 1-4.
[http://dx.doi.org/10.1172/JCI92035] [PMID: 28045402]

[38]   Lee L, Sanders RA. Metabolic syndrome. Pediatr Rev 2012; 33(10): 459-66.
[http://dx.doi.org/10.1542/pir.33.10.459] [PMID: 23027600]

[39]   World Health Organization W. Geneva: Global Recommendations on Physical Activity for Health 2010.

[40]   Segura-Jiménez V, Parrilla-Moreno F, Fernández-Santos JR, *et al.* Physical fitness as a mediator between objectively measured physical activity and clustered metabolic syndrome in children and adolescents: The UP&DOWN study. Nutr Metab Cardiovasc Dis 2016; 26(11): 1011-9.
[http://dx.doi.org/10.1016/j.numecd.2016.07.001] [PMID: 27519284]

[41]   Hallal PC, Andersen LB, Bull FC, Guthold R, Haskell W, Ekelund U. Global physical activity levels: surveillance progress, pitfalls, and prospects. Lancet 2012; 380(9838): 247-57.
[http://dx.doi.org/10.1016/S0140-6736(12)60646-1] [PMID: 22818937]

[42]   Koren D, Dumin M, Gozal D. Role of sleep quality in the metabolic syndrome. 2016; 281-310.

[43]   National Sleep Foundation. National Sleep Foundation Recommends New Sleep Durations. 2016. Available online at https://sleepfoundation.org/press- release/national-sleep-foundation-recomme-ds-new-sleep-times

[44]   Ramírez-Vélez R, García-Hermoso A, Agostinis-Sobrinho C, *et al.* Cycling to School and Body

Composition, Physical Fitness, and Metabolic Syndrome in Children and Adolescents. J Pediatr 2017; 188: 57-63.
[http://dx.doi.org/10.1016/j.jpeds.2017.05.065] [PMID: 28651798]

[45]   Schaan CW, Cureau FV, Salvo D, Kohl HW III, Schaan BD. Unhealthy snack intake modifies the association between screen-based sedentary time and metabolic syndrome in Brazilian adolescents. Int J Behav Nutr Phys Act 2019; 16(1): 115.
[http://dx.doi.org/10.1186/s12966-019-0880-8] [PMID: 31775773]

[46]   Wang J, Perona JS, Schmidt-RioValle J, Chen Y, Jing J, González-Jiménez E. Metabolic syndrome and its associated early-life factors among chinese and spanish adolescents: A pilot study. Nutrients 2019; 11(7): 10-5.
[http://dx.doi.org/10.3390/nu11071568] [PMID: 31336790]

[47]   Langley-Evans SC. Developmental programming of health and disease. Proc Nutr Soc 2006; 65(1): 97-105.
[http://dx.doi.org/10.1079/PNS2005478] [PMID: 16441949]

[48]   Vääräsmäki M, Pouta A, Elliot P, *et al.* Adolescent manifestations of metabolic syndrome among children born to women with gestational diabetes in a general-population birth cohort. Am J Epidemiol 2009; 169(10): 1209-15.
[http://dx.doi.org/10.1093/aje/kwp020] [PMID: 19363101]

[49]   Begum G, Davies A, Stevens A, *et al.* Maternal undernutrition programs tissue-specific epigenetic changes in the glucocorticoid receptor in adult offspring. Endocrinology 2013; 154(12): 4560-9.
[http://dx.doi.org/10.1210/en.2013-1693] [PMID: 24064364]

[50]   González-Jiménez E, Montero-Alonso MA, Schmidt-RioValle J, García-García CJ, Padez C. Metabolic syndrome in Spanish adolescents and its association with birth weight, breastfeeding duration, maternal smoking, and maternal obesity: a cross-sectional study. Eur J Nutr 2015; 54(4): 589-97.
[http://dx.doi.org/10.1007/s00394-014-0740-x] [PMID: 25052543]

[51]   Shannalee R. Martinez, Maresha S. Gay and LZ. Mother's Pre-pregnancy BMI is an Important Determinant of Adverse Cardiometabolic Risk in Childhood. Physiol Behav 2016; 176(1): 139-48.

[52]   Kautzky-Willer A, Harreiter J, Winhofer-Stöckl Y, *et al.* [Gestational diabetes mellitus (Update 2019)]. Wien Klin Wochenschr 2019; 131(S1) (Suppl. 1): 91-102.
[http://dx.doi.org/10.1007/s00508-018-1419-8] [PMID: 30980150]

[53]   Boney CM, Verma A, Tucker R, Vohr BR. Metabolic syndrome in childhood: association with birth weight, maternal obesity, and gestational diabetes mellitus. Pediatrics 2005; 115(3): e290-6.
[http://dx.doi.org/10.1542/peds.2004-1808] [PMID: 15741354]

[54]   García-Hermoso A, Ramírez-Vélez R, Saavedra JM. Exercise, health outcomes, and pædiatric obesity: A systematic review of meta-analyses. J Sci Med Sport 2019; 22(1): 76-84.
[http://dx.doi.org/10.1016/j.jsams.2018.07.006] [PMID: 30054135]

[55]   Stabelini Neto A, de Campos W, Dos Santos GC, Mazzardo Junior O. Metabolic syndrome risk score and time expended in moderate to vigorous physical activity in adolescents. BMC Pediatr 2014; 14(1): 42.
[http://dx.doi.org/10.1186/1471-2431-14-42] [PMID: 24529305]

[56]   De Jesus JM. Expert panel on integrated guidelines for cardiovascular health and risk reduction in children and adolescents: Summary report. Pediatrics 2011; 128(SUPP.5)

[57]   Styne DM, Arslanian SA, Connor EL, *et al.* Pediatric obesity-assessment, treatment, and prevention: An endocrine society clinical practice guideline. J Clin Endocrinol Metab 2017; 102(3): 709-57.
[http://dx.doi.org/10.1210/jc.2016-2573] [PMID: 28359099]

[58]   World Health Organization. Interim Report of the Commission on Ending Childhood Obesity. World Heal Organ 2015; pp. 1-30.

[59]   Ranucci C, Pippi R, Buratta L, *et al.* Effects of an intensive lifestyle intervention to treat overweight/obese children and adolescents. BioMed Res Int 2017; 2017: 8573725.
[http://dx.doi.org/10.1155/2017/8573725] [PMID: 28656151]

[60]   Pyper E, Harrington D, Manson H. The impact of different types of parental support behaviours on child physical activity, healthy eating, and screen time: a cross-sectional study. BMC Public Health 2016; 16(1): 568.
[http://dx.doi.org/10.1186/s12889-016-3245-0] [PMID: 27554089]

[61]   Brand C, Lima RA, Silva TF, *et al.* Effect of a multicomponent intervention in components of metabolic syndrome: a study with overweight/obese low-income school-aged children. Sport Sci Health 2019; 16(1): 137-45.
[http://dx.doi.org/10.1007/s11332-019-00590-w]

[62]   Al-Hamad D, Raman V. Metabolic syndrome in children and adolescents. Transl Pediatr 2017; 6(4): 397-407.
[http://dx.doi.org/10.21037/tp.2017.10.02] [PMID: 29184820]

[63]   Papalou O, Kandaraki EA, Papadakis G, Diamanti-Kandarakis E, Papalou O, *et al.* Endocrine Disrupting Chemicals: An Occult Mediator of Metabolic Disease. Front Endocrinol (Lausanne) 2019; 10: 112.
[http://dx.doi.org/10.3389/fendo.2019.00112] [PMID: 30881345]

[64]   Kelishadi R, Mirghaffari N, Poursafa P, Gidding SS, Kelishadi R, *et al.* Lifestyle and environmental factors associated with inflammation, oxidative stress and insulin resistance in children. Atherosclerosis 2009; 203(1): 311-9.
[http://dx.doi.org/10.1016/j.atherosclerosis.2008.06.022] [PMID: 18692848]

[65]   Poursafa P, Dadvand P, Amin MM, *et al.* Association of polycyclic aromatic hydrocarbons with cardiometabolic risk factors and obesity in children. Environ Int 2018; 118: 203-10.
[http://dx.doi.org/10.1016/j.envint.2018.05.048] [PMID: 29886236]

CHAPTER 5

Updates on Pediatric Epilepsy Syndromes

Ahmed Nugud[1,*], Alaa Nugud[2], Assmaa Nugud[3] and **Shomous Nugud[4]**

[1] *Al Jalila Children's Specialty Hospital, Dubai, UAE*

[2] *Latifa Women's and Children's Hospital, Dubai Health Authority, Dubai, UAE*

[3] *Ras Al Khaimah Medical and Health Sciences University, Ras Al Khaimah, UAE*

[4] *University of Sharjah, Sharjah, UAE*

Abstract: This chapter examines the basics of pediatric epilepsy syndromes and the new factors in the field that lead to and result from the disturbed function. Some disorders such as febrile seizures and idiopathic seizure disorders are fairly common in children, and pediatricians should be familiar with the approaches used to investigate such disorders. However, others, such as rare genetic diseases, are increasing in incidence due to the recent advances in genetic testing and personalized medicine. Nevertheless, epilepsy syndromes carry significant morbidity and even mortality in children. The advent of new genetic discoveries has also brought forth new lines of management for previously refractory diseases. The truly intractable epilepsy syndromes might be managed with surgery as a final resort.

Keywords: Absence seizures, Aura, Childhood epilepsy, Developmental delay, Dravet syndrome, Electrolyte disturbance, Encephalitis, Epilepsy neurosurgery, Febrile seizures, Generalized seizures, Genetic epilepsy, Metabolic epilepsy, Movement disorders, Non-epileptic seizures, Neurological evaluation, Partial seizures, Seizures syndromes, Seizures investigations, Seizures management, Status epilepticus.

INTRODUCTION

Diagnosing seizures is a challenge and should be considered with diligence, as in most cases, it confers a lifelong treatment and, in some cultures, is considered a stigma. A thorough and detailed medical history is paramount for the diagnosis of seizures and is the first step towards a detailed neurological assessment. Thus, history is the first step towards diagnosing pediatric movement disorders along

* **Corresponding author Ahmed A. Nugud:** Department of medical affairs, Al Jalila Children's Specialty Hospital, PO Box 7662, Dubai, UAE; Tel: +971509973764; E-mail: a7md13@gmail.com

Nima Rezaei and Noosha Samieefar (Eds.)

with physical examination that guides the clinicians towards a diagnostic approach and eventually the formulation of a management plan.

The history should provide a chronological timeline to the chief complaint, focusing on signs and symptoms associated with the suspected seizure, duration of the episode, any possible post-seizure symptoms, events leading to the episode, and any alleviating or aggravating elements. Whenever possible, clinicians should seek video recording of alleged episodes to further look into the condition, as even a short film would carry more information for the trained eyes than a lengthy description by a parent or a caregiver [1].

An integral part of the complete history of newly onset seizures is a review of systems, specifically looking for; 1) history of other symptoms that might be misattributed to other systems (*e.g.*, vomiting, fatigue, aura), 2) systemic illness that might lead to central nervous system manifestations (*e.g.*, lupus, metabolic diseases, mitochondrial disorders), 3) Possible infectious etiologies (*e.g.*, rheumatic fever, respiratory infections, urinary tract infections), 4) possible toxins exposure/poisoning (*e.g.*, lead exposure, pesticide exposure, neuropsychiatric medications ingestion). Auras can present in different formats, including 1) visual (color changes, flashing lights, seeing floaters and visual hallucinations), 2) tactile, 3) auditory, 4) olfactory, 5) others (*e.g.*, déjà vu, vestibular changes)

Detailed birth history must be obtained; this will further elucidate any risk of perinatal acquired conditions. This part starts with history prior to conception and follows till the end of the neonatal period. Clinicians should ask specifically about common pregnancy-related complications, including 1) adequate supplements intake during pregnancy, 2) perinatal follow up (and whether any concerns were raised about pregnancy-induced hypertension, preeclampsia, gestational diabetes, and infections), 3) gestational age at delivery and mode of delivery, 4) admission to neonatal intensive care and the reasons (if any), 5) quantify drug intake during pregnancy (including alcohol, prescription and illicit drugs, smoking, and any herbal remedies usage during pregnancy), 6) nature of fetal movement during pregnancy, 7) birth parameters (weight, length, and head circumference) should be noted, 8) if the patient had developed neonatal jaundice (in such case the clinician should inquire about the highest recorded level of bilirubin and mode of treatment), and 9) newborn screening results can also provide clues to neurological manifestations of metabolic disease. Obtaining medical records of patients might provide further insight into past medical history and possible etiologies for newly onset seizures [2].

A developmental history is an important tool in the diagnostic approach to newly onset seizures, especially if there are concerns about delay in acquiring skills or, more ominously, if a patient has lost skills. The knowledge about the range of time to skill acquisition and mastery are indispensable tools to correct diagnosis of newly onset seizures. Table **1** summarizes developmental milestones for the first 2 years.

Table 1. Expected developmental milestones and age of acquisition in the first two years of life.

Age	Gross Motor	Fine Motor	Speech / Language	Cognitive / Problem Solving	Social / Emotional
Newborn	Primitive reflexes – steps, place, Moro, Babinski, ATNR, Flexor posture	Primitive reflexes – grasp	Primitive reflexes – root, suck Alerts to sound Startles to loud sounds Variable cries	Visual focal length – 10 degrees Fix and follow slow horizontal arc Prefers contrast, colours, face Prefers high pitched voice	Bonding (parent -> child) Self-regulation/soothing
2 months	Head steady when held Head up 45 degrees prone	Hands open half of the time Bats at objects	Turns to voice Cooing	Prefers usual caregiver Attends to moderate novelty Follows past midline	Attachment (child -> parent) Social smile
4 months	Sits with support Head up 90 degrees prone, arms out Rolls front -> back	Palmar grasp Reaches and obtains items Brings object to the midline	Laugh, razz, "ga", squeal	Anticipates routines Purposeful sensory exploration of objects (eyes, hands, mouths)	Turn-taking conversations Explores parent's face
6 months	Postural reflexes Sits tripod Rolls both ways	Raking grasp Transfers hand to hand	Babbles (nonspecific)	Stranger anxiety Looks for dropped or partially hidden object	Expresses emotions: happy, sad, mad Memory lasts – 24 hours

(Table 1) cont.....

Age	Gross Motor	Fine Motor	Speech / Language	Cognitive / Problem Solving	Social / Emotional
9 months	Gets from all 4s -> sitting Sits well with hands free Pulls to stand Creeps on hands and knees	Inferior pincer grasp Pokes at objects	"Mama", "dada" (specific) Gestures "bye bye", "up" Gestures games ("pattycake")	Object permanence Uncover toy "peek-a-boo"	Separation anxiety
12 months	Walks a few steps Wide-based gait	Fine pincer(fingertips) Voluntary release throws objects Finger-feeds self cheerios	1 word with meaning (besides mama, dada) Inhibits with "no!" Responds to own name 1-step command with gesture	Cause and effect Trial and error Imitates gestures and sounds Uses objects functionally, *e.g.* rolls toy car	Explore from a secure base Points at wanted items Narrative memory begins
15 months	Walks well	Uses spoon, opens top cup Tower of 2 blocks	Points to 1 body part 1-step command no gesture 5 words Jargoning	Looks for moved hidden object if saw it being moved Experiments with toys to make them work	Shared attention: points at interesting items to show to a parent Brings toys to parent
18 months	Stoops and recovers Run	Carries toys while walking Removes clothing Tower of 4 blocks Scribbles fisted pencil grasp	Points to object, 3 body parts 10-25 words Embedded jargoning Labels familiar objects	Imitates housework Symbolic play with doll or bear, *e.g.* "Give teddy a drink"	Increased independence Parallel play
2 years	Jumps on two feet Up and down stair "marking time"	Handedness established Uses fork Tower of 6 blocks Imitates vertical stroke	Follows 2-step command 50+ words, 50% intelligible 2 word phrases "1", "me", "you", plurals	New problem-solving strategies without rehearsal Searches for hidden object after multiple displacements	Testing limits, tantrums Negativism ("no!") Possessive ("mine!")

In addition, questions about the general well-being of the child, sleep patterns, and level of activity should be asked. Also, family history should be sought, including; 1) history of central nervous system (CNS) pathologies, 2) history of consanguinity, and 3) genetic or metabolic abnormalities identified in either the maternal or paternal side of the family.

Once a detailed history is obtained, a general examination, as well as a focused neurological physical examination, should be obtained. The general exam should, as in history, look for systemic causes that might affect the CNS and Dysmorphic features of possible underlying genetic disorders. The overall general status of the child might give an indication of the child overall health status and might guide the clinician's physical examination. On the other hand, some specific signs might indicate a systemic disorder leading to movement disorders. For example, hepatosplenomegaly might indicate an underlying neurometabolic issue or a heart murmur that could be a sign of congenital heart disease or rheumatic fever. Table 2 summarizes cranial nerves examination.

Table 2. Cranial nerves examination with important maneuvers and findings.

Cranial Nerve	Component	Main Action	Examination Command	Normal	Abnormal
CN I. Olfactory	Smell- sensory	Smell in each nostril	*Use a common odour *One nostril then the other.	*Recognizes odour	Cannot recognize odour.
CN II. Optic	Vision- sensory	Afferent pupillary function, funduscopic examination, visual acuity, visual fields and structural eye movement.	*V. acuity - Eye chart	*20/20 or 6/6 vision	*Decreased.
			*V. field – confrontation	*Full field	*Field defect
			*V. reflexes (2-3) & accommodation reflex	*Reactive to light	*Fixed to light Stimulus
			*Colour vision	Normal vision for red blue and green in Ishihara's Test	Distorted vision to the wavelength / colour Blindness
			*Fundoscopy		

(Table 2) cont.....

Cranial Nerve	Component	Main Action	Examination Command	Normal	Abnormal
CN III oculomotor, IV trochlear & VI abducens	Ocular gaze and Posture - Motor	Smooth pursuit and saccadic eye, nystagmus, efferent pupillary function, and eyelid opening.	*Following finger/object	*Single image,	*Diplopia
			*Smooth pursuit	*Conjugate eye movements	*Disconjugate eye movements Nystagmus
CN V Trigeminal	Facial sensation-mixed	Jaw jerk, facial sensation, afferent corneal reflex, and muscles of mastication,	*Touch & Pain V1, V2, V3	*Normal sensations	Decreased or Absent sensation.
			*Muscles of Mastication	*Normal & Symmetrical	Asymmetrical
			*Corneal Reflex (5-7)	Present	Absent
			*Jaw Jerk	Present,	Exaggerated
CN VII Facial	Facial expression - Motor	Efferent corneal reflex, facial expression, eyelid closure, nasolabial folds, and power bulk	Facial Expression: Ask the patient to -To look up -To frown -To close eyes tightly -To smile -To blow -To Whistle	Symmetrical	Asymmetrical
CN VIII Vestibulocochlear	Acoustic(Hearing)- Sensory	Nystagmus, speech discrimination, Weber's test and Rinne's test	*Whisper in each ear.	Equal sound	*Unequal sound
			*Rinne's and Weber Tests.	Positive	*Negative
CN IX Glossopharyngeal / X Vagus	Voice control and swallowing – Mixed	Afferent and efferent gag reflex and uvula position	Inspect Palate & Uvula	Symmetric	Asymmetric
			Test together	GAG response.	No GAG response.
			Gag Reflex (9-10) Voice, Cough & Swallowing	Normal voice	Husky voice, recent change
CN XI	Spinal accessory (neck rotation & shoulder elevation)- Mixed	Power and bulk of sternocleidomastoid and Trapezii muscles.	Turn chin against resistance to check. STCLM & shoulder shrugging for Trapezius	Equal motor Power in both Sternocleido-Mastoids and Trapezii	Unequal power In these muscles.

Cranial Nerve	Component	Main Action	Examination Command	Normal	Abnormal
CN XIII Hypoglossal	Tongue – Motor	Position, bulk and fasciculation of tongue	Inspect tongue whilst inside mouth	Central and strong.	Wasting, Fasciculation
			Protrude tongue. "Tongue-in-Cheek" test	Strong.	Deviates to one side. Weak.

DIAGNOSTIC PROCEDURES

Lumbar Puncture

Cerebrospinal fluid (CSF) assessment *via* lumbar puncture can present an invaluable amount of information and is considered an integral part of basic workup in newly onset seizures, especially if associated with fever. Opening pressure is obtained that can help in diagnosing idiopathic intracranial hypertension. CSF is the cornerstone in the diagnosis of meningitis and encephalitis. It also has an important role in the diagnosis of other etiologies, including 1) demyelinating disorders, 2) collagen vascular disease, and 3) autoimmune encephalopathies.

The clinical utility of CSF examination in the initial evaluation of a newly onset non-febrile illness is of low yield unless a high index of suspicion on an autoimmune or an infectious etiology. Multiple reports have identified elevated protein and lactate levels in CSF postictal in patients with first unprovoked seizures. The elevated protein levels were hypothesized to be epileptogenic as it was correlated with blood-brain barrier disruption and possibly a marker for inflammation [3].

Electroencephalogram

The normal electroencephalogram (EEG) waves are categorized based on frequency to 1) β (13-20 Hz), 2) α waves (8-12 Hz), 3) θ (4-7 Hz), and 4) δ (1-3 Hz). Abnormalities in electroencephalogram can be generally categorized into two broad categories; 1) slowing and 2) epileptiform discharges. The disruption leads to background brain activity interruption; this can be focal, multifocal, or generalized in origin. There are many factors that might predispose a person to develop epileptiform electrical activity, such as photo-stimulation, sleep deprivation, and hyperventilation. Focal discharges are usually associated with an underlying structural abnormality. In contrast, diffuse discharge is associated with encephalopathies, intoxication and metabolic disorders.

Radiological Investigations

Table **3** highlights the important radiological investigations and its utility for different central nerves system pathologies.

Table 3. Important radiological investigations and their utility in different CNS pathologies.

Disease	Radiological Investigation	For Which Patient	Findings
Ischemic infarction or transit ischemic attack	Magnetic resonance imaging (MRI) or MRA for head and neck with or without gadolinium	In case CT is not available	Both CT and MRI can detect infracts more than 24hr old; nonetheless, MRI is advised as it limits ionizing radiation exposure.
	CT/ CTA head and neck	Unstable or potential candidates for tissue plasminogen activator or other acute interventions	
Intraparaenchymal hemorrhage	CT	More than 24 hrs	N/A
	MRI	Less than 24 hrs	Evaluate underlying vascular malformation, tumor, *etc.*
	MRA or catheter angiography if MRA is non-diagnostic	N/A	
Arteriovenous malformation	CT	Acute hemorrhage	N/A
	MRI and MRA with or without gadolinium	As soon as possible	N/A
	Catheter angiography	No diagnosis with non-invasive imaging	N/A
Cerebral aneurysm	CT without contrast	N/A	Acute subarachnoid hemorrhage
	MRA or CTA	N/A	Aneurysm identification
	Catheter angiography	Needed in some cases	N/A
	TDC	N/A	Vasospasm detection
Hypoxic- ischemic brain injury	U/S	For infants	N/A
	MRI	in case us is not diagnostic, older children or unstable infants	N/A
	CT	Unstable infants	N/A
	MRS	-	Can indicate lactate peak even if no structural abnormalities

(Table 3) cont.....

Disease	Radiological Investigation	For Which Patient	Findings
Metabolic disorders	MRI, mainly T2-weighted and FLAIR images	N/A	N/A
	Diffusion-weighted images	N/A	Useful for acute and chronic changes identification
	MRS, SPECT and PET	Useful in certain disorders	N/A
Hydrocephalus	US, CT with or without contrast or MR with gadolinium	US in infants	Communicating hydrocephalus diagnosis
	MR with or without gadolinium	N/A	Non-communicating hydrocephalus diagnosis
	CT	N/A	Follow-up after treatment for ventricular size
Headache	CT with or without contrast	N/A	N/A
	MRI with and without gadolinium	Suspicion of Structural disorder	Provides a better view for the parenchyma
Head trauma	CT without contrast	Primarily	N/A
	MRI	After initial assessment and treatment if clinically indicated	N/A
	Diffusion tensor imaging and or diffusion kurtosis sequences	N/A	White matter abnormalities detection
	MRI with and without gadolinium	N/A	N/A
	MRS	N/A	N/A
	PET	N/A	N/A
Multiple sclerosis	MRI with and without gadolinium	N/A	N/A
	Sagittal FLAIR images	N/A	N/A
Meningitis or encephalitis	CT with and without contrast	Before lumbar puncture, where there were signs of raised ICP on examination	N/A
	MRI with and without gadolinium	After initial evaluation treatment of complicated case	N/A

(Table 3) cont.....

Disease	Radiological Investigation	For Which Patient	Findings
Brain abscess	MRI with and without gadolinium	N/A	N/A
	Diffusion-weighted images	N/A	Can identify brain abscess from necrotic tumor
	MRS	N/A	
	CT with and without contrast	Unstable patients	N/A
Movement disorders	MRI with and without gadolinium	N/A	N/A
	PET	N/A	N/A
	DaTscan (SPECT scan using ioflupane iodine-123 as a contrast agent	When parkinsonian syndrome suspicion	Dopamine transporters detection

PEDIATRIC EPILEPSY

As classified by the "International League Against Epilepsy" in 2017 [4], seizures can be divided into: 1) focal, 2) generalized, and 3) unknown onset. Focal seizures can be motor or non-motor; this is further sub-categorized based on the level of consciousness to impaired and preserved consciousness. Henceforth, the nomenclature of seizures has been changed to focal awareness seizures, previously known as simple partial seizures, and focal seizures with impaired awareness of the surrounding environment, previously known as complex partial seizures. In contrast, seizures of unknown onset denote seizures with insufficient information to know the type of seizure. It is worth noting that febrile seizures are considered a separate category.

Febrile Seizures

Considered a separate entity, seen between 6 months to 6 years, febrile seizures are tonic-clonic episodes associated with an elevated core body temperature above 38°C that occurs in the absence of CNS structural abnormalities, infection of metabolic dysregulation, and the absences of other afebrile seizures. Simple febrile seizures last a maximum of 15 minutes and are not expected to recur within 24 hours, while complex seizures have a prolonged duration, lateralization of symptoms, recurrence occurs within 24 hours, and an increased risk of mortality is expected compared to simple seizures. Most patients with febrile seizures return to baseline activity within a short duration after the seizure has subsided. Seizure recurrence occurs around 30% after one episode and more than 50% with subsequent episodes.

With some genetic components seen in febrile seizures, some reports of autosomal dominance inheritance with single gene and polygenetic etiology are proposed. Other causes appear to be due to dysregulation inflammatory cascades, with decreased interleukin -1 to interleukin-8 ratio, leading to a generalized pro-inflammatory status. This correlates with hippocampal abnormalities identified on MRI scans in febrile status epilepticus.

Febrile Infection-related/refractory Epilepsy

Febrile infection-related/refractory epilepsy (FIRES) is a devastating epilepsy syndrome usually progressing to status epilepticus, preceded by a febrile illness without an identifiable source of infection. Seen in patients older than 5 years of age, usually with male predominance, patients present with the encephalitis-like presentation. Prior to the presentation, patients usually have normal development. Unfortunately, the majority will develop epilepsy that is resistant to conventional therapy. With the pathophysiology of this entity not fully understood, multiple other names have been proposed, including; 1) new-onset refractory status epilepticus and2) devastating epileptic encephalopathy in school children.

Recent reports have shown female predominance, in addition to liver function abnormalities at the time of seizure onset. Arrhythmias, initially thought to be in direct relation to multiple antiepileptic administrations, has been noted by Lee *et al.* in 2018 to be in direct relation to the frequency of seizures; this is thought to be due to autonomic dysfunction [5]. The authors also found hypersensitive skin reactions that increased in severity which is thought to be due to a combination of antiepileptic therapy and liver dysfunction [2].

In most cases, seizures are focal that might progress to generalized and require multiple medications to manage, including 1) antiepileptic drugs, 2) immune modulators, and 3) ketogenic diet and in some extreme cases, a burst suppression medical induced coma. Abnormal MRI findings can be detected in the majority of patients, mainly in the temporal region, basal ganglia, and bilateral thalami. In contrast, follow-up MRI findings usually show findings suggestive of brain atrophy. Hence, in most FIERS cases, severe neurological devastation and skill regression are seen on long-term follow-up.

Dravet Syndrome

Known also as severe myoclonic epilepsy of infancy, Dravet syndrome presents as generalized epilepsy with febrile seizures. On the spectrum of febrile epilepsy seizure syndromes, Dravet syndrome is considered the most severe, characterized by unilateral clonic seizures that occur monthly or every other month. With prolonged, frequent episodes seen in clusters, Dravet syndrome evolved as a separate entity from febrile seizures and is currently associated with *de novo* SCN1A gene mutation and reports of autosomal dominant inheritance. Initially, seizures are seen with fevers that ensue with a lower temperature threshold. Other types of seizures are seen with age, including absence and myoclonus seizures. Eventually, developmental delay is seen with time due to the nature of intractable epilepsy. Milder phenotypes of Dravet syndrome are associated with other genetic mutations, including GABRG2 and SCN2A.

Developmental and behavioral associated changes are commonly seen in a patient with Dravet syndrome, such as intellectual disability, autism spectrum disorder features including language and communication impairment, attention deficit, with higher prevalence than the general population. It has been reported that behavioral and communication problems are the main areas of concern for parents of Dravet syndrome patients [6]. Also, it was found that difficulties in behavior are strongly associated with reduced quality of life in Davert patients, as the overwhelming majority of patients have low scores on cognitive and adaptive behavior scores. Recently Devinsky *et al.*, found that in patients with Dravet syndrome drug-resistant seizures, cannabidiol had an increased reduction of seizure frequency, yet unfortunately, this intervention was associated with increased risk of adverse events including; 1) nausea and vomiting, 2) pyrexia, 3) seizures and 4) somnolence and lethargy, which led some patients to withdraw from the trial [7].

Focal Seizures

Preceded as a usually short lived, focal seizures are usually seen in children younger than 7 years of age without an aura while more likely with aura in the older age group. Such seizures are described as a state of decreased responsiveness to the surrounding environment and automatic semi purposeful movement known as "Automatisms". Usually, patients do not remember events around the seizures and might develop transient neurological deficits postictally, including memory impairment and motor weakness. Patients might also become sleepy after a seizure. Sleep-deprived video-assisted EEG usually helps in the diagnosis of such types of seizures. In addition, brain imaging studies are quite helpful in exploring underlying structural abnormalities.

Benign Epilepsy Syndromes with Focal Seizures

Benign childhood epilepsy with centrotemporal spikes (BECTS) is by far considered the most common entity in this group. It usually presents in the childhood response to antiepileptic medications, *e.g.* carbamazepine, and patients usually outgrow this disease by adolescence. EEG tracing shows wide-based centrotemporal spikes, while the radiological investigation is usually normal.

While atypical BETCS presents with multiple seizure types can be seen at younger ages and can be associated with developmental delays, with bilateral synchrony usually found on EEG studies.

Severe Epilepsy Syndromes with Focal Seizures

Epilepsy secondary to structural or metabolic causes confers a higher risk of being severe and resistant to medical therapy compared to idiopathic (genetic) epilepsy, (Table **4**). In infancy, refractory focal epilepsy is likely a result of severe metabolic issues, congenital anomalies, or ischemic insult. A notable cause in infancy leading to severe, intractable epilepsy is Epilepsy of Infancy with Migrating Focal Seizures (EIMFS), which leads to regression in developmental milestones and brain parenchymal atrophy. There are ample causes of intractable focal epilepsy, including; genetic causes, for example, KCNT1 channel mutations (calcium-potassium channels), structural malformations like focal cortical dysplasia, tuberous sclerosis lesions and tumors. Intractable seizures can be associated with awareness impairment; also, they might lead to secondary generalization. In cases where the secondary generalization takes the form of absence or atonic seizures, it is given the name pseudo–Lennox-Gastaut syndrome due to the similarity with Lennox-Gastaut syndrome. Another form of focal seizures in the temporal lobe is epilepsy, which can be due to any pathology in the temporal lobe, for example, tumors and mesial temporal lobe sclerosis (also known as hippocampal sclerosis), in which patients develop atrophy and cortical dysplasia of the hippocampus that might extend to the amygdala in severe cases. It is worth noting that medial temporal epilepsy is the most common surgically treated cause of focal epilepsy. Landau-Kleffner syndrome, also known as Landau-Kleffner aphasia syndrome, occurs due to temporal lobe abnormal continuous discharges during sleep leading to verbal agnosia and loss of speech. Landau-Kleffner syndrome is associated with a more severe form of global delay due to the nature of the continuous discharge during sleep.

Generalized Motor Seizures

The most common form in this category is the generalized tonic-clonic seizures; these are either primary or occur secondary to a focal seizure. In this type of seizure, the beginning of manifestations is usually by loss of consciousness, then the classic findings of eyes up rolling and generalized repetitive tonic-clonic movements ensue. The post-ictal phase is usually characterized by sleepiness, weakness and headaches, associated with ataxia and incontinence and usually lasts a few hours on average.

Table 4. Common pediatric epilepsy syndrome by the age of presentation and significant genetic association and treatment strategies [8, 9].

Age of Onset	Syndrome	Prognosis	Genetic Mutation	Suggested Treatment	Treatment Considerations
Neonatal	Benign neonatal seizures	Good	KCNQ2 KNCQ3	LEV, TPM, PB	N/A
	Early myoclonic encephalopathy and Ohtahara syndrome	Ominous	SCN8A	PB, steroids, VGB	Ketogenic diet, LEV High-dose phenytoin
	Benign familial neonatal convulsions	Good	N/A	LEV, TPM, PB	N/A
Infancy	Benign (nonfamilial) infantile seizures	Good	SCN8A	LEV, TPM, PB	High-dose phenytoin -
	Benign familial infantile convulsions	Good	N/A	LEV, TPM,OXC, CPZ, PB	N/A
	Epilepsy of infancy with migrating focal seizures	Ominous	KCNT1	LEV, PB, OXC, CBZ, PHT, TPM, QND	NZF, bromides Quinidine for gain-for-function mutations
	West syndrome	Variable	N/A	ACTH, steroids, VGB	BZD, TPM, ketogenic diet
	Dravet syndrome (sever myoclonic epilepsy in infancy)	Severe	SCN1A SCN2A	CLB, stiripintol, VPA(only after 2 yrs of age)	BZD, ZON, ketogenic diet Avoid using sodium blockers and vigabatrin Phenytoin and carbamazepine
	Benign myoclonic epilepsy in infancy	Variable	N/A	LEV,TPM,BZD	VPA, ZON
Early Childhood	Autosomal dominant nocturnal frontal lobe epilepsy	Variable	CHRNA4 CHRNAB2 CHRNA2 CRH DEPDC5 KCNT1	OXC, CBZ, LEV	CLB, PB, LAC

(Table 4) cont.....

Age of Onset	Syndrome	Prognosis	Genetic Mutation	Suggested Treatment	Treatment Considerations
Early Childhood	Familial lateral temporal lobe epilepsy	Variable	N/A	OXC, CBZ, LEV	CLB, PB, LAC
	Generalized epilepsies with febrile seizures plus	Variable	SCN1A SCN1B GABRG2 SCN2A	ESM, LTG, LEV, VPA (depending on seizure type)	CLB,TPM,PER
	Mesial temporal lobe epilepsy with hippocampal sclerosis	Variable	N/A	OXC, CBZ, LEV	GBP, PHT, PER
	Rasmussen syndrome	Ominous	N/A	LEV, OXC, CBZ, plasmaperesis, immunoglobulins	LAC,PB, PHT
	Hemiconvulsion-hemiplegia syndrome	Severe	N/A	OXC, CBZ, LEV	GBP, PER, ZON
	Epilepsy with myoclonic astatic seizures	Variable	N/A	ESM, TPM, VPA, LEV, ZON	BZD, ketogenic diet, LTG
	Childhood absence epilepsy	Good	N/A	ESM, LTG, VPA	Acetazolamide, CZP, ketogenic diet
	Epilepsy with myoclonic absences	Guarded	GATM	ESM, VPA, CZP	ZON, LTG
	Lennox-Gastaut syndrome	Severe	N/A	CLB, LTG, RFD, TPM, VPA	BZD, FBM, steroid
	Landau-Kleffner syndrome	Guarded	N/A	Nocturnal DZP, steroids, VPA, LEV	CLB, ESM, IVIG
	Epilepsy with continuous spike waves during slow-wave sleep	Guarded	N/A	Nocturnal DZP, steroids, VPA, LEV	CLB, ESM, IVIG
	Other visual-sensitive epilepsies	Variable	N/A	VPA	BZD, LEV, ZON
	Febrile seizures	Good	N/A	BZD (only as needed for febrile periods if frequent febrile seizures)	N/A

(Table 4) cont.....

Age of Onset	Syndrome	Prognosis	Genetic Mutation	Suggested Treatment	Treatment Considerations
Late Childhood	Benign childhood epilepsy with centrotemporal spikes	Good	N/A	OXC, CBZ, LEV, VPA	LAC, PER
	Early and late-onset idiopathic occipital epilepsy	Good	N/A	OXC, CBZ, LEV, VPA	LAC, PER
	Juvenile absence epilepsy	Good	N/A	ESM, LTG, VPA	Same as in childhood absence epilepsy
	Juvenile myoclonic epilepsy	Good	EFHC1 CACNB4 GABRA1	LEV, TPM, VPA	BZD, LTG, PB
	Epilepsy with generalized tonic-clonic seizures only	Good	N/A	LEV, LTG, TPM, VPA	BZD, CBZ, PER
	Idiopathic photosensitive occipital lobe epilepsy	Variable	N/A	VPA, LEV	BZD, LTG, ZON
	Progressive myoclonic epilepsies (Unverricht-Lundborg, Lafora, ceroid lipofuscinoses, *etc.*)	Ominous	ATN1(DRPLA) CSTB CLN1-14 EPM2A EPM2B/NHLRC1 GOSR2 PRICKLE1 SCARB2	TPM, VPA, ZON, LEV	BZD, PB, ketogenic diet
Miscellaneous	Mesial temporal lobe epilepsy defined by location and cause	Variable	N/A	LEV, OXC, CBZ, TPM, VPA	PHT, PB, CLB
	Mesial temporal lobe epilepsy defined by specific causes	Variable	N/A	LEV, OXC, CBZ, TPM, VPA	CLB, GBP, LAC
	Startle epilepsy	Guarded	N/A	OXC, CBZ, LEV, TPM, VPA	CLB, LEV, PB
	Reflex seizures	N/A	N/A	LEV, VPA	LTG, ZON
	Drug or other chemical induced seizure	N/A	N/A	Withdraw offending agent	N/A
	Immediate and early posttraumatic seizures	N/A	N/A	LEV, PHT	N/A

Benign Generalized Epilepsies

The most common example of this category is absence seizure, which usually starts in early to mid-childhood and has a good prognosis overall as most children outgrow it by late adolescents to early adulthood. Around a quarter of patients with absence seizures will go on to develop generalized tonic-clonic seizures.

Infantile benign myoclonic epilepsy is another example, typically occurs in the first year of life and is associated with generalized slow-wave discharges on EEG. While the most common cause of generalized epilepsy in the adolescent and young adults age group is Juvenile myoclonic epilepsy, also known as Janz syndrome, it accounts for about five percent of all epilepsy syndromes in this age group. The typical natural history of Janz syndrome is in early adolescences with the complaint of clumsiness prior to generalized seizures starting; seizures are noted early in the morning upon awakening from sleep. Janz syndrome is associated with generalized polyspike, and slow-wave discharges on EEG. Sleep deprivation, sensory stimulation (*e.g.* lights), illicit drugs, and alcohol can precipitate a seizure in susceptible individuals.

Severe Generalized Epilepsies

Such pathologies are associated with developmental delay and refractory seizures. For example, myoclonic infantile encephalopathy manifests in the first few months of life. It is usually the result of an inborn error of metabolism, including nonketotic hyperglycinemia, and is associated with burst suppression in EEG. These findings are also seen in early infantile epileptic encephalopathy, also known as Ohtahara syndrome, which is caused by mutations in gene encoding syntaxin-binding protein-1. The term early infantile epileptic encephalopathy has been used to describe multiple other genetic-epileptic encephalopathies due to different genetic mutations, all of which are characterized by the early development of epileptic encephalopathies and developmental delays and regression.

West Syndrome

Manifesting between 12 to 24 months of age, west syndrome is characterized by a triad of clusters of epileptic infantile spasms that are predominantly noticed in drowsiness or upon awakening, developmental regression and hypsarrhythmia on EEG, (Fig. **1**). Cryptogenic, also known as idiopathic, west syndrome usually has normal development and attain milestones within time prior to manifestations of the symptoms. ARX gene mutations can lead to the west syndrome, ambiguous genitalia, and cortical migration abnormalities in males. In contrast, in most cases of the syndrome, no underlying genetic mutations can be identified. In most cases, identification of symptoms is late, as parents and physicians confuse infantile spasms with jitters or startles.

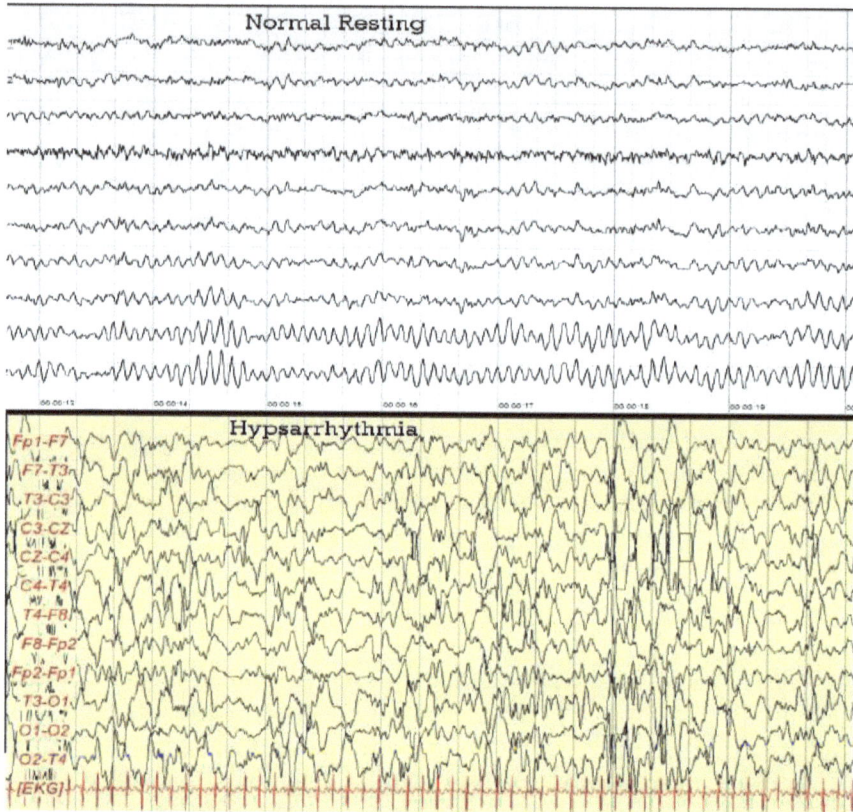

Fig. (1). Hypsarrhythmia is a high-voltage, slow, chaotic background with multifocal spikes [10].

Lennox-Gastaut Syndrome

Manifesting between two to ten years of age, Lennox-Gustaut syndrome is a triad of developmental delay, more than one type of seizures (tonic, myoclonic, astatic, and atypical absence), and characteristic EEG changes (one to two Hz spike and slow waves with slow background waves during arousal state and polyspike burst activity during sleep). Most patients will have long term neuro-cognitive sequelae. A small subset of patients initially manifest Ohtahara syndrome, then progress to West syndrome and finally develop Lennox-Gastaut syndrome.

A milder form of Lennox-Gastaut syndrome is known as Doose syndrome, Myclonic astatic epilepsy, characterized by no tonic seizures and no polysipke burst in sleep EEG tracing, and usually confers a better prognosis.

Landau-Kleffner Syndrome

This is a rare epileptic syndrome of unknown pathophysiology but a strong correlation with genetic mutation of GRIN2A and possibly autoimmune etiology. It is by developmental regression in a previously healthy child leading to deterioration in language skills and verbal/auditory agnosia. Multiple seizures can be seen in Landau-Kleffner syndrome with and without awareness impairment, including atypical absence, tonic-clonic and myoclonic seizures. Around 70% of the patients with Landau-Kleffner syndrome are presumed to develop clinically identifiable seizure disorders. Abnormalities in EEG include bitemporal predilection with high amplitude spike and wave pattern, more pronounced in rapid-eye-movement sleep. Radiological investigations typically yield normal findings.

Epilepsy syndrome with continuous spikes in slow-wave sleep is a related clinical entity to Landau-Kleffner syndrome, which manifests with electrical status epilepticus during sleep. The electrical discharge is typically originating from the frontal lobe

Medical treatment with Sodium Valproate is often the main therapeutic approach, combined with early speech therapy to halt the development of aphasia. Valproic acid combination with clobazam is needed to control seizures in a subset of cases, while nocturnal diazepam and oral steroids have been used to medically manage aphasia. Early management of aphasia is imperative, as once aphasia develops, it might take long-time periods to reacquire lost skills.

METABOLIC EPILEPSY SYNDROMES

Typically presenting in neonatal or early infantile age group, metabolic epilepsy syndromes typically present with intractable epilepsy with possibly rapid onset of encephalopathy with treatment targeting the supplementation or reduction of the burden of specific metabolites within the affected pathway. The most common cause is pyridoxine-dependent epilepsy; this type can present as early as in the fetal stage with utero seizures that can be mistaken as increased fetal activity. It can present with multiple seizure types, typically focal motor recurrent seizures, and will progress to status epilepticus if pyridoxine is not administered to abort the seizures. Elevated α-aminoadipic semialdehyde in serum, urine and CSF, along with elevated pipecolic acid levels in serum and CSF, confirm the diagnosis. Genetic mutation in ALDH7A1gene, which encodes antiquitin protein, is usually confirmatory of the condition. It is inherited in a homozygous or combined heterozygous manner. Other genetic mutations can present with pyridoxine-dependent epilepsy plus a spectrum of other findings; for example, PROSC gene mutations lead to pyridoxine epileptic encephalopathy without gastrointestinal manifestations. CSF studies will likely show elevated suppressed levels of homovanillic acid and 5-hydroxyindoleacetic acid with burst suppression patterns on EEG.

Folinic acid-responsive seizures can be considered in the same clinical spectrum as pyridoxine-dependent epilepsy, as it has a similar metabolic diagnostic profile and genetic mutations. In this syndrome, clinical response is noticed only with folinic acid supplementation along with pyridoxine. It can progress to intractable epilepsy as late as the infantile age group. It is associated with intellectual impairment, developmental regression, and an autism spectrum disorder.

Biotinidase deficiency presents with developmental delay, alopecia, and skin rash, in addition to a seizure disorder. Metabolic studies show lactic and propionic academia and respond to biotin administration.

Metabolic Epilepsy Related to Insulin/energy Regulation Disorders

Mutations in adenosine triphosphate–sensitive potassium channels lead to neonatal diabetes, seizure disorder and developmental delay. The use of sulfonylurea to improve glycemic control might positively impact neurological development in such cases. GLUT-1 deficiency leads to infantile epilepsy with complex movement disorders and microcephaly. Typically diagnosed with low CSF to plasma glucose ratio and low CSF lactate can be managed with a ketogenic diet.

Hyperinsulinism–hyperammonemia syndrome presents hypoglycemic seizures and elevated ammonia levels following a protein-rich meal. Such disorder can be managed with protein-restricted diet, antiepileptic drugs, and potassium channel agonists to decrease insulin release.

APPROACHES TO EPILEPSY SURGERY

Childhood refractory epilepsy can be defined as a persistent occurrence of unprovoked seizures after maximum medical therapy with two or more antiepileptic drugs. The chances of epilepsy management decrease with add-on therapy; it is estimated that the chance of seizure control with three antiepileptics is less than 10 percent, henceforth, the importance of proper patient selection and evaluation prior to surgery. Surgeries performed early in life, *i.e.*, before five years of age, will allow for the new center of function to emerge in other areas of the brain. The area of discharge should be carefully identified with the help of a specialized team *via* the means of inter-ictal EEG, prolonged video EEG, functional MRI, and neurophysiological analysis. PET scans, invasive EEG and stereo EEG can identify epileptiform areas in or near to the cortex. Epilepsy surgery is used in the management of drug-resistant epilepsy that can result from a number of etiologies, including; anatomical malformations like cortical dysplasia's, tumors, in specific syndromes like tuberous sclerosis and sturge-weber syndrome. An important facet for the success of the surgery is choosing the patient who will benefit from such intervention, *e.g.* intractable seizure due to metabolic etiology, will not benefit from surgical intervention. Ideal candidates for surgical intervention should have proven refractory epilepsy to medical therapy and proper identification of discharge area. Other considerations are anesthesia risk and cardiac involvement. For suitable surgical candidates, early surgical intervention can be proven to be life-changing. Unfortunately, the referral time is still lengthy. Pestana Knight *et al.*, in 2015, found that only one-third of patients who were referred for epilepsy surgery between 1997 and 2009 underwent a surgical procedure [11].

Classification of complex underlying etiologies might aid in choosing the right surgical approach; for example, in patients with Lennox-Gastaut syndrome vagus, nerve stimulation has been tried with overall good reports thus far, also, hemispherectomy for epileptic Rasmussen encephalitis and corpus callosotomy in cases of mesial temporal sclerosis.

Neurodevelopmental and Behavioral Health Evaluation

Evaluation of various cognitive and neurodevelopmental aspects of surgical candidates is important; such evaluation should be specifically tailored to the individual undergoing the surgical intervention; and include examination of intellectual abilities and intellectual quotient, mental health comorbidities, for example, depression, attention deficit hyperactive disorder, and neuropsychological areas like memory and comprehension. This evaluation helps the surgeons in possibly pinpointing the area of abnormality, and also it can be compared with post-operative evaluation to assess for possible areas of improvement.

Surgical Outcomes

Reports of postoperative seizure control show a dramatic decrease in seizure frequency as high as 80% in some reports. Yet, there is no general consensus about post-surgical seizure control in literature at this point [12].

The current body of evidence is inconsistent regarding cognitive and neurodevelopmental post-operatively, with some reports failing to identify any noticeable improvement in the intelligence of memory functions, while others reported a decline in language acquisition. In specific situations, good outcomes post-surgery were observed; for example, Skirrow *et al.*, in 2011, reported improvement in the intelligence quotient with around 10 points following successful temporal lobectomy in temporal lobe epilepsy [13].

Thus far, there have not been many studies investigating emotional and behavioral outcomes in the pediatric population, with the majority of evidence from the adult population, yet Andresen *et al.*, 2014, reported parental reports of behavioral improvements [14]. In contrast, other reports showed post-operative clinical depression and anxiety.

CONCLUSION

Epilepsy syndromes carry significant morbidity and even mortality in children. The advent of new genetic discoveries has also brought forth new lines of management for previously refractory diseases. In contrast, the truly intractable epilepsy syndromes might be managed with surgery as a final resort.

LIST OF ABBREVIATIONS

ACTH	Adrenocorticotropic hormone
BZD	Benzodiazepine
BECTS	Benign childhood epilepsy with centrotemporal spike
CT	Computed Topography
CTA	Computed Angiography
CSF	Cerobro-Spinal fluid.
CN	Cranial Nerves
CNS	Central Nerves System
CBZ	Carbamazepine
CLB	Clobazam
DZP	Diazepam
ESM	Ethosuximide
EEG	Electro-Encephalo-Gram
EIMFS	Epilepsy of Infancy with Migrating Focal Seizures
FBM	Felbamate
FIRES	Febrile infection related/refractory epilepsy
GBP	Gabapentin
Hz	Hertz
IVIG	Intravenous immunoglobulin
LAC	Lacosamide
LEV	Levetiracetam

LTG	Lamotrigine
MRI	Magnetic Resonance Imaging
N/A	Not applicable
OXC	Oxcarbazepine
PB	Phenobarbital
PET	Positron emission tomography
PER	Perampanel
PHT	Phenytoin
PRM	Primidone
QND	Quinidine
RFD	Rufinamide
TDC	Diffusion weighted scan
TPM	Topiramate
US	Ultrasonography
VGB	Vigabatrin
VPA	Valproic acid
ZON	Zonisamide

CONSENT FOR PUBLICATION

Not Applicable.

CONFLICT OF INTEREST

The authors declare no conflict of interest, financial or otherwise.

ACKNOWLEDGEMENT

Declared none.

REFERENCES

[1]   Nugud AA, Nugud S, Nugud A, Nugud AA, Kathamuthu R, Jalal M. Perinatal risk factors for development of retinopathy of prematurity in a tertiary neonatal intensive care unit. J Taibah Univ Med Sci 2019; 14(3): 306-11.
[http://dx.doi.org/10.1016/j.jtumed.2019.05.001] [PMID: 31435422]

[2]   Alwahab A, Kharsa A, Nugud A, Nugud S. Occipital Meningoencephalocele case report and review of current literature. Chinese Neurosurgical Journal 2017; 3(1): 40.
[http://dx.doi.org/10.1186/s41016-017-0104-5]

[3]   Zisimopoulou V, Mamali M, Katsavos S, Siatouni A, Tavernarakis A, Gatzonis S. Cerebrospinal fluid analysis after unprovoked first seizure. Funct Neurol 2016; 31(2): 101-7.
[http://dx.doi.org/10.11138/FNeur/2016.31.2.101] [PMID: 27358223]

[4]   Fisher RS, Cross JH, French JA, *et al.* Operational classification of seizure types by the International League Against Epilepsy: Position Paper of the ILAE Commission for Classification and Terminology. Epilepsia 2017; 58(4): 522-30.
[http://dx.doi.org/10.1111/epi.13670] [PMID: 28276060]

[5]   Lee HF, Chi CS. Febrile infection-related epilepsy syndrome (FIRES): therapeutic complications, long-term neurological and neuroimaging follow-up. Seizure 2018; 56: 53-9.
[http://dx.doi.org/10.1016/j.seizure.2018.02.003] [PMID: 29453111]

[6]   Jansson JS, Hallböök T, Reilly C. Intellectual functioning and behavior in Dravet syndrome: A systematic review. Epilepsy Behav 2020; 108107079
[http://dx.doi.org/10.1016/j.yebeh.2020.107079] [PMID: 32334365]

[7]   Devinsky O, Cross JH, Laux L, *et al.* Trial of Cannabidiol for Drug-Resistant Seizures in the Dravet Syndrome. N Engl J Med 2017; 376(21): 2011-20.
[http://dx.doi.org/10.1056/NEJMoa1611618] [PMID: 28538134]

[8]   McTague A, Howell KB, Cross JH, Kurian MA, Scheffer IE. The genetic landscape of the epileptic encephalopathies of infancy and childhood. Lancet Neurol 2016; 15(3): 304-16.
[http://dx.doi.org/10.1016/S1474-4422(15)00250-1] [PMID: 26597089]

[9]   Nelson W, Kliegman R, St Geme J, Behrman R, Tasker R, Shah S, *et al.* Nelson textbook of pediatrics. Philadelphia: Elsevier 2020.

[10]   Used under creative common license link: Retrieved 5 September. 2020. from https://upload.wikimedia.org/wikipedia/commons/c/cd/Human_EEG_Comparison.jpg

[11]   Pestana Knight EM, Schiltz NK, Bakaki PM, Koroukian SM, Lhatoo SD, Kaiboriboon K. Increasing utilization of pediatric epilepsy surgery in the United States between 1997 and 2009. Epilepsia 2015; 56(3): 375-81.
[http://dx.doi.org/10.1111/epi.12912] [PMID: 25630252]

[12]   Kellermann TS, Wagner JL, Smith G, Karia S, Eskandari R. Surgical Management of Pediatric Epilepsy: Decision-Making and Outcomes. Pediatr Neurol 2016; 64: 21-31.
[http://dx.doi.org/10.1016/j.pediatrneurol.2016.06.008] [PMID: 27568292]

[13]   Skirrow C, Cross JH, Cormack F, Harkness W, Vargha-Khadem F, Baldeweg T. Long-term intellectual outcome after temporal lobe surgery in childhood. Neurology 2011; 76(15): 1330-7.
[http://dx.doi.org/10.1212/WNL.0b013e31821527f0] [PMID: 21482948]

[14]   Andresen EN, Ramirez MJ, Kim KH, *et al.* Effects of surgical side and site on mood and behavior outcome in children with pharmacoresistant epilepsy. Front Neurol 2014; 5: 18.
[http://dx.doi.org/10.3389/fneur.2014.00018] [PMID: 24600433]

CHAPTER 6

Updates on Pediatric Genetic Epileptic Encephalopathies: A Diagnostic Algorithmic Approach

Vikas Dhiman[1,*], Shwetha Chiplunkar[2] and Rajnarayan R Tiwari[3]

[1] *Department of Environmental Health and Epidemiology, ICMR-National Institute for Research in Environmental Health (NIREH), Bhopal, Madhya Pradesh-462030, India*

[2] *Department of Pediatrics, Maidstone and Tunbridge Wells NHS Trust, Kent county-ME16 9QQ, United Kingdom*

[3] *ICMR-National Institute for Research in Environmental Health (NIREH), Bhopal, Madhya Pradesh-462030, India*

Abstract: Epileptic Encephalopathies (EEs) are a heterogeneous group of epilepsy syndromes predominantly seen in neonatal, infantile, and childhood age groups. EEs present with varied signs and symptoms often pose a diagnostic dilemma for the treating physician. The diagnostic complexities imposed by variable age of presentation and overlapping clinical signs and symptoms in EEs are further increased by exhaustive new information from advanced molecular genetic techniques like next-generation sequencing. Taking into account all these challenges, the main objective of this chapter is to briefly outline important diagnostic signs and symptoms, EEG, imaging and genetic findings of common neonatal, infantile and childhood-onset genetic epileptic encephalopathies, and secondly, to draw a simple and pragmatic diagnostic algorithm for the diagnosis of genetic epileptic encephalopathies by the treating physicians. Systematic diagnostic algorithms of commonly occurring EEs would not only guide physicians regarding the management of the patients but also help to counsel parents regarding the prognosis, risk of inheritance, and prenatal testing.

Keywords: Algorithm, Diagnostic, Dravet, Drug-resistant, Epileptic, Encephalopathies, Febrile, Genetics, Infantile, Landau-Kleffner, Lennox-Gastaut, Molecular, Myoclonic, Neonatal, Ohtahara, Pediatric, Semiology, Syndrome, Treatment, West-syndrome.

---

* **Corresponding author Vikas Dhiman:** Department of Environmental Health and Epidemiology, ICMR-National Institute for Research in Environmental Health (NIREH), Bhopal, Madhya Pradesh, India; Tel: +919501074334
Emails: drvikasdhiman.nimhans@gmail.com, dhiman.vikas@icmr.gov.in

Nima Rezaei and Noosha Samieefar (Eds.)

INTRODUCTION

Seizures in childhood are one of the commonest neurological symptoms encountered in clinical practice, and they range from a benign single seizure episode to intractable epilepsy and encephalopathy [1]. Epileptic encephalopathies (EEs) are devastating conditions characterized by drug-resistant generalized or focal seizures, electroencephalographic (EEG) abnormalities, and impaired cognitive, sensory, and motor development. It is reported that 40% of all seizures during first three years of age are due to EEs. The majority of children with EEs become resistant to available antiepileptic drugs (AEDs) and are prone to premature deaths, injuries, and poor quality of life. The underlying etiologies of EEs remain heterogeneous, ranging from idiopathic to potentially morbid genetic variants.

It has been found in a recent study that a genetic cause could be attributed in 28% of the children with EEs based on the diagnostic genetic testing [2], highlighting the complexity involved in making the diagnoses of EEs. Early diagnosis and therapeutic interventions are vital as these can alter the course of the disease and improve the final outcome. Considering a significant overlap and complexity among signs and symptoms seen in children with EEs and the difficulties associated with making an early diagnosis of EE, the main objectives of this chapter are a) to briefly outline important signs and symptoms, EEG, imaging, and genetic findings of common neonatal, infantile and childhood genetic epileptic encephalopathies, and b) to draw a simple and pragmatic algorithm for the diagnosis of genetic epileptic encephalopathies.

NEONATAL EPILEPTIC ENCEPHALOPATHIES

Neonatal Epileptic Encephalopathies (NEE) is an autosomal dominant, severe form of encephalopathy where seizures start as early as the first week of life [3]. Infants predominantly develop tonic seizures with associated autonomic features that remain recurrent and refractory to conventional antiepileptic medications. Sodium channel blockers like carbamazepine and phenytoin have shown some benefits and are considered first-line treatment. Ictal EEG typically shows a burst suppression pattern or multifocal epileptiform activity. Brain imaging shows hyperintensities in bilateral basal ganglia and thalamus that usually resolve by the age of three. Seizure cessation occurs anytime between nine months to four years of age but ensues a lasting neurological sequel with moderate to severe developmental delay in all domains [4]. EEG usually becomes normal with control in seizures [5]. *KCNQ2* (voltage-gated potassium channel) is implicated in this disorder harboring a heterozygous missense pathogenic mutation.

Another EE subtype, Benign Familial Neonatal Epilepsies (BFNE), is a rare form of epilepsy presenting in the early neonatal period. The onset is typically between the second to the eighth day of life. These infants develop brief but sometimes recurrent seizures that include tonic or apneic seizures, focal clonic activity, and autonomic symptoms. They are amenable to conventional antiepileptic medications and leave no neurological sequel. All laboratory investigations, including brain imaging, are normal [6]. Ictal EEG shows focal discharges that may secondarily generalize. Inter-ictal EEG is usually normal, rarely it shows 'theta pointu alternant' activity, characterized by dominant theta activity, non-reactive, inter-hemispheric asynchrony, and sharp waves. BFNE is autosomal dominant genetic epilepsy with mutations in *KCNQ2*, coding for a subunit of the voltage-gated potassium channel in the brain [7]. A heterozygous pathogenic variant (60-80% cases) [8] or deletion/duplication (20-40% cases) [9] in *KCNQ2* can cause the disease with a penetrance of 77-85% [5]. A minority of infants with BFNE harbored mutations in *KCNQ3,* a close homolog of *KCNQ2,* and one family harbored pericentric inversion of chromosome 5 [10]. BFNE has a good prognosis with spontaneous resolution of seizures by twelve months of age with no lasting sequel.

Ohtahara Syndrome

The seizure onset is specifically in the neonatal or early infantile period. The majority of seizures are present in the first month of life with recurrent episodes of tonic spasms, sometimes in clusters. There can also be associated generalized seizures, hemiconvulsions, and focal seizures but tonic spasms are more consistently observed in Ohtahara syndrome. Interestingly, myoclonic epilepsy has not been associated with Ohtahara syndrome [11]. The seizures can be similar to West syndrome (see below), but the age at onset, occurrence of seizures in both awake and sleep states, and specific EEG changes, differentiate it from West syndrome [12]. Clinically, Ohtahara syndrome is characterized by daily, recurrent seizures, with significant psychomotor delay and a poor prognosis. The characteristic EEG abnormality is the suppression burst pattern with sudden high voltage bursts alternating with flat records denoting the suppression. These alternations occur periodically in both awake and sleep states, differentiating it from West syndrome, which shows remarkable periodicity in sleep. The most common underlying pathology has been structural brain abnormalities like cerebral dysgenesis and cortical malformations. Ohtahara syndrome in a majority of cases progresses to West syndrome, as reported by a longitudinal study [13]. Ohtahara syndrome has poor prognosis with intractable seizures and significant psychomotor delay. Treatment trials with ACTH injections, clonazepam, ketogenic diet, and vitamin B6 supplementation have not shown any significant benefit [14].

Early Myoclonic Encephalopathy (EME)

EME is a severe form of epilepsy characterized by fragmentary, erratic myoclonus that eventually evolves into focal seizures and infantile spasms. The onset is typically in the first month of life. Eventually, infantile spasms appear by three to four months of age. Burst suppression pattern on EEG in both sleep and awake states is an essential finding for the diagnosis [13]. The prognosis of infants with EME is poor, with a high death rate in the first few years of life, or they lapse into a vegetative state [11].

INFANTILE EPILEPTIC ENCEPHALOPATHIES

Benign Familial Infantile Seizures (BFIS)

The onset is between four to seven months of life. Seizure semiology is characterized by psychomotor arrest, cyanosis, a tonic extension of limbs, and deviation of eyes and neck to one side. Seizures occur in clusters and can last up to three days but would never evolve into true status epilepticus. The neurodevelopment of the infant remains unaffected. Ictal EEG shows fast activity localized to the occipital region. Postictally, delta waves and spikes are observed in the occipitoparietal region. Seizures usually resolve within first year of life and have a benign course [15]. The disease has an autosomal dominant inheritance with genetic loci mapped to chromosome 19q. There are reports of BFIS associated with other neurological disorders with distinct etiology. A subgroup of BFIS patients was found to develop choreoathetosis later in life, and this was termed as Familial Infantile convulsions and choreoathetosis (ICCA). This phenotype showed linkage to chromosome 16 with involvement of *PRRT2* and dominant inheritance. Similarly, BFIS patients were reported to develop familial hemiplegic migraine (FHM), and the etiology co-segregated to chromosome 1q23, suggesting association of BFIS with other neurological disorders [16].

Benign Familial Neonatal-infantile Seizures are an extended spectrum of BFIS, which is caused by mutations in SCN2A. SCN2A codes for the alpha subunit of the voltage-gated sodium channel. This autosomal dominant disease has an onset between two to seven months of age. Seizures are focal with eye and neck deviation to one side followed by secondary generalization into tonic-clonic movements of limbs. Nevertheless, infants are developmentally normal before and after the onset of seizures. Ictal EEG recordings show focal posterior onset epileptiform discharges. Due to the consistent finding of *SCN2A* mutation, it is concluded as a distinct channelopathy with overlapping features of BFIS [17, 18].

Generalized Epilepsy with Febrile Seizures Plus (GEFS+)

GEFS+ accounts for infantile-onset generalized seizures occurring during a febrile illness. The seizures continue to occur beyond six years of age, and children also develop other forms of seizures that may be afebrile. These include myoclonus, absence, and myoclonic-astatic seizures. GEFS+ disorder is caused by mutations in *SCN1A, SCN2A, SCN1B,* and *GABRG2* genes. GEFS+ usually has an unfavorable prognosis with cognitive impairment after seizure onset [19].

Dravet Syndrome

Dravet syndrome, or severe myoclonic epilepsy of infancy (SMEI), is a severe form of infantile-onset epilepsy [20]. It is characterized by hemiconvulsions or generalized seizures within the first year of life in an otherwise normal infant. The seizures are typically, but not always, triggered by fever. Gradually, afebrile seizures also occur. As the phenotype evolves, it is associated with myoclonus, atypical absence, and focal seizures and sometimes evolves into status epilepticus. Milestones develop normally during first years of life, but thereafter gait issues, language impairment, and gradual deterioration in cognition ensue [21]. Serial brain imaging has revealed hippocampal sclerosis in most patients [22]. In around 60% patients, mutations are identified in *SCN1A* coding for voltage-gated sodium channel, and most of the mutations are *de novo* [23, 24]. The best therapeutic response has been attained with benzodiazepines, sodium valproate, topiramate and stiripentol. Carbamazepine and lamotrigine are reported to worsen the seizures and should be avoided. The disease has definite and severe cognitive and behavioral consequences along with motor disability, language impairment and autistic traits [25].

West Syndrome

West syndrome is characterized by infantile spasms and hypsarrhythmic EEG patterns [12]. The spasms are typically sudden axial movements with either flexion or extension of limbs and occur in clusters. The age at onset is classically around 6 months of age. It is rare before three months and after one year of age. There could be a varied combination of generalized tonic-clonic, tonic and myoclonic seizures coexisting in these infants. The etiology for West syndrome is varied and includes structural brain malformations, neurometabolic disorders, and chromosomal abnormalities like Down's syndrome, neurocutaneous syndromes like tuberous sclerosis, hypoxic damage, or cryptogenic etiology [26].

Interictal EEG shows chaotic, disorganized background overlapping with large amplitude spikes and waves known as hypsarrhythmia [27]. Infants may have a normal development prior to the onset of spasms. Post onset, most of them tend to regress neurologically. So far, the best response has been reported with the use of steroids and vigabatrin [28] with potential adverse effects [28]. The outcome of the disease greatly depends on the etiology, and the extent of seizure control attained in the initial phase.

Myoclonic Encephalopathy in Non-progressive Disorders

Occasionally, infants can develop myoclonic status that could be long lasting, difficult to recognize and often refractory to medications. When it is seen in infants suffering from non-progressive encephalopathy of varied etiology like genetic disorders (Angelman syndrome, Rett syndrome), prenatal anoxic damage and cortical malformations like polymicrogyria, callosal agenesis, vermian hypoplasia or sometimes of unknown etiology, it could be categorized as myoclonic encephalopathy in non-progressive disorders [29]. Infants develop prolonged myoclonic status characterized by daily or frequent 'absences' associated with facial/perioral myoclonia and limb jerks. Children usually have coexisting mental retardation and involuntary movements, and the status episodes could be easily missed.

EEG shows diffuse slowing and poor reactivity even when awake, with paroxysmal events that include rhythmic delta waves with superimposed spikes and asynchronous delta theta activity in frontocentral regions. Rhythmic myoclonia shows paroxysmal bursts similar to myoclonic absence. During drowsiness and slow-wave sleep, spike waves become extremely continuous and sleep spindles are difficult to recognize [30]. The syndrome has poor neurological outcomes. Nevertheless, a combination of ethosuximide, sodium valproate and levetiracetam has shown some benefit. Many children die during the prolonged status, and lasting neurological deficits persist in those who survive [31].

Epilepsy of Infancy with Migrating Focal Seizures

Migrating Partial Seizures of Infancy (MPSI) is a severe form of epilepsy diagnosed by the following criteria: Normal development before the onset of the seizure, seizure onset before the age of six months, partial seizures with shifting focus at onset, eventually multifocal seizures becoming continuous, refractoriness, severe psychomotor delay and a lack of demonstrable etiology [32]. Recent studies have found MPSI associated with *SCN1A* and *KCNT1* mutations [33, 34]. The seizures are predominantly focal, with the focus often shifting sides. There is associated limb myoclonus and deviation of the head and eye to one side. The fragmentary myoclonus eventually becomes continuous and generalized. There could be associated autonomic symptoms like flushing the face, salivation, and apnea.

Ictal EEG shows focal epileptiform discharges with multifocal nature becoming evident on long-term video monitoring. There could be hemispheric asymmetry with eventual diffuse background slowing. Brain imaging studies, blood biochemistry, electrophysiological studies, and biopsies are usually normal [32]. MPSI has a poor prognosis with early deaths, gross developmental delay, hypotonia and microcephaly in survivors with poor quality of living. It is suggested that MPSI should be categorized as one of the catastrophic epilepsies of infancy [35].

EPILEPTIC ENCEPHALOPATHIES OF CHILDHOOD AND ADOLESCENCE

Benign Childhood Epilepsy with Centrotemporal Spikes (BCECTS)

BCECTS, also known as benign rolandic epilepsy, accounts for 6% to 10% of all childhood epilepsies and has an age of onset between 4 and 10 years with a male to female ratio of 3:2. In 80-90% of the cases, seizures are brief and occur in clusters during sleep, characterized by hemifacial motor signs (tonic or clonic contractions of one side of face), hypersalivation, speech arrest and swallowing disturbances, with somatosensory symptoms such as unilateral numbness of face [36]. Frequent seizures are seen in only 6%, while 13% to 21% have only a single seizure event.

The causal gene for BCECTS is unknown. A high incidence of positive family history of epilepsy and febrile convulsions seen in children with BCECTS, is linked to chromosome 15q14 [37]. The cornerstone in diagnosing BCECTS is the characteristic inter-ictal EEG abnormalities, showing broad, diphasic, high voltage spikes followed by a slow wave, typically seen in the centrotemporal or rolandic areas. These CTS are not enhanced by eye-opening or closure, hyperventilation or photic stimulation and sometimes appear only during sleep. It is to be noted that 0.7% of children with no history of seizures present with incidental findings of CTS. Neuroimaging is usually normal in children with BCECTS [38], but an MRI brain is usually advised to rule out any other abnormalities, as CTS can be seen in patients with cortical dysplasia and tumors.

Prophylactic medication may not be required in children with infrequent seizures, but some recommended treating BCECTS with AEDs for 1 year. The drug of choice is carbamazepine, valproic acid and benzodiazepines [39]. Remission occurs in most of the children: 50% by age 6 years, 92% by age 12 years, and 99.8% by age 18 years. Few children, who evolve into atypical phenotypes characterized by an increase in the frequency of seizures, worsening of EEG and evidence of neuropsychological problems, may require longer treatment and follow-up.

Early-onset Childhood Occipital Epilepsy (Panayiotopoulos Type)

Early-onset childhood occipital epilepsy or Panayiotopoulos syndrome (PS) occurs in children without any neurodevelopmental delay or milestone regression. Chrysostomos Panayiotopoulos described it for the first time in 1988. The prevalence of PS is 13% among early childhood epilepsies and incidence of 2-3 per 100,000 children in the general population. The age at onset of seizures is 1-14 years, but in the majority, the first seizure occurs during 4-5 years of age. Seizures predominantly occur at night, with ictal vomiting and unilateral deviation of eyes seen in about 80% of the patients [40]. Vomiting may occur once or repetitively during the seizure and is usually associated with autonomic manifestations, facial pallor being the most frequent symptom. Deviation of eyes is usually accompanied by head deviation, and seizures evolve into unilateral clonic or tonic-clonic seizures or generalized tonic-clonic seizures and sometimes to status epilepticus [41].

The etiopathogenesis of PS is currently not known, but mutations in the SCN1A gene have been associated with the severity of PS. A positive family history of epilepsy is found in 30% of children with PS [40]. The most useful laboratory test in children with PS is EEG, which shows occipital epileptiform discharges in two-third of the patients. There are two distinct patterns seen in EEG: during sleep, bilateral and synchronous spikes are visible in the occipital leads, while during awake EEG; these occipital spikes are seen intermixed with slow and sharp wave complexes that appear immediately after closing the eyes. The occipital paroxysms disappear after the eye-opening. This phenomenon, called fixation-off sensitivity, is seen in PS [42]. Brain imaging studies (CT and MRI) are usually normal in PS, but they can be useful for impaired neurological examination or neurocognitive or motor symptoms.

AEDs are usually not recommended after the first seizure unless the first seizure is prolonged or has evolved to status epilepticus. Carbamazepine and valproic acid are the drugs of choice. Remission usually occurs 1-2 years after the first seizure, and the overall prognosis is excellent in PS [43].

Late-onset Childhood Occipital Epilepsy (Gastaut Syndrome)

Gastaut syndrome is seen in children aged 4-13.2 years, with peak incidence at 8 years. The most common seizures in Gastaut syndrome are visual seizures, characterized by visual hallucinations; illusions of ocular movements, tonic deviation of eyes, and eyelid fluttering with usually preserved consciousness. The seizure may progress to hemiclonic or generalized tonic-clonic seizures and are usually followed by headache, nausea or vomiting.

A family history of epilepsy has been reported in 33% to 43% of patients, but no genes have been implicated so far [44]. Inter-ictal EEG shows spikes or sharp waves in the occipital and posterior portion of the temporal lobe. Like PS, fixation-off sensitivity is also seen in the Gastaut type. Ictal EEG is characterized by fast spike discharges in either one or both occipital lobes. Visual-evoked potentials (VEPs) and somatosensory-evoked potentials (SEPs) abnormalities have been reported in patients with Gastaut syndrome [45]. Though Gastaut syndrome can be differentiated from PS on clinical manifestations, as many as 50% of children with occipital spikes can present mixed symptoms. Neuroimaging findings are normal. Treatment is usually indicated in Gastaut syndrome, with carbamazepine and clobazam being preferred. The prognosis of Gastaut syndrome is variable, mostly having a favorable outcome [46].

Epilepsy with Myoclonic Atonic (Astatic) Seizures (Doose Syndrome)

Epilepsy with myoclonic atonic seizures (EMAS) is a rare childhood epilepsy syndrome affecting 1-2% of children with epilepsy. It begins in early childhood, between 2-5 years of age, and is characterized by myoclonic atonic (astatic) seizures and other generalized seizure types like absence, tonic-clonic and myoclonic seizures. The astatic attack is a brief generalized myoclonic jerk affecting proximal muscles, which is followed by an atonic component resulting in drop attacks, which are very debilitating and can cause multiple injuries. In addition to seizures, the child may develop ataxia, dyspraxia, speech difficulties and attention deficit hyperactivity. Non-convulsive status epilepticus is seen in about 40% of the affected children.

The children with EMAS have a positive family history of either epilepsy (15-37%) or febrile seizures (50%) [8]. The inter-ictal EEG shows slowing (theta rhythm) and generalized spike and wave activity, especially during sleep. Since myoclonic and atonic seizures are common and responsible for drops attacks, video-EEG with EMG recordings are very useful in diagnosing. Imaging findings are normal. *SLC2A1* gene has been implicated in a few patients with EMAS [47].

AEDs like valproic acid, lamotrigine, ethosuximide, benzodiazepines, and levetiracetam are usually recommended. Carbamazepine and vigabatrin are known to aggravate EMAS. The prognosis is highly variable with total recovery within a few months to persistent behavioral problems later in adolescence [48].

Lennox-Gastaut Syndrome

Lennox-Gastaut syndrome (LGS) is a rare epilepsy encephalopathy with an incidence of 1.9 – 2 per 100,000 children. It is a severe childhood encephalopathy a triad of symptoms characterizes that: a) multiple seizure types like tonic-clonic, tonic, clonic, absences and myoclonus (tonic seizure during sleep is a consistent feature), b) diffuse slow spike-wave complexes on EEG, c) cognitive decline. The age at onset is between 1-15 years with a peak between 3-5 years with a slight male preponderance. The seizures are accompanied by severe psychological, behavioral, and personality changes (*e.g.* delay in psychomotor development, anger, cognitive disabilities), usually permanent.

Various pathogenic copy number variants and mutations involving genes such as GABRB3, ALG13, SCN8A, STXBP1, DNM1, FOXG1, or CHD2 have been seen in children with LGS. The mutations in the *XLIS* gene have been identified in patients with LGS, who has polymicrogyria on the brain MRI [49]. A sleep EEG usually shows slow diffuse spike and wave discharges or fast activity (10-12 Hz) [50]. Video-EEG with EMG electrodes is recommended if available in the resource setting. Brain imaging varies from normal (cryptogenic) to extensive lesions such as cortical malformations, lissencephaly or polymicrogyria, tuberous sclerosis complex, or neoplasia. Advanced investigations like Positron Emission Tomography (PET) scan, functional MRI, or single-photon emission computed tomography (SPECT) might be useful for pre-surgical evaluation.

LGS is highly drug-resistant [51]. AEDs of different mechanisms of action should be recommended, *e.g.*, levetiracetam, clobazam, and valproate. Topiramate and valproate combination is usually recommended for drop attacks. For intractable cases, surgical treatments like corpus callosotomy and alternative treatment modalities like vagal nerve stimulation or ketogenic diet have been tried with variable results [52]. The long prognosis of LGS is poor, with complete seizure freedom being rare. Behavioral and psychiatric symptoms pose major additional challenges for treating clinicians, especially during advanced age.

Landau-Kleffner Syndrome

Landau-Kleffner syndrome (LKS) is acquired epileptic aphasia, which occurs between 3-8 years of age in an otherwise normally developing child. The true incidence and prevalence of LKS are unknown. The child typically presents with a sudden loss of language, which in due course develop into verbal and/or verbal agnosia. Other typical signs are difficulties with articulation, fluency and word retrieval. The seizures may not be clinically apparent in all cases but if present (70-80%), they are characterized by rapid eye blinking, automatisms and brief ocular movements. Absence seizures, tonic seizures and generalized tonic-clonic seizures are also seen. The child usually has associated behavioral problems like attention deficit hyperactivity, aggression, depression, anxiety, social withdrawal and emotional lability.

A family history of epilepsy is present in about 3% of the patients. There is evidence of the implication of the *GRIN2A* gene in patients of LKS [53]. A continuous 1.5 to 5 Hz spike and wave activity is seen in slow sleep in the posterior temporal regions on EEG. But these activities occupy less than 85% of the slow sleep record and hence differentiated from Epileptic encephalopathy with continuous spike waves during sleep (CSWS) [54] (see below). Neuroimaging is usually normal.

The main of the treatment is to restore the language skills and to achieve seizure freedom. Clinical seizures are usually mild and respond to most of the available AEDs. Valproate, clobazam (or other benzodiazepines), levetiracetam, ethosuximide are the most frequently used antiepileptic drugs. If epileptic activity persists in EEG, oral corticosteroids may be given along with AEDs, showing a favorable outcome. The long-term prognosis for the seizure is good. However, the neuropsychological problems and aphasia may persist for longer [55].

Continuous Spike-wave During Sleep (CSWS)

CSWS is an age-related, self-limited epileptic encephalopathy, with most cases presenting after 9 years of age. It is characterized by a typical bilateral 1.5-5 Hz spike and wave activity strongly activated by Non-REM sleep and occupies>85% of the sleep record [56]. REM sleep and wakefulness interrupt this EEG activity. It is accompanied by mild and subtle seizures like focal motor, absence, hemiclonic and partial seizures. In addition, the child presents with profound cognitive disturbances like aphasia, apraxia, mental retardation and even dementia [57].

The treatment goal in CSWS is improved seizure control and reduction in inter-ictal seizure abnormalities. High-dose benzodiazepines or steroids are often used as first-line treatment. Similar to LKS, seizures usually respond to conventional AEDs, but cognitive and psychiatric symptoms are more difficult to treat. In addition, unlike LKS, the long-term outcome in CSWS, especially in children with late age of onset and with neuro-behavioral problems, remains poor [56].

EPILEPTIC ENCEPHALOPATHIES OF VARIABLE AGE

Progressive Myoclonic Epilepsies

Progressive myoclonic epilepsies (PME) are a heterogeneous group of disorders characterized by the presence of stimulus-sensitive myoclonus, progressive neurological deterioration, and seizures in childhood or adolescence. PMEs are rare epilepsy syndromes accounting for less than 1% of all epilepsies [58]. Myoclonic jerks are characterized by arrhythmic, asymmetric, and asynchronous jerks and usually show a focal or segmental distribution. Neurological deficits include progressive dementia, neuropathy and ataxia. They have multiple seizure types, *e.g.*, complex or simple partial seizures, absences, tonic or clonic or generalized tonic-clonic seizures.

Most of the PMEs follows an autosomal recessive pattern of inheritance. The molecular genetics and underlying biochemistry of most of PMEs are now known. Unverricht-Lundborg disease (ULD) is the most common PME characterized bystimulus-sensitive myoclonus and tonic-clonic generalized seizures. It is caused by a loss-of-function mutation in the *CSTB* gene located on chromosome 21q22.3 [59]. Lafora disease, another very debilitating PME, is caused by mutations in the EPM2 gene, which encodes for Lafora associated tyrosine phosphatase [60]. Lafora disease is diagnosed by the presence of typical clinical symptoms, genetic testing, and the presence of periodic acid-Schiff-positive intracellular inclusion bodies (Lafora bodies) in axillary skin biopsies.

Neuronal ceroid lipofuscinosis (NCLs) are another group of neurodegenerative encephalopathies characterized by progressive neurological and psychiatric manifestations, seizures, vision failure and the presence of autofluorescent lipopigment in neurons and other cell types. Curvilinear inclusions in electron microscopic examination of skin biopsy are diagnostic. Different subtypes of NCLs (CLN1-8) have been identified based on the age of onset, seizure types, and the type of storage material identified in tissues. Various chromosomal loci have been mapped for different subtypes of NCLs [61]. The details of other PMEs are beyond the scope of this review.

The treatment and prognosis are disease-specific. In most, the myoclonic jerks are treated with valproate and clonazepam; other AEDs are used depending on the seizure type. Usually, a high-dose polytherapy is required, which becomes more resistant as the disease progresses. Lafora disease and NCLs have a very poor prognosis. Patients usually become bedridden and die within a decade of the onset of first symptom [62]. On the other hand, Unverricht-Lundborg disease has a slower progression. Most patients with ULD can lead a normal life if adequate medical and ancillary care is provided [63]. Important clinical features of common EEs are depicted in Table **1**.

Table 1. Summary of various pediatric epileptic encephalopathies.

S. No.	Disorder/ Syndrome	Age at Onset	Predominant Seizure Type	Milestones Delay	Causes	Family History	EEG Changes	Imaging	Gene Implicated	Prognosis
1.	Benign Familial Neonatal Epilepsy (BFNE)	2-8th day of life	Brief tonic or aponeic seizures, focal clonic	No	Genetic	Usually present, autosomal dominant	Focal discharges, 'theta pointu alternant'	Normal	*KCNQ2*	Good

(Table 1) cont.....

S. No.	Disorder/ Syndrome	Age at Onset	Predominant Seizure Type	Milestones Delay	Causes	Family History	EEG Changes	Imaging	Gene Implicated	Prognosis
2.	Ohtahara syndrome	First month of life	Tonic spasms, in clusters, No myoclonic seizures	Yes	Secondary*	Usually absent	Suppression-burst pattern in both sleep and awake record	Cortical malformations	Not known	Poor
3.	Early myoclonic encephalopathy (EME)	First month of life	Fragmentary, erratic myoclonus, spasms	Yes	Cryptogenic and secondary*	May be present, autosomal recessive	Suppression-burst pattern in both sleep and awake record	Normal/ab-normal	Not known	Poor
4.	Benign Familial Infantile Epilepsy (BFIE)	4-7 months	Focal, sometimes secondarily generalized, cyanotic spells	No	Genetic	Usually present, autosomal dominant	Fast activity in occipital region, delta waves and spikes in occipito-parietal region post ictally	Normal	Chr. 19q, *PRRT2, SCN1A*	Good
5.	Generalized Epilepsy with Febrile seizure plus	6 months - > 6 years	Generalized seizures during febrile illness, afebrile seizures uncommon	No	Genetic	Usually present	Generalized as well as focal epileptiform discharges	Normal	*SCN1A, SCN2A, SCN1B,GABRG2*	Variable
6.	Dravet syndrome	4-8 months	Hemiconvulsions, myoclonus, atypical absence and focal seizures	Yes	Genetic	Usually present	Generalized as well as focal epileptiform discharges	Hippocampal sclerosis on serial imaging	*SCN1A*	Poor
7.	West syndrome	3 months – 1 year	Tonic spasms, generalized tonic clonic, tonic and myoclonic seizures	Yes	Genetic and Secondary*	May be present X-linked recessive	Chaotic disorganized background overlapping with large amplitude spikes and waves known as hypsarrhythmia	Cortical malformations	*CDKL5*	Poor
8.	Myoclonic encephalopathy in non-progressive disorders	1 month – 5 years	Prolonged myoclonic status, absences, facial/perioral myoclonia	Yes	Secondary*	Absent	Rhythmic delta waves with superimposed spikes	Cortical malformations, leucomalacia	Absent	Poor
9.	Epilepsy of infancy with migrating focal seizures	< 6 months of age	Partial seizures with shifting focus and sides, autonomic symptoms	Yes	Not known	Absent	Focal discharges, hemispheric asymmetry	Normal	Not known	Poor
10.	Benign childhood epilepsy with centro-temporal spikes (BCECTS)	4-10 years	Hemifacial motor, hypersalivation, speech arrest, swallowing disturbances & somatosensory symptoms, associated with sleep	No	Genetic	Usually present	Centrotemporal spikes (CTS)	Normal	15q14	Good
11.	Early onset childhood occipital epilepsy (Panayiotopoulos type)	4-5 years	Ictal vomiting and unilateral deviation of eyes, autonomic manifestations, predominantly at night	No	Genetic	Usually present	Bilateral and synchronous spikes in occipital leads, fixation of sensitivity phenomena	Normal	Not known yet	Good
12.	Late onset childhood occipital epilepsy (Gastaut syndrome)	4-13.2 years (maximum incidence: 8 years)	Visual seizures, visual hallucinations, tonic deviation of eyes and eyelid fluttering, hemiclonic or generalized tonic clonic	No	Genetic	Usually present	Dyphasic spike and wave discharges, spikes or sharp waves in the occipital and temporal lobe, fixation of sensitivity phenomena	Normal	Not known yet	Variable

(Table 1) cont.....

S. No.	Disorder/ Syndrome	Age at Onset	Predominant Seizure Type	Milestones Delay	Causes	Family History	EEG Changes	Imaging	Gene Implicated	Prognosis
13.	Epilepsy with myoclonic atonic (astatic) seizures	2-5 years	Myoclonic atonic (astatic) seizures, drop attacks	Yes	Genetic	Not known	Slowing and generalized spike and wave activity during sleep	Normal	SLC2A1	Variable
14.	Lennox-Gastaut syndrome	3-5 years	Multiple seizure types, tonic seizures during sleep is constant	Yes	Genetic	Usually present	Sleep EEG: slow diffuse spike and wave discharges or 10-12 Hz fast activity	Normal to cortical lesions	XLIS	Poor
15.	Landau-Kleffner syndrome	3-8 years	Eye blinking, automatisms and brief ocular movements, focal seizures	Yes with aphasia	Genetic	Usually present	1.5 to 5 Hz spike and wave activity is seen in slow sleep in temporal region	Normal	GRIN2A	Good
16	Epileptic encephalopathy with continuous spike wave during sleep (CSWS)	> 9 years of age	Eye blinking, automatisms and brief ocular movements, focal seizures	Yes with aphasia	Genetic	Usually present	Bilateral 1.5-5 Hz spike and wave activity strongly activated by sleep and occupying >85% of the sleep record	Normal	GRIN2A	Poor
17.	Progressive Myoclonic Epilepsies	Variable age	Stimulus sensitive myoclonus, progressive neurological deterioration, and seizures	Yes	Genetic	Usually present, mostly autosomal recessive	Multiphasic spike and wave discharges	Normal to cortical lesions	Unverricht-Lundborg disease: CSTB	Variable but mostly poor

*Secondary causes: Epilepsy secondary to other genetic disorders, infections, and anoxic damage

DIAGNOSTIC ALGORITHMS

In this chapter, we present a diagnostic algorithm for EEs based mainly on four clinical criteria: age at onset of seizures, seizure type, presence of any associated neurodevelopmental delay/regression and specific EEG findings. Figs. (1 - 3) summarize the algorithmic approach to neonatal, infantile and childhood EEs. Beginning with age at onset of seizures and following steps in sequence, a clinician can reach a probable diagnosis of EE. In infantile-onset seizures, treatable causes like infection, hypoglycemia, and electrolyte disturbances should be excluded. It is also recommended that a trial of pyridoxal phosphate or folic acid be initiated before considering genetic EEs. Further, a detailed biochemical evaluation includes serum amino acids and acylcarnitine profiles, urine organic acids, biotinidase levels, analysis of various neurotransmitters, lactate, pyruvate, and glucose levels in the cerebrospinal fluid become important in all age groups that can help exclude other metabolic causes of EEs. Any associated neurodevelopmental delay, regression of milestones, vision-hearing impairments, neurocutaneous markers, and congenital malformations can help differentiate various EEs. Video-EEG is considered the gold standard in classifying the type of seizure. Further, visual inspection of a seizure episode in the clinic and home videos could also significantly aid in characterizing the seizures. Finally, a technically accurate EEG can help localize seizure focus and characterizing patterns, which may help arrive at the final diagnosis.

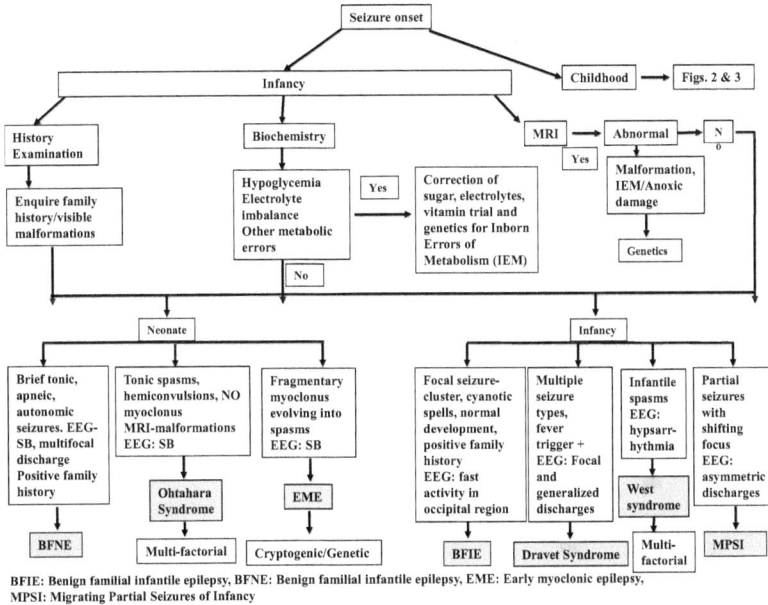

Fig. (1). Algorithmic approach to infantile and neonatal EEs.

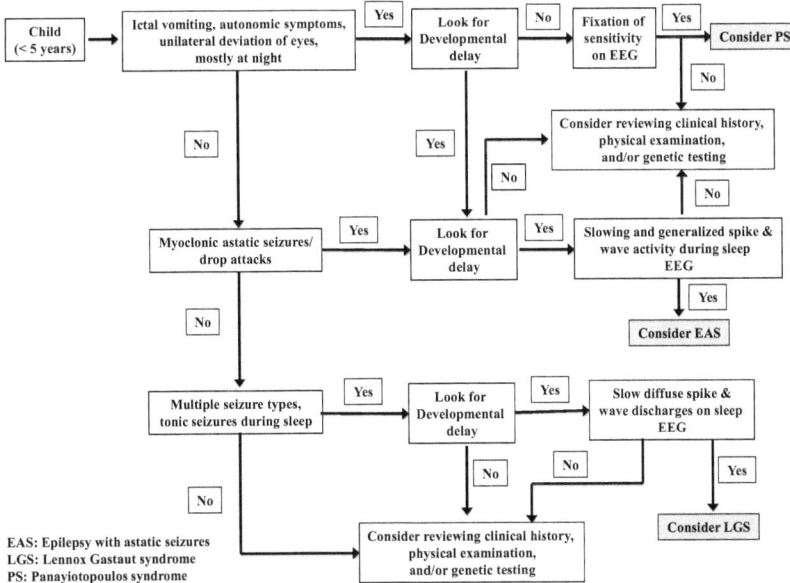

Fig. (2). Algorithmic approach to childhood EEs (< 5 years).

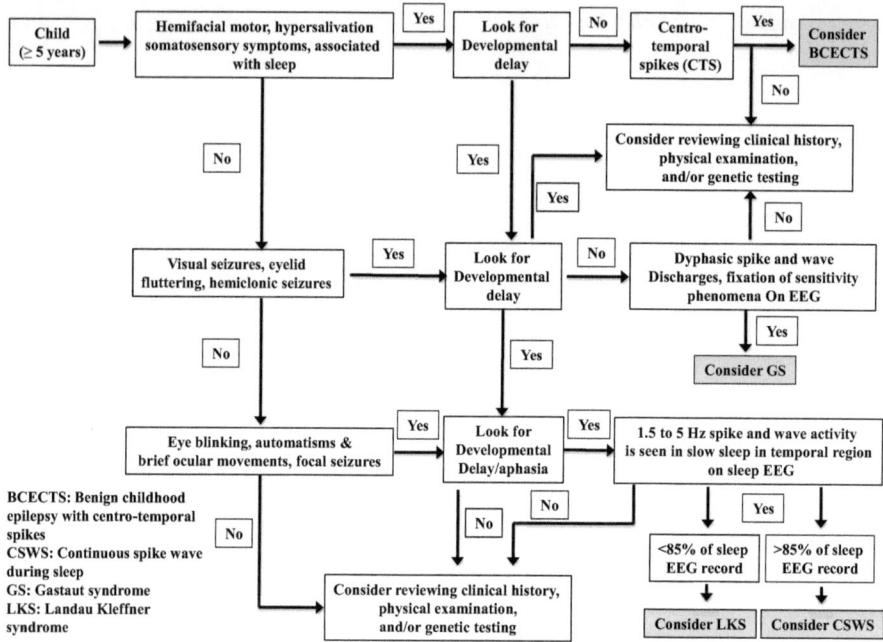

Fig. (3). Algorithmic approach to infantile and neonatal EEs (≥ 5 years).

Once a particular diagnosis is anticipated based on the diagnostic algorithm, evaluation of possible underlying etiologies should be undertaken. Targeted genetic testing (gene panels or individual genes) should be considered to identify the most likely underlying gene. In case of negative results, whole-exome sequencing (WES) may be considered. It is now being understood that many of the EEs occur due to de novo mutations in various genes and also carry a lesser risk of inheritance.

CONCLUSION

EEs are one of the most devastating neurological disorders in the pediatric age group. Our understanding of the underlying etiopathogenesis and genetic basis of EEs has considerably improved over the last decade. A systematic and methodological approach based on clinical and investigational findings like age at onset of a seizure, type of seizure, EEG findings, associated neurodevelopmental delay and genetic testing could help physicians and pediatricians to arrive at an early diagnosis. This aids the treating physician to counsel parents regarding the prognosis and risk of inheritance and offers prenatal testing. We propose that the diagnostic algorithms presented in this review be used as a general model by clinicians and pediatricians in daily practice. Further collaborative efforts are required to test the validity of these algorithms in a large population of children.

CONSENT FOR PUBLICATION

Not applicable.

CONFLICT OF INTEREST

The authors declare no conflict of interest, financial or otherwise.

ACKNOWLEDGEMENT

Declared none.

REFERENCES

[1]   Berg AT, Jallon P, Preux PM. The epidemiology of seizure disorders in infancy and childhood: definitions and classifications. In: Dulac O, Lassonde M, Sarnat HB, Eds. Handbook of Clinical Neurology. Elsevier B.V. 2013; pp. 391-8.

[2]   Hwang S-K, Kwon S. Early-onset epileptic encephalopathies and the diagnostic approach to underlying causes. Korean J Pediatr 2015; 58(11): 407-14.
[http://dx.doi.org/10.3345/kjp.2015.58.11.407] [PMID: 26692875]

[3]   Miceli F, Soldovieri MV, Joshi N, Weckhuysen S, Cooper E, Taglialatela M. KCNQ2-Related Disorders GeneReviews. Seattle: University of Washington 1993.

[4]   Weckhuysen S, Mandelstam S, Suls A, *et al.* KCNQ2 encephalopathy: emerging phenotype of a neonatal epileptic encephalopathy. Ann Neurol 2012; 71(1): 15-25.
[http://dx.doi.org/10.1002/ana.22644] [PMID: 22275249]

[5]   Berkovic SF. Genetics of Epilepsy in Clinical Practice. Epilepsy Curr 2015; 15(4): 192-6.
[http://dx.doi.org/10.5698/1535-7511-15.4.192] [PMID: 26316866]

[6]   Berg AT, Berkovic SF, Brodie MJ, *et al.* Revised terminology and concepts for organization of seizures and epilepsies: report of the ILAE Commission on Classification and Terminology, 2005-2009. Epilepsia 2010; 51(4): 676-85.
[http://dx.doi.org/10.1111/j.1528-1167.2010.02522.x] [PMID: 20196795]

[7]   Singh NA, Charlier C, Stauffer D, *et al.* A novel potassium channel gene, KCNQ2, is mutated in an inherited epilepsy of newborns. Nat Genet 1998; 18(1): 25-9.
[http://dx.doi.org/10.1038/ng0198-25] [PMID: 9425895]

[8]   Weckhuysen S, Ivanovic V, Hendrickx R, *et al.* Extending the KCNQ2 encephalopathy spectrum: clinical and neuroimaging findings in 17 patients. Neurology 2013; 81(19): 1697-703.
[http://dx.doi.org/10.1212/01.wnl.0000435296.72400.a1] [PMID: 24107868]

[9]   Heron SE, Cox K, Grinton BE, *et al.* Deletions or duplications in KCNQ2 can cause benign familial neonatal seizures. J Med Genet 2007; 44(12): 791-6.
[http://dx.doi.org/10.1136/jmg.2007.051938] [PMID: 17675531]

[10]   Concolino D, Iembo MA, Rossi E, *et al.* Familial pericentric inversion of chromosome 5 in a family with benign neonatal convulsions. J Med Genet 2002; 39(3): 214-6.
[http://dx.doi.org/10.1136/jmg.39.3.214] [PMID: 11897828]

[11]   Ohtahara S, Yamatogi Y. Ohtahara syndrome: with special reference to its developmental aspects for differentiating from early myoclonic encephalopathy. Epilepsy Res 2006; 70 (Suppl. 1): S58-67.
[http://dx.doi.org/10.1016/j.eplepsyres.2005.11.021] [PMID: 16829045]

[12]   Pavone P, Striano P, Falsaperla R, Pavone L, Ruggieri M. Infantile spasms syndrome, West syndrome and related phenotypes: what we know in 2013. Brain Dev 2014; 36(9): 739-51.

[http://dx.doi.org/10.1016/j.braindev.2013.10.008] [PMID: 24268986]

[13]   Beal JC, Cherian K, Moshe SL. Early-onset epileptic encephalopathies: Ohtahara syndrome and early myoclonic encephalopathy. Pediatr Neurol 2012; 47(5): 317-23.
[http://dx.doi.org/10.1016/j.pediatrneurol.2012.06.002] [PMID: 23044011]

[14]   Deprez L, Jansen A, De Jonghe P. Genetics of epilepsy syndromes starting in the first year of life. Neurology 2009; 72(3): 273-81.
[http://dx.doi.org/10.1212/01.wnl.0000339494.76377.d6] [PMID: 19153375]

[15]   Singhi P. Childhood Electroclinical Syndromes: a diagnostic and therapeutic algorithm. Indian J Pediatr 2014; 81(9): 888-97.
[http://dx.doi.org/10.1007/s12098-014-1529-x] [PMID: 25100198]

[16]   Olson HE, Poduri A, Pearl PL. Genetic forms of epilepsies and other paroxysmal disorders. Semin Neurol 2014; 34(3): 266-79.
[http://dx.doi.org/10.1055/s-0034-1386765] [PMID: 25192505]

[17]   Berkovic SF, Heron SE, Giordano L, *et al*. Benign familial neonatal-infantile seizures: characterization of a new sodium channelopathy. Ann Neurol 2004; 55(4): 550-7.
[http://dx.doi.org/10.1002/ana.20029] [PMID: 15048894]

[18]   Heron SE, Crossland KM, Andermann E, *et al*. Sodium-channel defects in benign familial neonatal-infantile seizures. Lancet 2002; 360(9336): 851-2.
[http://dx.doi.org/10.1016/S0140-6736(02)09968-3] [PMID: 12243921]

[19]   Polizzi A, Incorpora G, Pavone P, *et al*. Generalised epilepsy with febrile seizures plus (GEFS(+)): molecular analysis in a restricted area. Childs Nerv Syst 2012; 28(1): 141-5.
[http://dx.doi.org/10.1007/s00381-011-1592-9] [PMID: 22011963]

[20]   Dravet C. The core Dravet syndrome phenotype. Epilepsia 2011; 52(s2) (Suppl. 2): 3-9.
[http://dx.doi.org/10.1111/j.1528-1167.2011.02994.x] [PMID: 21463272]

[21]   Brunklaus A, Zuberi SM. Dravet syndrome--from epileptic encephalopathy to channelopathy. Epilepsia 2014; 55(7): 979-84.
[http://dx.doi.org/10.1111/epi.12652] [PMID: 24836964]

[22]   Camfield P, Camfield C, Nolan K. Helping Families Cope with the Severe Stress of Dravet Syndrome. Can J Neurol Sci 2016; 43(S3) (Suppl. 3): S9-S12.
[http://dx.doi.org/10.1017/cjn.2016.248] [PMID: 27264140]

[23]   Gürsoy S, Erçal D. Diagnostic Approach to Genetic Causes of Early-Onset Epileptic Encephalopathy. J Child Neurol 2016; 31(4): 523-32.
[http://dx.doi.org/10.1177/0883073815599262] [PMID: 26271793]

[24]   Harkin LA, McMahon JM, Iona X, *et al*. The spectrum of SCN1A-related infantile epileptic encephalopathies. Brain 2007; 130(Pt 3): 843-52.
[http://dx.doi.org/10.1093/brain/awm002] [PMID: 17347258]

[25]   Wirrell EC. Treatment of Dravet Syndrome. Canadian Journal of Neurological Sciences. 2016; 43: pp. (S3)S13-8.
[http://dx.doi.org/10.1017/cjn.2016.249]

[26]   Galanopoulou AS, Moshé SL. Pathogenesis and new candidate treatments for infantile spasms and early life epileptic encephalopathies: A view from preclinical studies. Neurobiol Dis 2015; 79: 135-49.
[http://dx.doi.org/10.1016/j.nbd.2015.04.015] [PMID: 25968935]

[27]   Panzica F, Binelli S, Canafoglia L, *et al*. ICTAL EEG fast activity in West syndrome: from onset to outcome. Epilepsia 2007; 48(11): 2101-10.
[http://dx.doi.org/10.1111/j.1528-1167.2007.01264.x] [PMID: 17825076]

[28]   Pellock JM, Faught E, Sergott RC, *et al*. Registry initiated to characterize vision loss associated with vigabatrin therapy. Epilepsy Behav 2011; 22(4): 710-7.

[http://dx.doi.org/10.1016/j.yebeh.2011.08.034] [PMID: 21978471]

[29]   Elia M. Myoclonic status in nonprogressive encephalopathies: an update. Epilepsia 2009; 50 (Suppl. 5): 41-4.
[http://dx.doi.org/10.1111/j.1528-1167.2009.02119.x] [PMID: 19469845]

[30]   Caraballo RH, Cersósimo RO, Espeche A, Arroyo HA, Fejerman N. Myoclonic status in nonprogressive encephalopathies: study of 29 cases. Epilepsia 2007; 48(1): 107-13.
[http://dx.doi.org/10.1111/j.1528-1167.2006.00902.x] [PMID: 17241216]

[31]   Caraballo R, Vilte C, Chamorro N, Fortini P, Ramirez B, Cersósimo R. Myoclonic status in non-progressive encephalopathies or Dalla Bernardina syndrome. J Pediatr Epilepsy 2015; 03(03): 173-80.
[http://dx.doi.org/10.3233/PEP-14088]

[32]   McTague A, Appleton R, Avula S, et al. Migrating partial seizures of infancy: expansion of the electroclinical, radiological and pathological disease spectrum. Brain 2013; 136(Pt 5): 1578-91.
[http://dx.doi.org/10.1093/brain/awt073] [PMID: 23599387]

[33]   Barcia G, Fleming MR, Deligniere A, et al. De novo gain-of-function KCNT1 channel mutations cause malignant migrating partial seizures of infancy. Nat Genet 2012; 44(11): 1255-9.
[http://dx.doi.org/10.1038/ng.2441] [PMID: 23086397]

[34]   Carranza Rojo D, Hamiwka L, McMahon JM, et al. De novo SCN1A mutations in migrating partial seizures of infancy. Neurology 2011; 77(4): 380-3.
[http://dx.doi.org/10.1212/WNL.0b013e318227046d] [PMID: 21753172]

[35]   Bearden D, Strong A, Ehnot J, DiGiovine M, Dlugos D, Goldberg EM. Targeted treatment of migrating partial seizures of infancy with quinidine. Ann Neurol 2014; 76(3): 457-61.
[http://dx.doi.org/10.1002/ana.24229] [PMID: 25042079]

[36]   Verrotti A, Latini G, Trotta D, et al. Typical and atypical rolandic epilepsy in childhood: a follow-up study. Pediatr Neurol 2002; 26(1): 26-9.
[http://dx.doi.org/10.1016/S0887-8994(01)00353-8] [PMID: 11814731]

[37]   Neubauer BA, Fiedler B, Himmelein B, et al. Centrotemporal spikes in families with rolandic epilepsy: linkage to chromosome 15q14. Neurology 1998; 51(6): 1608-12.
[http://dx.doi.org/10.1212/WNL.51.6.1608] [PMID: 9855510]

[38]   Gelisse P, Genton P, Raybaud C, Thiry A, Pincemaille O. Benign childhood epilepsy with centrotemporal spikes and hippocampal atrophy. Epilepsia 1999; 40(9): 1312-5.
[http://dx.doi.org/10.1111/j.1528-1157.1999.tb00864.x] [PMID: 10487198]

[39]   Veggiotti P, Beccaria F, Gatti A, Papalia G, Resi C, Lanzi G. Can protrusion of the tongue stop seizures in Rolandic epilepsy? Epileptic disorders: international epilepsy journal with videotape 1999; 1(4): 217-0.

[40]   Caraballo R, Cersosimo R, Medina C, Fejerman N. Panayiotopoulos-type benign childhood occipital epilepsy: a prospective study. Neurology 2000; 55(8): 1096-100.
[http://dx.doi.org/10.1212/WNL.55.8.1096] [PMID: 11071484]

[41]   Oguni H, Hayashi K, Imai K, Hirano Y, Mutoh A, Osawa M. Study on the early-onset variant of benign childhood epilepsy with occipital paroxysms otherwise described as early-onset benign occipital seizure susceptibility syndrome. Epilepsia 1999; 40(7): 1020-30.
[http://dx.doi.org/10.1111/j.1528-1157.1999.tb00812.x] [PMID: 10403229]

[42]   Panayiotopoulos CP. Inhibitory effect of central vision on occipital lobe seizures. Neurology 1981; 31(10): 1330-3.
[http://dx.doi.org/10.1212/WNL.31.10.1331] [PMID: 6810202]

[43]   Verrotti A, Domizio S, Guerra M, Sabatino G, Morgese G, Chiarelli F. Childhood epilepsy with occipital paroxysms and benign nocturnal childhood occipital epilepsy. J Child Neurol 2000; 15(4): 218-21.
[http://dx.doi.org/10.1177/088307380001500403] [PMID: 10805186]

[44]   Beaumanoir A. Infantile epilepsy with occipital focus and good prognosis. Eur Neurol 1983; 22(1): 43-52.
        [http://dx.doi.org/10.1159/000115535] [PMID: 6404635]

[45]   Gökçay A, Gökçay F, Ekmekçí O, Ulkü A. Occipital epilepsies in children. European journal of paediatric neurology: EJPN: official journal of the European Paediatric Neurology Society 2002; 6(5): 261-8.

[46]   Mennink S, van Nieuwenhuizen O, Jennekens-Schinkel A, van der Schouw YT, van der Meij W, van Huffelen AC. Early prediction of seizure remission in children with occipital lobe epilepsy. European journal of paediatric neurology: EJPN: official journal of the European Paediatric Neurology Society 2003; 7(4): 161-5.
        [http://dx.doi.org/10.1016/S1090-3798(03)00059-X]

[47]   Larsen J, Johannesen KM, Ek J, *et al.* The role of SLC2A1 mutations in myoclonic astatic epilepsy and absence epilepsy, and the estimated frequency of GLUT1 deficiency syndrome. Epilepsia 2015; 56(12): e203-8.
        [http://dx.doi.org/10.1111/epi.13222] [PMID: 26537434]

[48]   Kaminska A, Ickowicz A, Plouin P, Bru MF, Dellatolas G, Dulac O. Delineation of cryptogenic Lennox-Gastaut syndrome and myoclonic astatic epilepsy using multiple correspondence analysis. Epilepsy Res 1999; 36(1): 15-29.
        [http://dx.doi.org/10.1016/S0920-1211(99)00021-2] [PMID: 10463847]

[49]   Guerrini R. Genetic malformations of the cerebral cortex and epilepsy. Epilepsia 2005; 46(s1) (Suppl. 1): 32-7.
        [http://dx.doi.org/10.1111/j.0013-9580.2005.461010.x] [PMID: 15816977]

[50]   Archer JS, Warren AEL, Jackson GD, Abbott DF. Conceptualizing lennox-gastaut syndrome as a secondary network epilepsy. Front Neurol 2014; 5: 225.
        [http://dx.doi.org/10.3389/fneur.2014.00225] [PMID: 25400619]

[51]   Genton P. When antiepileptic drugs aggravate epilepsy. Brain Dev 2000; 22(2): 75-80.
        [http://dx.doi.org/10.1016/S0387-7604(99)00113-8] [PMID: 10722956]

[52]   Hancock EC, Cross JH. Treatment of Lennox-Gastaut syndrome. In: Hancock EC, Ed. Cochrane Database of Systematic Reviews. Chichester, UK: John Wiley & Sons, Ltd 2013; p. CD003277.

[53]   Gao K, Tankovic A, Zhang Y, *et al.* A de novo loss-of-function GRIN2A mutation associated with childhood focal epilepsy and acquired epileptic aphasia. PLoS One 2017; 12(2): e0170818.
        [http://dx.doi.org/10.1371/journal.pone.0170818] [PMID: 28182669]

[54]   Patry G, Lyagoubi S, Tassinari CA. Subclinical "electrical status epilepticus" induced by sleep in children. A clinical and electroencephalographic study of six cases. Arch Neurol 1971; 24(3): 242-52.
        [http://dx.doi.org/10.1001/archneur.1971.00480330070006] [PMID: 5101616]

[55]   Deonna T, Peter C, Ziegler AL. Adult follow-up of the acquired aphasia-epilepsy syndrome in childhood. Report of 7 cases. Neuropediatrics 1989; 20(3): 132-8.
        [http://dx.doi.org/10.1055/s-2008-1071278] [PMID: 2476680]

[56]   Galanopoulou AS, Bojko A, Lado F, Moshé SL. The spectrum of neuropsychiatric abnormalities associated with electrical status epilepticus in sleep. Brain Dev 2000; 22(5): 279-95.
        [http://dx.doi.org/10.1016/S0387-7604(00)00127-3] [PMID: 10891635]

[57]   Veggiotti P, Bova S, Granocchio E, Papalia G, Termine C, Lanzi G. Acquired epileptic frontal syndrome as long-term outcome in two children with CSWS. Neurophysiol Clin 2001; 31(6): 387-97.
        [http://dx.doi.org/10.1016/S0987-7053(01)00280-5] [PMID: 11810988]

[58]   Acharya JN, Satishchandra P, Shankar SK. Familial progressive myoclonus epilepsy: clinical and electrophysiologic observations. Epilepsia 1995; 36(5): 429-34.
        [http://dx.doi.org/10.1111/j.1528-1157.1995.tb00482.x] [PMID: 7614918]

[59]   Lalioti MD, Scott HS, Antonarakis SE. What is expanded in progressive myoclonus epilepsy? Nat Genet 1997; 17(1): 17-7.
[http://dx.doi.org/10.1038/ng0997-17] [PMID: 9288090]

[60]   Minassian BA, Lee JR, Herbrick JA, *et al.* Mutations in a gene encoding a novel protein tyrosine phosphatase cause progressive myoclonus epilepsy. Nat Genet 1998; 20(2): 171-4.
[http://dx.doi.org/10.1038/2470] [PMID: 9771710]

[61]   Mole SE, Williams RE, Goebel HH. Correlations between genotype, ultrastructural morphology and clinical phenotype in the neuronal ceroid lipofuscinoses. Neurogenetics 2005; 6(3): 107-26.
[http://dx.doi.org/10.1007/s10048-005-0218-3] [PMID: 15965709]

[62]   Shahwan A, Farrell M, Delanty N. Progressive myoclonic epilepsies: a review of genetic and therapeutic aspects. Lancet Neurol 2005; 4(4): 239-48.
[http://dx.doi.org/10.1016/S1474-4422(05)70043-0] [PMID: 15778103]

[63]   Kälviäinen R, Khyuppenen J, Koskenkorva P, Eriksson K, Vanninen R, Mervaala E. Clinical picture of EPM1-Unverricht-Lundborg disease. Epilepsia 2008; 49(4): 549-56.
[http://dx.doi.org/10.1111/j.1528-1167.2008.01546.x] [PMID: 18325013]

CHAPTER 7

Updates on Pediatric Demyelinating Disorders

Amit Agrawal[1,*] and **Umesh Pandwar**[1]

[1] *Department of Pediatrics, Gandhi Medical College & Hamidia Hospital, Bhopal, MP 462001, India*

Abstract: Myelin is a protective layer that enwraps the axonal terminals and is an essential component of the central nervous system white matter. Loss of myelin leads to conduction block in the axon leading to demyelinating disorders. Inherited poor formation of myelin is known as *hypomyelination,* and abnormally formed myelin is called *dysmyelination.* Demyelinating disorders exclude diseases where degeneration of the axon is the initial event and myelin is degraded secondarily. Most neurologists use the term *demyelination only for* acquired forms of loss of myelin with relative preservations of axons due to inflammation such as multiple sclerosis. Demyelinating disease in children may be monophasic (*e.g.,* acute disseminated encephalomyelitis, optic neuritis, and transverse myelitis) or chronic (multiple sclerosis and neuromyelitis optica). Pediatric multiple sclerosis is the most common demyelinating disorder in children. Recent genetic and clinical researches have significantly improved our understanding of the diverse spectrum of pediatric demyelinating disorders. In this chapter, an updated summary of the current knowledge on the categories, diagnosis, as well as management of pediatric demyelinating disorders has been presented.

Keywords: Adolescent, Central Nervous System/immunology, Central Nervous System/pathology, Child, Demyelinating Diseases/diagnosis, Demyelinating Diseases/drug therapy, Demyelinating Diseases/immunology, Demyelinating Diseases/pathology, Encephalomyelitis, Acute Disseminated / cerebrospinal fluid, Encephalomyelitis, Acute Disseminated/diagnosis, Humans, Magnetic Resonance Imaging, Multiple Sclerosis/cerebrospinal fluid, Multiple Sclerosis/diagnosis, Multiple Sclerosis/drug therapy, Myelin-Oligodendrocyte Glycoprotein / immunology, Neuromyelitis Optica/cerebrospinal fluid, Neuromyelitis Optica/diagnosis, Neuromyelitis Optica/drug therapy, Serologic Tests, Treatment Outcome.

* **Corresponding author Amit Agrawal:** Department of Pediatrics, Gandhi Medical College & Hamidia Hospital, Bhopal, MP 462001, India; Tel: +91-9826616019; E-mail: agrawaldramit@yahoo.co.in

Nima Rezaei and Noosha Samieefar (Eds.)

INTRODUCTION

Axonal terminals, cylindrical processes that arise from the axon hillock of every neuron, have synaptic connections with other neurons. Myelin is a protective layer that enwraps these axonal terminals and is an essential component of the central nervous system (CNS) white matter. Myelin is an extended component of the cell membrane in the nervous system and is divided into segments over the length of specialized nerve fibers. It works as an insulator to prevent loss of action potential current and increases the transmission velocity of stimulus in nerve fibers by decreasing membrane capacitance so that the charges are not able to accumulate at a point. The transmission speed of the action potential is faster in myelinated neurons as compared to unmyelinated ones. Myelin in CNS is produced by oligodendrocytes, and in PNS, it is produced by Schwann cells.

Myelin loss leads to conduction block in the axon by increasing membrane capacitance, accumulation of charges at the point of lost myelin, and slowing down the rate of nerve impulses transmission, thereby results in derangement of the neurologic functions [1]. The absence of myelin may be acquired or inherited. Inherited disorders of poorly formed myelin are known as hypomyelination disorders, and abnormally formed myelin is called dysmyelination [2].

Demyelinating disorders exclude those diseases where degeneration of axon is the initial event and myelin is degraded secondarily [3]. Most neurologists use the term *demyelination only for* acquired forms of myelin loss with relative preservations of axons due to inflammation such as multiple sclerosis [4]. Acquired disorders of demyelination are due to inflammation or immune-mediated destruction of normally formed myelin [5]. Poser also termed this group of myelin disorders as "demyelinating or myelinoclastic diseases" [6]. Acquired disorders of demyelination due to inflammation comprise both the central (CNS) and peripheral nervous system (PNS) myelin disorders. These are rare disorders with an incidence of 0.5-1.66 per 100,000 children per annum [7]. Demyelination is often preceded by an infectious illness, ischemic attack, or maybe due to a metabolic or hereditary defect. The cause of disorders that primarily affect myelin is idiopathic or unknown but may be due to the autoimmune process [8]. The wide spectrum of neurological signs and symptoms are covered by acquired demyelinating disorders due to myelin damage caused by inflammation (Table **1**).

Table 1. Causes of Acquired disorders of CNS demyelination.

Hypoxia and Ischemia	-
Nutritional Deficiencies	Vitamin B12 Deficiency

(Table 1) cont.....

Viral infection of CNS	Progressive multifocal leukoencephalopathy, Subacute sclerosing panencephalitis, Tropical spastic paraparesis/ HTLV-1–associated myelopathy
Primary demyelinating disorders	Monophasic - optic neuritis, acute transverse myelitis, acute disseminated encephalomyelitis Recurrent, progressive disorders – multiple sclerosis, neuromyelitis optica
Toxins and drugs	Alcohol, Carbon monoxide, Ethambutol

CLASSIFICATION OF PEDIATRIC DEMYELINATING DISEASES

Pediatric demyelinating disorders are generally classified as either monophasic (single episode) or polyphasic illness (relapses). In children, most of the demyelinating disorders present with monophasic illness are without any relapse. Monophasic forms of demyelinating disorders in children include acute disseminated encephalomyelitis, transverse myelitis, and optic neuritis. Multiple Sclerosis and neuromyelitis optica spectrum disorder are relapsing or polyphasic forms of demyelinating disorders. On the basis of signs and symptoms' localization, demyelinating disorders can be monofocal if a single lesion can be attributed for manifestations and polyfocal if multiple site lesions are required to explain signs and symptoms [9].

Acute Disseminated Encephalomyelitis

Acute Disseminated Encephalomyelitis (ADEM) is the clinical event of acute inflammatory demyelinating lesions on brain MRI with poly focal neurological deficits in nature and accompanying encephalopathy. ADEM usually presents in early childhood [10 - 12].

Epidemiology

The incidence is 0.1-0.6 per 100,000 per year in children. A study conducted on Canadian children showed an estimated annual incidence of 0.2 per 100,000 [13]. The seasonal pattern of ADEM is seen in North America, with a peak in winter and spring [14, 15]. There is a slight male predominance [16, 17]. The mean age of ADEM presentation is between 5 and 8 years but can occur at any age [18 - 20]. Recurrence is less common as the disease is usually monophasic. The term *multiphasic disseminated encephalomyelitis (MDEM) is used when recurrence occurs after 3 months of the first event.* In ADEM, Myelin oligodendrocyte glycoprotein antibodies (MOG- Ab) are present in the serum of 50% of children [21 - 23]. MOG-Ab antibodies are present in the serum of all cases of MDEM. Multiple Sclerosis (MS) should be suspected if an episode of non- ADEM demyelination affecting a new location occurs after an episode of ADEM and serum is negative for MOG-Ab. Acute Disseminated Encephalomyelitis – Optic Nerve (ADEM-ON is the term used when relapse involves optic nerve (ON). The term Neuromyelitis optica spectrum disorder (NMOSD) is used when relapse involves the optic nerve and spinal cord. These two conditions are usually MOG-Ab positive.

Pathogenesis

Although unproven, CNS autoantigens are probably produced after exposure to infections or vaccines by the mechanism of molecular mimicry. There is an activation of microglial cells, macrophages, Th1 (T helper), and Th2 cells [24, 25]. There is a history of acute febrile illness in most of the patients about one month before the onset of ADEM [17]. Common infections linked with ADEM are influenza virus, Epstein-Barr virus, cytomegalovirus, varicella virus, enterovirus, measles, mumps, rubella, herpes simplex, and *Mycoplasma pneumoniae. Though rare,* vaccines associated with ADEM are rabies, smallpox, measles, mumps, rubella, Japanese encephalitis, pertussis, diphtheria–polio–tetanus, and influenza [26].

Clinical Manifestations

ADEM initially presents with fever, lethargy, vomiting, headache, signs of meningeal irritation, and seizures which may progress into status epilepticus, but about 25% of cases present with ill-defined prodrome [18, 27]. The hallmark of ADEM is encephalopathy, which can manifest as changes in behavior, irritability, or coma [9, 28]. Common focal neurological signs are loss of vision, cranial nerve palsies, ataxia, and the deficit in motor and sensory examination. Bladder/ bowel dysfunction may occur in cases of spinal cord simultaneous demyelination. There is a clinically rapid progression over a few days in most cases in the form of brainstem dysfunction or an increase in intracranial pressure.

Neuroimaging

CT scan head may have hypodense lesions or it may be normal [18]. The Neuroimaging modality of choice is MRI Brain, which in T2WI shows large, bilateral, multifocal lesions with a variable degree of enhancement within the gray and white matter of the cerebrum, cerebellum and brainstem (Fig. **1**). Other areas involved are structures of deep gray matter (thalamus, basal ganglia) (Fig. **2**) [16, 18, 27, 29].

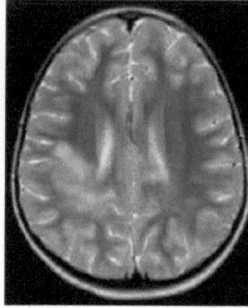

Fig. (1). T2WI sequence axial MRI of the brain demonstrates right-sided ill-defined high signal intensity lesion of white matter in peritrigonal region suggesting ADEM.

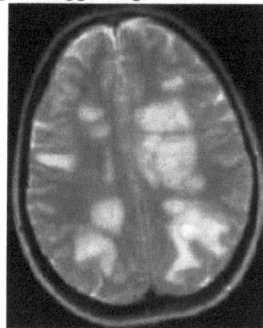

Fig. (2). MRI Brain T2WI sequence axial image demonstrates diffuse, bilateral, diffuse, ill-defined white matter lesions. Involvement of Gray matter including basal ganglia and thalamus is also seen.

Signs of improvement are seen in the form of complete resolution of abnormalities in T2WI in serial MRI after 3- 12 months. Acute hemorrhagic leukoencephalopathy, also known as Weston- Hurst disease, is a severe form of ADEM which is characterized by the large size of lesions with edema which results in mass effect, and pleocytosis (polymorphonucleated cell) in CSF while typical ADEM is characterized by the lymphocytic predominance in the CSF.

Laboratory Findings

For ADEM, no biological marker is available. CSF is mostly normal. It sometimes shows an increased number of lymphocytes or monocytes, in addition to increased levels of protein. Increased production of immune globulin in CSF can be present, too [30]. Rarely, CSF is also positive for Oligoclonal Bands. In electroencephalograms, usually, there is generalized slowing due to *encephalopathy, but sometimes epileptiform discharges of focal slowing.*

Differential Diagnosis

A wide range of disorders can mimic ADEM and antibiotics and antiviral treatment should be given empirically while investigations are pending especially in developing countries. If there is an enlarging or new lesion on Follow-up MRI after 3 to 12 mo of ADEM instead of signs of improvement then reevaluation to rule out other causes *e.g.* MS, tumors, immune-mediated disorders, leukodystrophies, vasculitis, metabolic disorders, mitochondrial disorders, or rheumatologic disorders [10].

Treatment

Corticosteroids in the form of high-dose intravenous methylprednisolone in the dose range of 20-30 mg/kg per day for 5 days (maximum - 1000 mg/day) followed by tapering dosage of prednisolone orally 1-2 mg/kg/day (max.40-60 mg/day) for 4-6 weeks, is the drug of choice in ADEM treatment. Other options are intravenous immunoglobulin (2 g/kg over 2-5 days) or plasmapheresis (5-7 exchanges every other day) for severe or unresponsive cases [31 - 33].

Prognosis

Recovery usually starts in days in most cases but sometimes it starts in weeks. Full recovery occurs in motor functions in most patients' recovery after ADEM. Sometimes residual defects persist. On a 10 year follow-up, the risk is about 25% for the development of multiple sclerosis [33]. Long term deficits in cognitive functions and changes in behavior are also other common sequelae.

Multiple Sclerosis

Multiple sclerosis (MS) is a chronic, autoimmune demyelinating disorder of CNS which is characterized by episodes of focal neurological events without encephalopathy [34 - 36]. The disease has typical relapsing-remitting courses. Different episodes are separated by more than one-month interval and involve different CNS regions. The disease is known as pediatric-onset MS (POMS) when the onset is before 18 years of age [37]. There is brain atrophy due to recurrent episodes of demyelination which in long term results in derangement of cognitive and motor functions.

Epidemiology

Multiple Sclerosis is rare in children. Incidence is 1 to 2 cases per million in western countries [38 - 41]. The disease predominantly affects females more than males (2:1) in postpubertal age groups, but there is no sex preference before puberty. Relapsing-remitting type is the typical presentation of POMS in almost every case, therefore, if the clinical presentation suggests the primary progressive type of MS, an alternative diagnosis should be sought for.

Risk Factors

Multiple factors, both genetic and environmental, and their interaction are responsible to make an individual susceptible to MS, particularly in adults. Environmental factors implicated are lack of exposure to sunlight, low level of vitamin D in the body, obesity, toxins, and infectious agents (*e.g.* Epstein-Barr virus) [42 - 45]. There is an increased risk in an individual with a positive family history. In an identical twin, relative risk is approximately 200 times more than that in the general population. HLADRB1*15:01 is the strongest genetic factor studied to date which is responsible for increased susceptibility to MS. It may be possible that environmental factors are more likely to play an important role than genetic factors in pediatric-onset MS.

Pathogenesis

There are multiple discrete areas of myelin and oligodendrocytes focal loss (with relative preservation of axons and neurons) within the white matter of the brain and spinal cord. Also, there is an infiltration of inflammatory cells, lymphocytes, and macrophages in the lesions. The lesions can occur at any site within the central nervous system, but they have a predilection for involvement of the periventricular white matter, the corpus callosum, optic nerves and the dorsal spinal cord.

Support for an autoimmune etiology for MS comes from animal studies. Depending on the animal model used, causative roles for T cells or B cells have been implicated. However, the evidence that MS is caused by either T-cell or B-cell auto-reactivity is limited [46]. Challenging the idea that MS plaques are caused by inflammatory-mediated tissue injury is through the fact that oligodendroglial cell loss can precede inflammatory infiltration and suggests that the inflammatory response is secondary to tissue injury of as yet an unknown etiology.

Clinical Manifestations

In more than 50% of pediatric MS patients, presentation is in form of polyfocal symptoms which includes paresthesia or focal sensory loss (39% - 63% patients), cerebellar symptoms such as ataxia or dysarthria (44% - 55% patients), pain in movement of the eye, often bilateral, and decreased visual acuity suggestive of optic neuritis (36% - 38% patients), symptoms related to brain stem involvement (30% - 31%), motor deficits (such as hemiparesis, or paraparesis in 29– 50% cases) and bowel/ bladder dysfunction (due to transverse myelitis or other lesions of the spinal cord) [18, 35, 47, 48]. Encephalopathy is not present except in the case of significant brainstem involvement.

Neuroimaging

Typical MS lesions in the T2WI sequence of Brain MRI are hyperintense, ovoid in shape, discrete and asymmetrically distributed in cerebral white matter (Fig. **3**). More commonly involved regions are periventricular, cortical, juxtacortical, brainstem and cerebellum [49]. The deep gray matter is the less commonly involved region. Spine MRI shows spinal cord lesions which typically involve partial-width of cord, and are limited to 1-2 segments of spine.

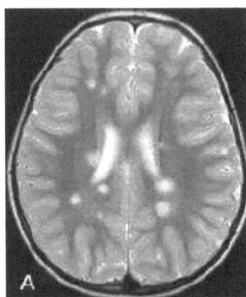

Fig. (3). T2-WI sequence of axial MRI brain MRI shows multiple hyperintense lesions.

Laboratory Findings

Leukocyte count in CSF in pediatric MS is elevated (more than 4 cells/μL) in approximately 66% of patients but it does not raise more than 30 cells/μL in typical presentations. If leucocyte count is higher than the number expected in vasculitis, infection or neuromyelitis optica should be suspected. There is predominantly neutrophilic leukocytosis and elevated IgG Index in CSF especially in children of more than 11 years of age [50, 51]. Besides, there is raised CSF protein level (100–720 mg/L). The presence of oligoclonal bands (OCBs) in CSF in about 90% of pediatric patients as compared to about 98% of adult patients is notable.

Other diagnostic modalities that are useful to confirm the presence of demyelination especially in clinically silent forms of the disease are Evoked potential testing (Brainstem Auditory-Evoked Potential, Visual Evoked Potential, and Somatosensory Evoked Potential).

Diagnosis

Usually, the diagnosis of pediatric MS can be made if there are at least two episodes of demyelination without encephalopathy in different locations of CNS. Each episode must last for more than 24 hours, and are more than 30 days apart. If there are no other reasonable explanations present, MS can be diagnosed on the basis of MRI only (both in adults and children) if it shows scattering in space (two or more lesions in T2WI involving periventricular, juxtacortical, infratentoria, or spinal regions) and time (presence of different lesions with gadolinium-enhancement and those without enhancement in the same scan).

Differential Diagnosis

Clinical presentation of ADEM is similar to MS except for encephalopathy and multifocal symptoms in ADEM. In NMOSD, there are concomitant severe optic neuritis and transverse myelitis (characterize by longitudinally extensive lesions in the spinal cord which involve more than 3 vertebral segments). Neurosarcoidosis, CNS vasculitis, Susac Syndrome, Hypoxic Ischemic vasculopathies, Cerebral autosomal dominant arteriopathy with subcortical infarcts and leukoencephalopathy (CADASIL), Connective tissue disorders, Neuro-Behcet disease, Chronic lymphocytic inflammation with pontine perivascular enhancement responsive to steroids (CLIPPERS), Fabry disease and Leber hereditary optic neuropathy are other differential diagnoses to be considered [52].

Treatment

Injectable Methylprednisolone 20-30 mg/kg/day (maximum dose 1000 mg/day) for 3-5 days. It can also be used for relapses in MS. The frequency of relapse and lesions on T2WI can be reduced by Disease-Modifying Therapies (DMTs) which are immunosuppressive or immunomodulatory agents that act by altering the inflammatory response that occurs during the relapsing-remitting phase. Most of the Disease-Modifying Therapies used in children are not US FDA approved, except Fingolimod. In a clinical trial, Fingolimod decreased the rate of relapse in POMS by 82% in comparison with interferon-beta-1α [53].

Immunomodulatory Therapy

Interferons (beta 1a or 1b) or glatiramer acetate (GA) are usually the first-line agents in children [54 - 58]. These agents are safe and well-tolerated in children. The most frequent side effect of interferons is raised transaminase level and it can be reduced by starting the one-fourth of the adult dose and gradual increase. Regular monitoring of peripheral blood leukocyte counts, liver function tests, and thyroid function tests should be done while the child is on interferon therapy. In addition, contraception should be advised in sexually active patients.

Second-Line Therapies

If frequent relapses occur despite treatment with interferon or glatiramer acetate, Immunosuppressive therapy should be offered. Proposed criteria to define inadequate responses to treatment require at least 6 months of optimum compliance and either relapse rate is increased/stable in comparison to that before treatment OR ≥2 events of demyelination (clinical/ MRI) within the last 12 months. Treatment options for inadequate response include change to another drug within first-line therapies or escalate to second-line therapy. Neutralizing antibodies may be responsible for frequent relapses in children on interferon therapy. Agents that can be used as second-line therapy are azathioprine, cyclophosphamide, methotrexate, rituximab, mitoxantrone, rituximab, and natalizumab [59 - 61]. Newer FDA approved oral agents in adults are dimethyl fumarate and teriflunomide (Table **2**).

Table 2. First-line therapy for pediatric-onset multiple sclerosis.

Drug	Dose	Route	Schedule
Interferon-beta 1a	30 µg	Intramuscular	Weekly
Pegylated Interferon beta 1a	125µg	Subcutaneous	Every 14days
Interferon beta 1b	0.25mg	Subcutaneous	Every 2 days
Glatiramer Acetate	20mg	Subcutaneous	Daily

Prognosis

Before the widespread use of DMT in pediatric MS patients, the relapse rate used to be higher. The rate of progression is lower in comparison to adults. Irreversible disability takes a long time to occur in pediatric MS (20-30 yr) but occurs at younger ages than adults because of the earlier age of onset. Permanent neurologic deficits are the visual defect and defect in the function of other cranial nerves, defect in motor and sensory function, defect in posture/balance and defect in bowel/bladder function. Children with MS have also been shown to have an overall smaller head size, brain volume, and thalamic volume in particular. As a result of gray matter degeneration, head size becomes smaller, and disability in cognition occurs in 30–50% of children with pediatric-onset MS [62 - 65]. Quality of life becomes poor because of fatigue which is a major symptom in pediatric MS. Other factors, which need attention, are quality of sleep, mood and hygiene of sleep.

Optic Neuritis

Unilateral or bilateral inflammation of optic nerves is known as optic neuritis which clinically manifests with dysfunction in vision. Etiology is usually idiopathic, and may be associated with generalized inflammatory conditions that involve multiple systems or inflammatory conditions restricted to CNS *e.g.* MS, ADEM, or NMOSD.

Clinical Presentation

It is among the few very common acquired forms of demyelination disorder. It constitutes almost one-fourth of all demyelination disorders present in children [13]. More commonly unilateral or sometimes bilateral loss of vision which can be severe is the typical presentation that takes hours to days to evolve and is preceded in most cases by viral infection [66, 67]. Besides, periocular pain, pain in movement of eyes, headache, abnormality in color vision, loss of visual field and afferent pupillary defect are other manifestations [68 - 71]. Unilateral involvement of ON can progress to bilateral involvement during the course of illness. Sometimes optic disc edema is seen on fundoscopy; however, it may be absent also. Therefore, the normal appearance of the optic nerve does not guarantee the absence of inflammation, as there might be retrobulbar optic nerve inflammation. The pale optic disc is seen after an initial episode or in the relapsing phase of ON.

Diagnosis

Prolonged latency is seen in visual evoked potentials (VEPs) [72]. Clinically silent inflammation in the other eye can be detected by VEPs in smaller children. Retinal structural changes, such as the thinning of the retinal nerve fiber layer (RNFL) which is helpful to monitor young children can be detected by Optical coherence tomography [73 - 75]. T1WI sequence of MRI orbits usually reveals thickening of the optic nerve with an increased intensity of signal on T2WI images but it may be normal (Fig. **4**). Demyelination which is induced by antibodies is more likely to be associated with a longitudinally extensive form of optic neuritis which involves optic chiasm, too [76]. Oligoclonal bands in CSF are useful to predict the risk of MS if MRI findings are also consistent with it. If brain MRI is normal and OCBs are absent in CSF; then, there is an extremely low risk to progress to MS.

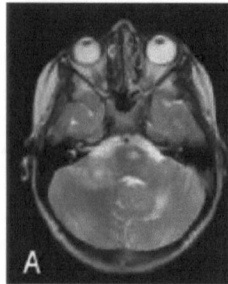

Fig. (4). T2WI sequence of axial flair weighted MRI brain shows bilateral Optic Neuritis.

Complete ophthalmologic evaluation with detailed history thorough clinical examination, and extensive investigations are essential for the exclusion of many conditions which are associated with optic neuritides such as systemic rheumatologic disorders (Behcet disease, sarcoidosis, systemic lupus erythematosus), infections (viral, tuberculosis, syphilis, Lyme disease), mitochondrial disorders (Leber hereditary optic neuropathy), toxic, metabolic, nutritional disorders or vascular events [77 - 79]. AQP4-Ab antibody level should be measured to take a decision to start prophylaxis as it is indicated in AQP4-b positive status. Similarly, MOG-Ab antibody level should also be measured to give counseling regarding recurrence of disease as MOG-Ab positive status indicates a higher risk of recurrence.

Treatment

Intravenous high dose corticosteroid therapy (methylprednisolone 20-30 mg/kg/day for 3 to 5 days, maximum dose-1000 mg per day) is the recommended first-line treatment. Although it leads to a speedy recovery, there is no difference in the long-term outcome as shown in the Optic Neuritis Treatment Trial (ONTT) done in adults [80 - 83]. Other treatment options are intravenous immunoglobulin (2 g/kg over 2 to 5 days) or plasmapheresis (5-7 exchanges every alternate day) [84 - 88]. Neuroprotection strategy consists of phenytoin which has a positive effect on RNFL thinning in cases of Acute Optic Neuritis.

Prognosis

Reassuringly, full recovery of High-contrast visual acuity (HCVA) usually occurs in children [87, 88]. Some damages in structural integrity (thinning of RNFL) are irreversible and are detected by Optical Coherence Tomography. Other defects that persist for lifelong are defects in color vision and low-contrast visual acuity (LCVA) impairment [89 - 91]. AQP4-antibody- positive status is usually the predictor of long-term defects in visual function in children.

Transverse Myelitis

Transverse myelitis (TM) is a condition with acute, partial, or complete demyelination of the spinal cord at any level with subsequent acute development of both motor and sensory deficits. There is a clear sensory level on examination with either unilateral or bilateral signs below the level of the lesion. A focal Hyperintense lesion is present in the T2WI image sequence of MRI spinal cord which is evidence of spinal cord inflammation [92]. Findings on examination of CSF are pleocytosis (more than 10 cells) and/or raised immunoglobulin G (IgG) index. It is a rapidly progressive disease and maximal disability occurs between 4 hr to 21 days.

Epidemiology

TM more commonly affects adults. Approximately 2 per million children per annum are affected by TM. A bimodal distribution of age is seen in children less than 5 yr of age and more than 10 yr of age [93]. The neurological deficits are usually severe and may be complete. In most cases, recovery is slow (takes weeks to months) and more likely to be incomplete. Approximately 40% of smaller children are likely to become ambulatory independently. Pathologically there is mononuclear cell infiltration in the perivascular area which indicates the infectious or inflammatory basis of disease. Sometimes spinal cord necrosis is seen that is more likely to be due to infections (enterovirus). In older children, the onset is rapid, with the most severe deficit in the neurologic function that occurs between 2 days to 2 weeks [94, 95]. In these children, recovery is more rapid, and is likely to be more complete as compared to younger children. In a few cases, necrosis and resultant permanent deficits may occur. Causes of TM are multiple but usually, it is idiopathic or may be due to immune-mediated damages to the spinal cord after an infection (viral or mycoplasma), or may be preceded by an immunization within few weeks before the onset of neurologic deficits [96]. Sometimes, direct infection of the cord may result in transverse myelitis. Other associated conditions with TM are Systemic vasculitis syndrome (SLE) and antibody-induced disorders of CNS (NMOSD associated with AQP4-Ab or MOG- Ab). Idiopathic forms of TM do not have a familial association or predisposition to a particular sex.

Acute flaccid myelitis is a variant of TM which is usually idiopathic or may be due to enterovirus D68 or D71) presents with weakness or paralysis, pleocytosis in CSF and features of myelitis and gray matter anterior horn abnormalities in MRI spine. There may be an asymmetric paralysis and it is usually not accompanied by deficits in the sensory part. Besides, the involvement of cranial nerves may occur and lead to facial muscle weakness, dysphagia, and dysarthria.

Clinical Manifestations

Pain in the neck or back is a common symptom. Other symptoms are anesthesia, numbness, areflexia, ataxia, or weakness in the parts below the level of lesion, priapism, and autonomic nervous system disturbances. These symptoms depend on the severity of lesions. Initially, there is flaccid paraplegia or quadriplegia due to spinal shock but it turns into spastic paralysis over a period of few weeks. Sometimes weakness is unilateral which suggests a hemicord lesion, which is more common in adolescents [97]. Another common finding is the retention of urine which occurs early in the course of the disease before incontinence which occurs later.

Early finding related to the sensory nervous system is due to the involvement of the posterior column, which can be elicited by examination of vibration and joint position sensation. Compromise in respiratory function may occur if the disease is very severe and involves higher levels of cord.

Diagnostic Evaluation and Differential Diagnosis

A complete evaluation is required to rule out etiologies before the diagnosis of acute TM is made. Other entities which can mimic acute TM are other disorder of demyelination, Guillain- Barré syndrome, Rheumatologic disorders, infectious myelitis and meningitis, abscess, trauma, spinal cord infarction, mass lesions arteriovenous malformations, distortion of the vertebral column and intervertebral disc and tumors of the spinal cord and spine [98, 99]. T1WI sequence of MRI spine (with/ without contrast enhancement) shows distension of the spinal cord at the level of involvement which mimics mass lesion. High intensity of signals involving multiple segments of the spinal cord is seen in the T2WI sequence of MRI spine in the infantile form of MS (Fig. **5**). Signal intensity is higher and located centrally which indicates an involvement of gray matter in addition to adjacent white matter in the T2WI sequence of MRI spine in the adolescent form of MS.

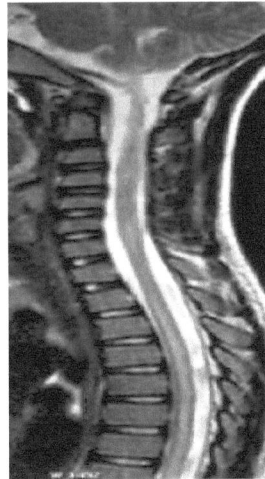

Fig. (5). T2WI sequence sagittal MRI spinal cord showing abnormal diffuse hyperintense lesion.

Usually, high signal intensity involves multiple segments but sometimes is restricted to one or two segments. Post gadolinium contrast enhancement in spine MRI that suggests inflammation is seen particularly in the infantile form of MS. The majority of acute MS lesions involve cervical and thoracic regions of the spinal cord. The diagnosis of MS suggested by the involvement of hemicord in axial section of spine MRI, while complete cord involvement with additional lesions in the brain and optic nerve suggests NMOSD. Vasculitic lesions (SLE) or infections (enterovirus) are suggested by the predominant involvement of gray matter. ADEM should be considered in patients with associated signs and symptoms of encephalopathy. Lumbar puncture should be done after excluding mass lesions on MRI.

There is pleocytosis (predominantly mononuclear cells infiltration) which is sometimes associated with elevated protein levels. All patients should be screened for AQP-4 and MOG antibodies to rule out NMOSD. Serological tests should be done to rule out the autoimmune conditions (*e.g.* SLE); especially, in older children.

Treatment

Standard treatment is not available for TM. The severity and duration of the disease can be decreased by modulating the immune response by using corticosteroids (methylprednisolone) in high dosage which is the initial treatment approach in children [100]. Intravenous immunoglobulin and plasma exchange are to be used in case of no response to corticosteroids [101]. Cyclophosphamide or rituximab are needed to be considered if the underlying disease process is antibody-mediated. Multiple Recurrences of the disease in children is an indication to start prophylactic therapy for the long term.

Neuromyelitis Optica Spectrum Disorders

Neuromyelitis optica spectrum disorders (NMOSDs) is characterized by the presence of Optic Neuritis with longitudinally extensive demyelinating spinal cord lesion which extends over three or more segments of the spinal cord. Also, there is the presence of antibodies to aquaporin-4 protein which is the protein linked to the astrocyte water channel.

Epidemiology

Adult patients with NMOSD are usually AQP4-Ab–positive while in children; NMOSD is more commonly associated with MOG-Ab status. The incidence of NMOSD in children is about 0.5% to 4.5%. Female sex preponderance is seen in both AQP4-Ab–positive NMOSD and MOG-Ab positive NMOSD. The Asian population is more predisposed to NMOSD as compared to the black or white population but mortality is higher in Africans as compared to others. NMOSD is mostly idiopathic but occasionally also has been reported in families. Genetic predisposition is also present in a few specific groups where the disease has been found to be associated with the HLADRB1* 0301 allele and a single-nucleotide polymorphism in CD58.

Pathogenesis

The aquaporin 4 water channels (which are targeted by mainly IgG1 subtype of IgG antibodies) are most abundantly found on the astrocyte foot processes within the optic nerve, periventricular area, brainstem, and spinal cord [102]. After the binding of these antibodies to extracellular loops of AQP4 protein, the classical complement pathway with C5b-C9 components gets activated, which leads to the attraction of leukocytes. Activation and degranulation of attracted leukocytes result in the death of astrocytes. Further in the process, simultaneous destruction of the oligodendrocytes and neurons also occurs by activated leukocytes and macrophages which have been attracted there by Chemokines released from degrading astrocytes. As a result of all these, the affected tissues become necrosed and cavitated.

Clinical Manifestations

Common signs and symptoms of NMOSD are those of Optic Neuritis such as pain in the eyes and diminished vision, due to Transverse Myelitis such as paresthesia and weakness below the level of lesion, or hiccups and intractable vomiting due to area postrema syndrome [103]. Optic Neuritis and Transverse Myelitis either present simultaneously or have separate occurrence weeks or years apart. Sometimes presentations with seizures and encephalopathy may be confused with ADEM.

Manifestations related to endocrine system disturbances in the form of diabetes insipidus, syndrome of inappropriate antidiuretic hormone secretion, obesity, disrupted puberty, hyperinsulinemia, diabetes mellitus, and thyroiditis may occur. Autoimmune disorders such as SLE, Sjogren syndrome, and other possible associations.

Imaging

MRI should include the optic nerve, entire spine, and brain. MRI Brain shows large, ill-defined demyelinating lesions that may be involving both white and gray matter (*e.g.* thalamus). Sometimes only subtle changes are visible in brain MRI, and occasionally, it may be normal. Demyelinating lesions in MRI are frequently found in the areas which are rich in aquaporin 4 channels (due to high antibody expression against AQP4 channels) *e.g.* the periventricular gray matter, hypothalamus and, dorsal brainstem [20].

Spine MRI shows longitudinally extensive TM where the demyelinating lesions involve three or more cord segments. Optic nerve MRI may reveal   longitudinally extensive Optic Neuritis in which the involvement of optic tract may be up to the optic chiasm. This is more commonly found in the MOG-Ab form of NMOSD.

Laboratory Findings

AQP4-Ab are present in the serum and CSF both, but more sensitive is the test for serum [104]. Similarly, MOG-Ab positivity is also more common in serum, probably because antibody production is extrathecal. Tests to detect antibody should be repeated if there is a high index of suspicion and initial tests were negative.CSF pleocytosis is often present but oligoclonal bands are absent in CSF.

Diagnosis

After exclusion of alternative diagnosis, NMOSD can be confirmed in an AQP4 antibody seropositive patient in presence of any one of the essential criteria which includes MRI findings compatible with Optic Neuritis, Transverse Myelitis, Narcolepsy, Area postrema Syndrome, and Diencephalic syndrome. The International Panel for NMO Diagnosis (IPND) now lays more emphasis on the AQP4 antibody status of patients diagnosed with NMOSD. If serological tests are negative for AQP4 antibody, then at least two of the essential criteria are needed to make a diagnosis of NMOSD [105].

Differential Diagnosis

Other disorders that are responsible for demyelinating lesions in CNS should be ruled out *e.g.* ADEM or Multiple Sclerosis. It is important to differentiate accurately NMOSD from MS because drugs used for long term treatment of MS may be ineffective for NMOSD or can exacerbate relapses.

Rheumatological or Vasculitis disorders (Behcet disease, Systemic Lupus Erythematosus. and Neurosarcoidosis) should be suspected if in presence of manifestations of other system involvement. The absence of antibodies related to NMOSD in CSF or serum is helpful to exclude viral encephalomyelitis, idiopathic Transverse Myelitis, and tropical spastic paraparesis. Genetic defects that can mimic NMOSD are DARS gene mutation or hemophagocytic lymphohistiocytosis (HLH). Metabolic disorders in the differential diagnosis are riboflavin responsive defects and biotinidase deficiency. Nutritional deficiencies such as deficiency of Vitamin B12 and Vitamin E, malignancies such as Langerhans cell histiocytosis and Lymphoma, and granulomatous inflammation such as tuberculosis can also have similar presentation; therefore, these need to be ruled out.

Treatment

Injectable methylprednisolone in high dosage (30mg per kg, max.1000mg) for 5 days or more depending on the severity of the disease is used to resolve initial acute attacks or relapses followed by tapering dosage of oral steroids for a few weeks. The course of injectable steroid may need to be repeated or plasmapheresis or intravenous immunoglobulins (2gm per kg for 2 to 5 days) may need to be considered in case of no response to initial treatment.

Disease-modifying therapy is effective to reduce the rate of relapses and needs to be started in NMOSD patients positive with AQP4-Ab. Agents used are Rituximab, mycophenolate mofetil (MMF), and azathioprine. Rituximab is also useful to treat acute attacks. A newer monoclonal antibody against complement protein C5, Eculizumab is found useful in adults to reduce relapses in severe forms of NMOSD. Another monoclonal antibody against IL-6, tocilizumab showed effectiveness in adults with AQP4 antibody-positive NMOSD. Satralizumab, a humanized monoclonal antibody against IL-6 is currently under trial.

Prognosis

Most of the patients of NMOSD with AQP4-antibody-positive status have frequent relapses that lead to the gradual deterioration in motor functions. MOG-Antibody-positive NMOSD is usually a monophasic illness and has a better prospectus for long-term prognosis. Irreversible deficits in neurological functions are related to vision (visual acuity, color vision and field of vision), sensory and motor function, posture/balance, and bladder or bowel control.

Schilder's Disease

It is also known as myelinoclastic diffuse sclerosis. For the first time, it was described in 1912 by Schilder and Poser further elaborated it in 1992. It is defined as a sub-acute disorder characterized by large bilateral and poorly symmetrical demyelinating lesions of the CNS.

Epidemiology

Etiology is not clear in most of the cases; however, it is shown to be associated with tuberculosis in some cases in a few studies [106]. Schilder's disease is mainly the disease of children with the peak age of presentation is 5-14 years.

Clinical Presentation

Affected children usually present with nonspecific signs and symptoms such as regression of milestones, seizures, movement disorder *e.g.* ataxia, and manifestations of increased intra cranial tension.

Diagnosis

In a Neuro-imaging study, the T2WI sequence of MRI brain shows large (at least 2 cm in size), confluent, the plaque-like hyperintense lesion (tumefactive demyelination) in the deep white matter which may be confused as abscess or neoplasm (Fig. **6**). It is important to differentiate demyelination neoplasm or infection early to avoid unnecessary chemotherapy/radiotherapy or surgery. T1WI MRI brain shows a lesion that is centrally hypointense and surrounded by a thick band of comparatively increased intensity. Gadolinium contrast-enhanced image shows an incomplete one side (rim facing lateral ventricles) limited enhancement. Schilder's disease can be differentiated from multiple sclerosis or ADEM by the absence of any additional lesions on neuroimaging of the brain and spine. CSF examination reveals raised protein and elevated IgG index in 50-60% of patients (Table **3**).

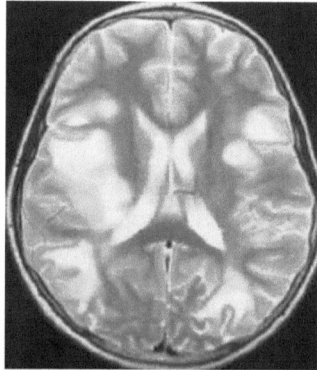

Fig. (6). T2WI sequence axial MRI brain showing hyper-intense, well defined, multiple lesions in the white matter surrounded by ill-defined areas of hyper-intensity.

T2WI sequence axial MRI brain demonstrates hyper-intense, well defined, multiple lesions of the white matter surrounded by ill-defined areas of hyper intensity consistent with Schilder's Disease.

Treatment

Rapid response is observed with a high dose of intravenous methylprednisolone which is the treatment of choice [17].

Table 3. Important Differential Diagnosis of acquired white matter disorder in children.

Disorder	Clinical Characteristics	Imaging
Infections		
- HIV Encephalopathy - Progressive Multifocal Leukoencephalopathy - Borreliosis - Sub-acute Sclerosing Panencephalitis - HTLV1 - Lymes Disease - Neurosyphillis	- Immunocompromised - Microcephaly - Pyramidal tracts sign - Developmental delay	- Cerebral atrophy - Bilateral symmetrical, confluent changes in white matter - Basal ganglia calcification - Multi-focal lesions with increased T2WI signal intensity mainly in frontal and parieto-occipital region - Involvement of subcortical U fibers
Vasculitides/Autoimmune		
- Systemic Lupus Erythematosus - Isolated CNS angiitis - CADASIL (Cerebral autosomal dominant arteriopathy with subcortical infarcts and leukoencephalopathy)	- Multi-system involvement - Antinuclear antibody positive - Rare in children	- Multi-focal lesions of increased signal intensity in T2WI/FLAIR - Infarcts - Contrast-enhanced active lesions
Tumors		
- Medulloblastoma - CNS Lymphoma - Astrocytoma	- Insidious onset - Presence of malignant cells in CSF	- Decreased intensity in T1WI - Increased intensity in T2WI - Frequent involvement of gray matter
Leukodystrophies		
- Adrenoleukodystrophy - Krabbe's Disease - Metachromatic Leukodystrophy - Alexander's disease	- Male sex - Skin hyperpigmentation - Problems in learning and behavior - Abnormally increased level of very long-chain fatty acids in the body	- Confluent symmetrical lesions - Predominant involvement of posterior part of the brain - Involvement of corticospinal tract and Splenium - Outer edge contrast enhancement
Mitochondrial		
Leigh's Disease	- Neurological regression - Ophthalmoplegia - Dystonia - Hyperlactatemia	- Bilateral symmetrical increased signal intensity of putamen and caudate nuclei in T2WI/FLAIR images - Diffuse hyperintensities in cortical white matter
Nutritional deficiencies		
- Vitamin B12 - Vitamin E - Folate	- Peripheral neuropathy - Anaemia - Myelopathy	Periventricular increased signal intensity in T2WI
Toxins/ Drugs/Radiation		

(Table 3) cont.....

Disorder	Clinical Characteristics	Imaging
Lead, Isoniazid, Radiation	Exposure History	- Bilateral, diffuse involvement of central and periventricular white matter with decreased T1WI and increased T2WI signal intensity - Sparing of Subcortical U fibers
Osmotic demyelination syndrome		
Osmotic demyelination syndrome	Rapid correction of Hyper or Hyponatremia	- Symmetrical changes in Basal Ganglia and cortical White Matter with decreased T1WI and increased FLAIR/T2WI signal intensity - Pons: centrally located lesion with sparing of corticospinal tracts
Infiltrative		
Sarcoidosis Histiocytosis	- Cranial nerve palsy - Visual disturbances - Aseptic meningitis - Hypothalamic dysfunction - Visual disturbances	- Discrete lesions in the periventricular area and contrast enhancement in meninges and hypothalamus - Decreased T1WI, and increased T2WI signal intensity in hypothalamus and cerebellum - Lesions in skull and mastoid

Table **4** highlights the differences among Important Acquired Demyelinating disorders in children.

Table 4. Differences among Important Acquired Demyelinating disorders in children.

-	ADEM	Multiple Sclerosis	Neuromyelitis Optica	Schilder's Disease
Age	Less than 10 years	More than 10 years	20 to 40 years	5 to 14 years
Gender	Male = Female	Female > Male	Female > Male	Male > Female
Encephalopathy	Essential	Rare	Not present	Not present
History of Flu- like Illness	Very Frequently present	Variably present	Frequently present	Not present
Course	Monophasic or Multiphasic	Relapsing Remitting, Primary Progressive, Secondary	Monophasic, Relapsing	Monophasic – not remitting, Remitting, Progressive
Common Area Involved	Basal Ganglia, Brainstem, Thalamus	Periventricular White Matter, Optic Nerve, Brain stem	Optic Nerve, Spinal cord	Central Semiovale, Parieto- occipital white matter

(Table 4) cont.....

-	ADEM	Multiple Sclerosis	Neuromyelitis Optica	Schilder's Disease
Neuroimaging (MRI)	Large, Symmetrical lesions	Small lesions	Nonspecific size of lesions	Large lesions
Spinal Cord	-	Limited to one segment	More than 3 segments involved	-
CSF Cells	Pleocytosis with lymphocyte predominance (> 50 cells)	Pleocytosis (lymphocytes less than 50)	Pleocytosis with polymorphs predominance	Normal
CSF Oligoclonal bands	Variable	Positive	Negative	Negative
-	-	Progressive, Clinically Isolated Syndrome	-	-
NMO IgG	-	In less than 10% of cases	In more than 70% of cases	-

CONCLUSION

In children, acquired disorders of demyelination are under-recognized and diverse conditions that impose challenges for both diagnosis and treatment. To reduce long-term disabilities and to improve prognosis, early recognition and optimum management of these conditions are essential, which is now becoming easier with recent advances in the neuroimaging modalities, revised definitions, and newer treatment options. Further studies are needed to understand more clearly some of the aspects of these conditions such as etiology, pathogenesis, biomarkers, and standardized protocols for treatment.

CONSENT FOR PUBLICATION

Not applicable.

CONFLICT OF INTEREST

The authors declare no conflict of interest, financial or otherwise.

ACKNOWLEDGEMENT

Declared none.

REFERENCES

[1]   Purves D, Augustine GJ, Fitzpatrick D, *et al.* Neuroscience. 2nd edition. Sunderland (MA): Sinauer

Associates; 2001. Increased conduction velocity as a result of myelination. 2001.
https://www.ncbi.nlm.nih.gov/books/NBK10921/

[2]   Duncan ID, Radcliff AB. Inherited and acquired disorders of myelin: The underlying myelin
        pathology. Exp Neurol 2016; 283(pt B): 452-75.
        [http://dx.doi.org/10.1016/j.expneurol.2016.04.002]

[3]   Love S. Demyelinating diseases. J Clin Pathol 2006; 59(11): 1151-9.
        [http://dx.doi.org/10.1136/jcp.2005.031195] [PMID: 17071802]

[4]   Haines , D. Jeffery, *et al.* Axonal damage in multiple sclerosis. The Mount Sinai journal of medicine,
        New York 2011; . 78,2(2011): 231-43.
        [http://dx.doi.org/10.1002/msj.20246]

[5]   Legido A, Tenembaum SN, Katsetos CD, Menkes JH. Autoimmune and postinfectious diseases.Child
        neurology. Philadelphia: Lippincott Williams & Wilkins 2006; pp. 561-3.

[6]   Van der Knaap MS, Valk J, Eds. Magnetic resonance of myelination and myelin disorders. New York:
        Springer 2005.
        [http://dx.doi.org/10.1007/3-540-27660-2]

[7]   Mehndiratta MM, Gulati NS. Central and peripheral demyelination. J Neurosci Rural Pract 2014; 5(1):
        84-6.
        [http://dx.doi.org/10.4103/0976-3147.127887] [PMID: 24741263]

[8]   Lassmann H. Classification of demyelinating diseases at the interface between etiology and
        pathogenesis. Curr Opin Neurol 2001; 14(3): 253-8.
        [http://dx.doi.org/10.1097/00019052-200106000-00001] [PMID: 11371746]

[9]   Krupp LB, Tardieu M, Amato MP, *et al.* International Pediatric Multiple Sclerosis Study Group
        criteria for pediatric multiple sclerosis and immune-mediated central nervous system demyelinating
        disorders: revisions to the 2007 definitions. Mult Scler 2013; 19(10): 1261-7.
        [http://dx.doi.org/10.1177/1352458513484547] [PMID: 23572237]

[10]   Rust RS. Multiple sclerosis, acute disseminated encephalomyelitis, and related conditions. Semin
        Pediatr Neurol 2000; 7(2): 66-90.
        [http://dx.doi.org/10.1053/pb.2000.6693] [PMID: 10914409]

[11]   Tenembaum S, Chitnis T, Ness J, Hahn JS. Acute disseminated encephalomyelitis. Neurology 2007;
        68(16) (Suppl. 2): S23-36.
        [http://dx.doi.org/10.1212/01.wnl.0000259404.51352.7f] [PMID: 17438235]

[12]   Dale RC. Acute disseminated encephalomyelitis. Semin Pediatr Infect Dis 2003; 14(2): 90-5.
        [http://dx.doi.org/10.1053/spid.2003.127225] [PMID: 12881796]

[13]   Banwell B, Kennedy J, Sadovnick D, *et al.* Incidence of acquired demyelination of the CNS in
        Canadian children. Neurology 2009; 72(3): 232-9.
        [http://dx.doi.org/10.1212/01.wnl.0000339482.84392.bd] [PMID: 19153370]

[14]   Leake JA, Albani S, Kao AS, *et al.* Acute disseminated encephalomyelitis in childhood:
        epidemiologic, clinical and laboratory features. Pediatr Infect Dis J 2004; 23(8): 756-64.
        [http://dx.doi.org/10.1097/01.inf.0000133048.75452.dd] [PMID: 15295226]

[15]   Pohl D, Hennemuth I, von Kries R, Hanefeld F. Paediatric multiple sclerosis and acute disseminated
        encephalomyelitis in Germany: results of a nationwide survey. Eur J Pediatr 2007; 166(5): 405-12.
        [http://dx.doi.org/10.1007/s00431-006-0249-2] [PMID: 17219129]

[16]   Murthy SN, Faden HS, Cohen ME, Bakshi R. Acute disseminated encephalomyelitis in children.
        Pediatrics 2002; 110(2 Pt 1): e21.
        [http://dx.doi.org/10.1542/peds.110.2.e21] [PMID: 12165620]

[17]   Kleiman M, Brunquell P. Acute disseminated encephalomyelitis: response to intravenous
        immunoglobulin. J Child Neurol 1995; 10(6): 481-3.

[http://dx.doi.org/10.1177/088307389501000612] [PMID: 8576561]

[18] Dale RC, de Sousa C, Chong WK, Cox TC, Harding B, Neville BG. Acute disseminated encephalomyelitis, multiphasic disseminated encephalomyelitis and multiple sclerosis in children. Brain 2000; 123(Pt 12): 2407-22.
[http://dx.doi.org/10.1093/brain/123.12.2407] [PMID: 11099444]

[19] Anlar B, Basaran C, Kose G, *et al.* Acute disseminated encephalomyelitis in children: outcome and prognosis. Neuropediatrics 2003; 34(4): 194-9.
[http://dx.doi.org/10.1055/s-2003-42208] [PMID: 12973660]

[20] McKeon A, Lennon VA, Lotze T, *et al.* CNS aquaporin-4 autoimmunity in children. Neurology 2008; 71(2): 93-100.
[http://dx.doi.org/10.1212/01.wnl.0000314832.24682.c6] [PMID: 18509092]

[21] Pröbstel AK, Dornmair K, Bittner R, *et al.* Antibodies to MOG are transient in childhood acute disseminated encephalomyelitis. Neurology 2011; 77(6): 580-8.
[http://dx.doi.org/10.1212/WNL.0b013e318228c0b1] [PMID: 21795651]

[22] Brilot F, Dale RC, Selter RC, *et al.* Antibodies to native myelin oligodendrocyte glycoprotein in children with inflammatory demyelinating central nervous system disease. Ann Neurol 2009; 66(6): 833-42.
[http://dx.doi.org/10.1002/ana.21916] [PMID: 20033986]

[23] Di Pauli F, Mader S, Rostasy K, *et al.* Temporal dynamics of anti-MOG antibodies in CNS demyelinating diseases. Clin Immunol 2011; 138(3): 247-54.
[http://dx.doi.org/10.1016/j.clim.2010.11.013] [PMID: 21169067]

[24] Ishizu T, Minohara M, Ichiyama T, *et al.* CSF cytokine and chemokine profiles in acute disseminated encephalomyelitis. J Neuroimmunol 2006; 175(1-2): 52-8.
[http://dx.doi.org/10.1016/j.jneuroim.2006.03.020] [PMID: 16697050]

[25] Franciotta D, Zardini E, Ravaglia S, *et al.* Cytokines and chemokines in cerebrospinal fluid and serum of adult patients with acute disseminated encephalomyelitis. J Neurol Sci 2006; 247(2): 202-7.
[http://dx.doi.org/10.1016/j.jns.2006.05.049] [PMID: 16784758]

[26] Sacconi S, Salviati L, Merelli E. Acute disseminated encephalomyelitis associated with hepatitis C virus infection. Arch Neurol 2001; 58(10): 1679-81.
[http://dx.doi.org/10.1001/archneur.58.10.1679] [PMID: 11594929]

[27] Hynson JL, Kornberg AJ, Coleman LT, Shield L, Harvey AS, Kean MJ. Clinical and neuroradiologic features of acute disseminated encephalomyelitis in children. Neurology 2001; 56(10): 1308-12.
[http://dx.doi.org/10.1212/WNL.56.10.1308] [PMID: 11376179]

[28] Alper G, Heyman R, Wang L. Multiple sclerosis and acute disseminated encephalomyelitis diagnosed in children after long-term follow-up: comparison of presenting features. Dev Med Child Neurol 2009; 51(6): 480-6.
[http://dx.doi.org/10.1111/j.1469-8749.2008.03136.x] [PMID: 19018840]

[29] Callen DJ, Shroff MM, Branson HM, *et al.* Role of MRI in the differentiation of ADEM from MS in children. Neurology 2009; 72(11): 968-73.
[http://dx.doi.org/10.1212/01.wnl.0000338630.20412.45] [PMID: 19038851]

[30] Rust RS Jr, Dodson WE, Trotter JL. Cerebrospinal fluid IgG in childhood: the establishment of reference values. Ann Neurol 1988; 23(4): 406-10.
[http://dx.doi.org/10.1002/ana.410230420] [PMID: 3382178]

[31] Nishikawa M, Ichiyama T, Hayashi T, Ouchi K, Furukawa S. Intravenous immunoglobulin therapy in acute disseminated encephalomyelitis. Pediatr Neurol 1999; 21(2): 583-6.
[http://dx.doi.org/10.1016/S0887-8994(99)00042-9] [PMID: 10465150]

[32] Keegan M, Pineda AA, McClelland RL, Darby CH, Rodriguez M, Weinshenker BG. Plasma exchange for severe attacks of CNS demyelination: predictors of response. Neurology 2002; 58(1): 143-6.

[http://dx.doi.org/10.1212/WNL.58.1.143] [PMID: 11781423]

[33]   Tenembaum S, Chamoles N, Fejerman N. Acute disseminated encephalomyelitis: a long-term follow-up study of 84 pediatric patients. Neurology 2002; 59(8): 1224-31.
[http://dx.doi.org/10.1212/WNL.59.8.1224] [PMID: 12391351]

[34]   McDonald WI, Compston A, Edan G, *et al.* Recommended diagnostic criteria for multiple sclerosis: guidelines from the International Panel on the diagnosis of multiple sclerosis. Ann Neurol 2001; 50(1): 121-7.
[http://dx.doi.org/10.1002/ana.1032] [PMID: 11456302]

[35]   Polman CH, Reingold SC, Edan G, *et al.* Diagnostic criteria for multiple sclerosis: 2005 revisions to the "McDonald Criteria". Ann Neurol 2005; 58(6): 840-6.
[http://dx.doi.org/10.1002/ana.20703] [PMID: 16283615]

[36]   Polman C H, Reingold S C, Banwell B, *et al.* Diagnostic criteria for multiple sclerosis revisions to the McDonald criteria Ann Neurol 2010; 69(2): 292-302.
[http://dx.doi.org/10.1002/ana.22366]

[37]   Krupp LB, Banwell B, Tenembaum S. Consensus definitions proposed for pediatric multiple sclerosis and related disorders. Neurology 2007; 68(16) (Suppl. 2): S7-S12.
[http://dx.doi.org/10.1212/01.wnl.0000259422.44235.a8] [PMID: 17438241]

[38]   Renoux C, Vukusic S, Mikaeloff Y, *et al.* Natural history of multiple sclerosis with childhood onset. N Engl J Med 2007; 356(25): 2603-13.
[http://dx.doi.org/10.1056/NEJMoa067597] [PMID: 17582070]

[39]   Chitnis T, Pirko I. Sensitivity vs specificity: progress and pitfalls in defining MRI criteria for pediatric MS. Neurology 2009; 72(11): 952-3.
[http://dx.doi.org/10.1212/01.wnl.0000344414.57976.97] [PMID: 19289735]

[40]   Ghezzi A, Deplano V, Faroni J, *et al.* Multiple sclerosis in childhood: clinical features of 149 cases. Mult Scler 1997; 3(1): 43-6.
[http://dx.doi.org/10.1177/135245859700300105] [PMID: 9160345]

[41]   Boiko A, Vorobeychik G, Paty D, Devonshire V, Sadovnick D. Early onset multiple sclerosis: a longitudinal study. Neurology 2002; 59(7): 1006-10.
[http://dx.doi.org/10.1212/WNL.59.7.1006] [PMID: 12370453]

[42]   Alotaibi S, Kennedy J, Tellier R, Stephens D, Banwell B. Epstein-Barr virus in pediatric multiple sclerosis. JAMA 2004; 291(15): 1875-9.
[http://dx.doi.org/10.1001/jama.291.15.1875] [PMID: 15100207]

[43]   Pohl D, Krone B, Rostasy K, *et al.* High seroprevalence of Epstein-Barr virus in children with multiple sclerosis. Neurology 2006; 67(11): 2063-5.
[http://dx.doi.org/10.1212/01.wnl.0000247665.94088.8d] [PMID: 17159123]

[44]   Banwell B, Krupp L, Kennedy J, *et al.* Clinical features and viral serologies in children with multiple sclerosis: a multinational observational study. Lancet Neurol 2007; 6(9): 773-81.
[http://dx.doi.org/10.1016/S1474-4422(07)70196-5] [PMID: 17689148]

[45]   Lünemann JD, Huppke P, Roberts S, Brück W, Gärtner J, Münz C. Broadened and elevated humoral immune response to EBNA1 in pediatric multiple sclerosis. Neurology 2008; 71(13): 1033-5.
[http://dx.doi.org/10.1212/01.wnl.0000326576.91097.87] [PMID: 18809840]

[46]   Banwell B, Bar-Or A, Cheung R, *et al.* Abnormal T-cell reactivities in childhood inflammatory demyelinating disease and type 1 diabetes. Ann Neurol 2008; 63(1): 98-111.
[http://dx.doi.org/10.1002/ana.21244] [PMID: 17932975]

[47]   Banwell B, Ghezzi A, Bar-Or A, Mikaeloff Y, Tardieu M. Multiple sclerosis in children: clinical diagnosis, therapeutic strategies, and future directions. Lancet Neurol 2007; 6(10): 887-902.
[http://dx.doi.org/10.1016/S1474-4422(07)70242-9] [PMID: 17884679]

[48]   Chabas D, Castillo-Trivino T, Mowry EM, Strober JB, Glenn OA, Waubant E. Vanishing MS T2-bright lesions before puberty: a distinct MRI phenotype? Neurology 2008; 71(14): 1090-3.
       [http://dx.doi.org/10.1212/01.wnl.0000326896.66714.ae] [PMID: 18824673]

[49]   Waubant E, Chabas D. Pediatric multiple sclerosis. Curr Treat Options Neurol 2009; 11(3): 203-10.
       [http://dx.doi.org/10.1007/s11940-009-0024-6] [PMID: 19364455]

[50]   Pohl D, Rostasy K, Reiber H, Hanefeld F. CSF characteristics in early-onset multiple sclerosis. Neurology 2004; 63(10): 1966-7.
       [http://dx.doi.org/10.1212/01.WNL.0000144352.67102.BC] [PMID: 15557527]

[51]   Chabas D J. Ness. Younger children with pediatric MS have a distinct CSF inflammatory profile at disease onset under review. 2009.

[52]   Hahn JS, Pohl D, Rensel M, Rao S. Differential diagnosis and evaluation in pediatric multiple sclerosis. Neurology 2007; 68(16) (Suppl. 2): S13-22.
       [http://dx.doi.org/10.1212/01.wnl.0000259403.31527.ef] [PMID: 17438234]

[53]   Banwell B, Arnold D, Bar-Or A, Ghezzi A, Greenberg B, Waubant E, *et al.* Effects of Fingolimod on MRI Outcomes in Patients with Pediatric Onset Multiple Sclerosis: Results from Phase 3 PARADIGMS Study. American Academy of Neurology (AAN) Annual Meeting. Los Angeles, CA. 2018.2018 Apr 27;

[54]   Thannhauser JE, Mah JK, Metz LM. Adherence of adolescents to multiple sclerosis disease-modifying therapy. Pediatr Neurol 2009; 41(2): 119-23.
       [http://dx.doi.org/10.1016/j.pediatrneurol.2009.03.004] [PMID: 19589460]

[55]   Banwell B, Reder AT, Krupp L, *et al.* Safety and tolerability of interferon beta-1b in pediatric multiple sclerosis. Neurology 2006; 66(4): 472-6.
       [http://dx.doi.org/10.1212/01.wnl.0000198257.52512.1a] [PMID: 16505297]

[56]   Kornek B, Bernert G, Balassy C, Geldner J, Prayer D, Feucht M. Glatiramer acetate treatment in patients with childhood and juvenile onset multiple sclerosis. Neuropediatrics 2003; 34(3): 120-6.
       [http://dx.doi.org/10.1055/s-2003-41274] [PMID: 12910434]

[57]   Ghezzi A. Immunomodulatory treatment of early onset multiple sclerosis: results of an Italian Co-operative Study. Neurol Sci 2005; 26(S4) (Suppl. 4): S183-6.
       [http://dx.doi.org/10.1007/s10072-005-0512-8] [PMID: 16388355]

[58]   Ghezzi A, Amato MP, Capobianco M, *et al.* Disease-modifying drugs in childhood-juvenile multiple sclerosis: results of an Italian co-operative study. Mult Scler 2005; 11(4): 420-4.
       [http://dx.doi.org/10.1191/1352458505ms1206oa] [PMID: 16042224]

[59]   Ghezzi A, Pozzilli C, Grimaldi LM, *et al.* Safety and efficacy of natalizumab in children with multiple sclerosis. Neurology 2010; 75(10): 912-7.
       [http://dx.doi.org/10.1212/WNL.0b013e3181f11daf] [PMID: 20820002]

[60]   Yeh EL. Krupp *et al.* Breakthrough disease in pediatric MS patients: a pediatric network experience. Annual Meeting of the American Academy of Neurology. Seattle, WA.

[61]   Karenfort M, Kieseier BC, Tibussek D, Assmann B, Schaper J, Mayatepek E. Rituximab as a highly effective treatment in a female adolescent with severe multiple sclerosis. Dev Med Child Neurol 2009; 51(2): 159-61.
       [http://dx.doi.org/10.1111/j.1469-8749.2008.03246.x] [PMID: 19191848]

[62]   Kaufman J, Birmaher B, Brent D, *et al.* Schedule for Affective Disorders and Schizophrenia for School-Age Children-Present and Lifetime Version (K-SADS-PL): initial reliability and validity data. J Am Acad Child Adolesc Psychiatry 1997; 36(7): 980-8.
       [http://dx.doi.org/10.1097/00004583-199707000-00021] [PMID: 9204677]

[63]   Amato MP, Goretti B, Ghezzi A, *et al.* Cognitive and psychosocial features in childhood and juvenile MS: two-year follow-up. Neurology 2010; 75(13): 1134-40.

[http://dx.doi.org/10.1212/WNL.0b013e3181f4d821] [PMID: 20876467]

[64]   Banwell BL, Anderson PE. The cognitive burden of multiple sclerosis in children. Neurology 2005; 64(5): 891-4.
[http://dx.doi.org/10.1212/01.WNL.0000152896.35341.51] [PMID: 15753431]

[65]   Cardoso M, Olmo NR, Fragoso YD. Systematic Review of Cognitive Dysfunction in Pediatric and Juvenile Multiple Sclerosis. Pediatr Neurol 2015; 53(4): 287-92.
[http://dx.doi.org/10.1016/j.pediatrneurol.2015.06.007] [PMID: 26233264]

[66]   Bonhomme GR, Waldman AT, Balcer LJ, *et al.* Pediatric optic neuritis: brain MRI abnormalities and risk of multiple sclerosis. Neurology 2009; 72(10): 881-5.
[http://dx.doi.org/10.1212/01.wnl.0000344163.65326.48] [PMID: 19273821]

[67]   Waldman AT, Stull LB, Galetta SL, Balcer LJ, Liu GT. Pediatric optic neuritis and risk of multiple sclerosis: meta-analysis of observational studies. J AAPOS 2011; 15(5): 441-6.
[http://dx.doi.org/10.1016/j.jaapos.2011.05.020] [PMID: 22108356]

[68]   Alper G, Wang L. Demyelinating optic neuritis in children. J Child Neurol 2009; 24(1): 45-8.
[http://dx.doi.org/10.1177/0883073808321052] [PMID: 18936195]

[69]   Lucchinetti CF, Kiers L, O'Duffy A, *et al.* Risk factors for developing multiple sclerosis after childhood optic neuritis. Neurology 1997; 49(5): 1413-8.
[http://dx.doi.org/10.1212/WNL.49.5.1413] [PMID: 9371931]

[70]   Lana-Peixoto MA, Andrade GC. The clinical profile of childhood optic neuritis. Arq Neuropsiquiatr 2001; 59(2-B): 311-7.
[http://dx.doi.org/10.1590/S0004-282X2001000300001] [PMID: 11460171]

[71]   Wilejto M, Shroff M, Buncic JR, Kennedy J, Goia C, Banwell B. The clinical features, MRI findings, and outcome of optic neuritis in children. Neurology 2006; 67(2): 258-62.
[http://dx.doi.org/10.1212/01.wnl.0000224757.69746.fb] [PMID: 16864818]

[72]   Voitenkov V, Skripchenko N, Klimkin A. Visual pathways involvement in clinically isolated syndrome in children. Int J Ophthalmol 2015; 8(2): 382-4.
[PMID: 25938060]

[73]   Yilmaz Ü, Gücüyener K, Erin DM, *et al.* Reduced retinal nerve fiber layer thickness and macular volume in pediatric multiple sclerosis. J Child Neurol 2012; 27(12): 1517-23.
[http://dx.doi.org/10.1177/0883073812447683] [PMID: 22752482]

[74]   Yeh EA, Marrie RA, Reginald YA, *et al.* Functional-structural correlations in the afferent visual pathway in pediatric demyelination. Neurology 2014; 83(23): 2147-52.
[http://dx.doi.org/10.1212/WNL.0000000000001046] [PMID: 25361777]

[75]   Yeh EA, Weinstock-Guttman B, Lincoff N, *et al.* Retinal nerve fiber thickness in inflammatory demyelinating diseases of childhood onset. Mult Scler 2009; 15(7): 802-10.
[http://dx.doi.org/10.1177/1352458509104586] [PMID: 19465453]

[76]   Ramanathan S, Prelog K, Barnes EH, *et al.* Radiological differentiation of optic neuritis with myelin oligodendrocyte glycoprotein antibodies, aquaporin-4 antibodies, and multiple sclerosis. Mult Scler 2016; 22(4): 470-82.
[http://dx.doi.org/10.1177/1352458515593406] [PMID: 26163068]

[77]   Pittock SJ, Lennon VA, de Seze J, *et al.* Neuromyelitis optica and non organ-specific autoimmunity. Arch Neurol 2008; 65(1): 78-83.
[http://dx.doi.org/10.1001/archneurol.2007.17] [PMID: 18195142]

[78]   Petzold A, Wattjes MP, Costello F, *et al.* The investigation of acute optic neuritis: a review and proposed protocol. Nat Rev Neurol 2014; 10(8): 447-58.
[http://dx.doi.org/10.1038/nrneurol.2014.108] [PMID: 25002105]

[79]   Fernández Carbonell C, Benson L, Rintell D, Prince J, Chitnis T. Functional relapses in pediatric

multiple sclerosis. J Child Neurol 2014; 29(7): 943-6.
[http://dx.doi.org/10.1177/0883073813501873] [PMID: 24065582]

[80]   Beck RW, Cleary PA, Anderson MM Jr, *et al.* A randomized, controlled trial of corticosteroids in the treatment of acute optic neuritis. N Engl J Med 1992; 326(9): 581-8.
[http://dx.doi.org/10.1056/NEJM199202273260901] [PMID: 1734247]

[81]   Beck RW, Cleary PA, Trobe JD, *et al.* The effect of corticosteroids for acute optic neuritis on the subsequent development of multiple sclerosis. N Engl J Med 1993; 329(24): 1764-9.
[http://dx.doi.org/10.1056/NEJM199312093292403] [PMID: 8232485]

[82]   Gal RL, Vedula SS, Beck R. Corticosteroids for treating optic neuritis. Cochrane Database Syst Rev 2015; 8(8): CD001430.
[PMID: 26273799]

[83]   Jayakody H, Bonthius DJ, Longmuir R, Joshi C. Pediatric optic neuritis: does a prolonged course of steroids reduce relapses? A preliminary study. Pediatr Neurol 2014; 51(5): 721-5.
[http://dx.doi.org/10.1016/j.pediatrneurol.2014.07.020] [PMID: 25152962]

[84]   Ruprecht K, Klinker E, Dintelmann T, Rieckmann P, Gold R. Plasma exchange for severe optic neuritis: treatment of 10 patients. Neurology 2004; 63(6): 1081-3.
[http://dx.doi.org/10.1212/01.WNL.0000138437.99046.6B] [PMID: 15452303]

[85]   Koziolek MJ, Tampe D, Bähr M, *et al.* Immunoadsorption therapy in patients with multiple sclerosis with steroid-refractory optical neuritis. J Neuroinflammation 2012; 9(1): 80.
[http://dx.doi.org/10.1186/1742-2094-9-80] [PMID: 22537481]

[86]   Bigi S, Banwell B, Yeh EA. Outcomes after early administration of plasma exchange in pediatric central nervous system inflammatory demyelination. J Child Neurol 2015; 30(7): 874-80.
[http://dx.doi.org/10.1177/0883073814545883] [PMID: 25246301]

[87]   Malik MT, Healy BC, Benson LA, *et al.* Factors associated with recovery from acute optic neuritis in patients with multiple sclerosis. Neurology 2014; 82(24): 2173-9.
[http://dx.doi.org/10.1212/WNL.0000000000000524] [PMID: 24850491]

[88]   Absoud M, Cummins C, Desai N, *et al.* Childhood optic neuritis clinical features and outcome. Arch Dis Child 2011; 96(9): 860-2.
[http://dx.doi.org/10.1136/adc.2009.175422] [PMID: 20554767]

[89]   The clinical profile of optic neuritis. Experience of the Optic Neuritis Treatment Trial. Arch Ophthalmol 1991; 109(12): 1673-8.
[http://dx.doi.org/10.1001/archopht.1991.01080120057025] [PMID: 1841573]

[90]   Baier ML, Cutter GR, Rudick RA, *et al.* Low-contrast letter acuity testing captures visual dysfunction in patients with multiple sclerosis. Neurology 2005; 64(6): 992-5.
[http://dx.doi.org/10.1212/01.WNL.0000154521.40686.63] [PMID: 15781814]

[91]   Balcer LJ, Baier ML, Pelak VS, *et al.* New low-contrast vision charts: reliability and test characteristics in patients with multiple sclerosis. Mult Scler 2000; 6(3): 163-71.
[http://dx.doi.org/10.1177/135245850000600305] [PMID: 10871827]

[92]   Alper G, Petropoulou KA, Fitz CR, Kim Y. Idiopathic acute transverse myelitis in children: an analysis and discussion of MRI findings. Mult Scler 2011; 17(1): 74-80.
[http://dx.doi.org/10.1177/1352458510381393] [PMID: 20858691]

[93]   Pidcock FS, Krishnan C, Crawford TO, Salorio CF, Trovato M, Kerr DA. Acute transverse myelitis in childhood: center-based analysis of 47 cases. Neurology 2007; 68(18): 1474-80.
[http://dx.doi.org/10.1212/01.wnl.0000260609.11357.6f] [PMID: 17470749]

[94]   De Goede CG, Holmes EM, Pike MG. Acquired transverse myelopathy in children in the United Kingdom--a 2 year prospective study. Eur J Paediatr Neurol 2010; 14(6): 479-87.
[http://dx.doi.org/10.1016/j.ejpn.2009.12.002] [PMID: 20089428]

[95]   Thomas T, Branson HM, Verhey LH, *et al.* The demographic, clinical, and magnetic resonance imaging (MRI) features of transverse myelitis in children. J Child Neurol 2012; 27(1): 11-21.
[http://dx.doi.org/10.1177/0883073811420495] [PMID: 21968984]

[96]   Kerr DA, Ayetey H. Immunopathogenesis of acute transverse myelitis. Curr Opin Neurol 2002; 15(3): 339-47.
[http://dx.doi.org/10.1097/00019052-200206000-00019] [PMID: 12045735]

[97]   Meyer P, Leboucq N, Molinari N, *et al.* Partial acute transverse myelitis is a predictor of multiple sclerosis in children. Mult Scler 2014; 20(11): 1485-93.
[http://dx.doi.org/10.1177/1352458514526943] [PMID: 24619933]

[98]   Messacar K, Schreiner TL, Maloney JA, *et al.* A cluster of acute flaccid paralysis and cranial nerve dysfunction temporally associated with an outbreak of enterovirus D68 in children in Colorado, USA. Lancet 2015; 385(9978): 1662-71.
[http://dx.doi.org/10.1016/S0140-6736(14)62457-0] [PMID: 25638662]

[99]   Rengarajan B, Venkateswaran S, McMillan HJ. Acute asymmetrical spinal infarct secondary to fibrocartilaginous embolism. Childs Nerv Syst 2015; 31(3): 487-91.
[http://dx.doi.org/10.1007/s00381-014-2562-9] [PMID: 25293530]

[100]   Defresne P, Meyer L, Tardieu M, *et al.* Efficacy of high dose steroid therapy in children with severe acute transverse myelitis. J Neurol Neurosurg Psychiatry 2001; 71(2): 272-4.
[http://dx.doi.org/10.1136/jnnp.71.2.272] [PMID: 11459911]

[101]   Scott TF, Frohman EM, De Seze J, Gronseth GS, Weinshenker BG. Evidence-based guideline: clinical evaluation and treatment of transverse myelitis: report of the Therapeutics and Technology Assessment Subcommittee of the American Academy of Neurology. Neurology 2011; 77(24): 2128-34.
[http://dx.doi.org/10.1212/WNL.0b013e31823dc535] [PMID: 22156988]

[102]   Banwell B, Tenembaum S, Lennon VA, *et al.* Neuromyelitis optica-IgG in childhood inflammatory demyelinating CNS disorders. Neurology 2008; 70(5): 344-52.
[http://dx.doi.org/10.1212/01.wnl.0000284600.80782.d5] [PMID: 18094334]

[103]   Kremer L, Mealy M, Jacob A, *et al.* Brainstem manifestations in neuromyelitis optica: a multicenter study of 258 patients. Mult Scler 2014; 20(7): 843-7.
[http://dx.doi.org/10.1177/1352458513507822] [PMID: 24099751]

[104]   Fryer JP, Lennon VA, Pittock SJ, *et al.* AQP4 autoantibody assay performance in clinical laboratory service. Neurol Neuroimmunol Neuroinflamm 2014; 1(1): e11.
[http://dx.doi.org/10.1212/NXI.0000000000000011] [PMID: 25340055]

[105]   Wingerchuk DM, Lennon VA, Pittock SJ, Lucchinetti CF, Weinshenker BG. Revised diagnostic criteria for neuromyelitis optica. Neurology 2006; 66(10): 1485-9.
[http://dx.doi.org/10.1212/01.wnl.0000216139.44259.74] [PMID: 16717206]

[106]   Pretorius ML, Loock DB, Ravenscroft A, Schoeman JF. Demyelinating Disease of the Schilder Type in 3 young SA children: dramatic response to Steroids. J Child Neurol 1998; 13: 197-201.
[http://dx.doi.org/10.1177/088307389801300501] [PMID: 9620009]

CHAPTER 8

Updates on Atopic Dermatitis

Edna Morán-Villaseñor[1] and **María Teresa García-Romero**[1,*]

[1] *Department of Dermatology, National Institute of Pediatrics, Insurgentes Sur 3700-C, Mexico City 04530, Mexico*

Abstract: Atopic dermatitis (AD) or atopic eczema is a complex and multifactorial chronic inflammatory skin disease that is characterized by intense itching and recurrent eczematous lesions. It is very frequent, affecting up to 20% of children in developed countries, and its prevalence has increased worldwide. Patients with AD have an increased risk of developing food allergy, allergic rhinitis, and asthma later in life; but may also present other comorbidities. The main symptom of AD is pruritus, which along with sleep disturbance, decreases the quality of life not only in patients but also in their families. Therapeutic options for AD have historically been limited, but recent advances have increased our understanding of its underlying mechanisms, contributing to the development of new therapies. In this chapter, we review the most recent knowledge about etiology, pathophysiology, clinical manifestations, comorbidities, and treatment options of AD.

Keywords: Atopic Dermatitides, Atopic Dermatitis, Atopic Eczema, Atopic Neurodermatitides, Atopic Neurodermatitis, Disseminated Neurodermatitides, Disseminated Neurodermatitis, Infantile Eczema, Pediatrics, Quality of life.

INTRODUCTION

Atopic dermatitis (AD) -also known as atopic eczema- is a chronic inflammatory skin disease that is characterized by intense itching and recurrent eczematous lesions. AD affects 10 to 20% of children in developed countries, and its prevalence has increased worldwide [1]. Several studies have demonstrated that the presence of AD increases the risk of developing food allergy, allergic rhinitis, and asthma later in life [2, 3]. Comorbidities, pruritus, and sleep disturbance significantly decrease quality of life not only in patients but in their families as well [4]. AD is complex and multifactorial, with historically limited therapeutic options, but significant recent advances have increased our understanding of the underlying mechanisms of AD, contributing to the development of new therapies.

---

* **Corresponding author María Teresa García-Romero:** Department of Dermatology, National Institute of Pediatrics, Insurgentes Sur 3700-C, Mexico City 04530, Mexico; Tel: 52-55-1084-0900; Ext. 2034; E-mail: teregarro@gmail.com

Nima Rezaei and Noosha Samieefar (Eds.)

EPIDEMIOLOGY

There are two main challenges when evaluating the epidemiology of AD: first, there are no widely accepted biomarkers or objective diagnostic tests for AD; and second, there is a lack of standardized nomenclature for AD which makes it difficult to develop consistent questionnaires for epidemiology research [5].

Overall, it is considered that AD affects 10 to 20% of children in developed countries and that its prevalence has increased worldwide in the past 30 years [1, 6, 7]. Prevalence estimates of childhood AD in the United States range from 6% to 12.97%, depending on the study design and approach used [5, 8, 9]. The International Study of Asthma and Allergies in Childhood (ISAAC) is the biggest and only study that has taken a global approach; it provided a global map of AD and found a wide variation in prevalence values worldwide, from 2.0% in Iran to 22.3% in Sweden at ages 6 to 7 years and from 1.4% in China to 21.8% in Morocco at ages 13 years to 14 years [6]. The ISAAC also found a global increase in the prevalence of symptoms of eczema from 1994-1995 to 2002-2003 [6]. Data from the National Health Interview Survey (NHIS), a US population-based household survey, indicates that the prevalence of childhood AD steadily increased from approximately 8% in 1997 to more than 12% in 2010 [5]. Many hypotheses have been explored to explain this increase, including modulation of immune priming by hygiene, gut microbiota diversity, exposure to endotoxins through farm animals, and the effects of pollution, climate, and diet [7].

ETIOLOGY

The pathophysiology of atopic dermatitis is complex and not fully understood yet. It is proposed to be the result of an interaction of genetic and environmental factors that ultimately leads to impaired epidermal barrier function and immune dysregulation (Fig. **1**) [10, 11].

IMPAIRED SKIN BARRIER FUNCTION

The most important function of the skin is to provide an effective barrier between the internal and external environments of an organism. The epidermal barrier limits passive water loss, restricts environmental chemical absorption, and prevents microbial infection. Therefore, any damage to the structure of the skin barrier enhances the penetration of allergens to the skin, increases transepidermal water loss (TEWL), and contributes to immune dysfunction [11, 12].

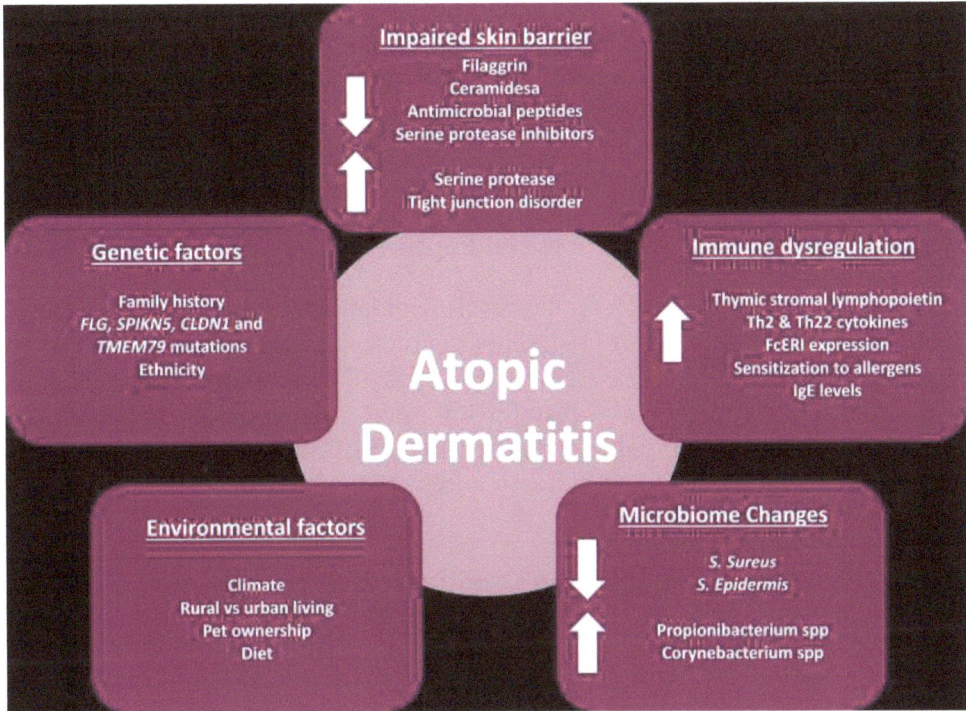

Fig. (1). Skin barrier abnormalities and immune dysfunction are the main features of atopic dermatitis (11).

Major contributors to an impaired skin barrier function include:

Decreased Filaggrin

Filaggrin (FLG) is a structural protein responsible for the keratinization, moisturization, and antimicrobial peptide functions of the skin. It is the main component of keratohyalin granules, and their breakdown products contribute to epidermal hydration and barrier function [13].

FLG can be broken down into free amino acids and converted into urocanic acid, which maintains the acidity level in the skin, and pyrrolidine carboxylic acid, which acts as a natural moisturizer. Mutations in FLG gene are associated with increased TEWL and dry skin in patients with AD [14].

However, 40% of FLG mutation carriers do not develop AD, and FLG mutations are only found in 10% of patients with AD [15]. Therefore, genetic abnormalities in FLG alone do not explain all the skin barrier dysfunctions of AD.

Decreased Ceramides

Decreased amounts of ceramides are also observed in patients with AD, both in lesional and non-lesional skins [16, 17]. An increased pH and an elevated serine proteinase activity promote inactivation and degradation of acid sphingomy-elinase and β-glucocerebrosidase, which are necessary enzymes for ceramide synthesis. Changes in the intercellular lipid composition contribute to the increased skin permeability seen in AD [18].

Decreased Production of Antimicrobial Peptides

Patients with AD have deficient expression of antimicrobial peptides (AMP) (cathelicidins and β-defensins) [19]. This decreased expression is due to altered filaggrin expression and decreased activity of toll-like receptors 2 (TLR2), which induce normal antimicrobial, β-defensin, and cathelicidin expression in keratinocytes [11]. A deficiency in the expression of antimicrobial peptides may account for the susceptibility of patients with AD to skin infection with *S.aureus* [19].

Decreased Serine Protease Inhibitors and Increased Serine Protease

An elevated serine proteinase activity reduces lamellar body secretion through plasminogen activator type 2 (PAR2) signaling. An increase in serine protease production is related to the reduced stratum corneum in skin of patients with AD. An elevated serine proteinase activity, as well as increased pH, promote inactivation and degradation of β-glucocerebrosidase and acid sphingomyelinase, both necessary for the adequate synthesis of ceramides [11].

Tight Junction Disorder

Tight junctions are complex intracellular barriers that control the permeability in the cell membranes of keratinocytes of the epidermal granular layer, and thus, they act as a second physical barrier. Knockout of claudin-1 (CLDN1), which is the most important adhesion protein in tight junctions, results in a critical lethal epidermal barrier defect in mice [20]. Reduced CLDN1 levels have also been detected in lesional AD skin with a significant decrease in tight junctions barrier function [21].

Immune Dysfunction

In the context of an altered epidermal barrier, antigens encounter epidermal Langerhans cell and inflammatory epidermal dendritic cells, bearing trimeric high-affinity receptor for IgE, culminating in IgE-mediated hypersensitivity, and alterations in Th1- and Th2- mediated immune responses (Fig. **2**) [11].

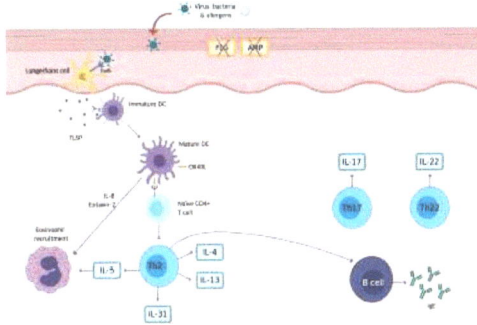

Fig. (2). Pathophysiology of atopic dermatitis.

Increased Thymic Stromal Lymphopoietin.

Thymic stromal lymphopoietin (TSLP) is a proinflammatory cytokine produced by epithelial cells. Keratinocytes in AD skin express high levels of TSLP, contributing to the initiation and exacerbation of immune responses [22]. TSLP initiates the innate and adaptative phases of immune responses in the skin by inducing the maturation of dendritic cells to express OX40L, which in turn differentiates naïve CD4+ T cells into Th2 cells to produce Th2 cytokines such as IL-4, IL-5 and IL-13, leading to the secretion of IgE from B cells [23, 24] (Fig. **2**). TSLP also activates other innate immune cells, such as natural killer T cells and selectively increases basophil hematopoiesis and promotes peripheral basophilia [25]. Therefore, TSLP may be considered and efficient therapeutic target to treat AD.

Increased Production of Th2 and Th22 Cytokines

Another key aspect of immune dysregulation is the increased production of Th2 and Th22 cytokines. AD is considered a model of imbalance between response of Th 1 and 2 lymphocytes, with predominance of Th2 response [26]. Strong activation of the Th2 and Th22 inflammatory responses are observed in lesional skin of children with AD [27].

Th2 lymphocytes produce IL-4 and IL-13, which inhibit the expression of FLG, and reduce production of antimicrobial peptides, thus establishing a relationship between immune dysfunction and disruption of barrier function typical in AD [28].

IL-4 and IL-13 are implicated in the synthesis of IL-31, a key participant in the induction of pruritus, and IL-15, which mediates recruitment of Th2 and eosinophils. In turn, pruritus leads to scratching, and scratching enhances skin barrier dysfunction and colonization by *Staphylococcus aureus*. Even though pathogenesis pivots around Th2/Th22 response, recent studies have found participation of Th17 and contribution from the Th1 axis in the chronic phase [29].

Altered Skin Microbiota

For decades, an association between *Staphylococcus aureus* (*S. aureus*) and AD has been known and has been the rationale for management options including topical and oral antibiotics, and dilute bleach baths. As the genomic revolution has exploded in the past few years, we have learned much more about the skin microbiota and the alterations, or dysbiosis, that occur in patients with AD. Approximately 70% of lesions of patients with AD are colonized by *S. aureus;* those with more severe disease having a higher incidence of colonization [30]. The types of *S. aureus* strains found on AD lesions are different than those found in the wider community, with strains from clonal complex 1 being particularly prevalent (whereas clonal complex 30 and others are more prevalent in nasal carriage during health) [31, 32].

In one of the first studies that characterized the skin microbiota in children with AD using 16s ribosomal RNA bacterial gene sequencing from serial skin samples, dramatic differences were identified at sites of active disease compared to controlled disease or healthy controls. The proportion of *S. aureus* was greater during disease flares than at baseline or post-treatment; and correlated with disease severity and a decreased diversity in other species. *Staphylococcus epidermidis* (*S. epidermidis*) also significantly increased during flares; but *Streptococcus, Propionibacterium and Corynebacterium* species increased only after therapy and disease improvement [33].

There is evidence to believe that *S. aureus* colonization contributes to inflammation that prolongs the course and/or increases severity of AD through its pro-inflammatory nature and toxin production [34]. It has been found that *S. aureus* increased in abundance prior to the onset of AD in infants, supporting a causal role [35].

However, there are many other species of bacteria that have been found to have an important role in AD pathogenesis. *S. epidermidis*, the predominant *Staphylococcus* species in the skin of healthy patients, has been considered to have the ability to inhibit *S. aureus* [36]. Both *S. aureus* and *S. epidermidis* may share a mutualistic or commensal relationship to enhance common resistance to antimicrobial peptides or enhance binding to exposed extracellular matrix proteins in inflamed AD skin [33].

These findings may provide the scientific fundamentals for new therapeutic options using topical probiotics with the purpose of decreasing abundance of *S. aureus* and/or increasing production of anti-inflammatory molecules. Nakatsuji T *et al* studied the effects of topical application of *S. hominis* and *S. epidermidis* to patients with AD, finding significant reductions in relative abundance of *S. aureus* after 24 hours [37].

Genetic Factors

The fact that the concordance rate for AD is higher among monozygotic twins (77%) than among dizygotic twins (15%) supports the importance of genetic factors [38].

Family History

Having a family history of food allergy, allergic rhinitis, asthma or AD is a risk factor for the development of AD. In these children, the risk of developing AD by 2 years is between 30 and 50% [39]. The odds of developing AD are 2- to 3-fold higher in children with one atopic parent, and this increases to 3-to 5-fold if both parents are atopic [40]. Maternal atopy may pose a higher risk for infantile AD than paternal atopy [41].

Genetic Mutations

Several genes have been associated with the development of AD. The strongest known genetic risk factor for AD is loss-of-function mutations in the FLG gene [42]. As mentioned previously, FLG plays a key role in the terminal differentiation of the epidermis and formation of the skin barrier, including the stratum corneum. *FLG* null mutations confer a risk for earlier-onset AD, and for more severe, persistent disease [40].

Single nucleotide polymorphisms in the serine peptidase inhibitor *SPINK5* and the SP *KLK7,* and mutations in *CLDN1, TMEM79* [43], the IgE receptor FceRb, the innate immunity-related *NOD1* and -2 and *TLR2, -4* and *-9,* and mutations in the acquired immunity-related genes *IL-4, -5, -9, -10, -12, -13, -18,* and *-31* and *TSLP* have also been described [11].

Race/ethnicity

Studies performed in the United States have shown that some sociodemographic groups seem to have a higher risk for childhood AD. A higher prevalence, as well as more severe AD, has been observed in African Americans/blacks, and in Hispanics [5].

Environmental Factors

Significant differences in AD prevalence, not only between but also within countries, suggest that environmental risk factors may play an important etiologic role [7]. The fact that migrant populations who move from areas of low to regions with high disease prevalence typically adopt the AD risk of their new environment supports this.

Climate

There is evidence that outdoor climate influences prevalence of childhood eczema. Significantly lower eczema prevalence was found in areas with higher relative humidity, higher UV index, higher mean temperatures and lower precipitation [44]. It is likely that higher humidity protects against eczema by improving skin barrier function.

As for higher UV index, it has been reported that ultraviolet radiation causes local cell-mediated immunosuppression [45]. In an open randomized-controlled study, Byremo *et al*, found a significant improvement in AD in children after a 4 weeks' stay in a warm subtropical climate; assessed objectively by SCORAD, a quality of life (QoL) index and skin bacterial colonization [45].

Pet Ownership

A cohort study found that dog ownership in early childhood might potentially protect children from the development of AD up to the age of 4 years, while cat ownership increased the risk [46]. Li *et al*, also found that early life exposure to dog significantly decreased the risk of AD, however in their study, the protective effect of pet exposure on the risk of AD, included dogs, cats and rabbits [47].

Rural *vs* Urban Living

In a systematic review of 26 studies, 19 found a higher risk of AD in a urbanized area, suggesting that there is evidence of higher disease burden in cities compared with the countryside [48]. The lower prevalence of AD in rural as compared with urban areas suggests a link to the "hygiene hypothesis", which postulates that the reduced of early childhood exposure to infectious agents increases susceptibility to allergic diseases [49]; the protective effect seen with early day care, unpasteurized farm milk and animal exposure is likely to be due to a general increase in exposure to non-pathogenic microbes [50].

Diet

The ISAAC Phase Three study found a consistent protective effect between frequent consumption of fresh fruits and vegetables (1-2x/week) and severe AD risk, whereas the opposite was true for fast-food consumption (>3x/week) [51]. Two studies found that the intake of fish during pregnancy lowers AD risk in the offspring, these results have been attributed to fish's rich content in anti-inflammatory n-3 polyunsaturated fatty acids (n-3 PUFA) [52, 53].

CLINICAL COURSE

AD is not clinically present at birth, but often develops during the first months of life. Approximately 45% of all cases of AD begin within the first 6 months of life, 60% during the first year, and 85% before 5 years of age [38]. However, it can start at any age, even in adults (late-onset AD) [1].

Fortunately, the disease is mild in about 67% of affected children, moderate in 26%, and severe only in 7% of the patients [9].

AD is often referred to as the "itch that rashes" because of the pruritus that patients experience. This hallmark symptom is responsible for its significant negative impact on QoL [4].

The earliest clinical signs are skin dryness and roughness, but eczematous lesions usually do not occur before the second month of life [1]. After this age, characteristic skin findings can be seen, including: dry skin; acute, subacute, or chronic eczematous lesions; (Fig. **3A-D**), erosions; and excoriations. These lesions can affect any part of the body, but they show a typically age-related morphology and distribution (Fig. **4A-I**), rarely they can generalize to secondary erythroderma. The hallmark of AD is the chronic and relapsing course of these lesions [38].

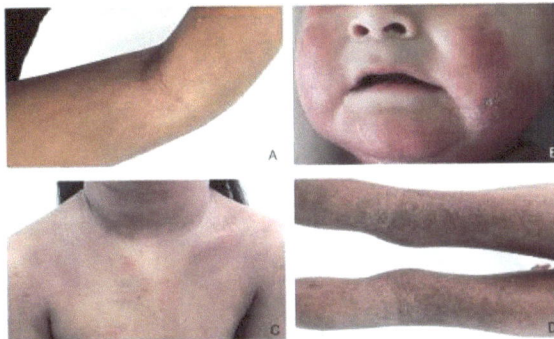

Fig. (3). Clinical findings in atopic dermatitis. **A:** dry skin, **B:** acute lesions, **C:** subacute lesions, **D:** chronic eczematous lesions.

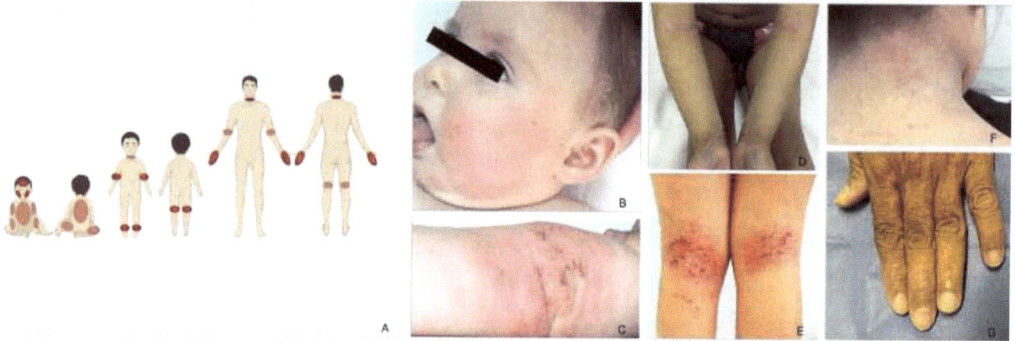

Fig. (4). A-I. Age-related distribution.

Age Related Distribution

Clinical manifestations of AD vary with age, and three stages can often be identified [1]:

Infantile

Up to 2 years. Infants tend to have red, crusted and weeping patches located on cheeks, scalp and extensor surfaces of the extremities. The midline of the face and the tip of the nose, in particular, are always spared (Fig. **4A-C**).

Childhood

Age 2-12 years. Lesions tend to localize to flexural surfaces, especially the cubital and knee folds, the wrists and ankles. Skin becomes thick and lichenified (Fig. **4D-F**).

Adult

In older children and adults, the flexural areas are still affected, and eczema is often present on the hands and feet (Fig. **4G-I**) [1, 38].

Morphological Variants

Although there are classic skin manifestations (dryness, roughness, eczematous lesions and lichenification), less common clinical manifestations of AD have been described, and they are considered morphological variants as shown in Fig. (5) [54].

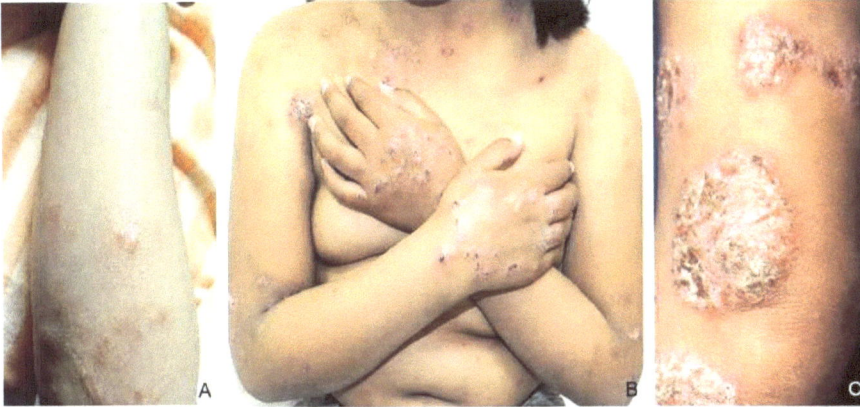

Fig. (5). Morphological variants in atopic dermatitis. **A**: follicular type, **B**: prurigo-like, **C**: nummular pattern.

Follicular Type

Characterized by densely aggregated follicular papules mainly on the lateral aspects of the trunk (Fig. **5A**). This variant is frequently seen in dark-skinned and Japanese patients [55]. It is thought to be more common in winter.

Papular-lichenoid

The juvenile papular dermatosis is localized mainly to the elbows and knees, and mainly occurs in spring and summer. It has been reported to be more frequent in infants [54].

Prurigo-like

Erythematous, excoriated papules and indurated nodules (Fig. **5B**). It is seen in patients with long-standing disease, and it is more frequent in preschool and school-aged children [54].

Nummular Pattern

Sharply demarcated patches and plaques of inflamed skin are characteristic of nummular or discoid eczema. These plaques are often colonized or infected with *S.aureus*. The extremities and the buttocks are the most commonly affected areas

(Fig. **5C**), and this variant is often difficult to treat [55]. As the prurigo like variant, nummular dermatitis is most common in preschool and school-aged children.

Erythroderma

This is a clinical presentation of severe AD that has generalized to affect all body sites, it is more common in preschool and school-aged children [54]. When a neonate or an infant presents erythroderma associated with failure to thrive, diarrhea and/or alopecia, a primary immunodeficiency must be ruled out [1].

Associated Clinical Features

Associated features of AD include pityriasis alba, keratosis pilaris, Dennie-Morgan fold, allergic salute, hyperlinearity of the palms and soles, ichthyosis vulgaris, Hertoghe's sign, circumoral pallor and white dermographism (Fig. **6**).

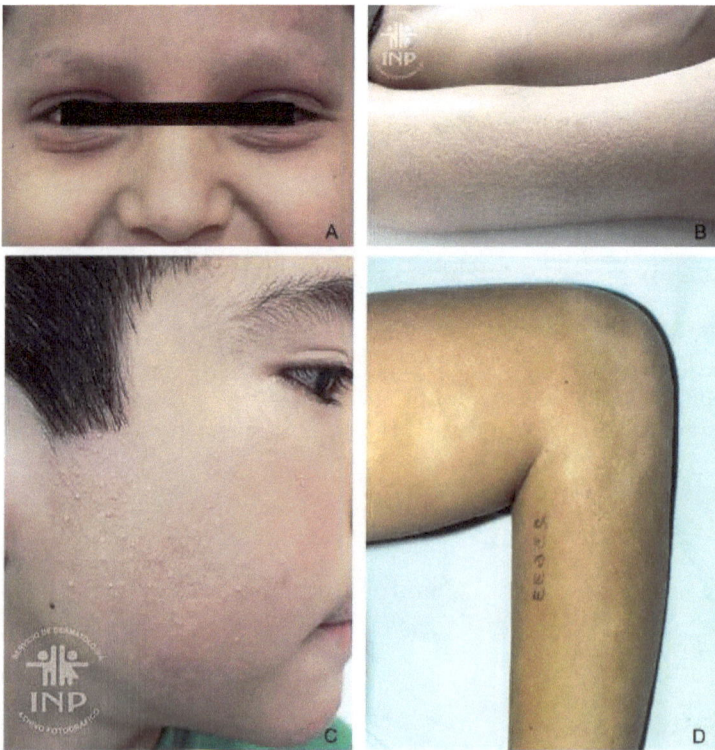

Fig. (6). Associated clinical features of atopic dermatitis. A: Dennie-Morgan fold, B: Ichthyosis vulgaris, C: Keratosis pilaris, D: Pityriasis alba.

COMORBIDITIES

There is growing evidence of comorbidities in both children and adults with AD [56, 57], which include other allergic diseases (allergic rhinitis, asthma and food allergy), cutaneous infections, sleep disturbances and mental health disorders [56, 58]. Recent studies have also found an association with osteoporosis [59, 60], fractures, anemia [61], obesity [62, 63], and cardiovascular disease [64], the association with the latter could be attributed to deterioration of QoL and the psychological aspects of AD, that could favor unhealthy habits, including a sedentary lifestyle and to chronic inflammation and the long-term use of immunosuppressants as systemic steroids [57].

Based on the presence of multiple comorbidities, AD cannot be considered just skin deep, and management of patients with AD must be multidisciplinary.

Association with Allergic Disease

Recent studies have demonstrated that the presence of AD increases the risk of developing food allergy, allergic rhinitis and asthma later in life [2, 9, 65]. This progression from AD to the manifestation of food allergy, allergic rhinitis, and asthma is often referred to the atopic or allergic march of childhood [2],and it is thought that AD is the "kick off" (Fig. **7**). Therefore, early diagnosis and management of AD may reduce the risk of developing other allergic diseases [3].

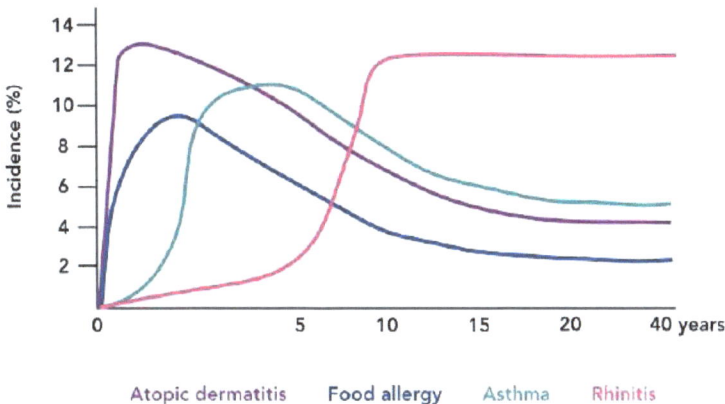

Fig. (7). The atopic march of childhood [2, 3].

Overall, infants with AD are approximately five times more likely to develop food allergy in comparison with infants without AD [9, 66]. However, the severity of skin disease directly correlates with the prevalence and severity of atopic comorbidities [9].

AD has been specifically associated with an increased risk of developing peanut allergy. Infants with eczema are 11 times more likely to develop peanut allergy through cutaneous exposure to environmental peanut allergens leading to development of food allergy through a broken-down skin barrier [66].

Nonetheless, current evidence suggests that strict diet management is not effective in the treatment of AD in the vast majority of patients [67, 68].

Contact Sensitizations

Patients with AD are more frequently sensitized against components of emollients such as preservatives, fragrances, emulsifiers, and antiseptics than are healthy individuals [69].

Depression, Anxiety and Attention Deficit Hyperactivity Disorder

The National Survey of Children's Health found statistically significant increases in the likelihood of autism, conduct disorder, attention deficit hyperactivity disorder, depression and anxiety in patients with AD [58].

A recent systematic review and meta-analysis found that almost 1 in 4 persons with AD had depressive symptoms, 1 in 6 had clinical depression, and 1 in 8 had suicidal ideation. Not only patients had a higher prevalence of depression, almost 1 in 3 parents of children with AD were depressed. Additionally, they evaluated effects of AD treatment on depression, and found that most studies showed improvement in depression scores when AD was treated [70].

Therefore, depression and other mental health disorders should be assessed in all patients with AD.

Sleep Disturbances

Severe eczema is associated with higher prevalence of sleep impairment [9, 71]. 47% to 89% of children with AD reporting sleep disturbance. The most commonly reported sleep problems include difficulty falling sleep, frequent nighttime awakenings, and excessive daytime sleepiness [71].

Parents of affected children also experience sleep loss during flare-ups [72]. Sleep disturbance not only impairs QoL, both of patients and their parents, it is also associated with higher rates of behavioral problems, impaired neurocognitive function, changes in mood, attention deficit hyperactivity disorder, and short stature, because sleep is essential for growth and development [73 - 76].

Pruritus and scratching movements disrupting sleep seem to be the most straightforward reason for sleep disturbance in children with AD, however new theories suggest that dysregulated levels of cytokines, could contribute to sleep disturbance [77].

An effective treatment plan is necessary in order to minimize the QoL impairment because of poor sleep in both affected patients and their caregivers.

COMPLICATIONS

Infections

Bacterial

S.aureus is the leading cause of skin and soft-tissue infections in patients with AD (Fig. **8C**). More than 75% of affected children are colonized by *S.aureus*, compared with <25% of healthy children in control groups [26]. Impaired TLR2 function and decreased antimicrobial peptide expression disrupt the normal immune response to *S. aureus* (10,11). The deficient epidermal barrier, with insufficient antimicrobial peptide upregulation, further contributes to *S. aureus* colonization. *S.aureus* contributes to exacerbations and chronification of disease through production of proteases, release of enterotoxins that act as T-cel- -activation superantigens, IgE-mediated sensitization and induction of mast cell degranulation [1]. It also causes activation of the NOD-, LRR- and pyring domain-containing protein 3 (NLRP3) inflammasome [10, 11].

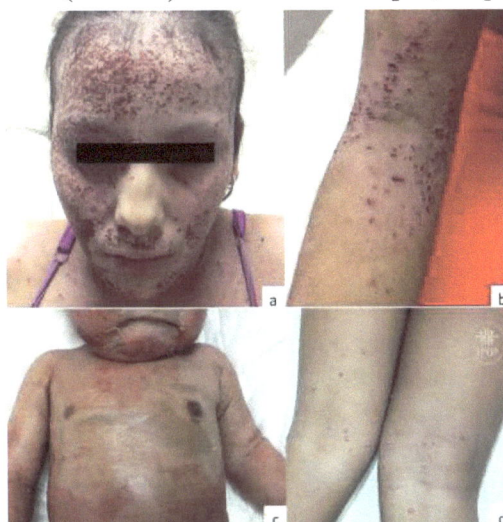

Fig. (8). Infectious complications of atopic dermatitis. a-b: Eczema herpeticum, c: *S.aureus* infection, d: Eczema molluscatum.

Viral

Patients with AD tend to have widespread disseminated viral infections, mostly due to herpes simplex virus, coxsackievirus and molluscum contagiosum virus. The disturbed skin barrier in AD might provide easier access for the virus, in addition Th2 cell predominance leads to production of IL-4, which induces IgE production and prevents differentiation of IFN-γ-producing Th1 cells, the lower levels of IFN-γ in the skin of patients with AD may allow the viruses to overgrow [78].

Eczema Herpeticum

Severe widespread skin infection with herpes simplex virus over AD lesions is called eczema herpeticum, and occurs in 3% of patients, particularly those with severe AD (Fig. **8A-B**) [1]. A decrease in CLDN1 expression in patients with AD is related to increased susceptibility to HSV-1 infection [11]. Prompt systemic antiviral therapy is required to limit disease duration and prevent further complications, such as herpes encephalitis or herpes keratitis [78, 79].

Eczema Coxsackium

In the past few years, atypical severe and extensive cases of hand, foot and mouth disease attributed to coxsackievirus A6 were reported, particularly in patients with previous AD. This eruption was termed eczema coxsackium and can have vesiculobullous, papular, petechial/purpuric manifestations. One characteristic feature is delayed onychomadesis [80].

Eczema Molluscatum

Patients with AD not only have more molluscum contagiosum virus infections than nonatopic individuals, but they also have more widespread disease, with up to several hundred lesions (Fig. **8D**). The itch and scratch cycle also contribute to molluscum dissemination and persistence [78].

Quality of Life

AD can negatively affect the QoL of both the patient, as well as parents and other caregivers, to a greater extent than other chronic diseases of childhood. Taking care of a child with moderate-to-severe AD was found to have a significantly higher impact on the social, emotional, and financial aspects of family, compared to caring for a child with insulin-dependent diabetes [81].

QoL in children with AD is often markedly impaired [82] due to symptoms such's as extreme pruritus, scratching and sleep disturbances that affect productivity at school; but also due to negative emotions and an increased number of mental health comorbidities, as mentioned previously [58]. Children often feel socially isolated because they cannot participate in all activities, and because of negative comments from others [4].

Patients' parents also experience decreased QoL caused by their children's sleep disorders and daytime tiredness. Parents can suffer emotional distress because treatment can be time consuming and expensive [4, 82].

Assessment of Quality of Life

Many AD-specific, dermatology specific and generic scales have been developed to measure QoL in patients with AD, including the Dermatology Life Quality Index (DQLQI), the Infants' and Toddlers' Dermatology Quality of Life (InTODermQoL), the Children's Dermatology Life Quality Index (CDLQI) and the Childhood Atopic Dermatitis Impact Scale (CADIS) [83]. These scales are not generally designed for use in routine clinical practice; they are mostly used in clinical trials for the assessment of treatment efficacy; however, impact of AD on QoL should be addressed in each visit [40].

DIAGNOSIS

To date no reliable biomarker can distinguish the disease from other entities, therefore the diagnosis is based on clinical history and physical findings [40].

Diagnostic Criteria

Due to the lack of definitive biomarkers for AD, it is difficult to set up standard diagnostic criteria for AD which cover the entire spectrum. Several sets of diagnostic criteria have been proposed for diagnosis of AD, some are more suitable for hospital settings and others for community settings [84].

The first diagnostic criteria were established in 1980 by Hanifin and Rajka, requiring that 3 of 4 major criteria and 3 of 23 minor criteria be met (Table **1**) [85]. While still considered reference diagnostic criteria due to their high sensitivity (96%) and specificity (93.7%) [86], such a large number of criteria are difficult to use in clinical practice. Moreover, some of the minor criteria are poorly defined or nonspecific, such as pityriasis alba or keratosis pilaris.

Table 1. Hanifin and Rajka diagnostic criteria [85].

Hanifin and Rajka Diagnostic Criteria	
Major criteria	Must have three or more major features: 1. Pruritus 2. Typical morphology and distribution Flexural lichenification in adults Facial and extensor eruptions in infants and children 3. Chronic or chronically relapsing dermatitis 4. Personal or family history of atopy (asthma, allergic rhinitis, atopic dermatitis)
Minor criteria	Must have three or more following minor features: 1. Xerosis 2. Ichthyosis/palmar hyperlinearity, keratosis pilaris 3. Immediate (type I) skin test reaction 4. Elevated serum IgE 5. Early age of onset 6. Tendency toward cutaneous infections (especially *S.aureus* and *herpes simplex*), impaired cell-mediated immunity. 7. Tendency toward non-specific hand and foot dermatitis 8. Nipple eczema 9. Cheilitis 10. Recurrent conjunctivitis 11. Dennie-Morgan infraorbital fold 12. Keratoconus 13. Anterior subcapsular cataracts 14. Orbital darkening 15. Facial pallor, facial erythema 16. Pityriasis alba 17. Anterior neck folds 18. Itch when sweating 19. Intolerance to wool and lipid solvents 20. Perifollicular accentuation 21. Food intolerance 22. Course influenced by environmental and emotional factors 23. White dermographism, delayed blanch

In 1994, Williams *et al*, attempted to refine the original Hanifin and Rajka criteria in order to establish a more practical diagnostic tool, and they developed the United Kingdom Working Party's diagnostic criteria (UK criteria) (Table **2**), which include a minimum set of valid and reliable diagnostic criteria for use in both hospital and community settings. These consist of 1 mandatory and 5 major criteria and do not require any laboratory testing [87]. However, even if they are more practical, they cannot be applied to very young children, and their sensitivity is lower than that of Hanifin and Rajka's criteria (86% *vs* 96%), making the latter more effective in diagnosing AD [86].

Table 2. The United Kingdom Working Party's diagnostic criteria [84, 87].

The United Kindomg Workin Party'S Diagnostic Criteria	
Major criteria	Must have one major criteria: 1. Itchy skin condition (or parental report of scratching or rubbing in a child)
Minor criteria	Must have three or more following minor criteria: 1. Onset under the age of 2 years 2. History of flexural involvement 3. History of asthma or hay fever (or a history of atopic disease in siblings and parents if the child is under 4 years) 4. History of a dry skin in the last year 5. Visible flexural dermatitis

In 2003, the American Academy of Dermatology suggested a set of criteria that are more streamlined and applicable to the full range of ages affected (Table **3**) [88]. The 3 most common diagnostic criteria are shown in Tables **1** - **3**.

Table 3. Diagnostic criteria by the American Academy of Dermatology [40, 88].

American Academy of Dermatology Diagnostic Criteria	
A. Essential features*	1. Pruritus 2. Eczema (acute, subacute, chronic) a. Typical morphology and age-specific patterns+ b. Chronic or relapsing history
B. Important features**	1. Early age at onset 2. Atopy a. Personal and/or family history b. IgE reactivity 3. Xerosis
C. Associated features	1. Atypical vascular responses (facial pallor, white dermographism, delayed blanch response) 2. Keratosis pilaris/hyperlinear palms/ichthyosis 3. Ocular/periorbital changes 4. Other regional findings (perioral changes/periauricular lesions) 5. Perifollicular accentuations/lichenification/prurigo lesions
Exclusionary conditions	It should be noted that a diagnosis of atopic dermatitis depends on excluding conditions, such as: scabies, seborrheic dermatitis, contact dermatitis, ichthyoses, cutaneous T-cell lymphoma, psoriasis, photosensitivity dermatoses, immune deficiency diseases and erythroderma of other causes.

(Table 3) cont.....

American Academy of Dermatology Diagnostic Criteria
* Must be present ** Seen in most cases, adding support to the diagnosis *** These clinical associations help to suggest the diagnosis of AD but are too nonspecific to be used for defining or detecting AD for research or epidemiologic studies. ⁺ Patterns include: 1. Facial, neck and extensor involvement in infants and children 2. Current or previous flexural lesions in any age group 3. Sparing of the groin and axillary regions

Finally, it would be worth mentioning the ISAAC criteria, which involved simple questionnaires that enabled the collection of comparable data from children throughout the world, facilitating the epidemiological surveys on childhood AD and other allergic diseases by international collaboration [89].

The ISAAC criteria might be considered the global standard for AD prevalence in a community setting [84]. According to ISAAC, eczema is diagnosed when answers to all three questions are positive [6]:

1. Have you (has your child) ever had a skin rash which was coming and going for at least 6 months?
2. Have you (has your child) had this itchy rash at any time in the past 12 months?
3. Has this itchy rash at any time affected any of the following places: the folds of the elbows; behind the knees, in front of the ankles; under the buttocks; or around the neck, ears, or eyes.

ISAAC was designed mainly to detect classic AD with flexural dermatitis and has the limitation that cannot differentiate from non-AD diseases with itchy skin eruptions. It was also designed to estimate AD prevalence in community setting. When validated based on the gold standard of skin examination twice a year, the sensitivity of the ISAAC was 68.8% and the PPV 56.4% in children aged 7-12 years, suggesting that the ISAAC has a limitation as a diagnostic tool at an individual level [84].

Laboratories

Patients with AD, compared to healthy controls, have high total and/or allergen-specific serum IgE concentrations, although their absence or their presence neither excludes nor confirms diagnosis, since normal IgE levels are present in nearly 20% of patients with AD and 55% of the US general population can have elevated allergen-specific IgE levels.

IgE levels are not a reliable indicator of disease severity therefore routine measurement is not recommended.

Serum immunoglobulin E, potassium hydroxide preparation, patch testing, and/or genetic testing may be helpful to rule out other skin conditions, but not for AD diagnosis [40].

Skin Biopsy

Skin biopsy is not routinely suggested. A biopsy is performed only when a differential diagnosis is considered.

Histologic features of acute eczematous plaques include epidermal intercellular edema (spongiosis) and a prominent perivascular infiltrate of lymphocytes, monocyte macrophages, dendritic cells and a few eosinophils in the dermis. In subacute and chronic lichenified, and excoriated plaques, the epidermis is thickened, and its upper layer is hypertrophied [38].

DISEASE SEVERITY

Around 30 methods have been established to measure disease severity [40, 90] (Table **4**). However validated measures to assess severity are not commonly used in the clinical practice, but mostly as tools for clinical research.

Table 4. Scoring systems for clinician assessment used in clinical research of atopic dermatitis [90].

Scoring System	Description	Severity Rating
Validated		
SCORing Atopic Dermatitis (SCORAD) [91]	3 components: (A) Extent (B) Intensity score (C) Subjective score	Mild = <25 Moderate = 25-50 Severe = >50
Eczema Area and Severity Index (EASI)	2 components: (1) Area score (2) Severity score	Mild = 1.1-7 Moderate = 7.1-21 Severe = 21.1-50 Very severe = 50.1-72
Patient-Oriented SCORAD (PO-SCORAD)	Adaptation of SCORAD for patients	Mild = <25 Moderate = 25-50 Severe = >50

(Table 4) cont.....

Scoring System	Description	Severity Rating
Patient-Oriented Eczema Measure (POEM)	7 questions regarding symptoms and their frequency over the past week.	Clear or almost clear = 0-2 Mild = 3-7 Moderate = 8-16 Severe = 17-24 Very severe = 25-28
Not validated		
Investigator Global Assessment (IGA) score	FDA categorization of atopic dermatitis severity based on investigator's subjective assessment of a representative lesions according to erythema, induration or papulation, and/or oozing or crusting.	0 = clear to 4 = severe
Six Signs Six Areas Atopic Dermatitis (SASSAD) scale	Subjective evaluation of extent of body surface area involved based on 6 signs at each of 6 sites	Each sign at each site is assessed using a scale: 0 = absent 1 = mild, 2 = moderate 3 = severe Maximum 108
Three Item Severity (TIS) scale	Subjective evaluation of a representative lesion based on erythema, edema or papulation, and excoriation	0 = none to 3 = severe
Pruritus (itch) score	Patient's subjective of itch using a VAS similar to pain scales.	VAS: 0 = none to 10 = severe

FDA: Food and Drug Administration, VAS: visual analog scale

The most commonly used disease severity scales are the Eczema Area and Severity Index (EASI), the SCORing of Atopic Dermatitis Index (SCORAD [91], the Patient-Oriented Eczema Measure (POEM) and the Investigator's Global Assessment (IGA). SCORAD index, the EASI score and POEM have been adequately tested and validated; therefore, their use can be considered when needed [40].

EASI score does not evaluate symptoms and objective estimate of the severity of area involved, while SCORAD incorporates both objective physician estimates of extent and severity and subjective patient assessment of itch and sleep loss [91].

Even if available disease severity scales and QoL severity scales are not recommended for routine clinical use [40]. it is mandatory to query about itch, sleep, impact on daily activity and disease persistence at every visit.

DIFFERENTIAL DIAGNOSIS

Other types of dermatitis can resemble AD, mainly inflammatory skin diseases, infections, nutritional deficiencies, primary immunodeficiencies, keratinization disorders, and malignant diseases. Main characteristics of each disease are shown in Table **5** [55, 92].

Table 5. Characteristics of common differential diagnosis of atopic dermatitis [55, 92].

Disease	Characteristics
Inflammatory Skin Diseases	
Seborrheic dermatitis [93].	It may be difficult to distinguish from AD. An early onset (first weeks of life), the presence of an adherent yellow greasy scale, rather than dry scaling skin, and the involvement of the scalp, eyebrows, and diaper area, can help differentiate them. However, they may also exist a continuum, with resolution of seborrheic dermatitis as clinical features of AD become more prominent.
Psoriasis [94].	Erythematous plaques with silvery-white scale typically involving the scalp, postauricular region, elbows, knees and umbilicus is characteristic of psoriasis. Opposed to AD, only one-third of psoriasis begins in childhood, and median age of childhood-onset psoriasis is between 7 and 10 years.
Irritant contact dermatitis [55].	Eczematous lesions confined to the site of exposure (specific localization) and history of locally applied irritants, can indicate an irritant contact dermatitis; however, it might coexist with AD.
Pityriasis lichenoides chronica [95].	Erythematous papules and plaques with a centrally adherent scale are most often seen in the trunk and extremities. Lesions resolve with postinflammatory hyper- or hypopigmentation. In contrast to AD, lesions are generally asymptomatic.
Infectious Skin Diseases	
Tinea corporis [92].	Well demarcated scaly plaques with central clearing, slightly raised reddened edge, and variable itch, are seen in tinea corporis. Potassium hydroxide preparation can be performed to confirm the diagnosis.
Impetigo [96].	Common cutaneous infection, especially prevalent in children. Scaly plaques with honey-yellow crusting are seen mostly on the face (around the nose) and in the limbs. Impetiginization may develop over plaques of AD.
Scabies [97].	Erythematous papules, pustules and burrows. Unlike AD, it can affect palms, soles, between fingers and genitalia. However, secondary eczematous changes can be seen. There is intense pruritus, as in AD, which can generate misdiagnosis.
Nutritional Deficiency	
Zinc deficiency (Acrodermatitis enteropathica) [98].	Erythematous scaly erosive patches and plaques are seen around the mouth and perianal area, along with alopecia and diarrhea, the latter are not seen in AD.

(Table 5) cont.....

Primary Immunodeficiencies	
Hyper-IgE syndrome [99, 100].	Hyper-IgE syndrome can present with severe eczematous lesions and infections of the skin, but it is also accompanied by recurrent pneumonia, a characteristic newborn rash, pathologic bone fractures and high serum IgE (>1,000 UI/mL)
Wiskott-Aldrich syndrome [101].	Is a rare x-linked primary immunodeficiency characterized by the triad of eczema, microthrombocytopenia, and severe and often recurrent infections.
Omenn syndrome [102].	Early-onset erythroderma, diffuse scaly rash, lymphadenopathy, hepatosplenomegaly, chronic diarrhea, eosinophilia, elevations in serum IgE and liver transaminase levels.
Keratinization Disorders	
Ichthyosis vulgaris [103].	Patients with ichthyosis vulgaris, as patients with AD, have loss-of-function mutations in the filaggrin gene. It is characterized by dry skin with fine scaling, particularly on extensor areas of extremities. Contrasting to AD, no erythema is seen. Patients with AD con also have ichthyosis vulgaris.
Netherton syndrome [104].	It is caused by mutations in the SPKINK5 gene. Typically, it manifests as congenital ichthyosiform erythroderma, hair shaft anomalies (bamboo hair), increased IgE and eosinophilia. After infancy, the characteristic skin features are eczematous lesions spread over the skin in a serpiginous linear pattern with double-edged scales (ichthyosis linearis circumflexa).
Malignant Diseases	
Mycosis fungoides [105].	Classic mycosis fungoides in children presents with eczematous patches and plaques on non-sun exposed areas. Hypopigmented plaques can also be seen in children. History, localization and a skin biopsy, may help differentiate them. Histopathology will reveal proliferation of mature CD4+ T lymphocytes with hyperchromatic cerebriform nuclei surrounded by clear cytoplasm.

AD: atopic dermatitis.

The characteristic features of AD, including age of onset, distribution, severe pruritus, xerosis, lichenification, and association with atopy, can help distinguish AD from common mimickers.

MANAGEMENT

Managing a patient with AD must take into account 5 aspects (Fig. **9**) [106].

Maintenance Skin Care

Baseline basic therapy for all patients with AD involves: Bath with warm water and a mild soap or a soap substitute, frequent and appropriate application of moisturizer, avoidance of clinically relevant triggers and educational programs [90, 107].

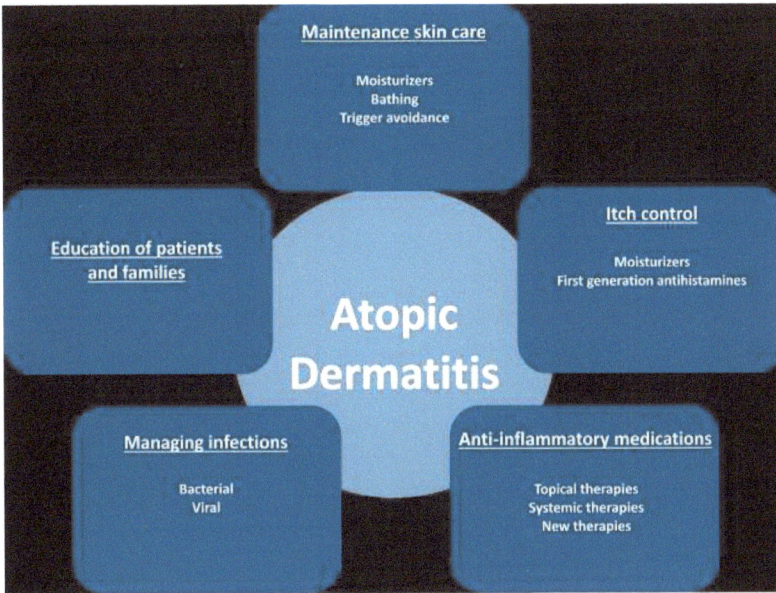

Fig. (9). Management of a patient with atopic dermatitis, must include 5 aspects.

Moisturizers

Skin hydration and frequent use of moisturizers are essential for all patients with AD both during flares and for maintenance. Adequate moisturization significantly decreases AD symptoms, including pruritus, and can even pathogenic bacterial colonization [108]. Emollient treatment can significantly reduce the need for high-potency topical corticosteroid consumption in infants with AD [109].

Appropriate application of moisturizer helps maintain adequate hydration of the epidermis, improves barrier function, decreases TEWL, and can even upregulate antimicrobial peptides and innate immune genes [110, 111]. Therefore, moisturizers themselves can reduce in inflammation and AD severity.

There is a lack of systematic studies to define an optimal amount or frequency of application, it is generally thought that liberal and frequent re-application is necessary such that xerosis is minimal [112].

Head-to-head trials between specific moisturizing products have not demonstrated one to be superior to others [113]. The ideal agent should be safe, effective, inexpensive; and free of additives, fragrances, perfumes, and other potentially sensitizing agents. Ideally, application of moisturizers should be made soon after bathing, which enhances skin hydration [112].

Bathing

Parents of children with AD often receive conflicting information about duration and frequency of bathing, leading to frustration and confusion. Partly, this is attributed to the lack of consensus in the different guidelines.

Daily bath with lukewarm water can hydrate the skin and remove potential skin exacerbating agents (bacteria, dirt, crusting, and other irritants and allergens), which can be helpful for patients with AD [90, 112].

A randomized, single-blind, crossover-controlled trial evaluated twice-daily soaking baths, followed by immediate application of an occlusive moisturizer (soak-and-seal) *versus* twice-weekly soak-and-seal baths, and found that the wet method (twice-daily) is superior to dry method (twice-weekly) at improving disease severity in moderate-to-severe pediatric AD, with a 30% SCORAD improvement [114]. Bath should always be followed by emollient application [107].

Soaps should be used minimally, and non-soap cleansers such as syndets should be considered in lieu of soaps in patients with AD [115].

Trigger Avoidance

A careful history should be taken to identify a relationship between suspected triggers and flares. The identification of individual trigger factors is crucial in the management of AD [107].

Younger children are more likely to have food allergy flares, while older children'sflares are more often triggered by aeroallergens [116]. Common non-specific provocation factors in all patients with AD include acids, bleaches, solvents, sweat, fragrances, preservatives, wool and occlusive fabrics [90, 107].

Trigger avoidance can greatly decrease the frequency and severity of flares [116].

Others

Bleach Baths

Bathing in dilute sodium hypochlorite has been suggested to have a therapeutic role in patients with moderate-to-severe AD who suffer from recurrent infections, possibly by decreasing bacterial colonization from *S.aureus* Wong *et al*, found that bleach baths containing 0.005% dilute hypochlorite solution, given for 5-10 min, 2-3 times per week, reduced AD severity and *S.aureus* density, which may contribute to AD flares [117].

However, a recent meta-analysis found that although they are effective in decreasing AD severity, they do not appear to be more effective than water baths alone, concluding that future larger-scale, well designed randomized controlled trials are needed [118].

Wet-wrap Therapy

Wet wrap therapy is a safe and efficacious intervention in children with severe or refractory AD [119, 120]. This therapy works by using water to promote skin hydration and increased absorption of topical treatments. Affected areas are treated by applying emollients or topical corticosteroids and then covered with wet and wringed tubular bandages, gauze or pajamas, followed by a second dry layer [119]. Patients can wear the wet wraps for a few hours or overnight a few days per week or even daily as tolerated.

Itch Control

Itch is the most bothersome symptom in AD.

Adequate moisturization and gentle skin care can significantly decrease pruritus [108]. However, some patients may need additional antipruritic therapy.

Topical corticosteroids (TCS) and topical calcineurin inhibitors (TCI) have an anti-inflammatory activity rather than acting as direct antipruritic agents, yet, they remain the most effective topical antipruritic agents in AD.

Topical antihistamines (5% doxepin), topical cannabinoid receptor agonists and topical capsaicin may improve pruritus, however, to date there is not enough randomized controlled trials to demonstrate their efficacy and therefore they cannot be recommended as an adjuvant antipruritic therapy in AD [107].

Short-term, intermittent use of sedating antihistamines may be beneficial in the setting of sleep loss secondary to itch, because of their sedative effect. Sedating therapies should only be used short-term, because long-term use can be detrimental to school performance.

Non-sedating antihistamines are not recommended as a routine treatment of AD, in the absence of urticaria or other atopic conditions such as rhinoconjunctivitis [121].

Anti-inflammatory Agents

Topical Therapies

Topical Corticosteroids

TCS remain first-line pharmacologic therapy for AD [107,122]. Twice-daily application of TCS for up to 4 weeks is commonly recommended for active inflammation [90]. For long-term maintenance or proactive therapy, application once or twice weekly to areas that commonly flare might be appropriate to stop relapse, with a low risk of adverse systemic or local effects [123].

Several factors should be considered when choosing a TCS, including potency, formulation, patient age and body area to which the medication will be applied. Treatment of the face (specially the eyelids) should be restricted to mild TCS, children should be treated with less potent TCS than adults, and patients should always be monitored for local and systemic adverse events [107].

Patient steroid phobia remains a concern and should be recognized and adequately addressed to improve adherence and avoid undertreatment [124].

Topical Calcineurin Inhibitors

TCI are alternatives to TCS for treatment of AD (steroid-sparing anti-inflammatory agents). TCI inhibit calcineurin-dependent T-cell activation, thereby impeding the transcription and release of proinflammatory cytokines and mediators [125]. Pimecrolimus, tacrolimus 0.03% ointment and tacrolimus 0.1% are licensed for AD treatment [107].

The anti-inflammatory potency of 0.1% tacrolimus ointment is similar to a TCS with intermediate potency [126], whereas the latter is clearly more effective than 1.0% pimecrolimus cream, however a meta-analysis found that TCI were associated with higher costs and a higher rate of skin burning and pruritus [122].

In contrast to TCS, none of TCI induces skin atrophy, therefore, they are specially indicated in sensitive skin areas (face, intertriginous sites, anogenital area) [107].

Traditionally they are indicated twice daily for exacerbations and proactive tacrolimus ointment (intermittent treatment 2 to 3 times weekly) has been shown to be safe and effective for up to 1 year in reducing the number of flares [127].

Topical Selective Phosphodiesterase 4 Inhibitors

Topical crisaborole is a new and effective treatment for AD lesions, approved by the US Food and Drug Administration (FDA) for the treatment of mild-t--moderate AD in patients 2 years of age and older. However, a recent study showed that twice daily topical crisaborole, is well tolerated and effective in infants (3 to <24 months) with mild-to-moderate AD with systemic exposures similar to patients aged >2 years [128].

Twice daily crisaborole has been shown to be effective and well tolerated compared to its vehicle [129, 130]. However, the efficacy of crisaborole in comparison with TCI or TCS is difficult to determine.

Other topical phosphodiesterase 4 inhibitors under investigation include OPA-15406 and E6005 [107].

Systemic Therapies

Phototherapy

Phototherapy has an immunosuppressive, immunomodulator and anti-inflammatory effect in AD, by reducing the expression of inflammatory cytokines [131]. It can reverse epidermal hyperplasia and thickening of the stratum corneum [132], and therefore is an effective therapeutic option for patients with moderate-to-severe AD.

Multiple forms of light therapy are beneficial for disease and symptom control including: natural sunlight, narrowband UVB, broadband UVB, UVA and topical and systemic psoralen plus UVA (PUVA) [121]. However medium-dose UVA1 (340-400 nm) and narrowband UVB (311-313 nm) are the most commonly recommended light treatment for AD in adult patients, PUVA therapy is not a first-choice therapy for safety profile reasons .

Although phototherapy is rarely used in prepubertal children, it is not contraindicated; its use depends rather on feasibility and equipment [107].

Major problem with phototherapy is that the patient must travel between 3 and 5 times per week for 6-12 weeks to a site that offers this therapy, which limits its use.

Systemic Immunomodulatory Agents

Systemic immunomodulatory agents are indicated in patients whom optimized topical regimens and/or phototherapy do not adequately control the disease, or when QoL is substantially impacted [121].

Cyclosporine A

Immunosuppressant of T cells and IL-2 production, it is an effective off-label treatment option for patients with AD refractory to conventional topical treatment [133]. Its short time to respond (average of 2 weeks) makes cyclosporine an effective treatment for acute flares [134].

Dosage and scheduling: 2.5 to 5 mg/kg/d, standardly 150 to 300 mg/d in adults. Cyclosporine A should be administered in divided doses twice daily. Higher initial dose result in more rapid control.

Adverse effects: Infection, nephrotoxicity, hypertension, tremor, hypertrichosis, headache, gingival hyperplasia, and increased risk of skin cancer and lymphoma [121].

Methotrexate

Methotrexate is an antifolate metabolite and blocks the synthesis of DNA, RNA and purines. It is FDA approved for oncologic and inflammatory disorders, including mycosis fungoides and psoriasis, however it is used off-label for AD [121].

Although is less effective than cyclosporine [135], it remains an important option for long-term maintenance of children with AD, with a favorable side effect profile, fewer adverse effects (compared to cyclosporine) and low cost [136, 137].

Dosage and scheduling: 7.5-25 mg/weekly and in children 0.2-0.7 mg/kg per week. It can be given as a single weekly dose or every 12 hours for 3 doses

Adverse effects: Nausea, ulcerative stomatitis, hepatotoxicity, myelosuppression and pulmonary fibrosis [121].

Azathioprine

Azathioprine is a purine analog that inhibits DNA production, thus affects cells with high proliferation rates, such as B cells and T cells during inflammatory disease. It is FDA approved for the treatment of rheumatoid arthritis and used off-label to treat other inflammatory disorders including AD [121]

As methotrexate, it can be used for long-term maintenance of AD [134].

Dosage and scheduling: 1-4 mg/kg/d.

Adverse effects: Myelosuppression, nausea, vomiting and hepatotoxicity. The metabolism of azathioprine is dependent on an individual's thiopurine methyltransferase levels (TPMT), genetic polymorphisms in TMPT activity are linked to a patient's susceptibility to azathioprine toxicity, therefore, baseline TMPT levels should be always performed before azathioprine initiation [121].

Mycophenolate Mofetil

Mycophenolate mofetil is an immunosuppressant that blocks the purine biosynthesis pathway of cells *via* the inhibition of inosine monophosphate dehydrogenase. It is FDA approved solely for solid organ transplant rejection prophylaxis, but it is used off-label as a therapeutic option in patients with AD [121], with a favorable side effect profile [134].

Dosage and scheduling: 30-50 mg/kg/d, in children the suggested dosing is based on body surface area (600-1200 mg/m2).

Adverse effects: Nausea, vomiting, abdominal cramping. Rarely anemia, leukopenia, thrombocytopenia and genitourinary symptoms have been reported [121].

Systemic Corticosteroids

Systemic corticosteroids are FDA approved to treat inflammatory skin disease (including AD) but they are not recommended as maintenance therapy. Systemic corticosteroids have a largely unfavorable risk/benefit ratio for long-term treatment of AD [134].

The anti-inflammatory effects of a short course (2-3 weeks) or parenteral or oral corticosteroids could help some patients with intermittent, severe, recalcitrant AD. However, rebound is often seen, and these agents should be used with extreme caution and in special circumstances [121].

Anti-IL-4 (Dupilumab)

Dupilumab is a human monoclonal antibody against the α-chain of the receptor of interleukin-4. It inhibits signaling of interlekin-4 and interleukin-13, type 2/Th2 cytokines. In phase 3 trials dupilumab has improved the signs and symptoms of AD, including pruritus, symptoms of anxiety and depression, and quality of life, as compared with placebo [138, 139]. In most trials published so far, up to 70% of patients achieve an EASI 75 or higher skin improvement, and it takes about 4 weeks to reach the full clinical outcome. The safety profile has been reported to be good, with conjunctivitis being the most frequently adverse event [134].

Since 2017, the FDA has approved dupilumab for the treatment of moderate-t--severe atopic dermatitis in adults [134], but it hasn't been until 2020 that it was approved for children 6 years and older [140].

New Therapies

Advances in our understanding of the pathogenesis of AD, beyond the Th2 axis have led to the development of new biologic and small molecules, administered both topically and systemically, that target key elements of inflammation. These new therapies under study are shown in Table **6** and new biologics are shown in Fig. (**10**) [29].

Table 6. Upcoming new therapies for atopic dermatitis.

Drug	Therapeutic Target	Evidence
Small Molecules		
Tofacitinib, baricitinib, upadacitinib, abrocitinib and ruxolitinib [141 - 144].	JAK inhibitors	A phase II study compared topical tofacitinib 2% *vs* placebo in 69 adults and showed significant improvements in EASI score compared with vehicle (-81.7% *vs* -29.9%; p <0.001). In a phase II study, 4 mg a day of oral baricitinib was associated with a higher proportion of patients achieving EASI-50 compared to placebo at 16 weeks with good tolerability.
Ominagan [145].	Antimicrobial peptide	Antimicrobial peptide therapies might improve the innate immune system and lead to a decreased cutaneous inflammation and epidermal barrier repair. Ominagan is currently being studied as a topical gel.
Tapinarof [145, 146].	Agonist of the aryl hydrocarbon receptor	In a phase II study, the use of tapinarof 1% twice a day reduced EASI and SCORAD compared with vehicle. Tapinarof cream is efficacious and well tolerated in adolescent and adult patients with AD however large confirmation trials are needed.
Biologic Agents		
Tezepelumab [147, 148].	Anti-thymic stromal lymphopoietin monoclonal antibody	A phase 2a study, randomized 113 patients to subcutaneous tezepelumab 280 mg or placebo every 2 weeks. Numerical improvements were seen in the tezepelumab group, however, none reached statistical significance.
Mepolizumab [149, 150].	Anti-IL-5 monoclonal antibody	Two RPCT have failed to demonstrate clinical improvement in adults with moderate to severe AD, despite a significant decrease in peripheral blood eosinophils.

(Table 6) cont.....

Drug	Therapeutic Target	Evidence
Nemolizumab [151 - 155].	Anti-IL-31 monoclonal antibody	Several studies in adults with moderate-to-severe AD, have found that subcutaneous nemolizumab improved EASI, IGA, and itch scores. It has been evaluated for up to 64 weeks showing that it is efficacious and overall well tolerated.
GBR 830 [156].	Anti-OX40	In a phase 2a study in 40 adults with moderate-to-severe AD, two doses of GBR 830 (10 mg/kg intravenous) administered 4 weeks apart were well tolerated and induced significant progressive tissue and clinical changes until day 71 (42 days after the last dose), compared to placebo.
Tralokinumab [157].	Anti-IL-13 monoclonal antibody	A phase IIb study including 204 adults with moderate-to-severe AD, found that at week 12, 300 mg of tralokinumab every 2 weeks significantly improved change from baseline in EASI score, SCORAD, DLQI, and pruritus numeric rating scale (7-day mean) scores *versus* placebo.
Lebrikizumab [158, 159].	Anti-IL-13 monoclonal antibody	A phase 2 study in 209 adults with moderate-to-severe AD reported that at week 12, significantly more patients achieved EASI-50 with lebrikizumab 125 mg every 4 weeks (82.4%; P = .026) than placebo every 4 weeks (62.3%). Another study including a total of 280 patients demonstrated that during 16 weeks of treatment, lebrikizumab provided rapid, dose-dependent efficacy across a broad range of clinical manifestations in adult patients with moderate to severe AD and demonstrated a favorable safety profile.
Secukinumab [160].	Anti-IL-17A antibody	A RPCT including 41 patients with moderate-to-severe AD found no improvement in reduction of epidermal thickness neither in clinical outcomes evaluated (SCORAD and EASI) with secukinumab. Concluding that IL-17 is not a valid therapeutic target in patients with AD.
Fezakinumab [161, 162].	Anti-IL-22 antibody	A phase 2a trial including 60 adult patients with moderate-t--severe AD compared IV fezakinumab monotherapy every 2 weeks for 10 weeks, *vs* placebo and found an improvement in SCORAD and in body surface area involvement in the drug-treated patients. Significance was primarily obtained in severe AD. Cellular and molecular effects of IL-22 blockade have been also studied in tissues form patients with AD finding greater reversal of the AD genomic profile with fezakinumab *versus* placebo.
Ustekinumab [163].	Anti-IL-12/23 monoclonal antibody	A systematic review including ten studies (eight case series and two RPCT), with a total of 107 patients, found that 58 patients (54.2%) gained an effective treatment with little adverse events, concluding that ustekinumab is a well-tolerated and safe treatment, however, no significant difference in effect from placebo was seen in patients with AD. Further, larger randomized controlled trials need to be conducted to identify a suitable regimen for AD and provide more evidence for clinical application.

(Table 6) cont.....

Drug	Therapeutic Target	Evidence
Omalizumab [164, 165].	Anti-IgE monoclonal antibody	Used in severe allergic asthma and in chronic urticaria. In single case studies, case series and small trials it appears to be safe and well-tolerated with some clinical benefit in AD patients, however, its efficacy has not been validated in phase III trials. A single-center RPCT including 62 patients aged 4 to 19 years found that omalizumab reduced AD severity and improved QoL in pediatric population with atopy and severe eczema.

EASI: Eczema Area and Severity Index, SCORAD:SCOring Atopic Dermatitis, AD: Atopic Dermatitis, RPCT: Randomized Placebo-Controlled Trial, IGA: Investigator's Global Assessment, DLQI: Dermatology Life Quality Index, QoL: quality of life,

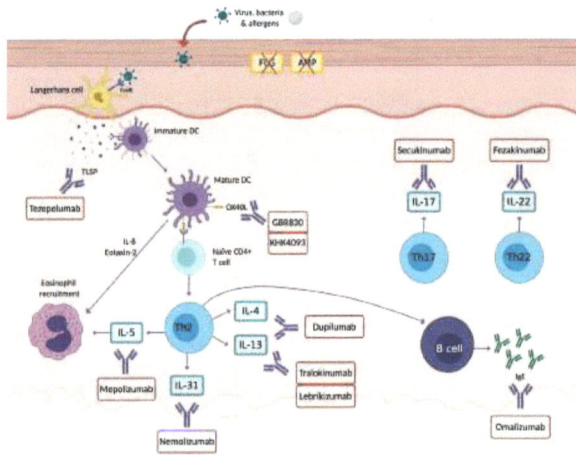

Fig. (10). Pathophysiology of atopic dermatitis and therapeutic targets of biologic agents.

Other Treatments

Oral Supplementation

Vitamin D

Vitamin D stimulates the expression of antimicrobial peptides, which are responsible for the prevention of skin infections, it decreases expression of proinflammatory cytokines and increases expression of regulatory cytokines, leading to reduced T-cell activation. It may also have a direct role in epidermal differentiation and skin barrier permeability [166].

In children, the majority of existing studies have shown a significant inverse correlation between vitamin D levels and SCORAD score (10 out 16 studies included in the systematic review made by Huang CM, *et al*).Besides the association of low vitamin D levels with more severe AD, 67% of studies have shown a significant improvement of AD when supplemented with vitamin D, although studies are inconsistent in terms of type of vitamin D used, dose and duration, mostly due to the fact that a regimen proven to show significant AD improvement has yet to be established [167].

This highlights the need for a large prospective RCT with the use of differing vitamin D doses and durations to establish the most effective supplementation regimen.

Therapeutic Patient Education

Therapeutic patient education (TPE), is defined by the World Health Organization as a continuous process of patient-centered medical care. It empowers patients to manage their disease by providing information and skill-acquisition techniques, which lead directly to better disease management. Patient education has been shown to contribute effectively to preventing complications and improving QoL and treatment adherence for numerous chronic illnesses, such as diabetes, asthma and cardiovascular disease. In dermatology, particularly for AD, TPE in diverse modalities has proven to be effective in improving treatment adherence and thus, severity of disease and QoL [168 - 172].

Interventions for ETP in AD can vary broadly from multidisciplinary sessions or support groups for patients and their families where there are playful activities related to AD management, educational sessions or programs, books, pamphlets or a specialized nurse that educates patients on an individual basis after consultations [168 - 172].

PREVENTION

Since AD is a chronic, relapsing inflammatory skin condition with a profound social, economic, and psychologic impact, an effective prevention strategy would have significant socioeconomic implications worldwide. Early interventions including neonatal emollient therapy, antihistamine use, and probiotic supplementation have been proposed as prevention strategies [173].

Emollient Use

Since new insights into the pathogenesis of AD have emerged indicating that skin barrier dysfunction plays a role in AD development, studies have tried to prove that emollient therapy from birth represents a safe and feasible approach [39, 174].

Simpson *et al*, found that applying emollient to 22 neonates at high risk for developing AD decreased the percentage of patients who developed AD when compared to historical statistics; however, no control group was included in the study [39]. Horimukai, *et al*. performed a prospective, randomized controlled trial including 118 neonates: they applied an emulsion-type moisturizer daily during the first 32 weeks of life to 59 neonates at high risk for AD, and found approximately 32% fewer neonates who received the moisturizer had AD/eczema by week 32 than control subjects (*p*=0.12) concluding that daily application of moisturizer reduces the risk of AD/eczema in infants [174]. Another randomized controlled study including 124 newborns at high risk of developing AD found a statistically significant protective effect with the use of daily emollients on the cumulative incidence of AD with a relative risk reduction of 50% (relative risk, 0.50; 95% CI, 0.28-0.9; P = .017). There were no emollient-related adverse events, suggesting that emollient therapy from birth represents a feasible, safe, low cost and effective approach for atopic dermatitis prevention [175].

Daily application of an emulsion-type moisturizer during the first weeks of life increased stratum corneum hydration at week 12 compared with that seen in infants who occasionally received the minimum amount of petroleum jelly (control subjects) [174].

Breastfeeding

There is evidence that exclusive breastfeeding for 3 to 4 months decreases the incidence of eczema in the first 2 years of life, there are no short- or long-term advantages for exclusive breastfeeding beyond 3 to 4 months for prevention of atopic disease [176]. However, for its multiple benefits in achieving optimal growth, development and health, the World's Health Organization recommends to exclusively breastfeed infants for the child's first six months and thereafter to give appropriate complementary foods and continue breastfeeding up to the age of two years or beyond.

Probiotic Supplementation

Other prevention strategies include probiotic supplementation and extensively hydrolyzed infant formulas, which have produced inconsistent results.

The intestinal microbiota has the ability to modulate the immune system and affect the risk of allergic diseases. AD has been associated with a decreased variety of gut microflora in infancy [173].

More than 15 randomized controlled trials have investigated the role of probiotics in the prevention of AD in high-risk infants. A systematic review and meta-analysis of 17 RCT with data from 4755 children found a significantly lower risk ratio of AD in infants treated pre-and postnatally with probiotics (RR 0.78 p=0.0003) [177]. Another meta-analysis including 28 studies and 6907 subjects (3595 receiving probiotics and 3312 controls), also found that the use of probiotic during both the prenatal and the postnatal period significantly reduced the incidence of AD.

Mixture of probiotics, including *Lactobacillus, Bifidobacterium* and *Propionibacterium* strains, significantly decreased the risk of AD [178].

Administering daily Lactobacillus rhamnosus HN001 to pregnant woman from 35 weeks' gestation until 6 months after delivery if breastfeeding and to infants from birth until 2 years resulted in a 50% decrease in AD prevalence at 2,4, and 6 years of age [173].

PROGNOSIS

Most patients will have resolution or improvement of AD by late childhood. Kim *et al* performed a meta-analysis including more than 110,000 subjects and found that 80% of childhood AD did not persist past 8 years of age, and only 5% of cases persisted by more than 20 years after diagnosis [179]. However other studies have found and increased prevalence of adult AD, which may reflect an increase in late-onset AD or that persistence of AD in adulthood is more common than previously reported [180].

Kim *et al* reported that children who developed AD by 2 years had less persistent disease (179). On the contrary, two studies found that persistent AD was significantly associated with early onset AD [181]. Therefore, more studies are required in order to elucidate factors associated with persistent disease.

CONCLUSION

AD is a complex and multifactorial chronic inflammatory skin disease characterized by intense itching and recurrent eczematous lesions. The main symptom of AD is pruritus, which along with sleep disturbance, decrease quality of life not only in patients but also their families. Therapeutic options for AD have historically been limited, but recent advances have increased our understanding of its underlying mechanisms, contributing to the development of new therapies.

CONSENT FOR PUBLICATION

Not applicable.

CONFLICT OF INTEREST

The authors declare no conflict of interest, financial or otherwise.

ACKNOWLEDGEMENT

Declared none.

REFERENCES

[1]   Weidinger S, Novak N. Atopic dermatitis. Lancet 2016; 387(10023): 1109-22.
        [http://dx.doi.org/10.1016/S0140-6736(15)00149-X] [PMID: 26377142]

[2]   Goksör E, Loid P, Alm B, Åberg N, Wennergren G. The allergic march comprises the coexistence of
        related patterns of allergic disease not just the progressive development of one disease. Acta Paediatr
        2016; 105(12): 1472-9.
        [http://dx.doi.org/10.1111/apa.13515] [PMID: 27381249]

[3]   Davidson WF, Leung DYM, Beck LA, *et al.* Report from the National Institute of Allergy and
        Infectious Diseases workshop on "Atopic dermatitis and the atopic march: Mechanisms and
        interventions". J Allergy Clin Immunol 2019; 143(3): 894-913.
        [http://dx.doi.org/10.1016/j.jaci.2019.01.003] [PMID: 30639346]

[4]   Blome C, Radtke MA, Eissing L, Augustin M. Quality of Life in Patients with Atopic Dermatitis:
        Disease Burden, Measurement, and Treatment Benefit. Am J Clin Dermatol 2016; 17(2): 163-9.
        [http://dx.doi.org/10.1007/s40257-015-0171-3] [PMID: 26818063]

[5]   Silverberg JI. Public Health Burden and Epidemiology of Atopic Dermatitis. Dermatol Clin 2017;
        35(3): 283-9.
        [http://dx.doi.org/10.1016/j.det.2017.02.002] [PMID: 28577797]

[6]   Asher MI, Montefort S, Björkstén B, *et al.* Worldwide time trends in the prevalence of symptoms of
        asthma, allergic rhinoconjunctivitis, and eczema in childhood: ISAAC Phases One and Three repeat
        multicountry cross-sectional surveys. Lancet 2006; 368(9537): 733-43.
        [http://dx.doi.org/10.1016/S0140-6736(06)69283-0] [PMID: 16935684]

[7]   Flohr C, Mann J. New insights into the epidemiology of childhood atopic dermatitis. Allergy 2014;
        69(1): 3-16.
        [http://dx.doi.org/10.1111/all.12270] [PMID: 24417229]

[8]   Shaw TE, Currie GP, Koudelka CW, Simpson EL. Eczema prevalence in the United States: data from
        the 2003 National Survey of Children's Health. J Invest Dermatol 2011; 131(1): 67-73.
        [http://dx.doi.org/10.1038/jid.2010.251] [PMID: 20739951]

[9]   Silverberg JI, Simpson EL. Association between severe eczema in children and multiple comorbid
        conditions and increased healthcare utilization. Pediatr Allergy Immunol 2013; 24(5): 476-86.
        [http://dx.doi.org/10.1111/pai.12095] [PMID: 23773154]

[10]   Kraft MT, Prince BT. Atopic Dermatitis Is a Barrier Issue, Not an Allergy Issue. Immunol Allergy
        Clin North Am 2019; 39(4): 507-19.
        [http://dx.doi.org/10.1016/j.iac.2019.07.005] [PMID: 31563185]

[11]   Yang G, Seok JK, Kang HC, Cho YY, Lee HS, Lee JY. Skin Barrier Abnormalities and Immune
        Dysfunction in Atopic Dermatitis. Int J Mol Sci 2020; 21(8): E2867.
        [http://dx.doi.org/10.3390/ijms21082867] [PMID: 32326002]

[12]   Cabanillas B, Brehler AC, Novak N. Atopic dermatitis phenotypes and the need for personalized
        medicine. Curr Opin Allergy Clin Immunol 2017; 17(4): 309-15.
        [http://dx.doi.org/10.1097/ACI.0000000000000376] [PMID: 28582322]

[13]　McLean WH. Filaggrin failure - from ichthyosis vulgaris to atopic eczema and beyond. Br J Dermatol 2016; 175 (Suppl. 2): 4-7.
[http://dx.doi.org/10.1111/bjd.14997] [PMID: 27667308]

[14]　Flohr C, England K, Radulovic S, *et al.* Filaggrin loss-of-function mutations are associated with early-onset eczema, eczema severity and transepidermal water loss at 3 months of age. Br J Dermatol 2010; 163(6): 1333-6.
[http://dx.doi.org/10.1111/j.1365-2133.2010.10068.x] [PMID: 21137118]

[15]　Palmer CN, Irvine AD, Terron-Kwiatkowski A, *et al.* Common loss-of-function variants of the epidermal barrier protein filaggrin are a major predisposing factor for atopic dermatitis. Nat Genet 2006; 38(4): 441-6.
[http://dx.doi.org/10.1038/ng1767] [PMID: 16550169]

[16]　Jungersted JM, Scheer H, Mempel M, *et al.* Stratum corneum lipids, skin barrier function and filaggrin mutations in patients with atopic eczema. Allergy 2010; 65(7): 911-8.
[http://dx.doi.org/10.1111/j.1398-9995.2010.02326.x] [PMID: 20132155]

[17]　Ishikawa J, Narita H, Kondo N, *et al.* Changes in the ceramide profile of atopic dermatitis patients. J Invest Dermatol 2010; 130(10): 2511-4.
[http://dx.doi.org/10.1038/jid.2010.161] [PMID: 20574438]

[18]　Elias PM, Wakefield JS. Mechanisms of abnormal lamellar body secretion and the dysfunctional skin barrier in patients with atopic dermatitis. J Allergy Clin Immunol 2014; 134(4): 781-791.e1.
[http://dx.doi.org/10.1016/j.jaci.2014.05.048] [PMID: 25131691]

[19]　Ong PY, Ohtake T, Brandt C, *et al.* Endogenous antimicrobial peptides and skin infections in atopic dermatitis. N Engl J Med 2002; 347(15): 1151-60.
[http://dx.doi.org/10.1056/NEJMoa021481] [PMID: 12374875]

[20]　Furuse M, Hata M, Furuse K, *et al.* Claudin-based tight junctions are crucial for the mammalian epidermal barrier: a lesson from claudin-1-deficient mice. J Cell Biol 2002; 156(6): 1099-111.
[http://dx.doi.org/10.1083/jcb.200110122] [PMID: 11889141]

[21]　Bergmann S, von Buenau B, Vidal-Y-Sy S, *et al.* Claudin-1 decrease impacts epidermal barrier function in atopic dermatitis lesions dose-dependently. Sci Rep 2020; 10(1): 2024.
[http://dx.doi.org/10.1038/s41598-020-58718-9] [PMID: 32029783]

[22]　Liu YJ. Thymic stromal lymphopoietin: master switch for allergic inflammation. J Exp Med 2006; 203(2): 269-73.
[http://dx.doi.org/10.1084/jem.20051745] [PMID: 16432252]

[23]　Liu YJ. Thymic stromal lymphopoietin and OX40 ligand pathway in the initiation of dendritic cell-mediated allergic inflammation. J Allergy Clin Immunol 2007; 120(2): 238-44.
[http://dx.doi.org/10.1016/j.jaci.2007.06.004] [PMID: 17666213]

[24]　Soumelis V, Reche PA, Kanzler H, *et al.* Human epithelial cells trigger dendritic cell mediated allergic inflammation by producing TSLP. Nat Immunol 2002; 3(7): 673-80.
[http://dx.doi.org/10.1038/ni805] [PMID: 12055625]

[25]　Siracusa MC, Saenz SA, Hill DA, *et al.* TSLP promotes interleukin-3-independent basophil haematopoiesis and type 2 inflammation. Nature 2011; 477(7363): 229-33.
[http://dx.doi.org/10.1038/nature10329] [PMID: 21841801]

[26]　Yang EJ, Sekhon S, Sanchez IM, Beck KM, Bhutani T. Recent Developments in Atopic Dermatitis. Pediatrics 2018; 142(4): e20181102.
[http://dx.doi.org/10.1542/peds.2018-1102] [PMID: 30266868]

[27]　Esaki H, Brunner PM, Renert-Yuval Y, *et al.* Early-onset pediatric atopic dermatitis is T_H2 but also T_H17 polarized in skin. J Allergy Clin Immunol 2016; 138(6): 1639-51.
[http://dx.doi.org/10.1016/j.jaci.2016.07.013] [PMID: 27671162]

[28]   Sullivan M, Silverberg NB. Current and emerging concepts in atopic dermatitis pathogenesis. Clin Dermatol 2017; 35(4): 349-53.
[http://dx.doi.org/10.1016/j.clindermatol.2017.03.006] [PMID: 28709564]

[29]   Munera-Campos M, Carrascosa JM. Innovation in Atopic Dermatitis: From Pathogenesis to Treatment. Actas Dermosifiliogr 2020; 111(3): 205-21.
[http://dx.doi.org/10.1016/j.ad.2019.11.002] [PMID: 31964499]

[30]   Totté JE, van der Feltz WT, Hennekam M, van Belkum A, van Zuuren EJ, Pasmans SG. Prevalence and odds of Staphylococcus aureus carriage in atopic dermatitis: a systematic review and meta-analysis. Br J Dermatol 2016; 175(4): 687-95.
[http://dx.doi.org/10.1111/bjd.14566] [PMID: 26994362]

[31]   Harkins CP, Pettigrew KA, Oravcová K, *et al.* The Microevolution and Epidemiology of Staphylococcus aureus Colonization during Atopic Eczema Disease Flare. J Invest Dermatol 2018; 138(2): 336-43.
[http://dx.doi.org/10.1016/j.jid.2017.09.023] [PMID: 28951239]

[32]   Clausen ML, Edslev SM, Andersen PS, Clemmensen K, Krogfelt KA, Agner T. Staphylococcus aureus colonization in atopic eczema and its association with filaggrin gene mutations. Br J Dermatol 2017; 177(5): 1394-400.
[http://dx.doi.org/10.1111/bjd.15470] [PMID: 28317091]

[33]   Kong HH, Oh J, Deming C, *et al.* Temporal shifts in the skin microbiome associated with disease flares and treatment in children with atopic dermatitis. Genome Res 2012; 22(5): 850-9.
[http://dx.doi.org/10.1101/gr.131029.111] [PMID: 22310478]

[34]   Byrd AL, Deming C, Cassidy SKB, *et al. Staphylococcus aureus* and *Staphylococcus epidermidis* strain diversity underlying pediatric atopic dermatitis. Sci Transl Med 2017; 9(397): eaal4651.
[http://dx.doi.org/10.1126/scitranslmed.aal4651] [PMID: 28679656]

[35]   Meylan P, Lang C, Mermoud S, *et al.* Skin Colonization by Staphylococcus aureus Precedes the Clinical Diagnosis of Atopic Dermatitis in Infancy. J Invest Dermatol 2017; 137(12): 2497-504.
[http://dx.doi.org/10.1016/j.jid.2017.07.834] [PMID: 28842320]

[36]   Iwase T, Uehara Y, Shinji H, *et al.* Staphylococcus epidermidis Esp inhibits Staphylococcus aureus biofilm formation and nasal colonization. Nature 2010; 465(7296): 346-9.
[http://dx.doi.org/10.1038/nature09074] [PMID: 20485435]

[37]   Nakatsuji T, Chen TH, Narala S, *et al.* Antimicrobials from human skin commensal bacteria protect against *Staphylococcus aureus* and are deficient in atopic dermatitis. Sci Transl Med 2017; 9(378): eaah4680.
[http://dx.doi.org/10.1126/scitranslmed.aah4680] [PMID: 28228596]

[38]   Bieber T. Atopic dermatitis. N Engl J Med 2008; 358(14): 1483-94.
[http://dx.doi.org/10.1056/NEJMra074081] [PMID: 18385500]

[39]   Simpson EL, Berry TM, Brown PA, Hanifin JM. A pilot study of emollient therapy for the primary prevention of atopic dermatitis. J Am Acad Dermatol 2010; 63(4): 587-93.
[http://dx.doi.org/10.1016/j.jaad.2009.11.011] [PMID: 20692725]

[40]   Eichenfield LF, Tom WL, Chamlin SL, *et al.* Guidelines of care for the management of atopic dermatitis: section 1. Diagnosis and assessment of atopic dermatitis. J Am Acad Dermatol 2014; 70(2): 338-51.
[http://dx.doi.org/10.1016/j.jaad.2013.10.010] [PMID: 24290431]

[41]   Ruiz RG, Kemeny DM, Price JF. Higher risk of infantile atopic dermatitis from maternal atopy than from paternal atopy. Clin Exp Allergy 1992; 22(8): 762-6.
[http://dx.doi.org/10.1111/j.1365-2222.1992.tb02816.x] [PMID: 1525695]

[42]   Irvine AD, McLean WH, Leung DY. Filaggrin mutations associated with skin and allergic diseases. N Engl J Med 2011; 365(14): 1315-27.

[http://dx.doi.org/10.1056/NEJMra1011040] [PMID: 21991953]

[43]   Cork MJ, Robinson DA, Vasilopoulos Y, *et al.* New perspectives on epidermal barrier dysfunction in atopic dermatitis: gene-environment interactions. J Allergy Clin Immunol 2006; 118(1): 3-21.
        [http://dx.doi.org/10.1016/j.jaci.2006.04.042] [PMID: 16815133]

[44]   Silverberg JI, Hanifin J, Simpson EL. Climatic factors are associated with childhood eczema prevalence in the United States. J Invest Dermatol 2013; 133(7): 1752-9.
        [http://dx.doi.org/10.1038/jid.2013.19] [PMID: 23334343]

[45]   Byremo G, Rød G, Carlsen KH. Effect of climatic change in children with atopic eczema. Allergy 2006; 61(12): 1403-10.
        [http://dx.doi.org/10.1111/j.1398-9995.2006.01209.x] [PMID: 17073869]

[46]   Epstein TG, Bernstein DI, Levin L, Khurana Hershey GK, Ryan PH, Reponen T, *et al.* Opposing effects of cat and dog ownership and allergic sensitization on eczema in an atopic birth cohort. J Pediatr 2011; 158(2): 265-71.

[47]   Li C, Chen Q, Zhang X, *et al.* Early Life Domestic Pet Ownership, and the Risk of Pet Sensitization and Atopic Dermatitis in Preschool Children: A Prospective Birth Cohort in Shanghai. Front Pediatr 2020; 8: 192.
        [http://dx.doi.org/10.3389/fped.2020.00192] [PMID: 32391295]

[48]   Schram ME, Tedja AM, Spijker R, Bos JD, Williams HC, Spuls PI. Is there a rural/urban gradient in the prevalence of eczema? A systematic review. Br J Dermatol 2010; 162(5): 964-73.
        [http://dx.doi.org/10.1111/j.1365-2133.2010.09689.x] [PMID: 20331459]

[49]   Patki A. Eat dirt and avoid atopy: the hygiene hypothesis revisited. Indian J Dermatol Venereol Leprol 2007; 73(1): 2-4.
        [http://dx.doi.org/10.4103/0378-6323.30642] [PMID: 17314438]

[50]   Flohr C, Yeo L. Atopic dermatitis and the hygiene hypothesis revisited. Curr Probl Dermatol 2011; 41: 1-34.
        [http://dx.doi.org/10.1159/000323290] [PMID: 21576944]

[51]   Ellwood P, Asher MI, García-Marcos L, *et al.* Do fast foods cause asthma, rhinoconjunctivitis and eczema? Global findings from the International Study of Asthma and Allergies in Childhood (ISAAC) phase three. Thorax 2013; 68(4): 351-60.
        [http://dx.doi.org/10.1136/thoraxjnl-2012-202285] [PMID: 23319429]

[52]   Sausenthaler S, Koletzko S, Schaaf B, *et al.* Maternal diet during pregnancy in relation to eczema and allergic sensitization in the offspring at 2 y of age. Am J Clin Nutr 2007; 85(2): 530-7.
        [http://dx.doi.org/10.1093/ajcn/85.2.530] [PMID: 17284754]

[53]   Romieu I, Torrent M, Garcia-Esteban R, *et al.* Maternal fish intake during pregnancy and atopy and asthma in infancy. Clin Exp Allergy 2007; 37(4): 518-25.
        [http://dx.doi.org/10.1111/j.1365-2222.2007.02685.x] [PMID: 17430348]

[54]   Julián-Gónzalez RE, Orozco-Covarrubias L, Durán-McKinster C, Palacios-Lopez C, Ruiz-Maldonado R, Sáez-de-Ocariz M. Less common clinical manifestations of atopic dermatitis: prevalence by age. Pediatr Dermatol 2012; 29(5): 580-3.
        [http://dx.doi.org/10.1111/j.1525-1470.2012.01739.x] [PMID: 22469300]

[55]   Deleuran M, Vestergaard C. Clinical heterogeneity and differential diagnosis of atopic dermatitis. Br J Dermatol 2014; 170 (Suppl. 1): 2-6.
        [http://dx.doi.org/10.1111/bjd.12933] [PMID: 24720512]

[56]   Oliveira C, Torres T. More than skin deep: the systemic nature of atopic dermatitis. Eur J Dermatol 2019; 29(3): 250-8.
        [PMID: 31122909]

[57]   Carrascosa JM, Morillas-Lahuerta V. Comorbidities in Atopic Dermatitis: An Update and Review of Controversies. Actas Dermosifiliogr 2020; 111(6): 481-6.

[http://dx.doi.org/10.1016/j.ad.2020.04.009] [PMID: 32401719]

[58]   Yaghmaie P, Koudelka CW, Simpson EL. Mental health comorbidity in patients with atopic dermatitis. J Allergy Clin Immunol 2013; 131(2): 428-33.
[http://dx.doi.org/10.1016/j.jaci.2012.10.041] [PMID: 23245818]

[59]   Haeck IM, Hamdy NA, Timmer-de Mik L, *et al.* Low bone mineral density in adult patients with moderate to severe atopic dermatitis. Br J Dermatol 2009; 161(6): 1248-54.
[http://dx.doi.org/10.1111/j.1365-2133.2009.09327.x] [PMID: 19673879]

[60]   Wu CY, Lu YY, Lu CC, Su YF, Tsai TH, Wu CH. Osteoporosis in adult patients with atopic dermatitis: A nationwide population-based study. PLoS One 2017; 12(2): e0171667.
[http://dx.doi.org/10.1371/journal.pone.0171667] [PMID: 28207767]

[61]   Drury KE, Schaeffer M, Silverberg JI. Association Between Atopic Disease and Anemia in US Children. JAMA Pediatr 2016; 170(1): 29-34.
[http://dx.doi.org/10.1001/jamapediatrics.2015.3065] [PMID: 26619045]

[62]   Zhang A, Silverberg JI. Association of atopic dermatitis with being overweight and obese: a systematic review and metaanalysis. J Am Acad Dermatol 2015; 72(4): 606-16.e4.
[http://dx.doi.org/10.1016/j.jaad.2014.12.013] [PMID: 25773409]

[63]   Silverberg JI, Becker L, Kwasny M, Menter A, Cordoro KM, Paller AS. Central obesity and high blood pressure in pediatric patients with atopic dermatitis. JAMA Dermatol 2015; 151(2): 144-52.
[http://dx.doi.org/10.1001/jamadermatol.2014.3059] [PMID: 25536049]

[64]   Silverberg JI. Association between adult atopic dermatitis, cardiovascular disease, and increased heart attacks in three population-based studies. Allergy 2015; 70(10): 1300-8.
[http://dx.doi.org/10.1111/all.12685] [PMID: 26148129]

[65]   Tran MM, Lefebvre DL, Dharma C, *et al.* Predicting the atopic march: Results from the Canadian Healthy Infant Longitudinal Development Study. J Allergy Clin Immunol 2018; 141(2): 601-607.e8.
[http://dx.doi.org/10.1016/j.jaci.2017.08.024] [PMID: 29153857]

[66]   Martin PE, Eckert JK, Koplin JJ, *et al.* Which infants with eczema are at risk of food allergy? Results from a population-based cohort. Clin Exp Allergy 2015; 45(1): 255-64.
[http://dx.doi.org/10.1111/cea.12406] [PMID: 25210971]

[67]   Bath-Hextall F, Delamere FM, Williams HC. Dietary exclusions for improving established atopic eczema in adults and children: systematic review. Allergy 2009; 64(2): 258-64.
[http://dx.doi.org/10.1111/j.1398-9995.2008.01917.x] [PMID: 19178405]

[68]   Lim NR, Lohman ME, Lio PA. The Role of Elimination Diets in Atopic Dermatitis-A Comprehensive Review. Pediatr Dermatol 2017; 34(5): 516-27.
[http://dx.doi.org/10.1111/pde.13244] [PMID: 28884902]

[69]   Heine G, Schnuch A, Uter W, Worm M. Type-IV sensitization profile of individuals with atopic eczema: results from the Information Network of Departments of Dermatology (IVDK) and the German Contact Dermatitis Research Group (DKG). Allergy 2006; 61(5): 611-6.
[http://dx.doi.org/10.1111/j.1398-9995.2006.01029.x] [PMID: 16629792]

[70]   Patel KR, Immaneni S, Singam V, Rastogi S, Silverberg JI. Association between atopic dermatitis, depression, and suicidal ideation: A systematic review and meta-analysis. J Am Acad Dermatol 2019; 80(2): 402-10.
[http://dx.doi.org/10.1016/j.jaad.2018.08.063] [PMID: 30365995]

[71]   Chang YS, Chiang BL. Sleep disorders and atopic dermatitis: A2-way street? J Allergy Clin Immunol 2018; 142(4): 1033-40.
[http://dx.doi.org/10.1016/j.jaci.2018.08.005] [PMID: 30144472]

[72]   Moore K, David TJ, Murray CS, Child F, Arkwright PD. Effect of childhood eczema and asthma on parental sleep and well-being: a prospective comparative study. Br J Dermatol 2006; 154(3): 514-8.
[http://dx.doi.org/10.1111/j.1365-2133.2005.07082.x] [PMID: 16445784]

[73]   Touchette E, Petit D, Séguin JR, Boivin M, Tremblay RE, Montplaisir JY. Associations between sleep duration patterns and behavioral/cognitive functioning at school entry. Sleep 2007; 30(9): 1213-9.
[http://dx.doi.org/10.1093/sleep/30.9.1213] [PMID: 17910393]

[74]   Sadeh A, Gruber R, Raviv A. Sleep, neurobehavioral functioning, and behavior problems in school-age children. Child Dev 2002; 73(2): 405-17.
[http://dx.doi.org/10.1111/1467-8624.00414] [PMID: 11949899]

[75]   Schmitt J, Chen CM, Apfelbacher C, *et al.* Infant eczema, infant sleeping problems, and mental health at 10 years of age: the prospective birth cohort study LISAplus. Allergy 2011; 66(3): 404-11.
[http://dx.doi.org/10.1111/j.1398-9995.2010.02487.x] [PMID: 21029113]

[76]   Silverberg JI, Paller AS. Association between eczema and stature in 9 US population-based studies. JAMA Dermatol 2015; 151(4): 401-9.
[http://dx.doi.org/10.1001/jamadermatol.2014.3432] [PMID: 25493447]

[77]   Chang YS, Chiang BL. Mechanism of Sleep Disturbance in Children with Atopic Dermatitis and the Role of the Circadian Rhythm and Melatonin. Int J Mol Sci 2016; 17(4): 462.
[http://dx.doi.org/10.3390/ijms17040462] [PMID: 27043528]

[78]   Wollenberg A, Wetzel S, Burgdorf WH, Haas J. Viral infections in atopic dermatitis: pathogenic aspects and clinical management. J Allergy Clin Immunol 2003; 112(4): 667-74.
[http://dx.doi.org/10.1016/j.jaci.2003.07.001] [PMID: 14564342]

[79]   Wollenberg A. Eczema herpeticum. Chem Immunol Allergy 2012; 96: 89-95.
[http://dx.doi.org/10.1159/000331892] [PMID: 22433376]

[80]   Mathes EF, Oza V, Frieden IJ, *et al.* "Eczema coxsackium" and unusual cutaneous findings in an enterovirus outbreak. Pediatrics 2013; 132(1): e149-57.
[http://dx.doi.org/10.1542/peds.2012-3175] [PMID: 23776120]

[81]   Su JC, Kemp AS, Varigos GA, Nolan TM. Atopic eczema: its impact on the family and financial cost. Arch Dis Child 1997; 76(2): 159-62.
[http://dx.doi.org/10.1136/adc.76.2.159] [PMID: 9068310]

[82]   Campos ALB, Araújo FM, Santos MALD, Santos AASD, Pires CAA. Impact of atopic dermatitis on the quality of life of pediatric patients and their guardiands. Rev Paul Pediatr 2017; 35(1): 5-10.
[http://dx.doi.org/10.1590/1984-0462/;2017;35;1;00006] [PMID: 28977306]

[83]   Chernyshov PV. The Evolution of Quality of Life Assessment and Use in Dermatology. Dermatology 2019; 235(3): 167-74.
[http://dx.doi.org/10.1159/000496923] [PMID: 30928986]

[84]   Lee SC. Various diagnostic criteria for atopic dermatitis (AD): A proposal of Reliable Estimation of Atopic Dermatitis in Childhood (REACH) criteria, a novel questionnaire-based diagnostic tool for AD. J Dermatol 2016; 43(4): 376-84.
[http://dx.doi.org/10.1111/1346-8138.13264] [PMID: 26813749]

[85]   Hanifin JM, Rajka G. Diagnostic features of atopic dermatitis. Acta Derm Venereol 1980; 92 (Suppl.): 44-7.

[86]   De D, Kanwar AJ, Handa S. Comparative efficacy of Hanifin and Rajka's criteria and the UK working party's diagnostic criteria in diagnosis of atopic dermatitis in a hospital setting in North India. J Eur Acad Dermatol Venereol 2006; 20(7): 853-9.
[http://dx.doi.org/10.1111/j.1468-3083.2006.01664.x] [PMID: 16898910]

[87]   Williams HC, Burney PG, Hay RJ, *et al.* The U.K. Working Party's Diagnostic Criteria for Atopic Dermatitis. I. Derivation of a minimum set of discriminators for atopic dermatitis. Br J Dermatol 1994; 131(3): 383-96.
[http://dx.doi.org/10.1111/j.1365-2133.1994.tb08530.x] [PMID: 7918015]

[88]   Eichenfield LF, Hanifin JM, Luger TA, Stevens SR, Pride HB. Consensus conference on pediatric

atopic dermatitis. J Am Acad Dermatol 2003; 49(6): 1088-95.
[http://dx.doi.org/10.1016/S0190-9622(03)02539-8] [PMID: 14639390]

[89]   Asher MI, Keil U, Anderson HR, *et al.* International Study of Asthma and Allergies in Childhood
       (ISAAC): rationale and methods. Eur Respir J 1995; 8(3): 483-91.
       [http://dx.doi.org/10.1183/09031936.95.08030483] [PMID: 7789502]

[90]   Boguniewicz M, Fonacier L, Guttman-Yassky E, Ong PY, Silverberg J, Farrar JR. Atopic dermatitis
       yardstick: Practical recommendations for an evolving therapeutic landscape. Ann Allergy Asthma
       Immunol 2018; 120(1): 10-22.e2.
       [http://dx.doi.org/10.1016/j.anai.2017.10.039] [PMID: 29273118]

[91]   Severity scoring of atopic dermatitis: the SCORAD index. Consensus Report of the European Task
       Force on Atopic Dermatitis. Dermatology 1993; 186(1): 23-31.
       [http://dx.doi.org/10.1159/000247298] [PMID: 8435513]

[92]   Barrett M, Luu M. Differential Diagnosis of Atopic Dermatitis. Immunol Allergy Clin North Am
       2017; 37(1): 11-34.
       [http://dx.doi.org/10.1016/j.iac.2016.08.009] [PMID: 27886900]

[93]   Dessinioti C, Katsambas A. Seborrheic dermatitis: etiology, risk factors, and treatments: facts and
       controversies. Clin Dermatol 2013; 31(4): 343-51.
       [http://dx.doi.org/10.1016/j.clindermatol.2013.01.001] [PMID: 23806151]

[94]   Eichenfield LF, Paller AS, Tom WL, *et al.* Pediatric psoriasis: Evolving perspectives. Pediatr
       Dermatol 2018; 35(2): 170-81.
       [http://dx.doi.org/10.1111/pde.13382] [PMID: 29314219]

[95]   Geller L, Antonov NK, Lauren CT, Morel KD, Garzon MC. Pityriasis Lichenoides in Childhood:
       Review of Clinical Presentation and Treatment Options. Pediatr Dermatol 2015; 32(5): 579-92.
       [http://dx.doi.org/10.1111/pde.12581] [PMID: 25816855]

[96]   Pereira LB. Impetigo - review. An Bras Dermatol 2014; 89(2): 293-9.
       [http://dx.doi.org/10.1590/abd1806-4841.20142283] [PMID: 24770507]

[97]   Banerji A. Scabies. Paediatr Child Health 2015; 20(7): 395-402.
       [http://dx.doi.org/10.1093/pch/20.7.395] [PMID: 26527041]

[98]   Lakdawala N, Grant-Kels JM. Acrodermatitis enteropathica and other nutritional diseases of the folds
       (intertriginous areas). Clin Dermatol 2015; 33(4): 414-9.
       [http://dx.doi.org/10.1016/j.clindermatol.2015.04.002] [PMID: 26051055]

[99]   Pichard DC, Freeman AF, Cowen EW. Primary immunodeficiency update: Part I. Syndromes
       associated with eczematous dermatitis. J Am Acad Dermatol 2015; 73(3): 355-64.
       [http://dx.doi.org/10.1016/j.jaad.2015.01.054] [PMID: 26282794]

[100] Woellner C, Gertz EM, Schäffer AA, *et al.* Mutations in STAT3 and diagnostic guidelines for hyper-
       IgE syndrome. J Allergy Clin Immunol 2010; 125(2): 424-432.e8.
       [http://dx.doi.org/10.1016/j.jaci.2009.10.059] [PMID: 20159255]

[101] Buchbinder D, Nugent DJ, Fillipovich AH. Wiskott-Aldrich syndrome: diagnosis, current
       management, and emerging treatments. Appl Clin Genet 2014; 7: 55-66.
       [http://dx.doi.org/10.2147/TACG.S58444] [PMID: 24817816]

[102] Chinn IK, Shearer WT. Severe Combined Immunodeficiency Disorders. Immunol Allergy Clin North
       Am 2015; 35(4): 671-94.
       [http://dx.doi.org/10.1016/j.iac.2015.07.002] [PMID: 26454313]

[103] Vahlquist A, Fischer J, Törmä H. Inherited Nonsyndromic Ichthyoses: An Update on Pathophysiology,
       Diagnosis and Treatment. Am J Clin Dermatol 2018; 19(1): 51-66.
       [http://dx.doi.org/10.1007/s40257-017-0313-x] [PMID: 28815464]

[104] Saral S, Vural A, Wollenberg A, Ruzicka T. A practical approach to ichthyoses with systemic

manifestations. Clin Genet 2017; 91(6): 799-812.
[http://dx.doi.org/10.1111/cge.12828] [PMID: 27377997]

[105] Jawed SI, Myskowski PL, Horwitz S, Moskowitz A, Querfeld C. Primary cutaneous T-cell lymphoma (mycosis fungoides and Sézary syndrome): part I. Diagnosis: clinical and histopathologic features and new molecular and biologic markers. J Am Acad Dermatol 2014; 70(2): 205.e1-205.e16.
[http://dx.doi.org/10.1016/j.jaad.2013.07.049] [PMID: 24438969]

[106] Tollefson MM, Bruckner AL, Dermatology SO. Atopic dermatitis: skin-directed management. Pediatrics 2014; 134(6): e1735-44.
[http://dx.doi.org/10.1542/peds.2014-2812] [PMID: 25422009]

[107] Wollenberg A, Barbarot S, Bieber T, *et al.* Consensus-based European guidelines for treatment of atopic eczema (atopic dermatitis) in adults and children: part I. J Eur Acad Dermatol Venereol 2018; 32(5): 657-82.
[http://dx.doi.org/10.1111/jdv.14891] [PMID: 29676534]

[108] Angelova-Fischer I, Neufang G, Jung K, Fischer TW, Zillikens D. A randomized, investigator-blinded efficacy assessment study of stand-alone emollient use in mild to moderately severe atopic dermatitis flares. J Eur Acad Dermatol Venereol 2014; 28 (Suppl. 3): 9-15.
[http://dx.doi.org/10.1111/jdv.12479] [PMID: 24702445]

[109] Grimalt R, Mengeaud V, Cambazard F, Group SI. The steroid-sparing effect of an emollient therapy in infants with atopic dermatitis: a randomized controlled study. Dermatology 2007; 214(1): 61-7.
[http://dx.doi.org/10.1159/000096915] [PMID: 17191050]

[110] Czarnowicki T, Malajian D, Khattri S, *et al.* Petrolatum: Barrier repair and antimicrobial responses underlying this "inert" moisturizer. J Allergy Clin Immunol 2016; 137(4): 1091-1102.e7.
[http://dx.doi.org/10.1016/j.jaci.2015.08.013] [PMID: 26431582]

[111] Simpson E, Trookman NS, Rizer RL, *et al.* Safety and tolerability of a body wash and moisturizer when applied to infants and toddlers with a history of atopic dermatitis: results from an open-label study. Pediatr Dermatol 2012; 29(5): 590-7.
[http://dx.doi.org/10.1111/j.1525-1470.2012.01809.x] [PMID: 22775151]

[112] Eichenfield LF, Tom WL, Berger TG, *et al.* Guidelines of care for the management of atopic dermatitis: section 2. Management and treatment of atopic dermatitis with topical therapies. J Am Acad Dermatol 2014; 71(1): 116-32.
[http://dx.doi.org/10.1016/j.jaad.2014.03.023] [PMID: 24813302]

[113] Miller DW, Koch SB, Yentzer BA, *et al.* An over-the-counter moisturizer is as clinically effective as, and more cost-effective than, prescription barrier creams in the treatment of children with mild-t--moderate atopic dermatitis: a randomized, controlled trial. J Drugs Dermatol 2011; 10(5): 531-7.
[PMID: 21533301]

[114] Cardona ID, Kempe EE, Lary C, Ginder JH, Jain N. Frequent Versus Infrequent Bathing in Pediatric Atopic Dermatitis: A Randomized Clinical Trial. J Allergy Clin Immunol Pract 2020; 8(3): 1014-21.
[http://dx.doi.org/10.1016/j.jaip.2019.10.042] [PMID: 31733336]

[115] Gittler JK, Wang JF, Orlow SJ. Bathing and Associated Treatments in Atopic Dermatitis. Am J Clin Dermatol 2017; 18(1): 45-57.
[http://dx.doi.org/10.1007/s40257-016-0240-2] [PMID: 27913962]

[116] Sidbury R, Tom WL, Bergman JN, *et al.* Guidelines of care for the management of atopic dermatitis: Section 4. Prevention of disease flares and use of adjunctive therapies and approaches. J Am Acad Dermatol 2014; 71(6): 1218-33.
[http://dx.doi.org/10.1016/j.jaad.2014.08.038] [PMID: 25264237]

[117] Wong SM, Ng TG, Baba R. Efficacy and safety of sodium hypochlorite (bleach) baths in patients with moderate to severe atopic dermatitis in Malaysia. J Dermatol 2013; 40(11): 874-80.
[http://dx.doi.org/10.1111/1346-8138.12265] [PMID: 24111816]

[118]   Chopra R, Vakharia PP, Sacotte R, Silverberg JI. Efficacy of bleach baths in reducing severity of atopic dermatitis: A systematic review and meta-analysis. Ann Allergy Asthma Immunol 2017; 119(5): 435-40.
[http://dx.doi.org/10.1016/j.anai.2017.08.289] [PMID: 29150071]

[119]   Devillers AC, Oranje AP. Wet-wrap treatment in children with atopic dermatitis: a practical guideline. Pediatr Dermatol 2012; 29(1): 24-7.
[http://dx.doi.org/10.1111/j.1525-1470.2011.01691.x] [PMID: 22256990]

[120]   González-López G, Ceballos-Rodríguez RM, González-López JJ, Feito Rodríguez M, Herranz-Pinto P. Efficacy and safety of wet wrap therapy for patients with atopic dermatitis: a systematic review and meta-analysis. Br J Dermatol 2016.
[PMID: 27861727]

[121]   Sidbury R, Davis DM, Cohen DE, *et al.* Guidelines of care for the management of atopic dermatitis: section 3. Management and treatment with phototherapy and systemic agents. J Am Acad Dermatol 2014; 71(2): 327-49.
[http://dx.doi.org/10.1016/j.jaad.2014.03.030] [PMID: 24813298]

[122]   Broeders JA, Ahmed Ali U, Fischer G. Systematic review and meta-analysis of randomized clinical trials (RCTs) comparing topical calcineurin inhibitors with topical corticosteroids for atopic dermatitis: A 15-year experience. J Am Acad Dermatol 2016; 75(2): 410-419.e3.
[http://dx.doi.org/10.1016/j.jaad.2016.02.1228] [PMID: 27177441]

[123]   Peserico A, Städtler G, Sebastian M, Fernandez RS, Vick K, Bieber T. Reduction of relapses of atopic dermatitis with methylprednisolone aceponate cream twice weekly in addition to maintenance treatment with emollient: a multicentre, randomized, double-blind, controlled study. Br J Dermatol 2008; 158(4): 801-7.
[http://dx.doi.org/10.1111/j.1365-2133.2008.08436.x] [PMID: 18284403]

[124]   Lee JY, Her Y, Kim CW, Kim SS. Topical Corticosteroid Phobia among Parents of Children with Atopic Eczema in Korea. Ann Dermatol 2015; 27(5): 499-506.
[http://dx.doi.org/10.5021/ad.2015.27.5.499] [PMID: 26512163]

[125]   Stuetz A, Baumann K, Grassberger M, Wolff K, Meingassner JG. Discovery of topical calcineurin inhibitors and pharmacological profile of pimecrolimus. Int Arch Allergy Immunol 2006; 141(3): 199-212.
[http://dx.doi.org/10.1159/000095289] [PMID: 16926539]

[126]   Reitamo S, Rustin M, Ruzicka T, *et al.* Efficacy and safety of tacrolimus ointment compared with that of hydrocortisone butyrate ointment in adult patients with atopic dermatitis. J Allergy Clin Immunol 2002; 109(3): 547-55.
[http://dx.doi.org/10.1067/mai.2002.121832] [PMID: 11898005]

[127]   Thaçi D, Reitamo S, Gonzalez Ensenat MA, *et al.* Proactive disease management with 0.03% tacrolimus ointment for children with atopic dermatitis: results of a randomized, multicentre, comparative study. Br J Dermatol 2008; 159(6): 1348-56.
[http://dx.doi.org/10.1111/j.1365-2133.2008.08813.x] [PMID: 18782319]

[128]   Schlessinger J, Shepard JS, Gower R, *et al.* Safety, Effectiveness, and Pharmacokinetics of Crisaborole in Infants Aged 3 to < 24Months with Mild-to-Moderate Atopic Dermatitis: A Phase IV Open-Label Study (CrisADe CARE 1). Am J Clin Dermatol 2020; 21(2): 275-84.
[http://dx.doi.org/10.1007/s40257-020-00510-6] [PMID: 32212104]

[129]   Bissonnette R, Pavel AB, Diaz A, *et al.* Crisaborole and atopic dermatitis skin biomarkers: An intrapatient randomized trial. J Allergy Clin Immunol 2019; 144(5): 1274-89.
[http://dx.doi.org/10.1016/j.jaci.2019.06.047] [PMID: 31419544]

[130]   Paller AS, Tom WL, Lebwohl MG, *et al.* Efficacy and safety of crisaborole ointment, a novel, nonsteroidal phosphodiesterase 4 (PDE4) inhibitor for the topical treatment of atopic dermatitis (AD) in children and adults. J Am Acad Dermatol 2016; 75(3): 494-503.e6.

[http://dx.doi.org/10.1016/j.jaad.2016.05.046] [PMID: 27417017]

[131] Gambichler T, Kreuter A, Tomi NS, Othlinghaus N, Altmeyer P, Skrygan M. Gene expression of cytokines in atopic eczema before and after ultraviolet A1 phototherapy. Br J Dermatol 2008; 158(5): 1117-20.
[http://dx.doi.org/10.1111/j.1365-2133.2008.08498.x] [PMID: 18363757]

[132] Tintle S, Shemer A, Suárez-Fariñas M, Fujita H, Gilleaudeau P, Sullivan-Whalen M, *et al.* Reversal of atopic dermatitis with narrow-band UVB phototherapy and biomarkers for therapeutic response. J Allergy Clin Immunol 2011; 128(3): 583-93.

[133] Sarıcaoğlu H, Yazici S, Zorlu Ö, Bülbül Başkan E, Aydoğan K. Cyclosporine-A for severe childhood atopic dermatitis: clinical experience on efficacy and safety profile. Turk J Med Sci 2018; 48(5): 933-8.
[http://dx.doi.org/10.3906/sag-1711-7] [PMID: 30384556]

[134] Wollenberg A, Barbarot S, Bieber T, *et al.* Consensus-based European guidelines for treatment of atopic eczema (atopic dermatitis) in adults and children: partII. J Eur Acad Dermatol Venereol 2018; 32(6): 850-78.
[http://dx.doi.org/10.1111/jdv.14888] [PMID: 29878606]

[135] Goujon C, Viguier M, Staumont-Sallé D, *et al.* Methotrexate Versus Cyclosporine in Adults with Moderate-to-Severe Atopic Dermatitis: A Phase III Randomized Noninferiority Trial. J Allergy Clin Immunol Pract 2018; 6(2): 562-569.e3.
[http://dx.doi.org/10.1016/j.jaip.2017.07.007] [PMID: 28967549]

[136] Anderson K, Putterman E, Rogers RS, Patel D, Treat JR, Castelo-Soccio L. Treatment of severe pediatric atopic dermatitis with methotrexate: A retrospective review. Pediatr Dermatol 2019; 36(3): 298-302.
[http://dx.doi.org/10.1111/pde.13781] [PMID: 30811669]

[137] Taieb Y, Baum S, Ben Amitai D, Barzilai A, Greenberger S. The use of methotrexate for treating childhood atopic dermatitis: a multicenter retrospective study. J Dermatolog Treat 2019; 30(3): 240-4.
[http://dx.doi.org/10.1080/09546634.2018.1508816] [PMID: 30109960]

[138] Simpson EL, Bieber T, Guttman-Yassky E, *et al.* Two Phase 3 Trials of Dupilumab *versus* Placebo in Atopic Dermatitis. N Engl J Med 2016; 375(24): 2335-48.
[http://dx.doi.org/10.1056/NEJMoa1610020] [PMID: 27690741]

[139] Blauvelt A, de Bruin-Weller M, Gooderham M, *et al.* Long-term management of moderate-to-severe atopic dermatitis with dupilumab and concomitant topical corticosteroids (LIBERTY AD CHRONOS): a 1-year, randomised, double-blinded, placebo-controlled, phase 3 trial. Lancet 2017; 389(10086): 2287-303.
[http://dx.doi.org/10.1016/S0140-6736(17)31191-1] [PMID: 28478972]

[140] Cork MJ, Thaçi D, Eichenfield LF, *et al.* Dupilumab in adolescents with uncontrolled moderate-t--severe atopic dermatitis: results from a phase IIa open-label trial and subsequent phase III open-label extension. Br J Dermatol 2020; 182(1): 85-96.
[http://dx.doi.org/10.1111/bjd.18476] [PMID: 31595499]

[141] He H, Guttman-Yassky E. JAK Inhibitors for Atopic Dermatitis: An Update. Am J Clin Dermatol 2019; 20(2): 181-92.
[http://dx.doi.org/10.1007/s40257-018-0413-2] [PMID: 30536048]

[142] Bissonnette R, Papp KA, Poulin Y, *et al.* Topical tofacitinib for atopic dermatitis: a phase IIa randomized trial. Br J Dermatol 2016; 175(5): 902-11.
[http://dx.doi.org/10.1111/bjd.14871] [PMID: 27423107]

[143] Guttman-Yassky E, Silverberg JI, Nemoto O, *et al.* Baricitinib in adult patients with moderate-t--severe atopic dermatitis: A phase 2 parallel, double-blinded, randomized placebo-controlled multiple-dose study. J Am Acad Dermatol 2019; 80(4): 913-921.e9.
[http://dx.doi.org/10.1016/j.jaad.2018.01.018] [PMID: 29410014]

[144] Mendes JT, Balogh EA, Strowd LC, Feldman SR. An evaluation of baricitinib as a therapeutic option for adult patients with moderate to severe atopic dermatitis. Expert Opin Pharmacother 2020; 21(9): 1027-33.
[http://dx.doi.org/10.1080/14656566.2020.1739268] [PMID: 32208940]

[145] Vakharia PP, Silverberg JI. New therapies for atopic dermatitis: Additional treatment classes. J Am Acad Dermatol 2018; 78(3) (Suppl. 1): S76-83.
[http://dx.doi.org/10.1016/j.jaad.2017.12.024] [PMID: 29248520]

[146] Peppers J, Paller AS, Maeda-Chubachi T, *et al.* A phase 2, randomized dose-finding study of tapinarof (GSK2894512 cream) for the treatment of atopic dermatitis. J Am Acad Dermatol 2019; 80(1): 89-98.e3.
[http://dx.doi.org/10.1016/j.jaad.2018.06.047] [PMID: 30554600]

[147] Simpson EL, Parnes JR, She D, *et al.* Tezepelumab, an anti-thymic stromal lymphopoietin monoclonal antibody, in the treatment of moderate to severe atopic dermatitis: A randomized phase 2a clinical trial. J Am Acad Dermatol 2019; 80(4): 1013-21.
[http://dx.doi.org/10.1016/j.jaad.2018.11.059] [PMID: 30550828]

[148] Parnes JR, Sullivan JT, Chen L, Dias C. Pharmacokinetics, Safety, and Tolerability of Tezepelumab (AMG 157) in Healthy and Atopic Dermatitis Adult Subjects. Clin Pharmacol Ther 2019; 106(2): 441-9.
[http://dx.doi.org/10.1002/cpt.1401] [PMID: 30779339]

[149] Oldhoff JM, Darsow U, Werfel T, *et al.* Anti-IL-5 recombinant humanized monoclonal antibody (mepolizumab) for the treatment of atopic dermatitis. Allergy 2005; 60(5): 693-6.
[http://dx.doi.org/10.1111/j.1398-9995.2005.00791.x] [PMID: 15813818]

[150] Kang EG, Narayana PK, Pouliquen IJ, Lopez MC, Ferreira-Cornwell MC, Getsy JA. Efficacy and safety of mepolizumab administered subcutaneously for moderate to severe atopic dermatitis. Allergy 2020; 75(4): 950-3.
[http://dx.doi.org/10.1111/all.14050] [PMID: 31515809]

[151] Ruzicka T, Hanifin JM, Furue M, *et al.* Anti-Interleukin-31 Receptor A Antibody for Atopic Dermatitis. N Engl J Med 2017; 376(9): 826-35.
[http://dx.doi.org/10.1056/NEJMoa1606490] [PMID: 28249150]

[152] Kabashima K, Furue M, Hanifin JM, *et al.* Nemolizumab in patients with moderate-to-severe atopic dermatitis: Randomized, phase II, long-term extension study. J Allergy Clin Immunol 2018; 142(4): 1121-1130.e7.
[http://dx.doi.org/10.1016/j.jaci.2018.03.018] [PMID: 29753033]

[153] Silverberg JI, Pinter A, Pulka G, *et al.* Phase 2B randomized study of nemolizumab in adults with moderate-to-severe atopic dermatitis and severe pruritus. J Allergy Clin Immunol 2020; 145(1): 173-82.
[http://dx.doi.org/10.1016/j.jaci.2019.08.013] [PMID: 31449914]

[154] Kabashima K, Matsumura T, Komazaki H, Kawashima M. Trial of Nemolizumab and Topical Agents for Atopic Dermatitis with Pruritus. N Engl J Med 2020; 383(2): 141-50.
[http://dx.doi.org/10.1056/NEJMoa1917006] [PMID: 32640132]

[155] Mihara R, Kabashima K, Furue M, Nakano M, Ruzicka T. Nemolizumab in moderate to severe atopic dermatitis: An exploratory analysis of work productivity and activity impairment in a randomized phase II study. J Dermatol 2019; 46(8): 662-71.
[http://dx.doi.org/10.1111/1346-8138.14934] [PMID: 31166620]

[156] Guttman-Yassky E, Pavel AB, Zhou L, *et al.* GBR 830, an anti-OX40, improves skin gene signatures and clinical scores in patients with atopic dermatitis. J Allergy Clin Immunol 2019; 144(2): 482-493.e7.
[http://dx.doi.org/10.1016/j.jaci.2018.11.053] [PMID: 30738171]

[157] Wollenberg A, Howell MD, Guttman-Yassky E, *et al.* Treatment of atopic dermatitis with tralokinumab, an anti-IL-13 mAb. J Allergy Clin Immunol 2019; 143(1): 135-41.
[http://dx.doi.org/10.1016/j.jaci.2018.05.029] [PMID: 29906525]

[158] Simpson EL, Flohr C, Eichenfield LF, *et al.* Efficacy and safety of lebrikizumab (an anti-IL-13 monoclonal antibody) in adults with moderate-to-severe atopic dermatitis inadequately controlled by topical corticosteroids: A randomized, placebo-controlled phase II trial (TREBLE). J Am Acad Dermatol 2018; 78(5): 863-871.e11.
[http://dx.doi.org/10.1016/j.jaad.2018.01.017] [PMID: 29353026]

[159] Guttman-Yassky E, Blauvelt A, Eichenfield LF, *et al.* Efficacy and Safety of Lebrikizumab, a High-Affinity Interleukin 13 Inhibitor, in Adults With Moderate to Severe Atopic Dermatitis: A Phase 2b Randomized Clinical Trial. JAMA Dermatol 2020; 156(4): 411-20.
[http://dx.doi.org/10.1001/jamadermatol.2020.0079] [PMID: 32101256]

[160] Ungar B, Pavel AB, Li R, Kimmel G, Nia J, Hashim P, *et al.* Phase 2 randomized, double-blind study of IL-17 targeting with secukinumab in atopic dermatitis. J Allergy Clin Immunol 2020.
[PMID: 32428528]

[161] Guttman-Yassky E, Brunner PM, Neumann AU, *et al.* Efficacy and safety of fezakinumab (an IL-22 monoclonal antibody) in adults with moderate-to-severe atopic dermatitis inadequately controlled by conventional treatments: A randomized, double-blind, phase 2a trial. J Am Acad Dermatol 2018; 78(5): 872-881.e6.
[http://dx.doi.org/10.1016/j.jaad.2018.01.016] [PMID: 29353025]

[162] Brunner PM, Pavel AB, Khattri S, *et al.* Baseline IL-22 expression in patients with atopic dermatitis stratifies tissue responses to fezakinumab. J Allergy Clin Immunol 2019; 143(1): 142-54.
[http://dx.doi.org/10.1016/j.jaci.2018.07.028] [PMID: 30121291]

[163] Pan Y, Xu L, Qiao J, Fang H. A systematic review of ustekinumab in the treatment of atopic dermatitis. J Dermatolog Treat 2018; 29(6): 539-41.
[http://dx.doi.org/10.1080/09546634.2017.1406894] [PMID: 29164954]

[164] Holm JG, Thomsen SF. Omalizumab for atopic dermatitis: evidence for and against its use. G Ital Dermatol Venereol 2019; 154(4): 480-7.
[http://dx.doi.org/10.23736/S0392-0488.19.06302-8] [PMID: 30717578]

[165] Chan S, Cornelius V, Cro S, Harper JI, Lack G. Treatment Effect of Omalizumab on Severe Pediatric Atopic Dermatitis: The ADAPT Randomized Clinical Trial. JAMA Pediatr 2019.
[PMID: 31764962]

[166] Borzutzky A, Camargo CA Jr. Role of vitamin D in the pathogenesis and treatment of atopic dermatitis. Expert Rev Clin Immunol 2013; 9(8): 751-60.
[http://dx.doi.org/10.1586/1744666X.2013.816493] [PMID: 23971753]

[167] Huang CM, Lara-Corrales I, Pope E. Effects of Vitamin D levels and supplementation on atopic dermatitis: A systematic review. Pediatr Dermatol 2018; 35(6): 754-60.
[http://dx.doi.org/10.1111/pde.13639] [PMID: 30284328]

[168] Staab D, von Rueden U, Kehrt R, *et al.* Evaluation of a parental training program for the management of childhood atopic dermatitis. Pediatr Allergy Immunol 2002; 13(2): 84-90.
[http://dx.doi.org/10.1034/j.1399-3038.2002.01005.x] [PMID: 12000479]

[169] Grillo M, Gassner L, Marshman G, Dunn S, Hudson P. Pediatric atopic eczema: the impact of an educational intervention. Pediatr Dermatol 2006; 23(5): 428-36.
[http://dx.doi.org/10.1111/j.1525-1470.2006.00277.x] [PMID: 17014636]

[170] Staab D, Diepgen TL, Fartasch M, *et al.* Age related, structured educational programmes for the management of atopic dermatitis in children and adolescents: multicentre, randomised controlled trial. BMJ 2006; 332(7547): 933-8.
[http://dx.doi.org/10.1136/bmj.332.7547.933] [PMID: 16627509]

[171] Weber MB, Fontes Neto PT, Prati C, *et al.* Improvement of pruritus and quality of life of children with atopic dermatitis and their families after joining support groups. J Eur Acad Dermatol Venereol 2008; 22(8): 992-7.
[http://dx.doi.org/10.1111/j.1468-3083.2008.02697.x] [PMID: 18422535]

[172] Shaw M, Morrell DS, Goldsmith LA. A study of targeted enhanced patient care for pediatric atopic dermatitis (STEP PAD). Pediatr Dermatol 2008; 25(1): 19-24.
[http://dx.doi.org/10.1111/j.1525-1470.2007.00575.x] [PMID: 18304147]

[173] Boulos S, Yan AC. Current concepts in the prevention of atopic dermatitis. Clin Dermatol 2018; 36(5): 668-71.
[http://dx.doi.org/10.1016/j.clindermatol.2017.03.004] [PMID: 30217281]

[174] Horimukai K, Morita K, Narita M, *et al.* Application of moisturizer to neonates prevents development of atopic dermatitis. J Allergy Clin Immunol 2014; 134(4): 824-830.e6.
[http://dx.doi.org/10.1016/j.jaci.2014.07.060] [PMID: 25282564]

[175] Simpson EL, Chalmers JR, Hanifin JM, *et al.* Emollient enhancement of the skin barrier from birth offers effective atopic dermatitis prevention. J Allergy Clin Immunol 2014; 134(4): 818-23.
[http://dx.doi.org/10.1016/j.jaci.2014.08.005] [PMID: 25282563]

[176] Greer FR, Sicherer SH, Burks AW, *et al.* The Effects of Early Nutritional Interventions on the Development of Atopic Disease in Infants and Children: The Role of Maternal Dietary Restriction, Breastfeeding, Hydrolyzed Formulas, and Timing of Introduction of Allergenic Complementary Foods. Pediatrics 2019; 143(4): e20190281.
[http://dx.doi.org/10.1542/peds.2019-0281] [PMID: 30886111]

[177] Zuccotti G, Meneghin F, Aceti A, *et al.* Probiotics for prevention of atopic diseases in infants: systematic review and meta-analysis. Allergy 2015; 70(11): 1356-71.
[http://dx.doi.org/10.1111/all.12700] [PMID: 26198702]

[178] Li L, Han Z, Niu X, *et al.* Probiotic Supplementation for Prevention of Atopic Dermatitis in Infants and Children: A Systematic Review and Meta-analysis. Am J Clin Dermatol 2019; 20(3): 367-77.
[http://dx.doi.org/10.1007/s40257-018-0404-3] [PMID: 30465329]

[179] Kim JP, Chao LX, Simpson EL, Silverberg JI. Persistence of atopic dermatitis (AD): A systematic review and meta-analysis. J Am Acad Dermatol 2016; 75(4): 681-687.e11.
[http://dx.doi.org/10.1016/j.jaad.2016.05.028] [PMID: 27544489]

[180] Mortz CG, Andersen KE, Dellgren C, Barington T, Bindslev-Jensen C. Atopic dermatitis from adolescence to adulthood in the TOACS cohort: prevalence, persistence and comorbidities. Allergy 2015; 70(7): 836-45.
[http://dx.doi.org/10.1111/all.12619] [PMID: 25832131]

[181] Wan J, Mitra N, Hoffstad OJ, Yan AC, Margolis DJ. Longitudinal atopic dermatitis control and persistence vary with timing of disease onset in children: A cohort study. J Am Acad Dermatol 2019; 81(6): 1292-9.
[http://dx.doi.org/10.1016/j.jaad.2019.05.016] [PMID: 31085263]

CHAPTER 9

Updates on Henoch-Schonlein Purpura

Patricia Morán-Álvarez[1], Guillermo Santos-Simarro[2] and Fernando Santos[3,4,*]

[1] *Department of Rheumatology Hospital Universitario Ramón y Cajal, Madrid, Spain*

[2] *Department of Pediatrics Hospital Universitario La Paz, Madrid, Spain*

[3] *Division of Pediatric Nephrology Hospital Universitario Central de Asturias, Oviedo, Asturias, Spain*

[4] *Department of Medicine University of Oviedo, Oviedo, Asturias, Spain*

Abstract: Henoch-Schönlein purpura (HSP), currently also known as immunoglobulin A (IgA) vasculitis, is the most common vasculitis in children. It is a systemic autoimmune disease mediated by complexes containing abnormal IgA. The cause of HSP is not well known, but the disease is often triggered by an upper respiratory infection in individuals with genetic susceptibility. The diagnosis relies on internationally agreed criteria, including palpable cutaneous purpura of orthostatic location associated with at least one of the following findings: arthralgia/arthritis, gastrointestinal manifestations, leukocytoclastic vasculitis with IgA deposits and/or renal involvement. The skin lesions are essential for the diagnosis. The digestive symptoms, mostly severe abdominal pain, intestinal bleeding, and more rarely, intussusception, maybe the initial and most worrisome clinical component of HSP during the acute presentation of the disease. Nephropathy determines the long-term prognosis. The clinical course of HSP is, in general, favorable. Bed rest results in remission of the purpura that often recurs as the child restarts standing and walking. Corticosteroids are effective, although not usually required, to treat abdominal pain and other severe manifestations. No medical treatment can avoid the possibility of renal involvement that may occur for several months after resolution of the skin lesions. Corticosteroids are used to treat severe forms of HSP nephropathy, which anatomopathologically corresponds to IgA glomerulonephritis. Active research studies are needed to clarify the pathogenesis, the prognostic factors, and the measures to be taken for the prevention and treatment of renal disease.

Keywords: Anaphylactoid purpura, Asialoglycoprotein receptor, ß1,3-galactosyltransferase, Childhood systemic vasculitis, Children, Galactose-deficient IgA1, Henoch-Schönlein purpura, IgA1 isoform, IgA vasculitis, IgA glomerulonephritis, IgAV nephropathy, IgG-Gd-IgA, Immune complexes, Leukocytoclastic vasculitis, Lower limb purpura, Non-granulomatous vasculitis,

---

* **Corresponding author Fernando Santos:** Nefrología Pediátrica, Pediatría. Hospital Universitario Central de Asturias, Avda de Roma s/n, 33011 Oviedo, Asturias, Spain; Tel: +34 985108237; E-mail: fsantos@uniovi.es

Nima Rezaei and Noosha Samieefar (Eds.)

Pediatric purpura, Pediatric vasculitis, Rheumatoid purpura, Small vessel vasculitis.

INTRODUCTION

Systemic vasculitides are characterized by blood vessel inflammation, leading to tissue injury from vascular stenosis, occlusion, aneurysm, and/or rupture. These entities are rare in childhood but are associated with significant morbidity and mortality. Only Henoch-Schönlein purpura (HSP) and Kawasaki disease are relatively common in pediatric patients. HSP is the most common primary systemic vasculitis in children. It is a non-granulomatous form of systemic vasculitis that affects small vessels predominantly.

The term HSP comes from Johann Schönlein and Eduard Henoch, two German doctors who first made a detailed description of the disease in the 1860s [1]. Recent consensus documents have proposed replacing the name HSP with that of IgA vasculitis (IgAV), based on the pathophysiological feature of the disease [2]. Both denominations will be used in this chapter, as the term HSP is widely extended in the medical community and is commonly used in everyday clinical practice. Other nomenclatures such as anaphylactoid purpura and rheumatoid purpura have also been utilized. The association of cutaneous, musculoskeletal, and renal manifestations has led to consider HSP as the cause of the composer Wolfgang Amadeus Mozart's death in 1791, although scientific evidence supporting this hypothesis is missing [3].

According to the internationally accepted classification of vasculitis in childhood [4], the diagnosis of HSP or IgAV includes the mandatory presence of purpura or petechia with lower limb predominance and at least one of the four following criteria: abdominal pain, arthritis or arthralgia, renal involvement (proteinuria, hematuria or red blood cell casts), histopathology findings showing leukocytoclastic vasculitis or glomerulonephritis with predominant IgA deposit.

A detailed description of these criteria will be provided in this chapter. In adults, unlike children, there are no internationally agreed-upon criteria for the diagnosis of IgAV.

EPIDEMIOLOGY

HSP is typical of the pediatric age, although it can also be seen in adults. It is the most common vasculitis among children, the annual incidence having been estimated from 3 to 26.7/100 000 for children and infants and 0.8-1.8/100 000 for adults [5]. The incidence peak stands around 4-6 years, 90% of cases are younger than 10 years of age, and it is rare in infants. HSP is found in both genders with a preponderance of males and in all races, being less frequent in black people with respect to white and Asian people [6]. There is seasonal variation likely linked to the variable incidence of upper respiratory tract infections [7].

PATHOGENESIS

HSP is a small vessel leukocytoclastic vasculitis of unclear pathogenic origin [8], the combination of genetic susceptibility and environmental risk factors (such as infections, food, vaccination, or drugs) being likely involved in the development of the disease [9].

Around 50% of HSP cases are preceded by an upper respiratory tract infection, suggesting this type of infection is the main trigger of the disease [10, 11], followed by gastrointestinal infections in 5-6% and urinary tract infections in 1%, approximately. Several infectious agents have been implicated, including *group A or B hemolytic Streptococcus, Staphylococcus aureus, parainfluenza, Helicobacter pylori, Parvovirus B19,* or *Epstein-Barr virus*, among others [11]. Some studies found *Streptococcus*, identified by anti-streptolysin (ASO) titer test and throat swab culture, as the most common infectious agent associated with HSP (around 30%) [9]. The relationship between several vaccines and HSP, including influenza A (H1N1) vaccination, has also been described [12].

As for the genetic component, HLA-DRB1*01, HLA-DRB1*11, and HLA-B*41:02 antigens have been proposed to be associated with an increased risk of developing HSP, whereas HLA-DRB1*07 has been conferred a protective effect [9, 13].

HSP is characterized by the deposition of IgA, mainly IgA1 isoform, immune complexes in the vessel walls of dermal capillaries, and in the renal mesangium. IgA-containing immune complexes and high blood levels of IgA in 50% of children can be observed during the acute phase of the illness. In addition, some studies have described the presence of IgA antineutrophil cytoplasmic antibodies (IgA-ANCA), IgA-rheumatoid factor (IgA-RF), or IgA-anti-cardiolipin antibodies (IgA-aCL) [11].

IgA is physiologically present in serum and mucosal secretions. Two IgA isoforms exist, IgA_1 and IgA_2, the former being the most prevalent (90%) in the circulation. In general, IgA_1 has a hinge region containing up to six O-linked glycan chains consisting of N-acetylgalactosamine (GalNAc), sialic acid, and galactose due to ß1,3-galactosyltransferase action [8, 10, 13]. This leads to the clearance of IgA_1 molecules through its interaction with the asialoglycoprotein receptor (ASGP-R) of the hepatocytes [10]. Nevertheless, reduced activity of ß1,3-galactosyltransferase, secondary to genetic predisposition, IL-6 production and/or infections, has been found in HSP patients. Consequently, aberrant glycosylation occurred, leading to galactose-deficient IgA1 (Gd-IgA1) [8, 10, 13]. These aberrantly glycosylated IgA1 molecules are recognized by IgG autoantibodies and soluble IgA Fc alpha receptor (sCD89), forming immune complexes. Some hypotheses about the source of these autoantibodies indicate that Gd-IgA1 itself could induce its production or be the result of cross-reactivity with GalNAc-containing molecules on pathogens or food [13]. These IgG-G--IgA1 immune complexes hamper its internalization and degradation by hepatic cells [10]. Deposition of IgA immune complexes produces the stimulation of alternative and lectin complement pathways; however, the classical route is not activated due to the lack of a C1q binding site [8, 13]. This results in the recruitment of polymorphonuclear leucocytes and the production of cytokines and chemokines, leading to inflammation and necrosis of vessel walls.

The suggested pathogenesis of HSP is graphically represented in Fig. (**1**).

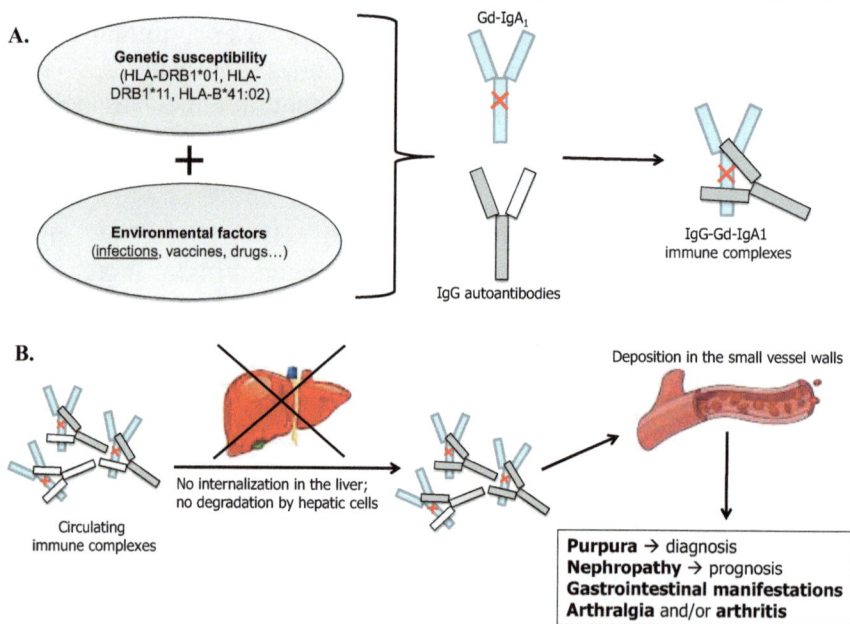

Fig. (1). Suggested pathogenesis of Henoch-Schönlein purpura. Production (A) and deposit (B) of immune complexes. IgA: immunoglobulin A. IgG: immunoglobulin G. Gd-IgA1: galactose-deficient IgA1.

CLINICAL FEATURES

Purpura

Skin involvement is present in all patients with HSP and usually is the initial manifestation. As mentioned above, purpura, commonly palpable and in crops or petechiae, with lower limb predominance is mandatory for diagnosis [4]. The cutaneous lesions may contain elements with different aspects, but the symmetric distribution of the rash in the buttocks and lower extremities is characteristic (Figs. **2** and **3**). Approximately one-third of patients may have purpuric elements in the trunk and upper extremities, mainly in the extensor surfaces and elbows. The lesions are orthostatic and may localize in the back when the child is in prolonged decubitus. Usually, with bed rest new lesions cease and the rash becomes progressively less noticeable, fades and disappears within a week to 10 days.

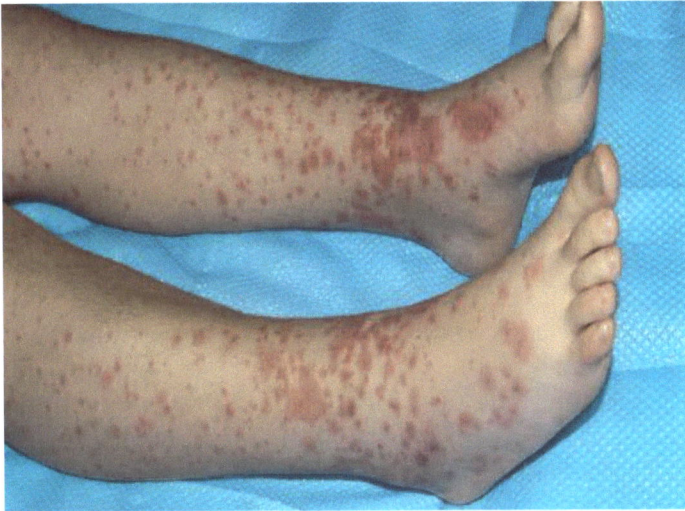

Fig. (2). Henoch-Schönlein purpura is characterized by palpable elements often grouped in confluent lesions, petechiae and lower limb predominance.

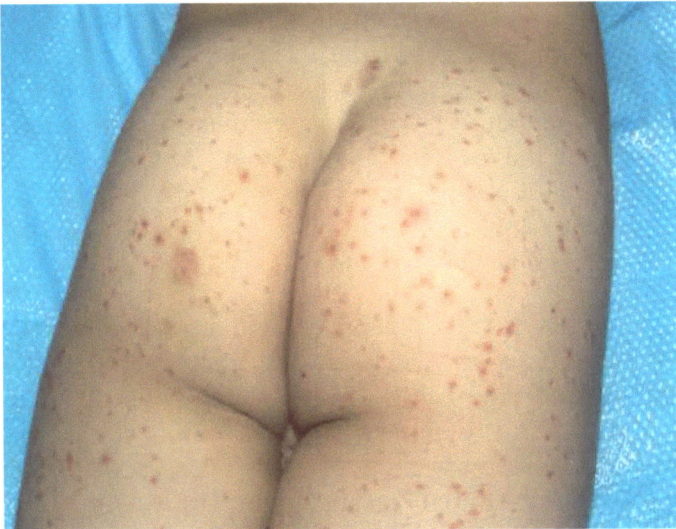

Fig. (3). Typical symmetric distribution of Henoch-Schönlein purpura lesions in both buttocks.

Articular Manifestations

Arthralgia and/or arthritis are the most frequent manifestations and affect 75-80% of HSP patients. Large joints are mostly involved, feet/ankles, knees, hands/wrists, and elbows in decreasing order of frequency. The articular manifestations can rarely precede the cutaneous rash, which poses initial diagnostic problems. They may have migratory character, are self-limited, and do not leave either deformities or functional sequelae.

Gastrointestinal Manifestations

Approximately 50-75% of HSP patients have acute gastrointestinal symptoms, mostly colicky abdominal pain, which may be severe and the dominant symptom of the disease. Intense abdominal pain preceding the cutaneous manifestations may lead to clinical confusion and the wrong diagnosis of acute appendicitis. Severe abdominal pain may be associated with hypoproteinemia caused by protein-losing enteropathy. Some form of intestinal bleeding is common, particularly if fecal occult blood is systematically searched. Severe complications include intussusception, bowel perforation, bowel gangrene, and massive hemorrhage [1]. Intussusception is the most common life-threatening gastrointestinal complication, affecting 3% to 4% of patients with HSP [10].

Nephropathy

Renal involvement should be searched systematically in pediatric patients with HSP because of its high frequency and prognostic significance [14]. Clinical manifestations of HSP nephropathy, currently known as IgAV nephropathy (IgAVN), are found in 20-60% of cases [15]. The most common features are isolated microscopic hematuria with or without proteinuria. Macroscopic hematuria may also be the presenting symptom. Acute nephritic syndrome, including renal failure and arterial hypertension, and nephrotic syndrome, are severe forms of manifestation, present in up to 6-7% of children with HSP, and they are associated with the worse outcome.

The risk of developing nephropathy reappears with each recurrence of cutaneous purpura. There is often days or weeks between the acute skin lesions and the beginning of renal signs, 91% of those who develop renal manifestations do so within 6 weeks and 97% within 6 months after the initial cutaneous manifestations. Therefore, urinary monitoring is necessary for at least six and optimally 12 months from the initial presentation of HSP.

Other Manifestations

HSP is a systemic disease involving small vessels so that it may cause symptoms in any organ. Urogenital involvement is relatively common. Up to 25% of HSP boys have scrotal pain that usually corresponds to orchitis but mimics testicular torsion and needs adequate exploration to differentiate. Central nervous system-related symptoms such as seizures, neuropathy, and headache may also be present in 2% of patients. Other manifestations of multiple organ systems, including pulmonary hemorrhage, have also been reported with less incidence.

DIFFERENTIAL DIAGNOSIS

Table **1** shows the internationally accepted classification of childhood vasculitis, mainly based on vessel size, proposed in 2006 [16] and further endorsed by the European League Against Rheumatism (EULAR), the Paediatric Rheumatology International Trials Organization (PRINTO), and the Paediatric Rheumatology European Society (PRES) in 2010 [4, 11].

Table 1. Childhood vasculitis classification [Ozen, 2006].

I. Predominantly large vessel vasculitis • Takayasu arteritis
II. Predominantly medium-sized vessel vasculitis • Childhood polyarteritis nodosa (PAN) • Cutaneous polyarteritis • Kawasaki disease
III. Predominantly small vessel vasculitis *Granulomatous:* • Wegener granulomatosis (WG, now referred to as granulomatosis with polyangiitis, GPA) • Churg-Strauss syndrome (CSS, now referred to as eosinophilic granulomatosis with polyangiitis, EGPA) *Non-granulomatous:* • Microscopic polyangiitis • Henoch-Schönlein purpura • Isolated cutaneous leucocytoclastic vasculitis • Hypocomplementaemic urticarial vasculitis
IV. Other vasculitides • Beçhet's disease • Vasculitis secondary to infection (including hepatitis B associated PAN), malignancies and drugs, including hypersensitivity vasculitis • Vasculitis associated with other connective tissue diseases • Isolated vasculitis of the central nervous system (Childhood Primary Angiitis of the central nervous system: cPACNS) • Cogan´s síndrome • Unclassified

The diagnosis of HSP requires the presence of purpura or petechia with lower limb predominance associated with one or more of the following: abdominal pain, arthritis or arthralgia, renal involvement, or compatible histopathology. Characteristic clinical features of children with HSP have also been discussed. The presence of articular, abdominal or, more rarely, renal manifestations preceding the cutaneous purpura may lead to initial diagnostic mistakes. Laboratory work-up showing normality of platelets and coagulation, elevation of serum IgA concentration, and negative immunologic studies such as complement, antinuclear antibodies, anti-double stranded normal deoxyribonuclease antineutrophil cytoplasmic antibodies may be of diagnostic help in a few selected cases. Skin biopsy is not usually indicated, but histopathological findings of small vessel leukocytoclastic vasculitis characterized by the presence of IgA-dominant immune deposits may also serve to support HSP diagnosis in a given individual [17].

TREATMENT

Most patients affected by HSP just need supportive care and symptomatic treatment based on bed rest, adequate analgesia, good hydration, and bowel rest, including sometimes the need for transient parenteral nutrition. Immunosuppressive treatments such as glucocorticoids, azathioprine, cyclosporine, or mycophenolate are required in selected patients. The reader is referred to SHARE (Single-Hub Access for Paediatric Rheumatology in Europe), European consensus-based guidance for the management of HSP in order to provide international, evidence-based recommendations optimizing the care of children with rheumatic diseases such as IgAV [18].

Treatment of Skin Involvement

Skin manifestations usually do not require specific treatment. In case of severe skin involvement, i.e., bullous or necrotic rash, therapies such as dapsone (an antibiotic with anti-inflammatory actions through myeloperoxidase inhibition), colchicine, rituximab (an anti-CD20 antibody, functioning as a B-cell inhibitor), or a short course of systemic corticosteroids (1 mg/ kg/day of oral prednisone) could be used on the basis of data published in small series or individual clinical reports [10, 11, 18, 19].

Treatment of Musculoskeletal Involvement

Expert opinion suggests non-steroidal anti-inflammatory drugs (NSAIDs) as the first line of treatment due to the good responses experienced by these patients. Treatment is usually well-tolerated; nevertheless, the use of NSAIDs is contraindicated if active gastrointestinal bleeding or nephritis exists (18). In case of failure, opioids or glucocorticoids at doses similar to those used in gastrointestinal or skin involvement may be an option [20].

Treatment of Gastrointestinal Involvement

Intense abdominal pain requires urgent ultrasonography to exclude intestinal intussusception, susceptible to surgical approach.Once this complication has been ruled out, corticosteroid treatment should be considered in children with bleeding or persistent severe abdominal pain. However, this treatment is not necessary since the majority improves spontaneously. Recommended doses of corticosteroids range from 1-2 mg/Kg/day of oral prednisone/prednisolone in mild cases to 10-30 mg/Kg of pulsed intravenous methylprednisolone with a maximum of 1g/day on three consecutive days for more severe cases [18]. There is no strong evidence about specific indications, dosage, and duration of corticosteroid administration. Ronkainen et al. (2006) demonstrated the efficacy of prednisone in terms of a decrease in the duration and the intensity of abdominal pain in a prospective randomized trial on 171 patients, 84 treated with prednisone vs. 87 receiving placebo [20]. By contrast, Huber et al. did not find significant differences between treatment and placebo groups [21]. Some studies have shown a significant reduction of intestinal intussusception in children treated with glucocorticoids [22]. Weiss et al. conducted a retrospective cohort study including 1895 children with new-onset HSP, in which they observed a significant reduction in the need for abdominal surgery among the patients who had been exposed to early period corticosteroids (day 1 and 2 from admission), compared with those with no corticosteroid exposure. Moreover, the former required less analgesia (NSAIDs and opioids) and abdominal imaging. However, the quality of evidence is poor [23].

Treatment of Renal Involvement

The nephropathy is not preventable by any treatment; that is, the prophylactic use of corticosteroids in extrarenal IgAV does not reduce the incidence of kidney involvement [24]. Even if it is true that nephritis determines the long-term consequences of HSP, it should be kept in mind that the renal involvement in pediatric patients is generally self-limited and of good prognosis.

Medical treatment of IgAVN requires the supervision and indication of a pediatric nephrologist. Persistent proteinuria, assessed by urinary protein/creatinine ratio > 0.2 mg/mg, for greater than three months, should be treated with angiotensin conversing enzyme inhibitor or angiotensin II receptor blocker in association with a low sodium diet. Suppose the patient develops nephrotic syndrome, or maintains nephrotic-range proteinuria, assessed by urinary protein/creatinine ratio > 2 mg/mg, or the glomerular filtration rate deteriorates. In that case, a kidney biopsy should be performed and treatment with oral prednisone/prednisolone and intravenous methylprednisolone should be used. A rapidly progressive IgVAN may require addition of cyclophosphamide. Novel biological agents may be tested in children with severe renal disease refractory to the above-mentioned treatments, but it should be emphasized that the vast majority of pediatric patients with HSP, even if they develop renal manifestations, have an excellent prognosis, and the aggressive therapies should be carefully evaluated for selected individual patients.

Miscellaneous Treatments

In case of orchitis, pulmonary hemorrhage, cerebral vasculitis or other severe organs- or life-threatening manifestations, corticosteroids should be considered in addition to other immunosuppressants or even plasma exchange [18].

PROGNOSIS

In the majority of children, the outcome is favorable, since most of them experiment a spontaneous resolution of symptoms. In general conditions, if renal involvement does not appear after the first episode of HSP, the resolution occurs within 1 month. In most cases, joint pain and uncomplicated abdominal pain usually resolve spontaneously within the first 48-72 hours, nevertheless, skin manifestations may last more time, being the last symptoms to remit [10].

Around one-third of patients recur at least once, mostly within 4 months of the initial presentation, although each episode is usually milder and shorter in duration than the previous ones [11, 17].

Long-term outcomes are determined by the degree of renal involvement [11, 25]. Pathological findings of IgAVN are indistinguishable from those of primary IgA nephropathy. The Oxford classification, including mesangial and endocapillary proliferation, lesions of glomerulosclerosis, tubular atrophy/interstitial fibrosis, and presence of crescents, is used to harmonize the microscopic features [26].

M – Mesangial cellularity, defined as more than four mesangial cells in any mesangial area of a glomerulus: M0 is mesangial cellularity in < 50% of glomeruli; M1 ≥50%.

E – Endocapillary proliferation, defined as hypercellularity due to an increased number of cells within glomerular capillary lumina: E0 is the absence of hypercellularity; E1 is hypercellularity in any glomeruli.

S – Segmental glomerulosclerosis, defined as adhesion or sclerosis (obliteration of capillary lumina by matrix) in part of but not the whole glomerular tuft: S0 is the absence of segmental glomerulosclerosis, S1 is the presence of segmental glomerulosclerosis in any glomerulus.

T – Tubular atrophy/interstitial fibrosis, defined as the estimated percentage of the cortical area showing tubular atrophy or interstitial fibrosis, whichever is greater: T0 is 0-25%; T1 is 25-50%; T2 is >50%.

C – Crescents: C0 (no crescents), C1 (crescents in less than one-fourth of glomeruli), and C2 (crescents in over one-fourth of glomeruli).

The Oxford MEST-C score based on the above punctuation has been validated as a prognostic tool in adults with primary IgA nephropathy, but there is insufficient evidence to support its use in HSP nephritis [27]. A recently published meta-analysis to identify risk factors associated with unfavorable outcomes in children found that older age at onset, lower glomerular filtration rate, initial renal features of nephrotic syndrome or nephritic-nephrotic syndrome, and renal biopsy with crescentic nephritis were predictive of poor prognosis in children with IgAVN [28].

A systematic review of studies of unselected children with HSP found that permanent renal impairment never developed after normal urinalysis; it occurred in 1.6% of those with isolated urinary abnormalities, and 19.5% of those who developed nephritic or nephrotic syndrome [29]. Children with initial presentation of IgAVN as renal failure, nephrotic or nephritic syndrome have the highest risk of developing chronic kidney disease, but, in general, the long-term prognosis of HSP nephropathy is favorable.

CONCLUSION

HSP is the most common vasculitis in children. It is a systemic disease that involves small vessels predominantly. The pathogenesis is unknown, mediated by IgA-containing immune complexes, and mostly triggered by upper respiratory infections. The diagnosis is based on the clinical presentation: characteristic purpura associated with gastrointestinal, articular, and/or renal manifestations. A typical anatomopathological finding is leukocytoclastic vasculitis with predominant IgA deposit. Severe acute abdominal pain may be the dominant presenting manifestation.

The long-term outcome is determined by renal involvement, which is not prevented by corticosteroid treatment, and the prognosis is usually favorable.

CONSENT FOR PUBLICATION

Not applicable.

CONFLICT OF INTEREST

The authors declare no conflict of interest, financial or otherwise.

ACKNOWLEDGEMENT

Declared none.

REFERENCES

[1]   Roache-Robinson P, Hotwagner DT. Henoch Schonlein Purpura (Anaphylactoid Purpura, HSP). 2018.

[2]   Jennette JC, Falk R, Bacon P, Basu N, Cid M, Ferrario F, *et al.* revised international chapel hill consensus conference nomenclature of vasculitides. 2013.

[3]   Guillery EN. Did Mozart die of kidney disease? A review from the bicentennial of his death. J Am Soc Nephrol 1992; 2(12): 1671-6.
[http://dx.doi.org/10.1681/ASN.V2121671] [PMID: 1498274]

[4]   Ozen S, Pistorio A, Iusan SM, *et al.* EULAR/PRINTO/PRES criteria for Henoch-Schönlein purpura, childhood polyarteritis nodosa, childhood Wegener granulomatosis and childhood Takayasu arteritis: Ankara 2008. Part II: Final classification criteria. Ann Rheum Dis 2010; 69(5): 798-806.
[http://dx.doi.org/10.1136/ard.2009.116657] [PMID: 20413568]

[5]   Piram M, Mahr A. Epidemiology of immunoglobulin A vasculitis (Henoch-Schönlein): current state of knowledge. Curr Opin Rheumatol 2013; 25(2): 171-8.
[http://dx.doi.org/10.1097/BOR.0b013e32835d8e2a] [PMID: 23318735]

[6]   Gardner-Medwin JM, Dolezalova P, Cummins C, Southwood TR. Incidence of Henoch-Schönlein purpura, Kawasaki disease, and rare vasculitides in children of different ethnic origins. Lancet 2002; 360(9341): 1197-202.
[http://dx.doi.org/10.1016/S0140-6736(02)11279-7] [PMID: 12401245]

[7]   Oni L, Sampath S. Childhood IgA Vasculitis (Henoch Schonlein Purpura)-Advances and Knowledge Gaps. Front Pediatr 2019; 7: 257.
[http://dx.doi.org/10.3389/fped.2019.00257] [PMID: 31316952]

[8]   Chen J-Y, Mao J-H. Henoch-Schönlein purpura nephritis in children: incidence, pathogenesis and management. World J Pediatr 2015; 11(1): 29-34.
[http://dx.doi.org/10.1007/s12519-014-0534-5] [PMID: 25557596]

[9]   Wang JJ, Xu Y, Liu FF, *et al.* Association of the infectious triggers with childhood Henoch-Schonlein purpura in Anhui province, China. J Infect Public Health 2020; 13(1): 110-7.
[http://dx.doi.org/10.1016/j.jiph.2019.07.004] [PMID: 31337540]

[10]   Trnka P. Henoch-Schönlein purpura in children. J Paediatr Child Health 2013; 49(12): 995-1003.
[http://dx.doi.org/10.1111/jpc.12403] [PMID: 24134307]

[11]   Brogan P, Ozen S, Eleftheriou D. Vasculitis. In: Martini A, Hachulla E, Eds. EULAR/PRES Textbook on Paediatric Rheumatology. London: BMJ Publishing Group Ltd. 2018.

[12]   Liu J-Y, Wu QS, Liu M, Wang L, Gao YH, Li SS. Henoch-Schönlein purpura nephritis following influenza vaccination: a case report and review of the literature. Southeast Asian J Trop Med Public Health 2016; 47(5): 945-50.
[PMID: 29620799]

[13]   Heineke MH, Ballering AV, Jamin A, Ben Mkaddem S, Monteiro RC, Van Egmond M. New insights in the pathogenesis of immunoglobulin A vasculitis (Henoch-Schönlein purpura). Autoimmun Rev 2017; 16(12): 1246-53.
[http://dx.doi.org/10.1016/j.autrev.2017.10.009] [PMID: 29037908]

[14]   Dyga K, Szczepańska M. IgA vasculitis with nephritis in children. Advances in clinical and experimental medicine: official organ Wroclaw Medical University 2020.
[http://dx.doi.org/10.17219/acem/112566]

[15]   Zaffanello M. Henoch-Schönlein Purpura Nephritis in Childhood. An Update on Glomerulopathies–Clinical and Treatment Aspects 2011; 209-30.

[16]   Ozen S, Ruperto N, Dillon MJ, *et al.* EULAR/PReS endorsed consensus criteria for the classification of childhood vasculitides. Ann Rheum Dis 2006; 65(7): 936-41.
[http://dx.doi.org/10.1136/ard.2005.046300] [PMID: 16322081]

[17]   Sohagia AB, Gunturu SG, Tong TR, Hertan HI. Henoch-Schonlein purpura—a case report and review of the literature. Gastroenterology research and practice 2010.

[18]   Ozen S, Marks SD, Brogan P, *et al.* European consensus-based recommendations for diagnosis and treatment of immunoglobulin A vasculitis-the SHARE initiative. Rheumatology (Oxford) 2019; 58(9): 1607-16.
[http://dx.doi.org/10.1093/rheumatology/kez041] [PMID: 30879080]

[19]   Hetland LE, Susrud KS, Lindahl KH, Bygum A. Henoch-Schönlein purpura: a literature review. Acta Derm Venereol 2017; 97(10): 1160-6.
[http://dx.doi.org/10.2340/00015555-2733] [PMID: 28654132]

[20]   Ronkainen J, Koskimies O, Ala-Houhala M, *et al.* Early prednisone therapy in Henoch-Schönlein purpura: a randomized, double-blind, placebo-controlled trial. J Pediatr 2006; 149(2): 241-7.
[http://dx.doi.org/10.1016/j.jpeds.2006.03.024] [PMID: 16887443]

[21]   Huber AM, King J, McLaine P, Klassen T, Pothos M. A randomized, placebo-controlled trial of prednisone in early Henoch Schönlein Purpura [ISRCTN85109383]. BMC Med 2004; 2(1): 7.
[http://dx.doi.org/10.1186/1741-7015-2-7] [PMID: 15059282]

[22]   Weiss PF, Feinstein JA, Luan X, Burnham JM, Feudtner C. Effects of corticosteroid on Henoch-Schönlein purpura: a systematic review. Pediatrics 2007; 120(5): 1079-87.
[http://dx.doi.org/10.1542/peds.2007-0667] [PMID: 17974746]

[23]   Weiss PF, Klink AJ, Localio R, *et al.* Corticosteroids may improve clinical outcomes during hospitalization for Henoch-Schönlein purpura. Pediatrics 2010; 126(4): 674-81.
[http://dx.doi.org/10.1542/peds.2009-3348] [PMID: 20855386]

[24]   Hahn D, Hodson EM, Willis NS, Craig JC. Interventions for preventing and treating kidney disease in Henoch☐Schönlein Purpura (HSP). Cochrane Database of Systematic Reviews 2015; (8):

[25]   Davin J-C, Coppo R. Henoch-Schönlein purpura nephritis in children. Nat Rev Nephrol 2014; 10(10): 563-73.
[http://dx.doi.org/10.1038/nrneph.2014.126] [PMID: 25072122]

[26]   Trimarchi H, Barratt J, Cattran DC, *et al.* Oxford classification of IgA nephropathy 2016: an update from the IgA nephropathy classification working group. Kidney Int 2017; 91(5): 1014-21.
[http://dx.doi.org/10.1016/j.kint.2017.02.003] [PMID: 28341274]

[27]   Jimenez A, Chen A, Lin J-J, South AM. Does MEST-C score predict outcomes in pediatric Henoch-Schönlein purpura nephritis? Pediatr Nephrol 2019; 34(12): 2583-9.
[http://dx.doi.org/10.1007/s00467-019-04327-2] [PMID: 31402405]

[28]   Shi D, Chan H, Yang X, *et al.* Risk factors associated with IgA vasculitis with nephritis (Henoch-Schönlein purpura nephritis) progressing to unfavorable outcomes: A meta-analysis. PLoS One 2019; 14(10): e0223218.

[http://dx.doi.org/10.1371/journal.pone.0223218] [PMID: 31574112]

[29]   Narchi H. Risk of long term renal impairment and duration of follow up recommended for Henoch-Schonlein purpura with normal or minimal urinary findings: a systematic review. Arch Dis Child 2005; 90(9): 916-20.
[http://dx.doi.org/10.1136/adc.2005.074641] [PMID: 15871983]

CHAPTER 10

Updates on Childhood-Onset Systemic Lupus Erythematosus

Selma Cecilia Scheffler Mendoza[1], Francisco Eduardo Rivas-Larrauri[1] and **Ana Luisa Rodríguez-Lozano[1,*]**

[1] *Immnunology Department, Instituto Nacional de Pediatría, Mexico City, Mexico*

Abstract: Systemic Lupus Erythematosus (SLE) is a chronic, autoimmune, and multisystem disease. Childhood-onset SLE (cSLE) contributes up to 20% of all cases of SLE and refers to patients who develop the disease before their 18th anniversary.

Impressive discoveries in all aspects of the disease emerge every day; one of the most interesting is whether cSLE is a single or a group of diseases, with diverse physiopathologic processes but sharing a rough phenotype. Patients with early onset disease (<5 years), with associated infections and severe disease manifestations, should urge the possibility of monogenic SLE, which represents a small proportion of all cSLE cases, but often with a more complicated clinical course.

Despite its being considered a rare disease, the clinical outcomes could be devastating. Patients with cSLE had higher disease activity indexes than adults. Although the survival has improved, it also implies that patients remain a longer period under the effects of the disease.

Enormous advances in the understanding of the physiopathological processes are helping to better diagnose children with lupus; still, we are distant to have a perfectly fitted therapy for all our patients. The outstanding efforts of clinicians and researchers to find new therapeutic strategies are encouraging.

In this chapter, you will find a concise description of the novel advancements concerning the disease pathogenesis, classification, assessment of disease activity, treatment, and outcomes.

Keywords: Autoimmune disease, Classification criteria, Childhood-onset, Clinical manifestations, Cyclophosphamide, Disease activity, Damage, Epidemiology, Genetics, Glucocorticoids, Monogenic lupus, Mycophenolate mofetil, Outcome, Pathogenesis, Pediatric, Photoprotection, Systemic lupus erythematosus, Targeted immunotherapy.

* **Corresponding author Ana Luisa Rodríguez-Lozano:** Immunology Department, Instituto Nacional de Pediatría, Mexico City, México; Tel: +52 (55) 1084 - 0900; Ext. 1579, 1337; E-mail: anarlozano@yahoo.com.mx

Nima Rezaei and Noosha Samieefar (Eds.)

INTRODUCTION

Systemic lupus erythematosus (SLE) is a complex, multisystem, chronic autoimmune disease [1] with the potential to involve any organ or system, with an unpredictable clinical course [2]. Characterized by the presence of numerous autoantibodies [3, 4], it commonly causes organ damage [5].

Childhood onset systemic lupus erythematosus (cSLE) is the preferred term to designate children who before their 18th birthday have met the classification criteria for systemic lupus erythematosus [6]. cSLE represents up to 20% of all patients with SLE [7]; other names as juvenile systemic lupus erythematosus, and pediatric systemic lupus erythematosus, are usually used in the literature.

Since the first cases were reported [8 - 13], impressive and continuous discoveries have been made in all aspects of the disease, one of the most exciting is whether cSLE is one disease or a group of diseases representing groups of patients with different physiopathologic processes, sharing several clinical manifestations and antibody profiles, that as a result, have allowed us to treat them more efficiently. There are many additional interesting aspects of the disease that will be reviewed in this chapter.

EPIDEMIOLOGY

cSLE is considered a rare disease, with higher frequency reported in Asians, African Americans, Hispanics, and Native Americans [14, 15]. The estimated incidence in England was 0.8 (0.5-1.2) per 100,000 children per year, but as mention previously, it varies depending on the ethnic origin. In Asia it was 5.6 (3.0-9.5) and in blacks 3.1 (0.6-9.1) while for whites was 0.4 (0.2-0.7) per 100,000 per year [16]. Australia has reported an annual incidence of 0.32 per 100,000 per year [17]. In the United States of America, the incidence was 2.2 per 100,000 Medicaid enrollees per year, while the prevalence was 9.73 per 100,000 [18]. More recently, an analysis of the online databank of the World Bank Group, taking into account 192 countries in 2017, estimated that there were over 200,000 children with cSLE, the majority concentrated in Asia and Africa, followed by the Americas, Europe, and Oceania with a prevalence of 113,176; 53,731; 24,315; 14,693 and 1,008; respectively [19]. Finally, in Korea, the prevalence was 5.35 per 100,000, and the incidence of 2.2 per 100,000 per year in patients between 5 and 18 years old. Interestingly, the authors noted an increase in the incidence and prevalence of girls age 14 and 15 years, observed in their change-point incidence graphics [20].

The median age at presentation is reported between 11 – 12 years, while the disease is very rare under the age of 5 years [15]. However, there is a tendency to separate patients by the pubertal stage. Smith and cols [21] resume the findings of Abdwani *et al.* [22], Pluchinotta *et al.* [23], Descloux *et al.* [24], and Gomes *et al.* [25], and the details are depicted in Table **1**.

Table 1. Number of cSLE patients by pubertal stage and gender distribution.

Author	Age Grouping			F:M
-	Prepubertal	Peripubertal	Postpubertal	-
Abdwani, N=103	39	29	35	83:20
Pluchinotta, N=53	13	11	29	38:15
Descloux, N=56	9	21	26	39:17
Gomes, N=847	39	395	413	726:121

There is a clear predominance of girls compared with boys; this tendency seems to increase along with age. In the prepubertal stage, it is about 2 girls for every boy affected (2:1), only Gomes *et al.* reported 4:1. On the peripubertal stage, the sex ratio is more variable, from 2:1 to 6:1, and for the postpubertal stage, it is from 3:1 to 11:1.

The predominance of females in autoimmune diseases, particularly in patients with lupus, does not totally elucidate; however, there is information regarding the role of sex hormones. The estrogen affects all cells of the immune system, resulting in enhancing INF-gamma and antibody production, and together with prolactin, may be implicated in cell survival [26 - 28].

GENETIC AND PATHOGENESIS

Systemic lupus erythematosus is considered a disease resulting from multiple interactions of factors [29]. Familial aggregation is frequent in patients with cSLE [30] who have more relatives with autoimmune diseases, particularly SLE and thyroid disease, than those without lupus [31]. Previous studies in twins indicate a large concordance between monozygotic twins, although it seems that this concordance is lower [32]. Some authors described 15% of SLE heritability. It shows not only the importance of the genetic basis of the disease [33 - 37] but many other factors involved as the epigenetic [38 - 43], ambient, diet, and infections [44 - 46], among many others.

In a recent and comprehensive review of the genetic etiology of SLE, the authors state: "*It was previously thought that the relevant genetic variants and the causal molecular pathway involved in lupus were associated with distinct clinical presentations. This simplification greatly underestimated the biological complexity of this disease. Mutations within the same gene and identical gene* variants have been associated with different clinical phenotypes, including lupus, type I interferonopathy, or familial chilblain lupus. Conversely, a significant clinical and molecular overlap has been observed between patients with mutations in different genes" [47].

A study of 117 unrelated cSLE patients from the UK Juvenile-onset SLE and French SLE GENIAL cohorts compared to 791 ethnically matched controls, aimed to analyze the contribution of genetic variations implicated in lupus pathogenesis, selected a set of genes (n=28) based on the mendeliome (mendelian forms of lupus) and defined causes of monogenic lupus in mouse models (n=64), or genes identified through Genome-wide association studies (GWAS) (n=67), 12 of them shared with mice models, the total number of genes analyzed were 147 [48]. The next-generation sequencing identified 30,955 variants in the 147 known genes. After filtering, 19 variants were identified in 15 children, 14 were heterozygous, ten of them were novel. Mendelian genotypes were confirmed in eight subjects, involving variants in C1QA, C1QC, C2, DNASE1L3, and IKZF1. Seven additional patients carried heterozygous variants in complement or type I interferon-associated autosomal recessive genes, with decreased concentrations of the encoded proteins C3 and C9 recorded in two patients. Inborn errors of immunity were estimated to account for 7% of cases of childhood-onset SLE. The authors discussed the possibility that a lupus phenotype might be driven by pathogenic variants in two or more genes; observed that the majority of Mendelian forms of cSLE in their study were related to anomalies in innate immunity genes, and an increased frequency of monoallelic variants described to cause lupus as an autosomal recessive trait. The authors' interpretation is that an accumulation of rare variants might contribute to disease expression and clinical heterogeneity.

Monogenic Lupus

The term monogenic lupus (mSLE) denotes an SLE patient with high-penetrance, either dominantly or recessively inherited pathogenic variants in a single gene [47]. Monogenic lupus constitutes only a small proportion of SLE cases [33]. However, most of them have been associated with a well-defined clinical presentation. Early onset disease (<5 years), associated infections, and severe disease manifestations as glomerulonephritis, cytopenias, neuropsychiatric disease, cutaneous manifestations, anti-dsDNA antibodies, and hemolytic anemia suggest mSLE [49].

There is a strong association between monogenic lupus with primary immunodeficiencies (PID) [50]. The most common form and also the first described, was the complement deficiencies being C2, C4 and C1q deficiencies, the commonest [51]. There are other forms much less frequent but associated with consanguinity as the protein kinase Cδ deficiency [52]. The most important genes related to monogenic SLE forms are depicted in Table **2** [34, 50 - 53].

Table 2. Single-gene defects, mechanisms and clinical manifestations associated with monogenic systemic lupus erythematosus (Fig. 1).

Protein/Defect	Inheritance	Mechanism	Clinical Manifestations
Complement deficiencies C1q, C1r/s, C2 and C4	AR	Impaired clearance of apoptotic cells and immune complexes	Recurrent infections Early onset Cutaneous manifestations Absence of anti-dsDNA antibodies
PKCδ deficiency	AR Consanguineous	Excessive B-cell proliferation (apoptosis)	Hepatosplenomegaly Lymphadenopathy EBV or CMV infection
Prolidase deficiency	AR	Alteration in C1q	Recurrent infections Elevated IgE Cutaneous manifestations (telangiectasias) Facial dysmorphia
Interferonopathy (TREX1, IFIH1, ADAR1, TRAP)	AR/AD, AD, AR/AD	Increase IFNα production	Aicardi-Goutières Syndrome (AGS) and AGS-like (Lupus pernio, Basal ganglia calcification) SLE SAVI SPENCD
RASopathy (RAS/MAPK pathway)	AD	Leukocyte proliferation Defective apoptosis	SLE Increase rate of pericarditis Splenomegaly, lymphadenopathy Noonan syndrome. Risk of malignancy transformation.
Mutation in DNASE1L3 DNASE1	AR/AD	Abnormal DNA degradation	SLE Sjögren Urticaria, cutaneous vasculitis. Recurrent abdominal pain. Uveitis and episcleritis. Glomerulonephritis with anti-C1q antibodies.

CMV, cytomegalovirus; dsDNA, double-stranded DNA; EBV, Epstein–Barr virus; SAVI (STING-associated vasculopathy with onset in infancy); SPENCD, Spondyloenchondrodysplasia; PKC, protein kinase C.

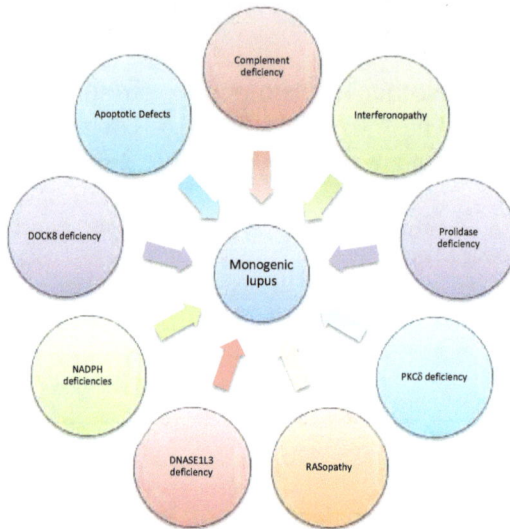

Fig. (1). Genetic defects related to monogenic lupus.

Complement Deficiency

In healthy individuals the complement system helps to decrease the autoantigen load by clearance of nucleolar proteins, C1q protein inhibits the Interferon alpha production by dendritic cells, C4 also helps the self-tolerance through complement receptor 1 and 2 [33].

A report of two siblings with recurrent infections and SLE features, demonstrated the insufficiency of C1q activity [54], since then, the study of complement deficiencies was initiated, nowadays, it is known, that deficiency in C1q, C1r, C1s, C2, C4a, and C4b predispose to SLE development. The prevalence of SLE in patients with homozygous C1q deficiency is about 90%, with many patients indicating a history of recurrent infections [55]; about 65% of patients with C1r/s defects also develop SLE. Defects in C1 and C2 receptors affect the immune tolerance induction, which can explain the higher frequency of SLE in patients with C1 or C4 deficiency [51].

Complement deficiencies drive autoimmunity through different mechanisms:

- Complement-mediated apoptosis induction.
- Negative selection of self-reactive B cells.
- Clearance of immune complexes.

The most frequent classical pathway complement deficiency is the homozygous C2 deficiency; the prevalence is about 1/10,000 in the European population. There are 2 types of C2 deficiency; in type 1 there is no translation of C2 protein, due to non-sense mutation, and in type 2 the protein is synthesized, but its secretion is impaired because of a missense mutation; up to 90% of C2 deficiencies are related to type 1. Deficiencies of C3 and C4 are less frequent than the deficiency of C1q [34].

Abnormal DNA Clearance and Interferonopathies

Type 1- Interferon (IFN-1) comprises 13 molecules produced by nucleated cells. IFN-1 plays an important role in immunity by detecting viruses and restricting viral replication. The relation between SLE and many monogenic conditions is associated with excessive IFN-1 production. *TREX1* mutations are one example of aberrant DNA degradation, this mutation causes familial chilblain lupus (FCL) an autosomal dominant disease associated with chilblain lesions in early childhood, Raynaud phenomenon, autoantibodies, and hypergammaglobulinemia, that evolve to SLE in 18% of cases [55].

Aicardi-Goutiéres syndrome (AGS) is an autosomal recessive disease with early onset encephalopathy, with matter calcifications, progressive neurologic dysfunction, cerebrospinal lymphocytosis, and chilblain lesions, in neonatal patients include hepatosplenomegaly and thrombocytopenia. AGS and FCL are associated with mutations in *TREX1* [53].

Ramantani *et al.* [56] report high prevalence (60%) of AGS patients with *TREX1* mutations, and present at least one of the following autoimmune features:

- Thrombocytopenia
- Leukopenia
- Antinuclear antibodies (ANA)
- Skin lesions
- Oral ulcers
- Arthritis
- Anti-dsDNA antibodies
- Antibodies to extractable nuclear antigens (ENA).

TREX1 deficiency triggers autoimmunity through the accumulation of self-DNA in the cytosol. When TREX1 is dysfunctional, the cytosolic DNA does not get degraded, thus producing damage-associated molecular pattern (DAMP), these activate the cyclic GMP-AMP (cGAMP synthase (cGAS))-STING-mediated INF-1 response and systemic inflammation [53].

DNASE1 (deoxyribonuclease 1) and DNASE1L3 genes encode proteins related to the nucleic acid degradation pathway. DNASE1L3 enzyme plays an important role in the clearance of DNA debris from apoptotic cells and exogenous DNA; the loss of this function may lead to a monogenic SLE and hypocomplementemic urticarial vasculitis syndrome [57].

There is another group of gene mutations related to Interferonopathies; the stimulator of interferon genes (STING), a transmembrane protein that resides in the endoplasmic reticulum of diverse cells like epithelial cells, macrophages, and dendritic cells. STING is very important for INF-1 production in response to pathogens related to double-stranded DNA [58]. STING mutations are associated with the development of vasculopathy with infant onset (SAVI), an autoinflammatory disease caused by its gain of function. Mutations affecting STING have been related to SLE [34, 51].

Prolidase Deficiency

Prolidase plays an important role in the activation of the INF-1 receptor. Its deficiency is a rare autosomal recessive defect, characterized by skin lesions, facial dysmorphia, mental retardation, splenomegaly, and multisystemic involvement; patients have high IgE levels and iminodipeptiduria; and present a higher susceptibility to recurrent severe infections, as for cytomegalovirus (CMV). There are reports in the literature of prolidase deficiency and SLE manifestations with the presence of anti-dsDNA antibodies [50].

Protein Kinase-Cδ Deficiency

This protein is a serine/threonine kinase involved in the control of cell proliferation and apoptosis. Its absence is related to an increase of B cell proliferation; there are reports of patients in different countries from endogamous communities with protein kinase-Cδ deficiency and SLE features [47, 50].

RASopathies

The RAS-associated autoimmune leukoproliferative disease has been associated with diverse human cancers. These patients presented with autoimmune cytopenias, hypergammaglobulinemia, lymphadenopathy, splenomegaly, and recurrent infections due to abnormal apoptosis (cell death). The RASopathies are a group of genetically well-defined diseases, such as Noonan syndrome (NS), among other conditions. There are cases of NS with SLE features reported in the literature [47].

Knowing the relationship between the immune system and the genes identified to cause monogenic lupus, would allow us to understand the intricate pathways and molecular mechanisms involved in the pathogenesis of SLE, which can be targeted for new treatments.

Today we know that several gene mutations can cause abnormal regulation and activation of sensing pathways of dsDNA, leading to dysregulation of IFN-1 production with the formation of autoantibodies and subsequent autoimmunity like SLE.

You should suspect mSLE in patients who have at least one of the following data:

1.- Early onset autoimmunity
2.- Family history of related monogenic disorders
3.- Autoimmune disease refractory to treatment
4.- Atypical autoimmune manifestations
5.- Consanguinity
6.- Severe recurrent infections

CLASSIFICATION AND DIAGNOSIS

Childhood onset systemic lupus erythematosus has probably the most variable clinical presentation amidst other diseases, from mild cutaneous involvement to almost-all organs and systems affected that can lead to death. Due to this variability, there have been many efforts to create tools that help recognize subjects with the illness. However, it is important to know that the classification criteria are not the same as the diagnostic criteria.

The classification criteria were created mainly for research purposes, are standardized definitions that are primarily intended to create well- defined, relatively homogenous cohorts for clinical research" [59], and are not intended for diagnosis.

Commonly, the classification criteria are used as diagnosis criteria; yet, there are no diagnostic criteria. The expertise of the physicians plays a primordial role in diagnosing patients who may not have enough classification criteria but may have a particular combination of clinical and laboratory manifestations. In 2017 a European group released the recommendations for diagnosis and treatment of childhood-onset systemic lupus erythematosus: The SHARE initiative, mainly focused on neuropsychiatric, cardiopulmonary involvement, and macrophage activation syndrome [60].

Up to date, there are none classification criteria made specifically for children, they are created for adults, and in the best case, validated for their use in children. See in Table **3**, the ACR classification criteria and, in Table **4**, a comparative resume of EULAR/ACR and SLICC classification criteria.

Table 3. The 1997 updated American College of Rheumatology classification criteria.

ACR[a]	Score
Malar rash	1
Discoid Lupus	1
Photosensitivity	1
Oral ulcers	1
Nonerosive arthritis (involving ≥2 joints)	1
Pleuritis or Pericarditis	1
Renal disorder (persistent proteinuria >0.5g/d, o > than 3+ dipstick. Or cellular casts)	1
Neurologic disorder (Seizures or Psychosis)	1
Hematologic disorder (Hemolytic anemia, or Leukopenia, or Lymphopenia, or thrombocytopenia)	1
Inmunologic disorder (anti-DNA or Anti-Sm, or Positive Antiphospholipid IgG or IgM ACL, LA, or a false-positive Treponema pallidum test.	1
Positive Antinuclear Antibody	1
SLE classification ≥4 criteria	

[a] [61]

Table 4. The 2019 European League Against Rheumatism/American College of Rheumatology Classification Criteria, and the 2012 Systemic Lupus International Collaborating Clinics Classification Criteria, for Systemic Lupus Erythematosus.

EULAR/ACR[a]		SLICC[b]
Entry Criterion		**Clinical Criteria**
Antinuclear Antibodies (ANA) at a titter of ≥1:80 on Hep-2 cells or an equivalent positive test (ever). If present, apply additive criteria		1. Acute cutaneous lupus Malar rash, Toxic epidermal necrolysis, Maculopapular lupus rash, Photosensitive rash
Additive criteria Do not count a criterion if there is a more likely explanation than SLE. Occurrence of a criterion on at least one occasion is sufficient. Criteria need not occur simultaneously. Within each domain, *only the highest weighted criterion is counted.*		2. Chronic cutaneous lupus Classic discoid rash, localized or generalized, Hypertrophic lupus, Panniculitis, Mucosal lupus, Lupus erythematosus timidus, Chilblain lupus, Discoid lupus/lichen planus overlap
Clinical Domains and Criteria	**Weight**	**3. Oral Ulcers or Nasal ulcers**

(Table 4) cont.....

Constitutional Fever (>38.3°C)	2	4. Nonscarring alopecia
Hematologic Leukopenia, <4,000/mm^3	- 3	5. Synovitis. Involving ≥2 joints or Tenderness in ≥2 joints and 30min of morning stiffness
Thrombocytopenia <100,000/mm^3	4	
Autoimmune hemolysis	4	
Neuropsychiatric	-	6. Serositis Typical pleurisy ≥1 day or pleural effusions or pleural rub. Typical pericardial pain ≥1 day or pericardial effusion, pericardial rub or pericarditis by electrocardiography
Delirium	2	
Psychosis	3	
Seizure	5	
Mucocutaneous*	-	7. Renal. Urine protein-to-creatinine ratio or 24-hour urine protein, representing 500 mg protein/24h or red blood cell cast
Non-scarring alopecia	2	
Oral Ulcers	2	
Subacute OR discoid lupus	4	
Acute cutaneous lupus	6	
Serosal	-	8. Neurologic Seizures, Psychosis, Mononeuritis multiplex, Myelitis, Peripheral or cranial neuropathy, Acute confusional state
Pleural or pericardial effusion	5	
Acute pericarditis	6	
Musculoskeletal Joint involvement	6	9. Hemolytic Anemia
RenaL	-	10. Leukopenia (<4,000/mm^3) or Lymphopenia (<1,000/mm^3) 11. Thrombocytopenia (<100,000/mm^3) Any of them at least once
Proteinuria >0.5g/24h	4	
Renal biopsy Class II or V LN	8	
Renal biopsy Class III or IV LN	10	
Immunology domains and criteria	-	**Immunologic Criteria**
Antiphospholipid antibodies ACL or anti-β2-GP1 or LA	2	1. ANA level above laboratory reference range
Complement proteins		2. Anti-DNA antibody level above laboratory reference range
Low C3 or low C4	3	
Low C3 and low C4	4	
SLE-specific antibodies Anti-dsDNA antibody or Anti-Smith antibody	6	3. Anti-Sm. Presence.
-	-	4. Antiphospholipid antibody *positivity* of any: LA, False-positive result test of rapid plasma reagin, ACL antibody IgA, IgG, or IgM (medium or high titer), anti-β2-GP1 (IgA, IgG, or IgM)

(Table 4) cont.....

Classify as SLE with a score ≥10 if entry criterion fulfilled	-	5. Low complement, Low C3, Low C4, Low CH50
-	-	6. Direct Coombs' test in the absence of hemolytic anemia
-	-	**SLE classification ≥4, but with at least one Clinical and one Immunologic criterion[§]**

*Observed by a clinician. [§]For the SLICC classification, a patient may not have the required 4 criteria, but the patient must have biopsy-proven lupus nephritis in the presence of ANA or anti-dsDNA antibodies to be classified. [a] [62] [b] [63]

The 2019 European League Against Rheumatism/American College of Rheumatology Classification Criteria for Systemic Lupus Erythematosus (EULAR/ACR) is the newer classification criteria [62]. The Systemic Lupus International Collaborating Clinics criteria (SLICC), was published in 2012 [63], and the most broadly known criteria are those created by the American College of Rheumatology, Table **3**. (ACR9 updated in 1997 [61].

One of the biggest changes made by the EULAR/ACR classification criteria in comparison to previous classifications is the reduction of the number of cutaneous manifestations, which have been criticized since the beginning (ACR 1997 update and before), arguing the overrepresentation of the cutaneous involvement. Nonetheless, the SLICC criteria far to reduce the items of mucocutaneous affection increased it. Another interesting change was the removal of the direct Coombs' test as an individual criterion of the SLICC classification criteria.

The efforts to update and create new classification criteria reflect, on one hand, the need to improve not only the sensitivity but the specificity of the classification, this goal seems to be accomplished by the 2019 EULAR/ACR classification criteria. On the other hand, the need to identify patients in the early stages of the disease seems to be decisive. The study of the impact of early *versus* late systemic lupus erythematosus diagnosis on clinical and economic outcomes [64] conducted in 4,166 adults with early diagnosis, and 4,166 with late diagnosis of SLE, reported lower rates of flares, use of healthcare resources, events of SLE-related comorbidities and costs in the former group. It is well known, that patients with adolescence-onset of the disease accrued more damage than adults [65]; therefore, it is critical to identify those children opportunely.

The results of the validation of the newest classification and the comparison made by other authors are depicted in Table **5**. It is important to mention that the studies of Rodrigues-Fonseca *et al.*, Sag *et al.*, and Fonseca *et al.,* were conducted in the pediatric population.

Table 5. Sensitivity and Specificity reported of the 3 systems used to classify patients with SLE.

Classification Criteria	Aringer *et al*[a]	Rodrigues-Fonseca *et al*[b]	Sag *et al*[c]	Fonseca *et al*[d]
	Sensitivity (%) / Specificity (%)			
ACR/EULAR 2019	96/93	87.7/67.4	N/A	N/A
SLICC 2012	97/84	89.3/80.9	98.7/85.3	82.7/93.5
ACR 1997	83/93	70.5/83.2	76.6/93.4	58/93.4

[a] [62] [b] [66] [c] [67] [d] [68]

The other aspect to take into account is, as previously mentioned, the fact that maybe, cSLE represent a group of patients with *different* diseases, that share some features, but are different, and try to include them all in one set of criteria, maybe is not the best approach.

It is a possibility that based on the clinical manifestations, the profile of cytokines, or genes, in near-future, new classification criteria could be created to identify all possible cases, to be treated, and to avoid the fear complications of the disease.

CLINICAL MANIFESTATIONS

The variability of the disease manifestations at presentation and during the disease course is a hallmark, there are patients with acute and fatal evolution, there are others with relapsing disease, and those with chronic intermittent or continuous activity; this is not a predictable disease. The wide-ranging clinical manifestations are, in part, due to the multiple organ affection and its severity. Usually, a patient with lupus will not appear with all the symptoms altogether, but they will be appearing along, in a variable period in which the manifestations can coincide.

Table **6** enlightens the most prevalent clinical features, such as mucocutaneous, musculoskeletal, constitutional symptoms (fever, fatigue, malaise, weight loss), and renal affection. Frequently, patients may have constitutional symptoms for several weeks to months before they develop more specific manifestations.

Table 6. Main clinical manifestations of patients with cSLE.

Clinical Manifestation	Massias *et al*[a] N= 418 (%)	Fonseca *et al*[b] N= 38 (%)	Sahin *et al*[c] N= 92 (%)	Abdwani *et al*[d] N=103 (%)
Constitutional	131(31.3)	N/A	51 (55.4)	66 (64)
Mucocutaneous	159 (38)	* (51.4)	90 (97.8)	65 (63.1)
Musculoskeletal	122 (29.2)	27 (70.9)	52 (65.5)	70 (67.9)
Hematological	106 (25.3)	* (32.6)	55 (59.8)	55 (53.4)

(Table 6) cont.....

Clinical Manifestation	Massias *et al*[a] N= 418 (%)	Fonseca *et al*[b] N= 38 (%)	Sahin *et al*[c] N= 92 (%)	Abdwani *et al*[d] N=103 (%)
Renal	137 (32.7)	19 (50)	27 (29.3)	38 (36.9)
Cardiorespiratory	49 (11.7)	8 (21)	15 (16.3)	28 (27.2)
Gastrointestinal	21 (5)	N/A	N/A	N/A
Neuropsychiatric	40 (9.5)	5 (13.1)	15 (16.3)	15 (14.5)

*These categories were reported by their components, for Mucocutaneous involvement, they reported malar rash, photosensitivity, discoid rash and oral ulcers in 30 (78.9%), 29 (76.3%), 2 (5.2%) and 17 (45.5%) patients respectively, for instance the total number exceeded the total number of patients. The same applies for the hematologic involvement, where they reported hemolytic anemia, leukopenia and thrombocytopenia in 9 (23.6%), 17 (46.1%) and 11 (28.9%) patients, again these numbers exceed the total number of patients because some patients have more than one manifestation in the same category, for that reason, we only presented the percentages. [a] [69] [b] [68] [c] [70] [d] [22]

The cutaneous affection is one of the commonest manifestations; its frequency varies from near to 50% to more than 90% [17, 70, 71]. There are two categories: 1) Lupus erythematosus specific skin lesions (acute and subacute cutaneous lupus erythematosus) and 2) Lupus erythematosus nonspecific skin lesions [72, 73].

1. Lupus Erythematosus Specific Skin Lesions

The most frequent is the malar rash; it is the first criterion of the American College of Rheumatology, has a sensitivity of 57% and specificity of 96%. It is a well-defined, symmetrical, erythematous rash located over the nasal bridge and malar area (butterfly rash), characteristically, the nasolabial folds remained unaffected; and are very sensitive to ultraviolet light. (Figs. **2** and **3**) show the characteristic malar rash in two different patients, in Fig. (**2**) an adolescent girl with the suspicion of monogenic lupus, who at the time had a severe flare, on the other hand, Fig. (**3**) shows the malar rash in an adolescent girl with a recent onset of the disease.

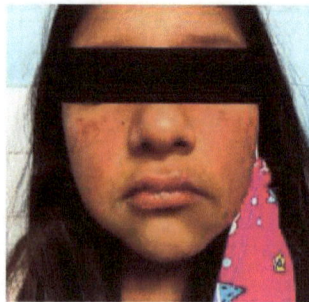

Fig. (2). Malar rash in a girl with suspicion of mongenic lupus.

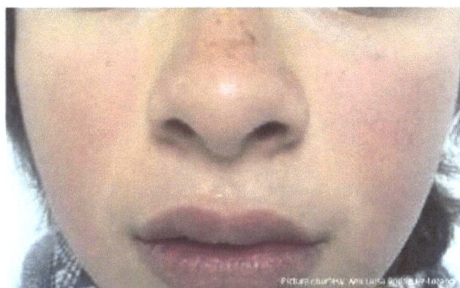

Fig. (3). Malar rash in a girl with a recent-onset of cSLE.

The discoid rash is less frequent than the malar rash, with a sensitivity of 18% and specificity of 59%, it usually presents as a disc-shaped, scarring, and indurated, erythematous-purplish papules, typically seen on the face and scalp (above the neck).

2. Lupus Erythematosus Nonspecific Skin Lesions

Photosensitivity can appear as any skin rash reacting to both UVA and UVB light, thus appearing on sun-exposed areas; it is the second criterion of the ACR, and has a sensitivity of 43% and specificity of 96%. Oral ulcers (including oral and nasopharyngeal ulcers) are classically painless; the most specific location for SLE is on the hard palate (erythematosus lesions); other oral ulcers can be painful (discoid lesions) and found all over the buccal mucosa. As some lesions could be asymptomatic, a careful physical examination is recommended.

Alopecia may be one of the firsts symptoms of the disease; it is common to observe thin and dry hair on the frontal and temporal regions, frequently accompanied by telogen effluvium; less frequently to observe are the "real" alopecia areas. Livedo reticularis and Raynaud's phenomenon are also often observed. Cutaneous vasculitis may be present as palpable purpura, papules, erythematous plaques, or macules, and urticarial vasculitis, which can be painful and lasts more than 24 hours; histologically, evidencing leukocytoclastic vasculitis [72, 73].

Fig. (**4**) shows palmar erythema accompanied by indurated and painful nodules in an adolescent boy with a recent-onset disease, he also presented with facial and lobular lesions showed in Fig. (**5**). He had a history of intense sun exposure when the cutaneous lesions started, was misdiagnosed and treated for acne for a few weeks before arriving at our Service.

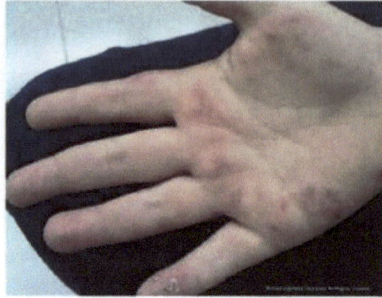

Fig. (4). Finger nodules and palmar erythema.

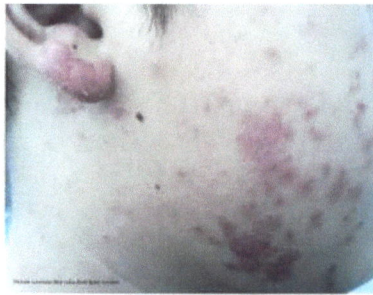

Fig. (5). Facial and lobular lesions.

Arthritis and arthralgia are the most common manifestations of the musculoskeletal apparatus, some authors report nearly 100% [65] while others the third part of patients [69]. Knees, ankles, and the small joints of the hands are frequently affected, in a mild to severe manner. Joint stiffness in the morning, and after inactivity periods are frequent [74]. Myositis is less frequent and must be distinguished from the post-infectious and the related to steroids.

The frequency of renal involvement varies among studies from 29% up to [70] 51 – 72.5% (22) [75]. In one study from Turkey, the frequency of nephritis was reported in 29%, the authors pointed out that nephritis was more prevalent in studies from around the world. Asia reported 71.7 to 82%, Africa 61 – 65.9% and Canada 55% [70]. Usually, it presents early in evolution and signifies an important cause of morbidity and mortality. In a recent study of 846 cSLE patients, 427 (50.5%) children presented with early onset lupus nephritis (ELN, active urinary sediment based on SLEDAI-2 K criteria, during the first six months of the diagnosis), the conclusions were that acute renal failure, arterial hypertension, hematuria, pyuria, urine casts, proteinuria, low C3, anti-dsDNA antibodies, damage accrual, and death were significantly higher in patients with ELN compared with those without [76]. Pyuria is not part of the classification criteria, but is frequent in patients with lupus nephritis even as unique finding, it is mandatory to exclude other causes like infection before to categorize this feature as a sign of renal activity.

A normal urinalysis does not exclude all cases of renal involvement, for that reason, not only the urinalysis but the creatinine, proteinuria and arterial tension should be examined during evolution. To quantify the proteinuria, it is preferable a 24-hour determination or a urinary protein to creatinine ratio, over dipstick. The gold standard for the diagnosis of lupus nephritis is a kidney biopsy [74]. There are six classes of lupus nephritis (LN); class I, minimal mesangial LN; class VI, advance sclerotic LN; but the classes II (mesangial proliferative LN), IV (diffuse LN) and V (membranous LN), are at immediate risk of chronic kidney disease progression [77]; so actively search for proteinuria, hematuria, and the presence of casts, must be monitored with serum creatinine, and arterial tension in every visit, as unrecognized renal affection could lead to an end renal disease. There are other causes of kidney injury, such as thrombotic microangiopathy, antiphospholipid nephropathy, non-immune complex podocytopathy, tubulointerstitial nephritis, acute tubular necrosis, renovascular disease, or nephrotoxicity from medications [78]; perhaps clinically very similar, but histologically different, which reflects the importance of the kidney biopsy.

The neuropsychiatric (NP) affection represents a diagnostic challenge [79]; there is a wide range of manifestations, from headache to seizures, psychosis, chorea, neuropathies, cranial nerve palsy, sinus thrombosis, cerebrovascular accidents, amaurosis fugax and psychiatric manifestations, amidst others. Depression is a commonly unrecognized manifestation of the disease, but it may be the first exhibition of lupus [80]. A recent report indicated a prevalence of 59% of depression, with 23% of children with suicidal ideation; the study did not distinguish predictive factors of depression, which could make the patient's identification difficult [81], with fatal implications. So an active search for clues indicating depression is highly recommended.

A study of 146 cSLE patients found that 41 (28%) had neuropsychiatric symptoms, the most frequent were headache, seizures and mood disorders; in their article, they reviewed many other studies with a similar proportion of neuropsychiatric manifestations. Interestingly, they did not find differences between patients with and without NP manifestations in terms of the group of age (<5, 5-10, an >10 years old), female to male ratio, mortality, and proportion of ANA ≥1:1280, but did find the anti-dsDNA elevation and thrombocytopenia more prevalent in the group of NP (82.9 vs. 66.7%, P=0.03 and 39 vs. 22.8%, P=0.02) [82]. They did not report the prevalence of antiphospholipid antibodies, that are known to be present in an important proportion of patients with NP manifestations [83 - 88]. In a previous extended and beautifully detailed report, the frequency of anticardiolipin (aCL) was 66%, although no association between the level of aCL and NP manifestations was found [86].

The presence of anti-phospholipids antibodies in patients with cSLE has been reported within 38-78% [83] and constituted a hallmark of the antiphospholipid syndrome (APS). In adults, is characterized by thrombosis and fetal loss in the presence of antiphospholipid antibodies, such as aCL IgG or IgM in medium or high titer (>40 GPL/MPL or >99th percentile), or anti-beta-2 glycoprotein I (β2GPI) IgG or IgM in titer >99th percentile, and/or positive lupus anticoagulant.

When APS is associated with other autoimmune diseases is called secondary APS; and is associated with older age at onset, higher frequency of venous thrombotic events, and hematologic and skin manifestations. When there is not a demonstrable cause, it is called primary APS, its presentation is usually in younger children and is associated with a higher frequency of arterial thrombosis [85, 87]. The distinct clinical manifestations between children and adults are notorious, mainly regarding the comorbidities, and to a lesser extent, pregnancy; however, there are not classification criteria for children APS. Usually, the evidence of thrombosis was a mandatory criterion to classify a patient with APS; nowadays, it is recognized that there are thrombotic and non-thrombotic manifestations [88]. The most frequent manifestations reported in children from China, and an International Registry [85, 89], are described below:

a) Thrombotic manifestations: venous thrombosis was present in 21% and 60%, and arterial thrombosis in 20% and 32%.

b) Non-thrombotic manifestations: Immune thrombocytopenia was present in 52 and 8%, autoimmune hemolytic anemia in 33 and 7%, skin lesions as Raynaud's phenomenon, acromelic gangrene, vasculitis rash, livedo reticularis, and skin ulcers of the lower limbs, in 26 and 18%, arthritis in 21%, pulmonary hypertension in 5%, and heart valve vegetations in 2%, respectively.

Some manifestations are more frequent in certain groups of age compared with others. A study of 88 children divided into preschoolers, scholars, and adolescents; found that arthritis was less prevalent (P=0.022) and hepatosplenomegaly was more prevalent (P=0.024), both in the preschoolers, and did not find any differences in the rest of the clinical manifestations between groups [90]. Conversely, patients with early disease commence (<6 years old) have more fever and reticuloentdothelial manifestations (P<0.0001) than their counterparts, children between 6 years and < 12 years and children >12 years. The neuropsychiatric involvement was significantly more frequent in children ≥6 years and < 12 years, P <0.0001 [91]. The identified manifestations in prepubertal children were higher renal disease rates compared with pubertal and postpubertal children (51% vs. 23% vs. 20%; p=0.039); greater frequency of cutaneous manifestation versus pubertal and postpubertal children (74% vs. 69% vs. 46%; p=0.029); and lower hematologic affection compared to the pubertal and postpubertal children (28% vs. 66% vs. 71%; p<0.001). Urticarial vasculitis was identified exclusively in the prepubertal group in the 53.8% [22].

The ocular involvement in patients with cSLE has received less attention than it deserves; the etiology, manifestations, and severity are widely variable. In adults, it can occur in one-third of patients [92]. The dry eye disease and retinal involvement are the most frequent; the neuro-ophthalmic manifestations, on the contrary, are less common, but the prognosis can be poorer. We must be aware, of the ocular toxicity related to treatment, such as the use of steroids, chloroquine, and hydroxychloroquine; that can be silent and still produce a visual loss if untreated.

Several clinical manifestations may precede the diagnosis of cSLE, providing us with warnings about the disease.

A study intended to identify those manifestations; divided them into two categories, whether they precede the diagnosis or were present within the first month; or if they were present 3 or more months between their initial symptoms and the cSLE diagnosis.

They found that the palate and buccal ulcers (P= 0.003 and P=0.032), pleuritis (P<0.0001), renal affection (P=0.009), proteinuria (P=0.002), neuropsychiatric involvement (P=0.008), leukopenia or lymphopenia (P<0.0001), and thrombocytopenia (P=0.037), precede the SLE diagnosis, compared to patients with 3 or more months of symptoms [93]. Synovitis is a common manifestation, but its frequency increased in the months following the diagnosis. There is a report of a 12-year-old girl with lupus enteritis, who arrived with abdominal pain as her unique symptom; after the biopsy discovered enteritis, she developed leucopenia, lymphopenia and an oral ulcer. The author recommends being alert of female adolescents with abdominal pain [94]. Acalculous and lithiasic cholecystitis, mesenteric vasculitis or thrombosis, and pancreatitis should also be considered in the study of abdominal pain.

DISEASE ACTIVITY AND DAMAGE ACCRUAL

Disease activity (DA) refers to the clinical and biochemical manifestations due to acute or subacute inflammation, which at least theoretically, responds to treatment without leading to organ damage. The constant or continuous inflammation can cause structural organ changes and/or loss of function, which is call damage and is at least theoretically, irreversible. In children, it may not be as determinant as in adults, specifically in terms of growth.

Measure DA enables to know the actual condition of the patients and to compare it with the last visit(s), to observe their evolution, which translates their response to therapy, or determine if the patient is having a flare, so it becomes relevant to clinical practice and decision making especially on treatment. To read more about the theoretical basis and methods of disease activity measures in pediatric rheumatology, please refer to Luca's review [95].

There is not a pathognomonic feature or a biomarker that decodes disease activity. Due to the variability of the manifestations, sometimes it is difficult to determine to what extent DA accounts for the clinical picture. Physician's Global Assessment (PGA) is based on a Likert scale, where 0 = none DA, 1 = mild DA, 2 = moderate DA, and 3 = severe DA; in expert hands could be very useful; otherwise, the variability between observers can hinder the real condition of the patients. Nonetheless, PGA is frequently used as a gold standard in clinical research mainly to validate new instruments. There are several tools to measure DA; most of them based their measures in the 2-weeks previous to the patient's clinical visit, while other tools extend the observation to the previous month.

There are not specific indices to measure global disease activity in children, but herein we will describe the most used, see Table 7. For detailed information about validity, clinical usability, and other important features regarding the indices, please refer to Lattanzi *et al.* review [96].

Table 7. Comparison of indices used to measure Disease Activity.

-	SLEDAI	SLEDAI-2K	BILAG-2004	SLAM-R	ECLAM	MEX-SLEDAI
Period assessed	10 days	10 or 30 days*	Last 4 weeks, compared to the previous 4 weeks	Last month	Last month	10 days
Items	24 items for 9 organ/systems	22 items for 8 organ systems. DNA and complement were dismiss	101 items for 9 systems	9 organs plus 7 laboratory items	12 categories 10 organs/systems, plus ESR and complement	22 items in 10 domains
Score	0-105	0-101	A, B, C, D and E	0-84	0-17.5	0-32

(Table 7) cont.....

-	SLEDAI	SLEDAI-2K	BILAG-2004	SLAM-R	ECLAM	MEX-SLEDAI
Disease Activity score	0= no activity 1= mild 2= activity, but improvement 3= Persistent 4= Flare 7= active disease >12 important flare	0= no activity 1= mild 2= activity, but improvement 3= Persistent 4= Flare 7= active disease >12 important flare	A= very active B=active C= mild persistent activity D=was active but not at the time E= never active	>7 considered relevant	complicated scoring scheme	>4
Time to Apply	10 minutes	10 minutes	20 minutes	15 minutes		10 minutes

*In a study comparing SLEDAI-2K 10 days versus SLEDAI-2K 30 days, scores were concordant [108].

Systemic Lupus Erythematosus Disease Activity Index (SLEDAI) is the most known and worldwide used tool [97]; SLEDAI-2K is an actualization of the original SLEDAI [98], but there are many others like the British Isles Lupus Assessment Group (BILAG) [99], the SLE Activity Measure (SLAM) [100], the European Consensus Lupus Activity Measurement (ECLAM) [101] and the MEX-SLEDAI [102] amidst many others.

A comparative study of SLEDAI, BILAG, and SLAM in children [103] analyzed the differences between the indices; for example, the time consumed applying SLEDAI was less than for BILAG, besides BILAG require more background knowledge and the kidney biopsy (performed within 3 months) result. Regarding the renal involvement, an important factor in children with lupus, SLEDAI score sums up to 16 in comparison to only 8, in SLAM. The authors conclude that three indices were comparable and can be used to measure DA and the clinical change in children with lupus. More recently, a study aimed to assess lupus activity with SLEDAI-2K and ECLAM over time, found a high correlation between them ($r=0.78$, $p<0.001$), the authors conclude that SLEDAI-2K and ECLAM are likewise to estimate longitudinal DA [104].

The BILAG-2004 index demonstrates its utility measuring disease activity in children [105]; however, formal training is needed, it can take more time to apply, and the glossary at hand may be necessary [106]; nonetheless, to research purposes, it is broadly used. A similar situation happens with ECLAM; it also demonstrates its validity; yet, there is a lack of information for some definitions, and the scoring system is complex and not consistently applied in the literature [107].

The MEX-SLEDAI was conceived with the purpose to be more accessible, mainly for countries with fewer technological advances and economically disfavors. The authors compared the SLEDAI-2K, the modified SLEDAI-2K, the SLAM-R and MEX-SLEDAI, and they found that all the tools had adequate convergence validity. When the SLEDAI-2K was the gold standard; SLAM-R, MEX-SLEDAI and the modified SLEDAI-2K had an overall accuracy of 66, 84, and 91%, respectively; when the PGA was used as the gold standard; then MEX-SLEDAI had an overall accuracy of 89%, the modified SLEDAI-2K 77%, and SLAM-R 63%. When only the costs of the laboratory were considered, the modified SLEDAI-2K and MEX-SLEDAI were 73% and 62%, less expensive than the SLEDAI-2K. The authors concluded that the instruments are adequate for assessment of disease activity, being the modified SLEDAI-2K the best option [109].

We conducted a study in 90 cSLE patients from a tertiary pediatric center in Mexico City to assess the factors associated to damage [110], when we compared SLEDAI-2K with MEX-SLEDAI we obtained a Spearman correlation of 0.914, p <0.000, and the reliability of 0.925 (95% CI 0.886 – 0.951; Chronbach' alpha coefficient), therefore, in our experience both instruments are adequate to measure disease activity.

All three instruments derived from the original SLEDAI, the similarities between them are evident, see Table **8**; nonetheless, the advantage of skip the immunologic studies in the modified SLEDAI-2K and MEX-SLEDAI had helped measure disease activity consistently in our clinical practice.

Table 8. Comparative table showing the descriptors of the original SLEDAI, the modified SLEDAI-2K, and the SLEDAI-MEX.

SLEDAI-2K		Modified SLEDAI-2K		MEX-SLEDAI	
Weight	Descriptor	Weight	Descriptor	Weight	Descriptor
8	Seizure	8	Seizure	8	Neurologic Disease
8	Psychosis	8	Psychosis	6	Renal Disorder
8	Organic Brain Syndrome	8	Organic Brain Syndrome	4	Vasculitis
8	Visual Disturbances	8	Visual Disturbances	3	Haemolysis Thrombocytopenia
8	Cranial Nerve Disorder	8	Cranial Nerve Disorder	3	Myositis
8	Lupus Headache	8	Lupus Headache	2	Arthritis
8	CVA	8	CVA	2	Mucocutaneous Disorder
8	Vasculitis	8	Vasculitis	2	Serositis

(Table 8) cont.....

SLEDAI-2K		Modified SLEDAI-2K		MEX-SLEDAI	
Weight	Descriptor	Weight	Descriptor	Weight	Descriptor
4	Arthritis	4	Arthritis	1	Fever Fatigue
4	Myositis	4	Myositis	1	Leucopenia Lymphopenia
4	Urinary Casts	4	Urinary Casts		
4	Hematuria	4	Hematuria	-	-
4	Proteinuria	4	Proteinuria	-	-
4	Pyuria	4	Pyuria	-	-
2	New Rash	2	New Rash	-	-
2	Alopecia	2	Alopecia	-	-
2	Mucosal Ulcers	2	Mucosal Ulcers	-	-
2	Pleurisy	2	Pleurisy	-	-
2	Pericarditis	2	Pericarditis	-	-
2	Low Complement	1	Fever	-	-
2	Increased DNA binding	1	Thrombocytopenia	-	-
1	Fever	1	Leukopenia	-	-
1	Thrombocytopenia	-	-	-	-
1	Leukopenia	-	-	-	-

SLEDAI, Systemic Lupus Erythematosus Disease Activity Index, MEX-SLEDAI, the Mexican version of the SLEDAI. CVA, cerebrovascular accident. DNA, Deoxyribonucleic acid.

Knowing the actual condition of the patients is relevant, but measure disease activity over time is important too, it results in the most important risk factor to damage in a study of 66 cSLE patients [111]. The disease pattern (chronic active, relapsing-remitting, and long quiescent activity) studied in 37 cSLE patients, was associated with damage and disease duration in nearly two-thirds of the children (p<0.0001); and those with the chronic active pattern evolve earlier to damage compared with the relapsing-remitting pattern [112]. In another study in cSLE patients, the frequency of severe/major flare was also associated with accruing more new damage [55].

Damage was recently defined as: *"Impairment of anatomy or physiology that may be associated with scarring, may accumulate, and is not completely reversible. Damage may be caused by disease, adverse effects of medication, or associated comorbidity. In children this may lead to stunted cognitive and physical development."* Besides, adult patients with damage will accumulate more damages, which means, previous damage is a significant predictor to accrue more damages [113]; it is probable that the same occurs to children; as they grow up, they are exposed to more time of disease, medication, and infections [114 - 116], all contributing to the development of more damage. Accordingly, efforts must be made to avoid damage accrual especially in children.

Recently, the assessment of damage in patients with cSLE was implemented, in 2003 an analysis of 387 patients was carried out [117], it revealed that 50.5% of cSLE patients had damage (SDI ≥1), the more affected organs were: renal (21.8%), neuropsychiatric (15.8%), musculoskeletal (11.7%), ocular (10.9%), and cutaneous (9.6%).

In 2006, a proposal for a pediatric version of the Systemic Lupus International Collaborating Clinics/American College of Rheumatology Damage Index (SDI), was published based on the analysis of 1,015 patients with cSLE [118]. The most important contribution to the creation of a pediatric version *versus* the adult instrument was the consideration of growth failure and delayed puberty. The new version of the SDI, to assess pediatric damage is depicted in Table **9**. A score equals to zero implies no damage while a score of 47 indicates the worst possible; the higher the score, the worse the disease damage. In their study, 405 (39.9%) cSLE patients had a score ≥ 1. The mean SDI score was 0.8, with a median of 0, range 0–12. They also found that the SDI score increase along with the disease duration. The most frequent organs damaged were renal (13%), neuropsychiatric (10.7%), musculoskeletal (10.7%), ocular (8.2%), and skin (7.6%). Growth failure was observed in 15.3% whereas delayed puberty in 11.3%. It is relevant, the observation that, in the first year of the disease, damage in the neuropsychiatric, renal, and musculoskeletal organ systems occurred at a high rate. The instrument includes a "Malignancy" domain, which had zero observations in the study.

Table 9. The pediatric version of the Systemic Lupus International Collaborating Clinics/American College of Rheumatology Damage Index (SDI).

Item	Possible Score
Ocular (either eye, by clinical assessment)	0 or 1
Any cataract ever	0 or 1
Retinal change or optic atrophy	

(Table 9) cont.....

Item	Possible Score
Neuropsychiatric Cognitive impairment (*e.g.* memory deficit, difficulty with calculation, poor concentration, difficulty in spoken or written language, impaired performance level) or major psychosis Seizures requiring therapy for 6 months Cerebrovascular accident ever (score 2 if >1), resection not for malignancy Cranial or peripheral neuropathy (excluding optic) Transverse myelitis	0 or 1 0 or 1 0, 1 or 2 0 or 1 0 or 1
Renal Estimated or measured glomerular filtration rate <50% Proteinuria ≥ 3.5g/24h or End-stage renal disease (regardless of dialysis or transplantation)	0 or 1 0 or 1
Pulmonary Pulmonary hypertension (right ventricular prominence or loud P2) Pulmonary fibrosis (by physical and radiographic examination) Shrinking lung (by radiographic examination) Pleural fibrosis (by radiographic examination) Pulmonary infarction (by radiographic examination) or resection not for Malignancy	0 or 1 0 or 1 0 or 1 0 or 1 0 or 1
Cardiovascular Angina or coronary artery bypass Myocardial infarction ever (score 2 if >1) Cardiomyopathy (ventricular dysfunction) Valvular disease (diastolic murmur, or systolic murmur >3/6) Pericarditis for ≥ 6 months or pericardiectomy	0 or 1 0, 1 or 2 0 or 1 0 or 1 0 or 1
Peripheral vascular Claudication for ≥ 6 months Minor tissue loss ever (pulp space) Significant tissue loss ever (*e.g.* loss of digit or limb, resection) (score 2 if >1) Venous thrombosis with swelling ulceration, or venous stasis	0 or 1 0 or 1 0, 1 or 2 0 or 1
Gastrointestinal Infarction or resection of bowel (below duodenum), spleen, liver, or gallbladder ever (score 2 if>1) Mesenteric insufficiency Chronic peritonitis Stricture or upper gastrointestinal tract surgery ever Pancreatic insufficiency requiring enzyme replacement or with Pseudocyst	0, 1 or 2 0 or 1 0 or 1 0 or 1 0 or 1

(Table 9) cont.....

Item	Possible Score
Musculoskeletal Muscle atrophy or weakness Deforming or erosive arthritis (including reducible deformities, excluding avascular necrosis) Osteoporosis with fracture or vertebral collapse (excluding avascular necrosis) Avascular necrosis (score 2 if >1) Osteomyelitis Rupture tendons	0 or 1 0 or 1 0 or 1 0, 1 or 2 0 or 1 0 or 1
Skin Scarring chronic alopecia Extensive scarring or panniculum other than scalp and pulp space Skin ulceration (excluding thrombosis) for ≥ 6 months	0 or 1 0 or 1 0 or 1
Diabetes (regardless of treatment)	0 or 1
Malignancy (exclude dysplasia) (score 2 if >1 site)	0, 1 or 2
Premature gonadal failure	0 or 1
Growth failure	0 or 1
Delayed puberty	0 or 1

There are criticisms [119] regarding the growth failure, as it well known, once the disease is controlled and the steroid doses reduced, patients can growth again, even reach a normal height; additionally, the delayed puberty could not be permanent. For those reasons, some authors suggest the reduced final height as the irreversible outcome and measure gonadotropin levels in patients meeting the SDI criterion for delayed puberty. In a recent study, the final adult height in patients with lupus diagnosed in childhood, mainly during puberty, was shorter than expected [120]. However, if we wait until patients reach adulthood to know if there is a problem in that aspect, we could miss important opportunities to treat them; so, it is a pending issue to resolve, like many others in cSLE.

The most recent study analyzing damage and its severity found 1,048 cSLE patients 463 (44.2%) with damage (SDI ≥1) at their last follow up, and was developed in average 3.8 years post-diagnosis. Independently of the disease duration, the organs most frequently damaged were the neuropsychiatric, kidney, skin, and musculoskeletal [5]. The authors considered that the pediatric adaptation of SDI [118] was not adequate to measure damage severity, that they defined as: *"Severity of damage is measured by the organs involved, and the extent of anatomical and physiologic derangement as judged by the expected impact on mortality, degree of support required, activity limitation, restriction in social participation, and patient- centered quality of life."* Discussing for example, that both stroke and cataracts, receive the same score, and certainly, have a different impact on patients. They suggest, add a Likert scale to items to better capture the impact on the organ damaged.

Damage occurring since diagnosis of systemic lupus erythematosus is ascertained by clinical assessment and defined as persistent changes in anatomy, physiology, pathology, or function, which may be the result of prior active disease, complications of therapy, or comorbid conditions, are not due to currently active disease, and have been present for at least 6 months. The same lesion cannot be scored twice. Damage is often irreversible and cumulative, and thus, damage scores are most frequently expected to increase or remain stable over time. However, because some forms of damage may improve or even resolve in pediatric patients, it is anticipated that in some cases scores may decline (*i.e.*, a manifestation that was previously present and has resolved would scored as "0" at the time of the present assessment). All items are defined according to the glossary of terms included with the original Systemic Lupus International Collaborating Clinics/American College of Rheumatology Damage Index. However, it is recommended that proteinuria be adjusted for height and weight in young children. Growth failure is defined as the presence of at least 2 of the following 3 features: 1) height below the third percentile for age; 2) growth velocity over 6 months below the third percentile for age; 3) crossing at least 2 percentiles (5%, 10%, 25%, 50%, 75%, 95%) on growth chart. In each patient, final height assessment is always needed to verify whether growth failure results in a permanently short height. Delayed puberty is defined as a delay in development of secondary sexual characteristics more than 2 SD below the mean for age by Tanner staging. For assessment of growth failure and delayed puberty, national standards or standards appropriate for the patient's racial or ethnic background should be used whenever available, instead of international standards.

There are few studies about the risk factors for the development of damage reported in the literature [111, 121]. Nevertheless, there is a concordance between studies regarding gender, ethnicity, and disease duration; surprisingly, kidney disease does not constitute a risk factor in these studies. Notably, the studies are different and not comparable. In the Asian study, the only risk factor associated was neuropsychiatric manifestations during the disease course, OR (95%CI) 14.59 (1.38-154.1), the authors referred that that group of patients had a low rate of damage accrual, which may explain their results. In the other study, the only important predictor of damage was cumulative disease activity over time.

In a study of 80 patients with cSLE, we found that SLEDAI >6, hemolytic anemia and proteinuria (>0.5g/day) at diagnosis were associated factors with damage (SDI $\geq$ 2) at the last visit, χ^2 (P-value) 11.9 (0.001), 9.39 (0.002), and nephritis 5.6 (0.18), respectively [110].

There are many factors why the studies report such different results, but coincided with the infection-hospitalization factor to the development of damage or death [91, 121 - 125], to keep in mind.

TREATMENT

The clinical manifestations in children are frequently more severe than in adults [78, 126, 127]. Diverse mechanisms are implicated in the pathogenesis and organ damage of the disease including dysregulated immune response, production of autoantibodies, activation and or complement deficiency, increase in the production of interferons, aberrant apoptosis, defects in lymphocyte signaling and immune complex deposition [50, 128].

The SLE treatment is based on specific manifestations and its severity, but also accordingly to each pathogenic mechanism [129]. The main goal of the treatment is to control disease activity, avoidance of flares, prevention of organ damage, minimization of the iatrogenic effects of medications, and the improvement of the quality of life. It is important to collaborate with multiple specialists in the case of multi-organ involvement, and we should individualize the treatment strategies for better control of the disease [74].

We listed a resume of the SHARE (Single Hub and Access point for pediatric Rheumatology in Europe) recommendations for the treatment of cSLE [60]:

1. All children should be on hydroxychloroquine treatment
2. Decisions on treatment changes or modifications should be actively examined
3. A Disease-modifying anti-rheumatic drugs (DMARD) should be added to therapy if it is not possible to taper the prednisone dose
4. For hematological involvement, a mild/moderate DMARD should be added
5. If Rituximab is required, the recommended dose is either 750 mg/m^2 at day 1 and day 15, or a 375 mg/m^2 once a week, for four doses
6. For neuropsychiatric manifestations, corticosteroids and immunosuppressants are indicated

Based on the pathogenesis of cSLE, we categorized the treatment in conventional immunomodulation and targeted immunotherapy (Fig. **6**).

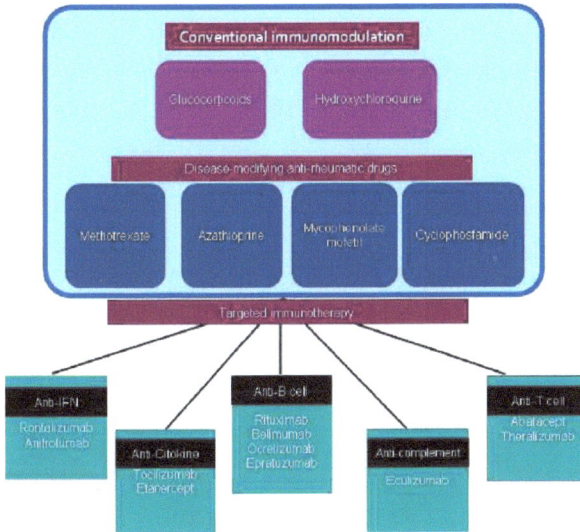

Fig. (6). Treatment options in cSLE.

Conventional Immunomodulation

Glucocorticoids (GC)

One of the main purposes to control the disease activity is the inhibition of prostaglandins and cytokine production, inhibition of cell proliferation, induction of apoptosis of B and T lymphocytes, and macrophages. The dose is decided according to the severity and organ involvement [21, 130].

A low dose of corticosteroids is recommended for mild to moderate disease activity and high dose, for severe manifestations [21]. The Childhood Arthritis and Rheumatology Research Alliance (CARRA), recommend a schema for the treatment of Proliferative Lupus Nephritis in children. For induction therapy, they presented different GC regimes; oral, intravenous, and combined. But they argue that the intravenous regime has the potential to eliminate the interferon-gamma signature; thus, three methylprednisolone pulses (30 mg/kg/dose up to 1000 mg/dose), at the time of induction therapy initiation, upon completion of the induction therapy after 24 weeks [131]. The goal is to achieve daily doses of oral GC between 10 and 20 mg per day, with the objective of minimizing the glucocorticoid dose but reaching a good control of the disease activity. For the immunosuppressant therapy, either cyclophosphamide or Mycophenolic acid, are used. *See the corresponding sections below.

We recommend the strict surveillance of the adverse effects of GC; due to high doses of GC may produce deleterious effects, such as myopathy, hyperlipidemia, Cushing syndrome, osteoporosis, and susceptibility to major infections. Whereas long-term, low doses, can produce skeletal growth inhibition, acne, cataracts, weight gain, osteonecrosis and also behavioral disorders [132]. For children taking GC for more than 3 months, the recommendation is to add calcium, in doses ranging from 1000 to 1200 mg/day; and daily 600 to 800 international units of vitamin D; to prevent or reverse bone loss.

Hydroxychloroquine

Hydroxychloroquine (HCQ) is an antimalarial agent, used as the first line therapy in SLE, is recommended in all SLE patients. The main action mechanisms are the inhibition of Toll-like receptor pathways, effects on phagocytosis, and leukocyte migration. Also, there are described other effects, like a cardiovascular protector and improving the lipid profiles. HCQ decreases flare rates and organ dam other age.

One of the adverse effects of HCQ is the retinal toxicity, therefore, a periodical ophthalmological examination at least annually is recommended. The risk of HCQ toxicity is minimized by dosing to a maximum of 5 mg/kg based on real body weight [74].

Disease-Modifying Anti-Rheumatic Drugs (DMARD)

A DMARD should be added to the therapy to help to taper the prednisone dose and to avoid severe organ damage [60].

Methotrexate (MTX)

MTX is a folic acid analog and inhibitor of dihydrofolate reductase and thymidylate synthase, in SLE is used as an alternative to azathioprine, the main indications are the mucocutaneous and the musculoskeletal disease.

Azathioprine (AZA)

AZA is a purine analog and a GC-sparing agent; its indications are the therapy of lupus nephritis, dermatologic and hematologic manifestations. The common side effects are hematological disturbances; as neutropenia and lymphopenia, myelotoxicity; other non-hematological effects are hepatotoxicity and susceptibility to infection [133].

Mycophenolate Mofetil (MMF)

MMF inhibits *de novo* synthesis of guanosine nucleotides; it has effect on B and T cells. The indications are moderate to severe disease manifestations, like hematological, cardiovascular, neuropsychiatric, and renal involvement [21]. MMF has lower rates of adverse effects in comparison to cyclophosphamide; the principal side effects are cytopenias, gastrointestinal symptoms and teratogenicity [74, 133].

Cyclophosphamide (CYC)

CYC is an alkylating agent used for the treatment of severe nephritis, neuropsychiatric, and hematological involvement.

In the case of lupus nephritis, the treatment has two phases; the induction and the maintenance. The induction therapy aimed to control disease activity has two different plans for the cyclophosphamide dosage, either the monthly administration of an initial dose of IV CYC 500 mg/m2 body surface area, with increments of subsequent doses to a maximum dose of 1,500 mg for 6 months; or a low dose of IV CYC, 500 mg every 2 weeks for 6 doses.

The other option, for the induction, is Mycophenolic acid, given PO 600 mg/m2/dose twice daily with a maximum dose of 1,500 mg.

The next phase is maintenance therapy, intended to avoid relapses and control disease activity [133, 134]. CYC is associated with increased risk of infections and hemorrhagic cystitis; whereas, large accumulate doses, are associated with malignancies [74].

The effectiveness of MMF *vs.* CYC as induction therapy in patients with lupus nephritis was analyzed in 51 children, 34/51 (67%) received MMF, and 17/51 (33%) intravenous CYC (IVCYC). There was no statistical difference in terms of DA, urine albumin/creatinine ratio, serum creatinine, erythrocyte sedimentation rate, anti-dsDNA antibodies, C3 levels, PGA and damage, or in the time for renal flare. The authors conclude that MMF and IVCYC appear to be comparably efficacious regarding the treatment response, damage accrual, and time to the next flare [135].

Targeted Immunotherapy

Based on the pathogenesis of cSLE, the targeted immunosuppression is more specific and directed to the different components of the immune system; including B and T lymphocytes, interferons, complement, and cytokines to prevent cell activation, differentiation, and survival. Almost all the experience on biologics for the treatment of cSLE is based on adult protocols, retrospective studies, and reports.

B-Cell

a) **Rituximab (RTX)** is a chimeric monoclonal anti-CD20 antibody against B cells. It is the most used biologic agent in patients with cSLE; nowadays there are no randomized controlled trials (RCTs) in children, but based on systematic reviews and other clinical studies, RTX seems to be a promising option [136 - 140]. The main indications are severe, refractory disease and organ involvement, especially renal, neuropsychiatric and hematologic. In the systematic review by Peterknecht *et al.* it was found a significant improvement in disease activity after RTX, but several patients also required antibiotic treatment for infectious complications [137]. Different treatments protocols used the recommendations of the SHARE initiative, either 750mg/m² doses on day 1 and day 15, or 375 mg/m²/dose once a week, for four doses [60]. One of the most common adverse side effects is infections and hypogammaglobulinemia; thus, levels of immunoglobulins (particularly IgG), vaccine titers, and peripheral blood lymphocytes, determined by flow cytometry are highly recommended before the treatment with RTX begins [133].

b) **Belimumab (BMB)** is a fully humanized monoclonal antibody (mAb) against the B-lymphocyte stimulator (BLyS), attenuating B cell survival and differentiation into plasma and memory cells. Since 2011, BMB is approved for the treatment of active SLE in adults with moderate disease activity but is not approved for severe lupus nephritis (LN) and/ or severe neuropsychiatric lupus (NPSLE) [21].

Recently, the FDA approved intravenous Belimumab for cSLE in patients ranging from 5 to 17 years old. The Pediatric Lupus Trial of Belimumab Plus Background Standard Therapy (PLUTO) included children with active disease and excluded patients with severe LN or NPSLE; the results showed good responses with an intravenous dose of 10 mg/kg. It was found a lower risk of severe flare and longer duration between flares, with the same safety profile as in adults. Currently, it is taking place a clinical trial with subcutaneous BMB in cSLE. The main adverse events are arthralgias, headache, infectious susceptibility, infusion reactions, and hypersensitivity [141].

A systematic review focused on the effectiveness and safety of biological therapeutics in cSLE found 498 studies eligible for analysis; only 9 had the qualitative synthesis required to be analyzed. There were 8 Rituximab studies and one of Belimumab. Eight out of 8 studies reported a long-term (≥12 months) improvement in disease activity, the authors conclude based on the evidence that the use of RTX is acceptable for refractory disease activity. RTX was also effective in reducing corticosteroids doses and in the treatment of hematological manifestations (persistent autoimmune thrombocytopenia (AITP) and autoimmune hemolytic anemia (AIHA). Regarding the adverse events, anaphylactic infusion-related reactions were reported at a frequency of 2-13%. Infections after RTX were reported from 2% to 25%. Hypogammaglobulinemia was common but transient, and intravenous immunoglobulin G (IVIG) replace therapy was indicated for 2-50% in 3/5 studies [137]. Regarding Belimumab, the PLUTO studies phase II, included 93 children, and the key results were 62% flares reduction and higher SLE responder index [141]. There is no updated information to issue a recommendation on Belimumab yet.

c) Other B cells targeted therapy

-**Ocrelizumab** is another anti-CD20 mAb. It demonstrated better response *versus* placebo in adults with LN, but with secondary severe infections, the trial was suspended [142].

-**Epratuzumab** is a humanized mAb against CD22, a receptor on the mature B cells. The clinical trials have demonstrated effective response, well-tolerated, but not yet approved [143].

-**Blisibimod** is a fusion protein that selectively binds the Fc portion of the IgG and the B Lymphocyte stimulator (BLys), acting as a selective antagonist of BLys. The clinical trials reported a good response to improving disease activity [144].

T-Cells

The inhibition of T cell activation is another strategy for the treatment of cSLE.

a) **Abatacept**, is a fusion protein directed to CTLA-4, preventing the T-cells co-stimulation; thus, B cells cannot respond. Currently, Abatacept has beneficial results in refractory Rhupus syndrome (overlap between arthritis and SLE), but also, in some clinical trials patients presented flares in the same proportion than the ones in the control group. Another option is the use of Abatacept in combination with RTX during the period of B cell depletion [145]. More studies are necessary to demonstrate its effectiveness and the applications in the treatment of cSLE patients [142].

Interferons (IFN)

IFN-α is a mediator in the pathogenesis of SLE, especially in children with Aicardi-Goutières syndrome and in patients with SAVI. Increased IFN-α levels correlate to disease activity and severity. The lupus patients have the up-regulation of IFN-α-dependent genes in peripheral blood mononuclear cells, constituting the IFN signature.

a) **Rontalizumab** is a mAb directed to neutralize all 12 subtypes of IFN-α. It has induced a rapid and sustained decline in the expression of IFN-regulated genes with a good safety profile but did not reduce the IFN signature to basal levels [146].

b) **Anifrolumab** is a mAb against the subunit 1 of the type I interferon receptor. This drug has demonstrated improvement in adults with organ damage, like skin and joints, and is the most promising agent of this group of drugs [147]. The common side effects are the susceptibility to viral infections, increasing the risk for influenza and herpes zoster infection [148].

Cytokines

Diverse cytokines are implicated in the immunopathogenesis of SLE, and they are associated with loss of tolerance and damage in organs. The main related cytokines are TNF, IL-4, IL-6, and IL-10; fortunately, with targeted immunotherapy, we can block some of them [128].

a. Tocilizumab (TCZ)

TCZ is a humanized mAb against the IL-6 receptor. IL-6 is a proinflammatory cytokine that is elevated in patients with active lupus. It induces differentiation of B cells into antibody-secreting cells [142]. One open-label trial demonstrated improvement in disease activity, arthritis, and autoantibodies in adult patients [148].

Other IL-6 mAb is the **sirukumab**. It has high affinity and specificity for IL-6. It has been studied in adult patients with mild to moderate SLE, and recently a Phase II trial for lupus nephritis with no significant changes in proteinuria, and with serious adverse events [142, 149].

b. Anti-TNF

According to Kleinmann *et al.* in the International and Multidisciplinary Expert Recommendations for the use of biologics in SLE, the blockade of TNF in adults with Rhupus is a therapeutic option, the drugs most reported are Adalimumab, Etanercept, Infliximab, Certolizumab pegol, and Golimumab, but with special surveillance of lupus flares [150].

c. Janus Kinase/Signal Transducer and Activator of Transcription Inhibition.

The JAK/STAT signaling pathway is dysregulated in SLE, and blocking its activity would be a therapeutic option. One of the drugs that block this activity is **Tofacitinib**, a pan-JAK inhibitor; in murine models, it reduces proteinuria, levels of dsDNA antibodies, and organ damage [148]. A phase Ib RCT of tofacitinib in patients with mild to moderate SLE is finished, but there are no results yet; and, and two Phase I/II trials are also currently recruiting [144].

Complement

Eculizumab is a humanized recombinant mAb and constitutes an important targeted therapy aimed to block the complement pathway; it blocks C5 from converting to C5a and C5b; consequently, preventing the formation of the membrane attack complex. Randomized trials using Eculizumab are still ongoing, but with promising results in other autoimmune diseases [130, 151].

Transplant

In patients with a severe, progressive, and therapy-resistant disease, the option of hematopoietic stem cell transplantation (HSCT) is available, especially for children with monogenic lupus [152, 153]. There are two forms of HSCT, the autologous and the allogeneic transplant; each one has specific indications.

There are few reported experiences with autologous HSCT in cSLE, Jayne *et al.* [154] performed 17 procedures with 33% of complete remission, and 7% of partial remission. In the case of monogenic lupus, there is one successful case of a male with C1q deficiency and severe phenotype with skin and renal damage [153]. And a report of a successful HSCT in one patient with PI3K delta syndrome and lupus phenotype [155].

Other Treatment Recommendations

Photoprotection must be part of the scheme of treatment for patients with cSLE [156, 157], photosensitivity can have a significant impact on disease activity and quality of life [158]; one study found [159] that patients that used sunscreen regularly had lower renal involvement, thrombocytopenia, and hospitalizations compared to those who did not use it (OR (95% CI) 0.22 (0.06 – 0.869), 0.22 (0.06 – 0.85), and 0.10 (0.03 – 0.35)), respectively. In patients in whom the photoprotection awareness is high, there was no association with disease activity or damage [160]; differences could be due to the disparity in the sun exposure and the use of sunscreen, in the first study up to 33.3% of patients reported an hour or more of daily exposure to sunlight, while in the last study up to 95.5% of patients used photoprotection methods.

A significant proportion of the requirements of **vitamin D** came from sun exposure; hence, patients with cSLE have to increase the intake of vitamin D, from the diet or supplementation, a daily intake of at least 400 UI for children older than 1 year could be enough, but the doses should be adjusted based on the serum 25-hydroxyvitamin D (25[OH]D) levels [157].

Recommendations [161] and guidelines [162] on vaccination for cSLE patients endorse that children should receive vaccines according to the recommendations and the schedules for the general public. Pneumococcal vaccination is recommended for all SLE patients; while, Influenza vaccination for the immunosuppressed SLE patients and case-to-case indication for live or live-attenuated vaccines.

Others

Intravenous Immunoglobulin G (IVIG)

Besides the use of IVIG as replacing therapy for secondary hypogammaglo-bulinemia due to the use of Rituximab [163], there are other indications for its use in pediatric rheumatology such as Kawasaki disease, chronic inflammatory demyelinating polyneuropathy, Guillain-Barrè syndrome and Inflammatory myopathies [164]. Specifically in cSLE, the most known indication is for patients with hematologic involvement as autoimmune hemolytic anemia; however, it has been used for many other indications as immune thrombocytopenia, chorea, myocarditis, lupus nephritis, neuropsychiatric involvement and catastrophic antiphospholipid syndrome [165, 166], but the most valuable advantage of IVIG over DMARD is, its use as an immunomodulator in patients with active disease an infection [167, 168].

We reviewed several treatment options for cSLE, a better understanding of the different pathogenic mechanisms will help to design a tailored treatment per each phenotype of cSLE. It is important to identify monogenic lupus in patients with early onset manifestations or with a particular presentation to offer targeted immunotherapy. More rigorous studies are necessary to establish better practices; and we should consider a multidisciplinary collaboration for the proper treatment of cSLE.

OUTCOME

A recent meta-analysis of survival [169] included 125 adult studies and 51 pediatric studies (except for neonatal lupus); 33 from high-income countries and 18 from low/middle-income countries. The authors found among the high-income countries an important increase in survival from the 1960s to 1970s, but after that, only a discrete improvement was observed; nevertheless, from 2008 to 2016, the 5-year and 10-year survival were 0.99 and 0.97, respectively. Conversely, in countries from low/middle income, the major increment in survival was between 1970 and 1990, and remain stable until 2016, the 5-year and 10-year survival were 0.85 and 0.79, respectively. Causes of death were available in 39 studies; in low/middle-income countries, the frequency of death due to cSLE tends to increase over time, with high rates of lupus nephritis. Conversely, in high-income countries, the most frequent causes of death were SLE in more than 50% and infections.

The RELESSER Registry recently informed the identification of 3 clusters of damage in cSLE patients [170]. In Table **10**, we resume the most relevant findings of the study.

Table 10. Clusters of cSLE with its main clinical features, damage and death.

-	Cluster 1	Cluster 2	Cluster 3
N (%)	251 (72.7)	50 (14.65)	44 (12.7)
Females, N (%)	220 (87.6)	43 (86)	43 (97.7)
Age at diagnosis, mean ± SD	14.34 ±2.97	13.65±3.06	14.45±2.17
Damage	Neuropsychiatric (9.2%) Peripheral vascular (4.8%) Cardiovascular (4%)	Renal (60%) Ocular (54%) Cardiovascular (20%)	Musculoskeletal (100%) Neuropsychiatric (18.2%) Peripheral vascular (15.9%) Renal (9%)
SDI score, mean ± SD	0.70 ± 1.18	2.90 ± 1.54	2.66 ± 1.87
Death, N (%)	5 (2)	5 (10)	2 (4.5)

[a] Extracted from (175) SD, standard deviation. The authors analyzed those children with disease duration less than five years (N=80 cSLE) and found that cluster 3 had the higher rate of damage 5/5 (100%), with SDI 2.6

± 2.07, and one death (5%), in comparison with cluster 1, 11/72 (15.3%), SDI 0.64 ± 1.27 and 2 deaths (2.8%), and cluster 2 with damage 3/3 (100%), SDI 1.67 ± 1.56, and no deaths.

Note that in cluster 1, some patients do not develop damage, and none of them had renal damage, both in the analysis of less than 5 years of disease duration and in the whole study. Conversely, patients in clusters 2 and 3, all children had a degree of damage, and particularly cluster 2 with renal affection in 60% and cardiovascular involvement in 20%, these patients had the higher rate of mortality. Another important observation of this study is that antimalarial use protected against the increase of damage.

The cardiovascular affection is not frequently seen in children; however, a study of 5,679 admissions in patients with cSLE, 705 with pericardial effusion and 4974 without pericardial effusion, reported more affection in blacks, infectious disease, renal disease, anemia, and mortality at discharge in patients with pericardial effusion; besides the in-hospital mortality was reported 2.5 times higher [171].

Another study [94] showed differences in mortality based on the beginning age of lupus, group A (<6 years, n=39), group B (≥6 <12 years, n= 395), and group C (≥12 < 18 years, n=413). They found in group 1 more fever (82%) and reticuloendothelial manifestations (54%) in comparison with group B and C (76%, 48% and 61%, 32%), respectively. They also accrued more damage in the neuropsychiatric (21%), skin (10%), Peripheral vascular (5%), and ocular (10%) compared with the other groups. However, the SDI was not statistically different nor the renal affection. Mortality was also more frequent in group A compared with group B and C (15% *vs.* 10% *vs.* 6%, p=0.028). Almost 50% (33/69) of deaths occurred in the first two years of diagnosis; 78% were due to infections, and 70% had disease activity.

Regarding the importance of infections and disease activity in mortality, a study of 71 cSLE patients followed-up for up to 10 years, based on the most recent hospitalization found that 53 children survived while 18 died. Severe sepsis OR (95%CI) 17.8 (4.5-70.9), general infection 6.1 (1.5 – 25), SLEDAI ≥8 7.6 (1.1-53.8), fungal infection 5.4 (3.2 -9), acute renal failure 5.1 (2.5-10.5), and acute thrombocytopenia 3.97 (1.9-8.4), were the risk factors associated to death in the univariate analysis. In the multivariate analysis, severe sepsis (OR = 98, CI = 16.3-586.2) was the only independent variable in death prediction [123].

CONCLUSION

cSLE is a complex disease, or should we say, an intricate and complex group of diseases sharing a roughly common phenotype. There is so much to learn in this field. But taking in mind the main clinical features in the different groups of age, and the new tools to classify and follow-up the clinical course of these patients will help you in your daily clinical practice. Herein you learn the treatment options, but it should be individualized, and require a group of specialists.

CONSENT FOR PUBLICATION

Not applicable.

CONFLICT OF INTEREST

The authors declare no conflict of interest, financial or otherwise.

ACKNOWLEDGEMENT

We are thankful for the valuable assistance of Carla Toledo Salinas MD for obtaining the permission to share pictures of our patients.

We also would like to thank to all our patients, who have instructed us not only in terms of medicine.

REFERENCES

[1]   Barsalou J, Levy DM, Silverman ED. An update on childhood-onset systemic lupus erythematosus. Curr Opin Rheumatol 2013; 25(5): 616-22.
[http://dx.doi.org/10.1097/BOR.0b013e328363e868] [PMID: 23836073]

[2]   Tselios K, Gladman DD, Touma Z, Su J, Anderson N, Urowitz MB. Monophasic disease course in systemic lupus erythematosus. J Rheumatol 2018; 45(8): 1131-5.
[http://dx.doi.org/10.3899/jrheum.171319] [PMID: 29858240]

[3]   Yaniv G, Twig G, Shor DB, *et al.* A volcanic explosion of autoantibodies in systemic lupus erythematosus: a diversity of 180 different antibodies found in SLE patients. Autoimmun Rev 2015; 14(1): 75-9.
[http://dx.doi.org/10.1016/j.autrev.2014.10.003] [PMID: 25449682]

[4]   Allam N, Gaber W, Helaly M. Antibody Clustering in Systemic lupus Erythematosus and their clinical correlates. EJAE 2017; 4: 218-26.

[5]   Holland MJ, Beresford MW, Feldman BM, *et al.* Measuring Disease Damage and Its Severity in Childhood-Onset Systemic Lupus Erythematosus. Arthritis Care Res (Hoboken) 2018; 70(11): 1621-9.
[http://dx.doi.org/10.1002/acr.23531] [PMID: 29409150]

[6]   Silva CA, Avcin T, Brunner HI. Taxonomy for systemic lupus erythematosus with onset before adulthood. Arthritis Care Res (Hoboken) 2012; 64(12): 1787-93.
[http://dx.doi.org/10.1002/acr.21757] [PMID: 22730317]

[7]   Klein-Gitelman M, Reiff A, Silverman ED. Systemic lupus erythematosus in childhood. Rheum Dis Clin North Am 2002; 28(3): 561-577, vi-vii.
[http://dx.doi.org/10.1016/S0889-857X(02)00015-7] [PMID: 12380370]

[8]   Zetterstrom R, Berglund G. Systemic lupus erythematosus in childhood; a clinical study. Acta Paediatr (Stockh) 1956; 45(2): 189-204.
[http://dx.doi.org/10.1111/j.1651-2227.1956.tb17690.x] [PMID: 13313143]

[9]   Kovacs L, Calder J, Matas M, Hanson S. Acute disseminated lupus erythematosus in a North

American Indian girl. Can Med Assoc J 1956; 74(7): 552-5.
[PMID: 13304805]

[10]   Arzt L. [Disseminated lupus erythematosus; malignant lupus erythematosus (Goldsmith-Bear); history and concept]. J Mt Sinai Hosp N Y 1952; 19(1): 19-29.
[PMID: 14938969]

[11]   Brito AdaR. [Case of febrile lupus-erythematous purpura haemorrhagica (malignant lupus erythemato-visceritis)]. Port Med 1951; 35(5): 265-81.
[PMID: 14911415]

[12]   Lian C, Siguier F, Lonjumeau B, Duperrat B, Lemenager . [Malignant lupus erythematosus visceritis with myositis, terminal cardiac insufficiency; anatomico-clinical study]. Bull Mem Soc Med Hop Paris 1950; 66: 467-76.
[PMID: 15414406]

[13]   Orr H. Acute disseminated lupus erythematosus. Can Med Assoc J 1950; 62(5): 432-7.
[PMID: 15411621]

[14]   Hiraki LT, Benseler SM, Tyrrell PN, Harvey E, Hebert D, Silverman ED. Ethnic differences in pediatric systemic lupus erythematosus. J Rheumatol 2009; 36(11): 2539-46.
[http://dx.doi.org/10.3899/jrheum.081141] [PMID: 19833755]

[15]   Levy DM, Kamphuis S. Systemic lupus erythematosus in children and adolescents. Pediatr Clin North Am 2012; 59(2): 345-64.
[http://dx.doi.org/10.1016/j.pcl.2012.03.007] [PMID: 22560574]

[16]   Gardner-Medwin JMM, Dolezalova P, Cummins C, Southwood TR. Incidence of Henoch-Schönlein purpura, Kawasaki disease, and rare vasculitides in children of different ethnic origins. Lancet 2002; 360(9341): 1197-202.
[http://dx.doi.org/10.1016/S0140-6736(02)11279-7] [PMID: 12401245]

[17]   Mackie FE, Kainer G, Adib N, *et al.* The national incidence and clinical picture of SLE in children in Australia - a report from the Australian Paediatric Surveillance Unit. Lupus 2015; 24(1): 66-73.
[http://dx.doi.org/10.1177/0961203314552118] [PMID: 25288030]

[18]   Hiraki LT, Feldman CH, Liu J, *et al.* Prevalence, incidence, and demographics of systemic lupus erythematosus and lupus nephritis from 2000 to 2004 among children in the US Medicaid beneficiary population. Arthritis Rheum 2012; 64(8): 2669-76.
[http://dx.doi.org/10.1002/art.34472] [PMID: 22847366]

[19]   Dave M, Rankin J, Pearce M, Foster HE. Global prevalence estimates of three chronic musculoskeletal conditions: club foot, juvenile idiopathic arthritis and juvenile systemic lupus erythematosus. Pediatr Rheumatol Online J 2020; 18(1): 49.
[http://dx.doi.org/10.1186/s12969-020-00443-8] [PMID: 32532304]

[20]   Kwak SG, Par S-H, Kim JY. Incidence and prevalence of juvenile systemic lupus erythematosus in Korea: data from the national health claims database 2017. J Rheumatol 2020; 191186
[http://dx.doi.org/10.3899/jrheum.191186] [PMID: 32358155]

[21]   Smith EMD, Lythgoe H, Midgley A, Beresford MW, Hedrich CM. Juvenile-onset systemic lupus erythematosus: Update on clinical presentation, pathophysiology and treatment options. Clin Immunol 2019; 209: 108274.
[http://dx.doi.org/10.1016/j.clim.2019.108274] [PMID: 31678365]

[22]   Abdwani R, Abdalla E, Al-Zakwani I. Unique Characteristics of Prepubertal Onset Systemic Lupus Erythematosus. Int J Pediatr 2019; 2019: 9537065.
[http://dx.doi.org/10.1155/2019/9537065] [PMID: 31263503]

[23]   Pluchinotta FR, Schiavo B, Vittadello F, Martini G, Perilongo G, Zulian F. Distinctive clinical features of pediatric systemic lupus erythematosus in three different age classes. Lupus 2007; 16(8): 550-5.
[http://dx.doi.org/10.1177/0961203307080636] [PMID: 17711887]

[24] Descloux E, Durieu I, Cochat P, *et al.* Influence of age at disease onset in the outcome of paediatric systemic lupus erythematosus. Rheumatology (Oxford) 2009; 48(7): 779-84.
[http://dx.doi.org/10.1093/rheumatology/kep067] [PMID: 19416945]

[25] Gomes RC, Silva MF, Kozu K, *et al.* Features of 847 Childhood-Onset Systemic Lupus Erythematosus Patients in Three Age Groups at Diagnosis: A Brazilian Multicenter Study. Arthritis Care Res (Hoboken) 2016; 68(11): 1736-41.
[http://dx.doi.org/10.1002/acr.22881] [PMID: 27014968]

[26] Selmi C, Brunetta E, Raimondo MG, Meroni PL. The X chromosome and the sex ratio of autoimmunity. Autoimmun Rev 2012; 11(6-7): A531-7.
[http://dx.doi.org/10.1016/j.autrev.2011.11.024] [PMID: 22155196]

[27] Lleo A, Battezzati PM, Selmi C, Gershwin ME, Podda M. Is autoimmunity a matter of sex? Autoimmun Rev 2008; 7(8): 626-30.
[http://dx.doi.org/10.1016/j.autrev.2008.06.009] [PMID: 18603021]

[28] Cattalini M, Soliani M, Caparello MC, Cimaz R. Sex Differences in Pediatric Rheumatology. Clin Rev Allergy Immunol 2019; 56(3): 293-307.
[http://dx.doi.org/10.1007/s12016-017-8642-3] [PMID: 28849549]

[29] Choi MY, Barber MRW, Barber CEH, Clarke AE, Fritzler MJ. Preventing the development of SLE: identifying risk factors and proposing pathways for clinical care. Lupus 2016; 25(8): 838-49.
[http://dx.doi.org/10.1177/0961203316640367] [PMID: 27252260]

[30] Walters HM, Pan N, Moorthy LN, Ward MJ, Peterson MG, Lehman TJ. Patterns and influence of familial autoimmunity in pediatric systemic lupus erythematosus. Pediatr Rheumatol Online J 2012; 10(1): 22.
[http://dx.doi.org/10.1186/1546-0096-10-22] [PMID: 22891746]

[31] Ashournia P, Sadeghi P, Rezaei N, Moradinejad M-H, Ziaee V. Prevalence of Family History of Autoimmune Disorders in Juvenile Systemic Lupus Erythematosus. Maedica (Buchar) 2018; 13(1): 21-4.
[http://dx.doi.org/10.26574/maedica.2018.13.1.21] [PMID: 29868136]

[32] Ulff-Møller CJ, Svendsen AJ, Viemose LN, Jacobsen S. Concordance of autoimmune disease in a nationwide Danish systemic lupus erythematosus twin cohort. Semin Arthritis Rheum 2018; 47(4): 538-44.
[http://dx.doi.org/10.1016/j.semarthrit.2017.06.007] [PMID: 28755788]

[33] Batu ED. Monogenic systemic lupus erythematosus: insights in pathophysiology. Rheumatol Int 2018; 38(10): 1763-75.
[http://dx.doi.org/10.1007/s00296-018-4048-7] [PMID: 29766256]

[34] Hiraki LT, Silverman ED. Genomics of Systemic Lupus Erythematosus: Insights Gained by Studying Monogenic Young-Onset Systemic Lupus Erythematosus. Rheum Dis Clin North Am 2017; 43(3): 415-34.
[http://dx.doi.org/10.1016/j.rdc.2017.04.005] [PMID: 28711143]

[35] Goulielmos GN, Zervou MI, Vazgiourakis VM, Ghodke-Puranik Y, Garyfallos A, Niewold TB. The genetics and molecular pathogenesis of systemic lupus erythematosus (SLE) in populations of different ancestry. Gene 2018; 668: 59-72.
[http://dx.doi.org/10.1016/j.gene.2018.05.041] [PMID: 29775752]

[36] Graham RR, Ortmann W, Rodine P, *et al.* Specific combinations of HLA-DR2 and DR3 class II haplotypes contribute graded risk for disease susceptibility and autoantibodies in human SLE. Eur J Hum Genet 2007; 15(8): 823-30.
[http://dx.doi.org/10.1038/sj.ejhg.5201827] [PMID: 17406641]

[37] Taylor KE, Chung SA, Graham RR, *et al.* Risk alleles for systemic lupus erythematosus in a large case-control collection and associations with clinical subphenotypes. PLoS Genet 2011; 7(2):

e1001311.
[http://dx.doi.org/10.1371/journal.pgen.1001311] [PMID: 21379322]

[38]   Wang Z, Chang C, Peng M, Lu Q. Translating epigenetics into clinic: focus on lupus. Clin Epigenetics 2017; 9(1): 78.
[http://dx.doi.org/10.1186/s13148-017-0378-7] [PMID: 28785369]

[39]   Scharer CD, Blalock EL, Mi T, *et al.* Epigenetic programming underpins B cell dysfunction in human SLE. Nat Immunol 2019; 20(8): 1071-82.
[http://dx.doi.org/10.1038/s41590-019-0419-9] [PMID: 31263277]

[40]   Farivar S, Shaabanpour Aghamaleki F. Effects of major epigenetic factors on systemic lupus erythematosus. Iran Biomed J 2018; 22(5): 294-302.
[http://dx.doi.org/10.29252/ibj.22.5.294] [PMID: 29803202]

[41]   Quiroz EN, Chavez-Estrada V, Macias-Ochoa K, Ayala-Navarro MF, Flores-Aguilar AS, Morales-Navarrete F, *et al.* Epigenetic mechanisms and posttranslational modifications in systemic lupus erythematosus. Int J Mol Sci 2019.
[http://dx.doi.org/10.3390/ijms20225679]

[42]   Breitbach ME, Ramaker RC, Roberts K, Kimberly RP, Absher D. Population-Specific Patterns of Epigenetic Defects in the B Cell Lineage in Patients With Systemic Lupus Erythematosus. Arthritis Rheumatol 2020; 72(2): 282-91.
[http://dx.doi.org/10.1002/art.41083] [PMID: 31430064]

[43]   Wardowska A. The epigenetic face of lupus: Focus on antigen-presenting cells. Int Immunopharmacol 2020; 81: 106262.
[http://dx.doi.org/10.1016/j.intimp.2020.106262] [PMID: 32045873]

[44]   Conde PG, Farhat LC, Braga ALF, Sallum AEM, Farhat SCL, Silva CA. Are prematurity and environmental factors determinants for developing childhood-onset systemic lupus erythematosus? Mod Rheumatol 2018; 28(1): 156-60.
[http://dx.doi.org/10.1080/14397595.2017.1332508] [PMID: 28696177]

[45]   Mu Q, Zhang H, Luo XM. SLE: Another autoimmune disorder influenced by microbes and diet? Front Immunol 2015; 6: 608.
[http://dx.doi.org/10.3389/fimmu.2015.00608] [PMID: 26648937]

[46]   Qiu CC, Caricchio R, Gallucci S. Triggers of Autoimmunity: The Role of Bacterial Infections in the Extracellular Exposure of Lupus Nuclear Autoantigens. Front Immunol 2019; 10: 2608.
[http://dx.doi.org/10.3389/fimmu.2019.02608] [PMID: 31781110]

[47]   Demirkaya E, Sahin S, Romano M, Zhou Q, Aksentijevich I. New Horizons in the Genetic Etiology of Systemic Lupus Erythematosus and Lupus-Like Disease: Monogenic Lupus and Beyond. J Clin Med 2020; 9(3): 712.
[http://dx.doi.org/10.3390/jcm9030712] [PMID: 32151092]

[48]   Belot A, Rice GI, Omarjee SO, *et al.* Contribution of rare and predicted pathogenic gene variants to childhood-onset lupus: a large, genetic panel analysis of British and French cohorts. Lancet Rheumatol 2020; 2(2): e99-e109.
[http://dx.doi.org/10.1016/S2665-9913(19)30142-0]

[49]   Webb R, Kelly JA, Somers EC, *et al.* Early disease onset is predicted by a higher genetic risk for lupus and is associated with a more severe phenotype in lupus patients. Ann Rheum Dis 2011; 70(1): 151-6.
[http://dx.doi.org/10.1136/ard.2010.141697] [PMID: 20881011]

[50]   Rivas-Larrauri F, Yamazaki-Nakashimada MA. Systemic lupus erythematosus: Is it one disease? Reumatol Clin 2016; 12(5): 274-81.
[http://dx.doi.org/10.1016/j.reuma.2016.01.005] [PMID: 26922326]

[51]   Costa-Reis P, Sullivan KE. Monogenic lupus: it's all new! Curr Opin Immunol 2017; 49: 87-95.
[http://dx.doi.org/10.1016/j.coi.2017.10.008] [PMID: 29100097]

[52] Belot A, Kasher P, Trotter E, Foray A, Debaud A, Rice G, *et al.* Protein Kinase Cδ Deficiency Causes Mendelian SLE with B cell-defective apoptosis and hyperproliferation.pdf. Arthritis Rheum 2013; 65: 2161-71.
[http://dx.doi.org/10.1002/art.38008] [PMID: 23666743]

[53] Alperin JM, Ortiz-Fernández L, Sawalha AH. Monogenic Lupus: A Developing Paradigm of Disease. Front Immunol 2018; 9: 2496.
[http://dx.doi.org/10.3389/fimmu.2018.02496] [PMID: 30459768]

[54] Moncada B, Day NK, Good RA, Windhorst DB. Lupus-erythematosus-like syndrome with a familial defect of complement. N Engl J Med 1972; 286(13): 689-93.
[http://dx.doi.org/10.1056/NEJM197203302861304] [PMID: 4110615]

[55] Lo MS. Monogenic Lupus. Curr Rheumatol Rep 2016; 18(12): 71.
[http://dx.doi.org/10.1007/s11926-016-0621-9] [PMID: 27812953]

[56] Ramantani G, Kohlhase J, Hertzberg C, *et al.* Expanding the phenotypic spectrum of lupus erythematosus in Aicardi-Goutières syndrome. Arthritis Rheum 2010; 62(5): 1469-77.
[http://dx.doi.org/10.1002/art.27367] [PMID: 20131292]

[57] Ghodke-Puranik Y, Niewold TB. Immunogenetics of systemic lupus erythematosus: A comprehensive review. J Autoimmun 2015; 64: 125-36.
[http://dx.doi.org/10.1016/j.jaut.2015.08.004] [PMID: 26324017]

[58] Kim H, Sanchez GAM, Goldbach-Mansky R. Insights from Mendelian Interferonopathies: Comparison of CANDLE, SAVI with AGS, Monogenic Lupus. J Mol Med (Berl) 2016; 94(10): 1111-27.
[http://dx.doi.org/10.1007/s00109-016-1465-5] [PMID: 27678529]

[59] Aggarwal R, Ringold S, Khanna D, *et al.* Distinctions between diagnostic and classification criteria? Arthritis Care Res (Hoboken) 2015; 67(7): 891-7.
[http://dx.doi.org/10.1002/acr.22583] [PMID: 25776731]

[60] Groot N, de Graeff N, Avcin T, *et al.* European evidence-based recommendations for diagnosis and treatment of childhood-onset systemic lupus erythematosus: the SHARE initiative. Ann Rheum Dis 2017; 76(11): 1788-96.
[http://dx.doi.org/10.1136/annrheumdis-2016-210960] [PMID: 28630236]

[61] Hochberg MC. Updating the American College of Rheumatology revised criteria for the classification of systemic lupus erythematosus. Arthritis Rheum 1997; 40(9): 1725.
[http://dx.doi.org/10.1002/art.1780400928] [PMID: 9324032]

[62] Aringer M, Costenbader K, Daikh D, *et al.* 2019 European League Against Rheumatism/American College of Rheumatology Classification Criteria for Systemic Lupus Erythematosus. Arthritis Rheumatol 2019; 71(9): 1400-12.
[http://dx.doi.org/10.1002/art.40930] [PMID: 31385462]

[63] Petri M, Orbai AM, Alarcón GS, *et al.* Derivation and validation of the Systemic Lupus International Collaborating Clinics classification criteria for systemic lupus erythematosus. Arthritis Rheum 2012; 64(8): 2677-86.
[http://dx.doi.org/10.1002/art.34473] [PMID: 22553077]

[64] Oglesby A, Korves C, Laliberté F, Dennis G, Rao S, Suthoff ED, *et al.* Impact of early versus late systemic lupus erythematosus diagnosis on clinical and economic outcomes. App Heal Econ Heal Policy 2014.
[http://dx.doi.org/10.1007/s40258-014-0085-x]

[65] Tucker LB, Uribe AG, Fernández M, *et al.* Adolescent onset of lupus results in more aggressive disease and worse outcomes: results of a nested matched case-control study within LUMINA, a multiethnic US cohort (LUMINA LVII). Lupus 2008; 17(4): 314-22.
[http://dx.doi.org/10.1177/0961203307087875] [PMID: 18413413]

[66]   Rodrigues Fonseca A, Felix Rodrigues MC, Sztajnbok FR, Gerardin Poirot Land M, Knupp Feitosa de Oliveira S. Comparison among ACR1997, SLICC and the new EULAR/ACR classification criteria in childhood-onset systemic lupus erythematosus. Adv Rheumatol 2019; 59(1): 20.
[http://dx.doi.org/10.1186/s42358-019-0062-z] [PMID: 31092290]

[67]   Sag E, Tartaglione A, Batu ED, *et al.* Performance of the new SLICC classification criteria in childhood systemic lupus erythematosus: a multicentre study. Clin Exp Rheumatol 2014; 32(3): 440-4.
[PMID: 24642380]

[68]   Fonseca AR, Gaspar-Elsas MI, Land MG, de Oliveira SK. Comparison between three systems of classification criteria in juvenile systemic lupus erythematous. Rheumatology (Oxford) 2015; 54(2): 241-7.
[http://dx.doi.org/10.1093/rheumatology/keu278] [PMID: 25125590]

[69]   Massias JS, Smith EMD, Al-Abadi E, *et al.* Clinical and laboratory characteristics in juvenile-onset systemic lupus erythematosus across age groups. Lupus 2020; 29(5): 474-81.
[http://dx.doi.org/10.1177/0961203320909156] [PMID: 32233733]

[70]   Sahin S, Adrovic A, Barut K, *et al.* Juvenile systemic lupus erythematosus in Turkey: demographic, clinical and laboratory features with disease activity and outcome. Lupus 2018; 27(3): 514-9.
[http://dx.doi.org/10.1177/0961203317747717] [PMID: 29233038]

[71]   Fonseca R, Aguiar F, Rodrigues M, Brito I. Clinical phenotype and outcome in lupus according to age: a comparison between juvenile and adult onset. Reum Clin 2018; 14(3): 160-3.
[http://dx.doi.org/10.1016/j.reumae.2016.10.010] [PMID: 28040420]

[72]   Chiewchengchol D, Murphy R, Edwards SW, Beresford MW. Mucocutaneous manifestations in juvenile-onset systemic lupus erythematosus: a review of literature. Pediatr Rheumatol Online J 2015; 13(1): 1-9.
[http://dx.doi.org/10.1186/1546-0096-13-1] [PMID: 25587243]

[73]   Uva L, Miguel D, Pinheiro C, Freitas JP, Marques Gomes M, Filipe P. Cutaneous manifestations of systemic lupus erythematosus. Autoimmune Dis 2012; 2012: 834291.
[http://dx.doi.org/10.1155/2012/834291] [PMID: 22888407]

[74]   Harry O, Yasin S, Brunner H. Childhood-Onset Systemic Lupus Erythematosus: A Review and Update. J Pediatr 2018; 196: 22-30.e2.
[http://dx.doi.org/10.1016/j.jpeds.2018.01.045] [PMID: 29703361]

[75]   Mohamed DF, Aziz ABEDA, Hassan SAM, Shedid NH, El-Owaidy RH, Teama MAEM. Juvenile lupus: Different clinical and serological presentations compared to adult lupus in Egypt. Egypt Rheumatol 2018; 40(1): 55-8.
[http://dx.doi.org/10.1016/j.ejr.2017.04.004]

[76]   Miguel DF, Terreri MT, Pereira RMR, *et al.* Comparison of urinary parameters, biomarkers, and outcome of childhood systemic lupus erythematosus early onset-lupus nephritis. Adv Rheumatol 2020; 60(1): 10.
[http://dx.doi.org/10.1186/s42358-020-0114-4] [PMID: 32005292]

[77]   Anders HJ, Saxena R, Zhao MH, Parodis I, Salmon JE, Mohan C. Lupus nephritis. Nat Rev Dis Primers 2020; 6(1): 7.
[http://dx.doi.org/10.1038/s41572-019-0141-9] [PMID: 31974366]

[78]   Parikh SV, Almaani S, Brodsky S, Rovin BH. Update on Lupus Nephritis: Core Curriculum 2020. AJKD 2020.
[http://dx.doi.org/10.1053/j.ajkd.2019.10.017]

[79]   AlE'ed A, Vega-Fernandez P, Muscal E, *et al.* Challenges of Diagnosing Cognitive Dysfunction With Neuropsychiatric Systemic Lupus Erythematosus in Childhood. Arthritis Care Res (Hoboken) 2017; 69(10): 1449-59.
[http://dx.doi.org/10.1002/acr.23163] [PMID: 27992660]

[80]   Monteiro DE Castro TC, Hsien HC. Depression as the First Manifestation in a Young Girl With Juvenile Systemic Lupus Erythematosus. Arch Rheumatol 2017; 33(1): 105-6.
[http://dx.doi.org/10.5606/ArchRheumatol.2018.6485] [PMID: 29901024]

[81]   Davis AM, Graham TB, Zhu Y, McPheeters ML. Depression and medication nonadherence in childhood-onset systemic lupus erythematosus. Lupus 2018; 27(9): 1532-41.
[http://dx.doi.org/10.1177/0961203318779710] [PMID: 29954282]

[82]   Khajezadeh MA, Zamani G, Moazzami B, Nagahi Z, Mousavi-Torshizi M, Ziaee V. Neuropsychiatric Involvement in Juvenile-Onset Systemic Lupus Erythematosus. Neurol Res Int 2018; 2018: 2548142.
[http://dx.doi.org/10.1155/2018/2548142] [PMID: 30002929]

[83]   Ahluwalia J, Singh S, Naseem S, *et al.* Antiphospholipid antibodies in children with systemic lupus erythematosus: a long-term clinical and laboratory follow-up status study from northwest India. Rheumatol Int 2014; 34(5): 669-73.
[http://dx.doi.org/10.1007/s00296-013-2736-x] [PMID: 23563494]

[84]   Sarecka-Hujar B, Kopyta I. Antiphospholipid syndrome and its role in pediatric cerebrovascular diseases: A literature review. World J Clin Cases 2020; 8(10): 1806-17.
[http://dx.doi.org/10.12998/wjcc.v8.i10.1806] [PMID: 32518771]

[85]   Avčin T, Cimaz R, Silverman ED, *et al.* Pediatric antiphospholipid syndrome: clinical and immunologic features of 121 patients in an international registry. Pediatrics 2008; 122(5): e1100-7.
[http://dx.doi.org/10.1542/peds.2008-1209] [PMID: 18955411]

[86]   Olfat MO, Al-Mayouf SM, Muzaffer MA. Pattern of neuropsychiatric manifestations and outcome in juvenile systemic lupus erythematosus. Clin Rheumatol 2004; 23(5): 395-9.
[http://dx.doi.org/10.1007/s10067-004-0898-3] [PMID: 15278752]

[87]   Soybilgic A, Avcin T. Pediatric APS: State of the Art. Curr Rheumatol Rep 2020; 22(3): 9.
[http://dx.doi.org/10.1007/s11926-020-0887-9] [PMID: 32124078]

[88]   Madison J, Zuo Y. JS K. Pediatric antiphospholipid syndrome. Eur J Rheumatol. 2020; 7(suppl 1:S3-12)

[89]   Ma J, Song H, Wei M, He Y. Clinical characteristics and thrombosis outcomes of paediatric antiphospholipid syndrome: analysis of 58 patients. Clin Rheumatol 2018; 37(5): 1295-303.
[http://dx.doi.org/10.1007/s10067-017-3776-5] [PMID: 28748509]

[90]   Zhu J, Wu F, Huang X. Age-related differences in the clinical characteristics of systemic lupus erythematosus in children. Rheumatol Int 2013; 33(1): 111-5.
[http://dx.doi.org/10.1007/s00296-011-2354-4] [PMID: 22228466]

[91]   Lopes SRM, Gormezano NWS, Gomes RC, *et al.* Outcomes of 847 childhood-onset systemic lupus erythematosus patients in three age groups. Lupus 2017; 26(9): 996-1001.
[http://dx.doi.org/10.1177/0961203317690616] [PMID: 28134038]

[92]   Conigliaro P, Cesareo M, Chimenti MS, *et al.* Take a look at the eyes in Systemic Lupus Erythematosus: A novel point of view. Autoimmun Rev 2019; 18(3): 247-54.
[http://dx.doi.org/10.1016/j.autrev.2018.09.011] [PMID: 30639641]

[93]   Novak GV, Molinari BC, Ferreira JC, *et al.* Characteristics of 1555 childhood-onset lupus in three groups based on distinct time intervals to disease diagnosis: a Brazilian multicenter study. Lupus 2018; 27(10): 1712-7.
[http://dx.doi.org/10.1177/0961203318787037] [PMID: 30020023]

[94]   Chowichian M, Aanpreung P, Pongpaibul A, Charuvanij S. Lupus enteritis as the sole presenting feature of systemic lupus erythematosus: case report and review of the literature. Paediatr Int Child Health 2019; 39(4): 294-8.
[http://dx.doi.org/10.1080/20469047.2018.1504430] [PMID: 30191770]

[95]   Luca NJFB, Feldman BM. Disease activity measures in paediatric rheumatic diseases. Int J Rheumatol

2013; 2013: 715352.
[http://dx.doi.org/10.1155/2013/715352] [PMID: 24089617]

[96]   Lattanzi B, Consolaro A, Solari N, Ruperto N, Martini A, Ravelli A. Measures of disease activity and damage in pediatric systemic lupus erythematosus: British Isles Lupus Assessment Group (BILAG), European Consensus Lupus Activity Measurement (ECLAM), Systemic Lupus Activity Measure (SLAM), Systemic Lupus Erythematosus Disease Activity Index (SLEDAI), Physician's Global Assessment of Disease Activity (MD Global), and Systemic Lupus International Collaborating Clinics/American College of Rheumatology Damage Index (SLICC/ACR DI; SDI). Arthritis Care Res (Hoboken) 2011; 63(S11) (Suppl. 11): S112-7.
[http://dx.doi.org/10.1002/acr.20623] [PMID: 22588739]

[97]   Bombardier C, Gladman DD, Urowitz MB, *et al.* Derivation of the SLEDAI. A disease activity index for lupus patients. Arthritis Rheum 1992; 35(6): 630-40.
[http://dx.doi.org/10.1002/art.1780350606] [PMID: 1599520]

[98]   Gladman DD, Ibañez D, Urowitz MB. Systemic lupus erythematosus disease activity index 2000. J Rheumatol 2002; 29(2): 288-91.
[PMID: 11838846]

[99]   Isenberg DA, Rahman A, Allen E, *et al.* BILAG 2004. Development and initial validation of an updated version of the British Isles Lupus Assessment Group's disease activity index for patients with systemic lupus erythematosus. Rheumatology (Oxford) 2005; 44(7): 902-6.
[http://dx.doi.org/10.1093/rheumatology/keh624] [PMID: 15814577]

[100]   Liang MH, Socher SA, Larson MG, Schur PH. Reliability and validity of six systems for the clinical assessment of disease activity in systemic lupus erythematosus. Arthritis Rheum 1989; 32(9): 1107-18.
[http://dx.doi.org/10.1002/anr.1780320909] [PMID: 2775320]

[101]   Vitali C, Bencivelli W, Isenberg DA, *et al.* Disease activity in systemic lupus erythematosus: report of the Consensus Study Group of the European Workshop for Rheumatology Research. II. Identification of the variables indicative of disease activity and their use in the development of an activity score. Clin Exp Rheumatol 1992; 10(5): 541-7.
[PMID: 1458710]

[102]   Guzmán J, Cardiel MH, Arce-Salinas A, Sánchez-Guerrero J, Alarcón-Segovia D. Measurement of disease activity in systemic lupus erythematosus. Prospective validation of 3 clinical indices. J Rheumatol 1992; 19(10): 1551-8.
[PMID: 1464867]

[103]   Brunner HI, Feldman BM, Bombardier C, Silverman ED. Sensitivity of the systemic lupus erythematosus disease activity index, British Isles Lupus Assessment Group Index, and Systemic Lupus Activity Measure in the evaluation of clinical change in childhood-onset Systemic Lupus Erythematosus. Arthritis Rheum 1999; 42(7): 1354-60.
[http://dx.doi.org/10.1002/1529-0131(199907)42:7<1354::AID-ANR8>3.0.CO;2-4]   [PMID: 10403262]

[104]   Sato JO, Corrente JE, Saad-Magalhães C. Correlation between the Modified Systemic Lupus Erythematosus Disease Activity Index 2000 and the European Consensus Lupus Activity Measurement in juvenile systemic lupus erythematosus. Lupus 2016; 25(13): 1479-84.
[http://dx.doi.org/10.1177/0961203316651737] [PMID: 27230556]

[105]   Marks SD, Pilkington C, Woo P, Dillon MJ. The use of the British Isles Lupus Assessment Group (BILAG) index as a valid tool in assessing disease activity in childhood-onset systemic lupus erythematosus. Rheumatology (Oxford) 2004; 43(9): 1186-9.
[http://dx.doi.org/10.1093/rheumatology/keh284] [PMID: 15226518]

[106]   Romero-Diaz J, Isenberg D, Ramsey-Goldman R. Measures of adult systemic lupus erythematosus. Arthritis Care Res (Hoboken) 2011; 63(S11) (Suppl. 11): S37-46.
[http://dx.doi.org/10.1002/acr.20572] [PMID: 22588757]

[107] Brunner HI, Silverman ED, Bombardier C, Feldman BM. European Consensus Lupus Activity Measurement is sensitive to change in disease activity in childhood-onset systemic lupus erythematosus. Arthritis Rheum 2003; 49(3): 335-41.
[http://dx.doi.org/10.1002/art.11111] [PMID: 12794788]

[108] Touma Z, Urowitz MB, Ibañez D, Gladman DD. SLEDAI-2K 10 days versus SLEDAI-2K 30 days in a longitudinal evaluation. Lupus 2011; 20(1): 67-70.
[http://dx.doi.org/10.1177/0961203310385163] [PMID: 21233149]

[109] Uribe AG, Vilá LM, McGwin G Jr, Sanchez ML, Reveille JD, Alarcón GS. The Systemic Lupus Activity Measure-revised, the Mexican Systemic Lupus Erythematosus Disease Activity Index (SLEDAI), and a modified SLEDAI-2K are adequate instruments to measure disease activity in systemic lupus erythematosus. J Rheumatol 2004; 31(10): 1934-40.
[PMID: 15468356]

[110] Rodriguez-Lozano A, Rivas-Larrauri F, García de la Puente S. Associated features to damage in 80 juvenile systemic lupus erythematosus patients from a tertiary pediatric center.

[111] Brunner HI, Silverman ED, To T, Bombardier C, Feldman BM. Risk factors for damage in childhood-onset systemic lupus erythematosus: cumulative disease activity and medication use predict disease damage. Arthritis Rheum 2002; 46(2): 436-44.
[http://dx.doi.org/10.1002/art.10072] [PMID: 11840446]

[112] Sato JO, Corrente JE, Saad-Magalhães C. Chronic active disease pattern predicts early damage in juvenile systemic lupus erythematosus. Lupus 2015; 24(13): 1421-8.
[http://dx.doi.org/10.1177/0961203315599449] [PMID: 26253073]

[113] Alarcón GS, Roseman JM, McGwin G Jr, et al. Systemic lupus erythematosus in three ethnic groups. XX. Damage as a predictor of further damage. Rheumatology (Oxford) 2004; 43(2): 202-5.
[http://dx.doi.org/10.1093/rheumatology/keg481] [PMID: 12923289]

[114] Lee PPW, Lee TL, Ho MHK, Wong WHS, Lau YL. Recurrent major infections in juvenile-onset systemic lupus erythematosus--a close link with long-term disease damage. Rheumatology (Oxford) 2007; 46(8): 1290-6.
[http://dx.doi.org/10.1093/rheumatology/kem102] [PMID: 17522097]

[115] Lilleby V, Flatø B, Førre O. Disease duration, hypertension and medication requirements are associated with organ damage in childhood-onset systemic lupus erythematosus. Clin Exp Rheumatol 2005; 23(2): 261-9.
[PMID: 15895902]

[116] Bandeira M, Buratti S, Bartoli M, et al. Relationship between damage accrual, disease flares and cumulative drug therapies in juvenile-onset systemic lupus erythematosus. Lupus 2006; 15(8): 515-20.
[http://dx.doi.org/10.1191/0961203306lu2316oa] [PMID: 16942004]

[117] Ravelli A, Duarte-Salazar C, Buratti S, et al. Assessment of damage in juvenile-onset systemic lupus erythematosus: a multicenter cohort study. Arthritis Rheum 2003; 49(4): 501-7.
[http://dx.doi.org/10.1002/art.11205] [PMID: 12910556]

[118] Gutiérrez-Suárez R, Ruperto N, Gastaldi R, et al. A proposal for a pediatric version of the Systemic Lupus International Collaborating Clinics/American College of Rheumatology Damage Index based on the analysis of 1,015 patients with juvenile-onset systemic lupus erythematosus. Arthritis Rheum 2006; 54(9): 2989-96.
[http://dx.doi.org/10.1002/art.22048] [PMID: 16947634]

[119] Hiraki LT, Hamilton J, Silverman ED. Measuring permanent damage in pediatric systemic lupus erythematosus. Lupus 2007; 16(8): 657-62.
[http://dx.doi.org/10.1177/0961203307078975] [PMID: 17711904]

[120] Heshin-Bekenstein M, Perl L, Hersh AO, et al. Final adult height of patients with childhood-onset systemic lupus erythematosus: a cross sectional analysis. Pediatr Rheumatol Online J 2018; 16(1): 30.

[http://dx.doi.org/10.1186/s12969-018-0239-8] [PMID: 29688869]

[121] Sit JKK, Chan WKY. Risk factors for damage in childhood-onset systemic lupus erythematosus in Asians: a case control study. Pediatr Rheumatol Online J 2018; 16(1): 56.
[http://dx.doi.org/10.1186/s12969-018-0271-8] [PMID: 30201026]

[122] Lee PPW, Lee T-L, Ho MH-K, Wong WHS, Lau Y-L. Recurrent major infections in juvenile-onset systemic lupus erythematosus--a close link with long-term disease damage. Rheumatology (Oxford) 2007; 46(8): 1290-6.
[http://dx.doi.org/10.1093/rheumatology/kem102] [PMID: 17522097]

[123] Faco MMM, Leone C, Campos LMA, Febrônio MV, Marques HHS, Silva CA. Risk factors associated with the death of patients hospitalized for juvenile systemic lupus erythematosus. Braz J Med Biol Res 2007; 40(7): 993-1002.
[http://dx.doi.org/10.1590/S0100-879X2006005000110] [PMID: 17653454]

[124] Aggarwal A, Phatak S, Srivastava P, Lawrence A, Agarwal V, Misra R. Outcomes in juvenile onset lupus: single center cohort from a developing country. Lupus 2018; 27(11): 1867-75.
[http://dx.doi.org/10.1177/0961203318791046] [PMID: 30071768]

[125] Lewandowski LB, Schanberg LE, Thielman N, *et al.* Severe disease presentation and poor outcomes among pediatric systemic lupus erythematosus patients in South Africa. Lupus 2017; 26(2): 186-94.
[http://dx.doi.org/10.1177/0961203316660625] [PMID: 27488473]

[126] Brunner HI, Gladman DD, Ibañez D, Urowitz MD, Silverman ED. Difference in disease features between childhood-onset and adult-onset systemic lupus erythematosus. Arthritis Rheum 2008; 58(2): 556-62.
[http://dx.doi.org/10.1002/art.23204] [PMID: 18240232]

[127] Aggarwal A, Srivastava P. Childhood onset systemic lupus erythematosus: how is it different from adult SLE? Int J Rheum Dis 2015; 18(2): 182-91.
[http://dx.doi.org/10.1111/1756-185X.12419] [PMID: 24965742]

[128] Tsokos GC, Lo MS, Costa Reis P, Sullivan KE. New insights into the immunopathogenesis of systemic lupus erythematosus. Nat Rev Rheumatol 2016; 12(12): 716-30.
[http://dx.doi.org/10.1038/nrrheum.2016.186] [PMID: 27872476]

[129] Tarvin SE, O'Neil KM. Systemic Lupus Erythematosus, Sjögren Syndrome, and Mixed Connective Tissue Disease in Children and Adolescents. Pediatr Clin North Am 2018; 65(4): 711-37.
[http://dx.doi.org/10.1016/j.pcl.2018.04.001] [PMID: 30031495]

[130] Pan L, Lu MP, Wang JH, Xu M, Yang SR. Immunological pathogenesis and treatment of systemic lupus erythematosus. World J Pediatr 2020; 16(1): 19-30.
[http://dx.doi.org/10.1007/s12519-019-00229-3] [PMID: 30796732]

[131] Mina R, von Scheven E, Ardoin SP, *et al.* Consensus treatment plans for induction therapy of newly diagnosed proliferative lupus nephritis in juvenile systemic lupus erythematosus. Arthritis Care Res (Hoboken) 2012; 64(3): 375-83.
[http://dx.doi.org/10.1002/acr.21558] [PMID: 22162255]

[132] Deng J, Chalhoub NE, Sherwin CM, Li C, Brunner HI. Glucocorticoids pharmacology and their application in the treatment of childhood-onset systemic lupus erythematosus. Semin Arthritis Rheum 2019; 49(2): 251-9.
[http://dx.doi.org/10.1016/j.semarthrit.2019.03.010] [PMID: 30987856]

[133] Thakral A, Klein-Gitelman MS. An Update on Treatment and Management of Pediatric Systemic Lupus Erythematosus. Rheumatol Ther 2016; 3(2): 209-19.
[http://dx.doi.org/10.1007/s40744-016-0044-0] [PMID: 27747587]

[134] Arıcı ZS, Batu ED, Ozen S. Reviewing the recommendations for lupus in children. Curr Rheumatol Rep 2015; 17(3): 17.
[http://dx.doi.org/10.1007/s11926-014-0489-5] [PMID: 25761924]

[135] Smith E, Al-Abadi E, Armon K, *et al.* Outcomes following mycophenolate mofetil versus cyclophosphamide induction treatment for proliferative juvenile-onset lupus nephritis. Lupus 2019; 28(5): 613-20.
[http://dx.doi.org/10.1177/0961203319836712] [PMID: 30871425]

[136] Mahmoud I, Jellouli M, Boukhris I, *et al.* Efficacy and Safety of Rituximab in the Management of Pediatric Systemic Lupus Erythematosus: A Systematic Review. J Pediatr 2017; 187: 213-219.e2.
[http://dx.doi.org/10.1016/j.jpeds.2017.05.002] [PMID: 28602379]

[137] Peterknecht E, Keasey MP, Beresford MW. The effectiveness and safety of biological therapeutics in juvenile-onset systemic lupus erythematosus (JSLE): a systematic review. Lupus 2018; 27(13): 2135-45.
[http://dx.doi.org/10.1177/0961203318804879] [PMID: 30336753]

[138] Watson L, Beresford MW, Maynes C, *et al.* The indications, efficacy and adverse events of rituximab in a large cohort of patients with juvenile-onset SLE. Lupus 2015; 24(1): 10-7.
[http://dx.doi.org/10.1177/0961203314547793] [PMID: 25117653]

[139] Basu B, Roy B, Babu BG. Efficacy and safety of rituximab in comparison with common induction therapies in pediatric active lupus nephritis. Pediatr Nephrol 2017; 32(6): 1013-21.
[http://dx.doi.org/10.1007/s00467-017-3583-x] [PMID: 28191596]

[140] Tambralli A, Beukelman T, Cron RQ, Stoll ML. Safety and efficacy of rituximab in childhood-onset systemic lupus erythematosus and other rheumatic diseases. J Rheumatol 2015; 42(3): 541-6.
[http://dx.doi.org/10.3899/jrheum.140863] [PMID: 25593242]

[141] Guzman M, Hui-Yuen JS. Management of pediatric systemic lupus erythematosus: Focus on Belimumab. Drug Des Devel Ther 2020; 14: 2503-13.
[http://dx.doi.org/10.2147/DDDT.S216193] [PMID: 32612353]

[142] Leone A, Sciascia S, Kamal A, Khamashta M. Biologicals for the treatment of systemic lupus erythematosus: current status and emerging therapies. Expert Rev Clin Immunol 2015; 11(1): 109-16.
[http://dx.doi.org/10.1586/1744666X.2015.994508] [PMID: 25511179]

[143] Traczewski P, Rudnicka L. Treatment of systemic lupus erythematosus with epratuzumab. Br J Clin Pharmacol 2011; 71(2): 175-82.
[http://dx.doi.org/10.1111/j.1365-2125.2010.03767.x] [PMID: 21219397]

[144] Klavdianou K, Lazarini A, Fanouriakis A. Targeted Biologic Therapy for Systemic Lupus Erythematosus: Emerging Pathways and Drug Pipeline. BioDrugs 2020; 34(2): 133-47.
[http://dx.doi.org/10.1007/s40259-020-00405-2] [PMID: 32002918]

[145] Speth F, Hinze CH, Schranz P, Miller-Wiegart E, Haefner R. Combination of rituximab and abatacept as an exit strategy for repetitive B-cell depletion in children with severe autoimmune diseases: a report of three cases. Lupus 2018; 27(12): 1996-8.
[http://dx.doi.org/10.1177/0961203318783057] [PMID: 29958501]

[146] Mathian A, Hie M, Cohen-Aubart F, Amoura Z. Targeting interferons in systemic lupus erythematosus: current and future prospects. Drugs 2015; 75(8): 835-46.
[http://dx.doi.org/10.1007/s40265-015-0394-x] [PMID: 25940912]

[147] Rodriguez-Smith J, Brunner HI. Update on the treatment and outcome of systemic lupus erythematous in children. Curr Opin Rheumatol 2019; 31(5): 464-70.
[http://dx.doi.org/10.1097/BOR.0000000000000621] [PMID: 31107290]

[148] Paley MA, Strand V, Kim AHJ. From mechanism to therapies in systemic lupus erythematosus. Curr Opin Rheumatol 2017; 29(2): 178-86.
[http://dx.doi.org/10.1097/BOR.0000000000000369] [PMID: 28118202]

[149] Thanarajasingam U, Niewold TB. Sirukumab : a novel therapy for lupus nephritis? Expert Opin Investig Drugs 2014; 23(10): 1449-55.
[http://dx.doi.org/10.1517/13543784.2014.950837] [PMID: 25189410]

[150] Kleinmann JF, Tubach F, Le Guern V, *et al.* International and multidisciplinary expert recommendations for the use of biologics in systemic lupus erythematosus. Autoimmun Rev 2017; 16(6): 650-7.
[http://dx.doi.org/10.1016/j.autrev.2017.04.011] [PMID: 28434948]

[151] Davis LS, Reimold AM. Research and therapeutics-traditional and emerging therapies in systemic lupus erythematosus. Rheumatology (Oxford) 2017; 56 (Suppl. 1): i100-13.
[http://dx.doi.org/10.1093/rheumatology/kew417] [PMID: 28375452]

[152] Su G, Luan Z, Wu F, *et al.* Long-term follow-up of autologous stem cell transplantation for severe paediatric systemic lupus erythematosus. Clin Rheumatol 2013; 32(12): 1727-34.
[http://dx.doi.org/10.1007/s10067-013-2324-1] [PMID: 23925552]

[153] Arkwright PD, Riley P, Hughes SM, Alachkar H, Wynn RF. Successful cure of C1q deficiency in human subjects treated with hematopoietic stem cell transplantation. J Allergy Clin Immunol 2014; 133(1): 265-7.
[http://dx.doi.org/10.1016/j.jaci.2013.07.035] [PMID: 24035158]

[154] Jayne D, Passweg J, Marmont A, *et al.* Autologous stem cell transplantation for systemic lupus erythematosus. Lupus 2004; 13(3): 168-76.
[http://dx.doi.org/10.1191/0961203304lu525oa] [PMID: 15119545]

[155] Nademi Z, Slatter MA, Dvorak CC, *et al.* Hematopoietic stem cell transplant in patients with activated PI3K delta syndrome. J Allergy Clin Immunol 2017; 139(3): 1046-9.
[http://dx.doi.org/10.1016/j.jaci.2016.09.040] [PMID: 27847301]

[156] Wan SJ, Lara-Corrales I. Sun Protection in Pediatric Patients With Rheumatic Disease. Clin Pediatr (Phila) 2019; 58(2): 140-5.
[http://dx.doi.org/10.1177/0009922818802632] [PMID: 30264580]

[157] Dayrit-Castro C, Tantuco K, Lara-Corrales I. Recommendations for photoprotection in pediatric rheumatology patients. Curr Opin Pediatr 2019; 31(4): 491-7.
[http://dx.doi.org/10.1097/MOP.0000000000000798] [PMID: 31299020]

[158] Rizwan M, Haylett AK, Richards HL, Ling TC, Rhodes LE. Impact of photosensitivity disorders on the life quality of children. Photodermatol Photoimmunol Photomed 2012; 28(6): 290-2.
[http://dx.doi.org/10.1111/j.1600-0781.2012.00691.x] [PMID: 23126289]

[159] Vilá LM, Mayor AM, Valentín AH, *et al.* Association of sunlight exposure and photoprotection measures with clinical outcome in systemic lupus erythematosus. P R Health Sci J 1999; 18(2): 89-94.
[PMID: 10461313]

[160] Abdul Kadir WD, Jamil A, Shaharir SS, Md Nor N, Abdul Gafor AH. Photoprotection awareness and practices among patients with systemic lupus erythematosus and its association with disease activity and severity. Lupus 2018; 27(8): 1287-95.
[http://dx.doi.org/10.1177/0961203318770016] [PMID: 29665756]

[161] Garg M, Mufti N, Palmore TN, Hasni SA. Recommendations and barriers to vaccination in systemic lupus erythematosus. Autoimmun Rev 2018; 17(10): 990-1001.
[http://dx.doi.org/10.1016/j.autrev.2018.04.006] [PMID: 30103044]

[162] Mathian A, Arnaud L, Adoue D, *et al.* [Prevention of infections in adults and adolescents with systemic lupus erythematosus: Guidelines for the clinical practice based on the literature and expert opinion]. Rev Med Interne 2016; 37(5): 307-20.
[http://dx.doi.org/10.1016/j.revmed.2016.01.005] [PMID: 26899776]

[163] Khojah AM, Miller ML, Klein-Gitelman MS, *et al.* Rituximab-associated Hypogammaglobulinemia in pediatric patients with autoimmune diseases. Pediatr Rheumatol Online J 2019; 17(1): 61.
[http://dx.doi.org/10.1186/s12969-019-0365-y] [PMID: 31462263]

[164] Mulhearn B, Bruce IN. Indications for IVIG in rheumatic diseases. Rheumatology (Oxford) 2015; 54(3): 383-91.

[http://dx.doi.org/10.1093/rheumatology/keu429] [PMID: 25406359]

[165] Prasad AN, Chaudhary S. Intravenous immunoglobulin in pediatrics: A review. Med J Armed Forces India 2014; 70(3): 277-80.
[http://dx.doi.org/10.1016/j.mjafi.2013.05.011] [PMID: 25378784]

[166] Rodriguez MM, Wagner-Weiner L. Intravenous immunoglobulin in pediatric rheumatology: When to use it and what is the evidence. Pediatr Ann 2017; 46(1): e19-24.
[http://dx.doi.org/10.3928/19382359-20161214-01] [PMID: 28079914]

[167] Sakthiswary R, D'Cruz D. Intravenous immunoglobulin in the therapeutic armamentarium of systemic lupus erythematosus: a systematic review and meta-analysis. Medicine (Baltimore) 2014; 93(16): e86.
[http://dx.doi.org/10.1097/MD.0000000000000086] [PMID: 25310743]

[168] Simoes J, Sciascia S, Camara I, *et al.* Use of intravenous immunoglobulin in patients with active vasculitis associated with concomitant infection. J Clin Rheumatol 2015; 21(1): 35-7.
[http://dx.doi.org/10.1097/RHU.0000000000000201] [PMID: 25539433]

[169] Tektonidou MG, Lewandowski LB, Hu J, Dasgupta A, Ward MM. Survival in adults and children with systemic lupus erythematosus: a systematic review and Bayesian meta-analysis of studies from 1950 to 2016. Ann Rheum Dis 2017; 76(12): 2009-16.
[http://dx.doi.org/10.1136/annrheumdis-2017-211663] [PMID: 28794077]

[170] Torrente-Segarra V, Salman Monte TC, Rúa-Figueroa I, *et al.* Relationship between damage and mortality in juvenile-onset systemic lupus erythematosus: Cluster analyses in a large cohort from the Spanish Society of Rheumatology Lupus Registry (RELESSER). Semin Arthritis Rheum 2019; 48(6): 1025-9.
[http://dx.doi.org/10.1016/j.semarthrit.2018.09.005] [PMID: 30344081]

[171] Dalby ST, Tang X, Daily JA, Sukumaran S, Collins RT, Bolin EH. Effect of pericardial effusion on outcomes in children admitted with systemic lupus erythematosus: a multicenter retrospective cohort study from the United States. Lupus 2019; 28(3): 389-95.
[http://dx.doi.org/10.1177/0961203319828523] [PMID: 30744520]

CHAPTER 11

Updates on Severe Combined Immunodeficiency

Fausto Cossu[1,*]

[1] *Pediatric Clinic of University, "Antonio Cao" Hospital, Cagliari, Sardinia, Italy*

Abstract: Mutations in any one of several genes essential for T lymphocyte development and function cause human Severe Combined Immunodeficiency (SCID), a heterogeneous group of monogenic inborn errors of immunity.

Newborns with SCID acquire multiple, persistent, and severe viral, bacterial, and fungal infections shortly after birth and rarely reach their first birthday. SCID is a pediatric emergency: with prompt diagnosis and treatment, essentially every baby with SCID could be cured by hematopoietic stem cell transplantation or gene therapy.

Most SCID newborns appear normal and healthy at birth, but SCID is always a prenatal disorder of the development of T lymphocytes, and it is already present at birth. Therefore, SCID is detected by newborn screening through measurement of TRECs (T cell receptor excision circles), which counts naïve T lymphocytes, already absent or markedly reduced.

The vast majority of newborns worldwide are not yet screened for SCID. The diagnostic approach and the 'natural history' of affected infants and their families are now completely different depending on whether or not neonatal screening for SCID is available, apart from the availability/unavailability of SCID therapies (hematopoietic stem cell transplantation, *etc.*).

Keywords: B-cell, Bubble boy, Gene therapy, Genetics, Genotype, Hematopoietic stem cell transplantation, Immunodeficiency, Leaky mutation, Lymphopenia, Maternal engraftment, Newborn screening, NK-cell, Null mutation, Omenn syndrome, Phenotype, SCID, T-cell, Thymus, TRECs, Viral vector.

INTRODUCTION

Mutations in any one of several genes essential for T lymphocyte development and function cause human SCID (Severe Combined Immunodeficiency), a heterogeneous group of monogenic inborn errors of immunity with an overall incidence of about 1 in 50,000 to 90,000 newborns [1 - 4]. The incidence is rema-

---

* **Corresponding author Fausto Cossu:** Pediatric Clinic of University, "Antonio Cao" Hospital, Via Jenner sn, 09121 Cagliari, Sardinia, Italy; Tel: (+39) 070 52965660; E-mail: fausto.cossu@unica.it

Nima Rezaei and Noosha Samieefar (Eds.)
All rights reserved-© 2022 Bentham Science Publishers

rkably higher in many ethnic groups due to the founder effect and common consanguineous marriage (AR, autosomal-recessive, SCID) [5 - 7].

Usually, "null" mutations of these genes with the absence of residual gene/protein function cause Typical SCID, while "non-null" ("hypomorphic", "leaky") mutations allowing some residual functions are associated with Atypical SCID.

"Typical/Atypical" refers to the clinical and immunological phenotype, "null/non-null, hypomorphic, leaky" to the molecular findings.

In 2008, Wisconsin, Massachusetts, and the Navajo Nation (USA) became the first states in the world to screen all newborns for SCID by measurement of T cell receptor excision circles, TRECs [8], and as of December 2018, all 50 states in the USA (plus the District of Columbia, Guam and Puerto Rico) performed universal Newborn Screening (NBS) for SCID. Similar NBS have been implemented in Taiwan, Israel, Iceland, New Zealand, Norway, Sweden, Switzerland, Lebanon, Germany, and some regions of Canada, Finland, Spain (Catalonia), Italy (Tuscany). Pilot programs have been completed or are ongoing in Iran, Brazil, Netherlands, Saudi Arabia, UK, France, and other countries [9, 10].

The diagnostic approach to SCID and the 'natural history' of SCID infants, their families, and their clinicians are now completely different in these two conditions: NO NBS for SCID *versus* YES NBS for SCID [11, 12].

The vast majority of newborns worldwide are not yet screened for SCID. This happens both in developing countries, where also hematopoietic stem cell transplantation (HSCT) is very rarely available [13], and for example, in most of Europe, where often SCID NBS is absent but, instead, whole-exome sequencing (WES) may be possible.

NO NEWBORN SCREENING FOR SCID

In the absence of NBS, the initial clinical manifestations of SCID are most frequently observed in the first few months of life, and the median age at diagnosis is 4-7 months; so, apart from families with a recognized positive history of SCID (<20 percent of cases), 'delayed diagnosis, harmful administration of contra-indicated live vaccines, delay in clinical management and poor outcome are still too frequent' [6].

To achieve a timely clinical/genetic diagnosis, it is essential to know and remember many aspects of SCID [3].

Children with SCID have absent or very low naïve CD3 T cells, do not produce T lymphocytes or, however, functional T lymphocytes, and acquire multiple, persistent and severe viral, bacterial and fungal infections shortly after birth.

Fever, cough, persistent thrush and mucocutaneous candidiasis, upper airway infections, bronchiolitis, pneumonia, skin infections, diarrhoea, meningitis, sepsis, systemic viral infections, disseminated fungal infection, *etc.* affect infants by common and opportunistic pathogens such as cytomegalovirus (CMV), Epstein-Barr virus (EBV), adenovirus, respiratory syncytial virus (RSV), herpes simplex virus (HSV), varicella zoster virus (VZV), rotavirus, norovirus, influenza and parainfluenza viruses, *Staphylococcus spp.*, *Streptococcus spp.*, *Pseudomonas spp.*, *Escherichia coli spp.*, other Gram- *spp.*, *Candida spp.*, *Pneumocystis jirovecii*, *Aspergillus spp.*, *etc* [14, 15].

Children fail to thrive and rarely reach their first birthday.

In SCID (or suspected SCID) infants, it is mandatory that all transfusions involve irradiated and preferably WBC-filtered blood products to avoid the transfusion of functional donor lymphocytes, which would certainly cause life-threatening Graft *versus* Host Disease (GvHD). In fact, this precaution should be used in all newborns as a general rule.

SCID is a pediatric emergency [16] with prompt diagnosis and treatment, and before acquiring an infection, including infections from "live" vaccines, *e.g.*, *Bacille Calmette-Guérin* (BCG), or rotavirus [17, 18], essentially every baby with SCID could be cured by HSCT or gene therapy (GT).

Most newborns with SCID appear normal and healthy at birth, but cutaneous signs similar to GvHD from engraftment of transplacentally derived maternal T lymphocytes are sometimes present.

Instead, low birth length and weight, microcephaly, dysmorphic facies, metaphyseal chondrodysplasia or other skeletal abnormalities, alopecia, congenital heart disease, *etc.* are nonimmunological manifestations of the less frequent forms of SCID in which cell types and organs other than lymphocytes and lymphoid organs are also affected by their genetic mutations ("syndromic SCIDs").

However, even if most newborns with SCID appear normal and healthy, SCID is always a prenatal disorder of the development of T lymphocytes, and it is already present at birth.

In all forms of SCID ("congenital severe T cell immunodeficiencies"), the development and function of T lymphocytes are severely compromised.

Usually, the thymus is dysplastic and atrophic (no thymic shadow on chest x-ray), with the absence of thymocytes, Hassall's corpuscles, and corticomedullary differentiation.

Mature T cells are also absent in the peripheral blood and lymphoid tissues: especially if B lymphocytes are also missing, tonsils and palpable peripheral lymph nodes are absent on clinical examination.

However, T lymphocytes, B lymphocytes, and NK (natural killer) lymphocytes share progenitors for cell lineages, signaling pathways in development and function, and metabolic pathways (note that NK cells, unlike T and B lymphocytes, do not rearrange their germline DNA to produce genes encoding antigen-specific receptors).

Therefore, B lymphocytes and/or NK cells are usually severely compromised in SCID. The distinct forms of SCID are characterized by different combinations of T/B/NK counts such as T⁻B⁻NK⁻ T⁻B⁺NK⁻, T⁻B⁻NK⁺, T⁻B⁺NK⁺ (⁻ means absence or severely reduced counts).

Moreover, without normal CD4 T helper lymphocytes [19], B lymphocytes, macrophages, and also eventual residual T lymphocytes cannot work even if present and "normal". Due to the absence or non-functioning of B cells, agammaglobulinemia is the rule (with rare exceptions) apart from maternal transplacental IgG.

In most SCID, the absence of T lymphocytes (and possibly of B or/and NK cells) causes marked lymphopenia.

Typical SCID is defined by an absolute lymphocyte count (ALC) <500 cells/μL, absence or a very low number of T cells (CD3 T cells <300/μL), and no or very low T-cell function with response to Phytohemagglutinin, PHA, <10% of normal [20].

So, a Typical T⁻ SCID could also be defined as a "T⁰ ⁽ᶻᵉʳᵒ⁾ SCID".

Note that in adults, lymphopenia means ALC <1,000/μL, but the normal lower limits are 2,000/μL in newborns and 4,000/μL in infants by 6 to 9 months of age [21, 22].

Therefore, in the first few months of life, any ALC <2,500/μL is potentially pathogenic and may indicate SCID. Similarly, note that the normal lower limit of CD3 T cell counts for age <2 years is 1,500/μL [20].

However, many infants with SCID have more than 300 T cells/μL, with possibly normal or high B or/and NK cell counts and a resulting "normal" ALC. So, a normal for age ALC/μL in the complete blood count (CBC) with differential white blood cell counts is insufficient to rule out SCID diagnosis.

Therefore, severe lymphopenia, a "cardinal" sign, is not present in many SCID infants.

Unlike T^0 Typical SCID, $T^{+/++}$ SCID (SCID with $T^{low/normal/high}$ counts) occurs in three conditions:

1) Atypical SCID by Leaky Mutations

Defined by CD3 T cells 300-1000/μL and response to PHA <30% of normal [20], it is caused by hypomorphic mutations ("leaky", non-null mutations, allowing residual function) of all genes whose null mutations cause typical SCID instead.

More often, T^- SCID newborns become $T^{+/++}$ SCID due to abnormal and oligoclonal T cells that modify counts from $T^-B^-NK^-$ to $T^+B^-NK^-$, from $T^-B^+NK^-$ to $T^+B^+NK^-$, from $T^-B^-NK^+$ to $T^+B^-NK^+$, or from $T^-B^+NK^+$ to $T^+B^+NK^+$.

These abnormal T lymphocytes (oligoclonal Vβ TCR families; very low naïve CD4 CD45RA T cells; high memory CD4 CD45RO T cells; high activated CD3DR$^+$ T cells; very low/absent *in vitro* mitogen-induced lymphocyte proliferation; and very low/absent TRECs, that is very useful regard to newborn SCID screening) are present in two other frequent conditions:

2) SCID with Massive Engraftment of Transplacentally Derived Maternal T Lymphocytes

Such maternal T lymphocytes are pathognomonic for the diagnosis of SCID (HLA typing of infant's peripheral blood, showing both maternal HLA haplotypes plus one paternal HLA haplotype; maternal DNA in infant's peripheral blood), and may also cause various manifestations, such as skin and liver disease similar to GvHD, with variable eruption (usually initial on the face, neck, palms, and soles, then generalized; maculopapular rash, fine exfoliation, xerotic skin, scaly erythematous plaques, *etc.*) and progressive increase of liver enzymes and bilirubin [23 - 25]; autoimmune thrombocytopenia or pancytopenia (pre- or post-HSCT), rejection of HSCT from father or donors other than mother [26]; monoclonal gammopathy (Fig. **1**) because of clonal expansion of maternal or newborn B cells in the absence of normal CD4 T_{REG} lymphocytes [3, 27]; attenuated clinical SCID if fetus/mother HLA compatibility [28]; increased risk of acute GvHD post-HSCT [29].

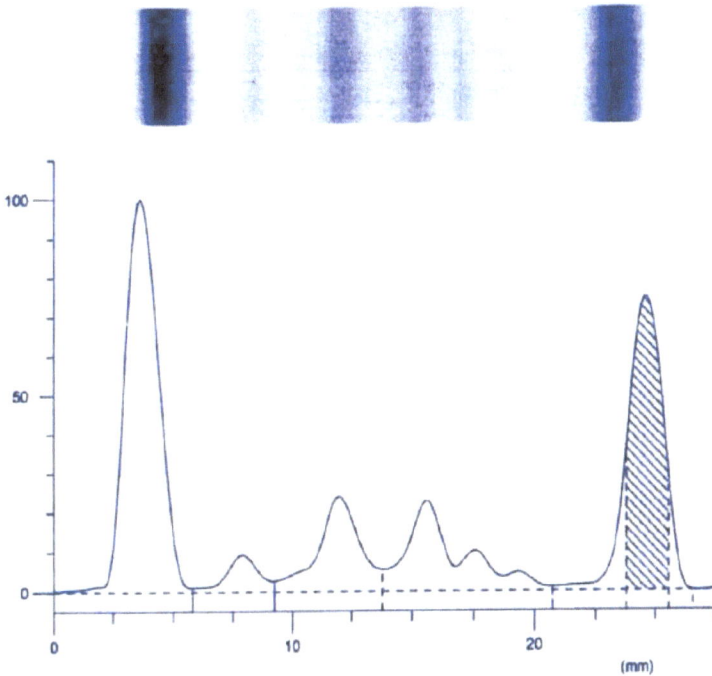

Fig. (1). Monoclonal IgG gammopathy in a 4-month-old female infant with AR $T^-B^-NK^+$ SCID, modified to $T^{++}B^-NK^+$ SCID by massive maternal T lymphocyte engraftment (Artemis deficiency by homozygous *DCLRE1C* exon 14 c.1217delT, p.fsPhe396X mutation (Cossu F. Genetics of SCID. Ital J Pediatr 2010; 36: 76).

3) Omenn Syndrome (OS)

Described in 1965 by Gilbert S. Omenn in an extraordinary Irish family with many marriages between cousins and twelve affected newborns [30], is a frequent SCID phenotype: *e.g.*, in Sardinia, Italy, 3 of the 7 SCID infants diagnosed from 1998 to 2019 showed OS phenotype.

OS is caused by hypomorphic, leaky mutations of all genes whose null mutations cause typical SCID instead [31].

Leaky mutations allow a little abnormal production of T pathogenic child's, not maternal, autologous oligoclonal hyper-autoreactive CD4 CD45RO DR^+ T_H2 lymphocytes. These T cells then expand and infiltrate and damage various organs by lack of immunological tolerance both central (dysplastic thymus, with markedly reduced expression of Autoimmune Regulator Element, AIRE, and

Tissue-Specific Antigens, TSA, by thymocyte-dependent epithelial and dendritic cells) and peripheral (absence of normal peripheral CD4 T_{REG} cells) [32, 33].

Usually, B cell counts are markedly reduced, but some abnormal and oligoclonal B cells are present: they show a restricted B cell receptor (BCR) repertoire and an increased frequency of switched IgE transcripts, with often elevated IgE unlike the other immunoglobulins [34].

In OS, *RAG1-RAG2* (recombination activating gene 1-2) is the first identified and most commonly mutated genes ("classic" OS), with infants, often compound heterozygous, carrying at least one hypomorphic variant that allows a little residual recombinase activity. Some mutations seem to be more frequent: *e.g.*, *RAG1* frameshift mutations that affect the N-terminus region of the protein, or missense mutations affecting the RAG2-PHD, plant homeodomain finger [35, 36].

Note that OS and non-OS SCID may occur in patients carrying identical *RAG1-RAG2* mutations, even within the same family [37, 38].

Less commonly, OS has been observed by leaky mutations of many other SCID genes: *IL2RG* [39], *IL7RA* [40], *DCLRE1C* [41], *LIG4* [42], *ZAP70* [43], *AK2* [44], *ADA* [45], Complete DiGeorge Syndrome [46, 47], *CHD7* [48], *RMRP* [49].

Clinically OS is an extremely serious SCID and has a very poor prognosis unless an early and definitive cure is provided, so it could be proposed to make the term "OS" mean "Omenn Syndrome" but also "**Omenn SCID**".

Besides the overwhelming and life-threatening infections typical of SCID, Omenn infants (Fig. **2**) present with aggressive tissue inflammation, rash evolving in exfoliative dermatitis and very severe erythroderma, alopecia and loss of eyebrows and eyelashes, mucositis, unmanageable diarrhoea, protein loss through the skin and the gut, generalized edema, metabolic alterations, raised serum IgE, hypereosinophilia, enlarged lymph nodes and hepatosplenomegaly.

Skin and mucosal barrier leakage cause an even higher risk of invasive bacterial and fungal infections.

Signs and symptoms do not appear simultaneously and evolve with time; *e.g.*, the rash usually is absent at birth but appears within the first weeks of life, unlike atopic dermatitis with which OS is often initially misdiagnosed.

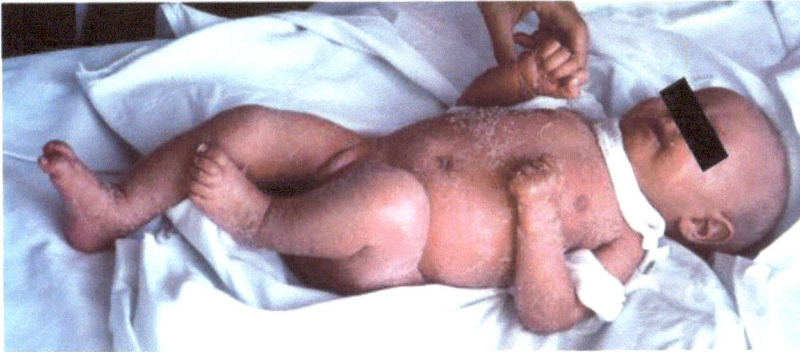

Fig. (2). Omenn Syndrome in a 5-month-old female infant (absence of *RAG1-RAG2* mutations, unidentified gene defect) (Cossu F. Genetics of SCID. Ital J Pediatr 2010; 36: 76).

OS infants need the usual "emergency" intensive treatment of SCID (urgent HSCT, allowed by antimicrobial drugs, immunoglobulin replacement, supportive treatment with parenteral nutrition, *etc.*) but in association with immuno-suppressive drugs: topical (skin) and systemic steroids, cyclosporine A, tacrolimus, and possibly Anti-thymocyte globulin, ATG, or alemtuzumab). These drugs suppress the autologous autoreactive T cell clones and their tissue infiltration and inflammation, *e.g.*, usually skin improves within 1 - 3 weeks of treatment.

Pharmacologic suppression of abnormal T cells, which will then be destroyed by conditioning pre-HSCT regimens, also facilitates engraftment of donor hematopoietic stem cells [31].

GENETICS

The latest classification of Human Inborn Errors of Immunity from the International Union of Immunological Societies Expert Committee, IUIS, lists 18 genes whose mutations cause T^-B^+ or T^-B^- SCID [50] (Table **1**).

The distinct forms of SCID can also be classified into four groups according to prevalent molecular pathogenetic mechanisms and other aspects:

- SCID caused by cytokine signaling defects;

- SCID caused by pre-T cell receptor defects:

defects in V(D)J recombination, or

impaired signaling through the pre-T cell receptor;

- SCID caused by metabolic disorders;

- other SCIDs.

Table 1. IUIS 2019 classification of SCID (Tangye *et al.* 2020).

Gene (see later in this Chapter)	Inheritance	OMIM number (Online Mendelian Inheritance in Man)
T⁻B⁺ SCID	-	-
IL2RG	XL	308380
JAK3	AR	600173
IL7RA	AR	146661
PTPRC	AR	151460
CD3D	AR	186790
CD3E	AR	186830
CD3Z	AR	186780
CORO1A	AR	605000
LAT	AR	602354
T⁻B⁻ SCID	-	-
RAG1	AR	179615
RAG2	AR	179616
DCLRE1C	AR	605988
PRKDC	AR	615966
NHEJ1	AR	601837
LIG4	AR	608958
ADA	AR	103020
AK2	AR	602049
RAC2	AD GOF	308230

SCID Caused by Cytokine Signaling Defects

Common Gamma Chain (γc) Deficiency ("SCIDX-1")

Only male infants are affected by common gamma chain (γc) deficiency, X-linked T⁻B⁺NK⁻ SCID caused by null mutations in *IL2RG* gene, located on chromosome Xq13.1 and encoding the γ chain (γc) of interleukin-2 (IL-2) receptor. The "bubble boy" David Phillip Vetter (September 21, 1971 - February 22, 1984) was affected by this SCID, with mutation *IL2RG* nonsense exon 7 C937A S308X, -62 aa. of 369 aa [51 - 54].

IL-2 deficient knockout mice and the rare interleukin-2 receptor α chain, IL2RA, deficient human patients do not present SCID but instead severe defect of CD4 T_{REG} and autoimmunity: this "bubble boy paradox" was resolved by the discovery that IL-2 receptor γ chain is shared (common γ chain) by the receptors of IL-4, IL-7, IL-9, IL-15 and IL-21 [55, 56].

Lack of IL-7 signaling causes an early block in T cell development, and lack of IL-15 signaling prevents NK cell development, while B cell differentiation and immunoglobulin production are compromised by defects in IL-4 and IL-21 signaling; thus, T and NK cells are almost completely absent, while B cells are present, sometimes in high numbers, but non-functioning: $T^-B^+NK^-$ SCID, with agammaglobulinemia.

At least in USA and Canada, SCIDX-1 is the most frequent SCID; it is an exclusively immunological form except that also cutaneous keratinocytes express γc-dependent cytokine receptors, especially IL-7R, and this is necessary for the local innate immunity against human papilloma virus (HPV); therefore, severe cutaneous HPV disease, including epidermodysplasia verruciformis, is a frequent late complication in common γc (and JAK3, and, less, IL7RA) SCID patients many years after successful HSCT [57].

IL2RG has 8 exons, encoding the 369-amino acid γ chain expressed within receptor complexes on the membrane of hematopoietic and lymphoid cells; exons 1-5 encode the extracellular domain, containing the four cysteines and the repeated tryptophan, serine (WSXWS) motifs; exon 6 encodes the transmembrane portion, and exons 7-8 encode the intracellular domain that associates with the JAK3 tyrosine kinase. About 200 *IL2RG* distinct mutations have been identified to date, more than half located in exon 3-5 and most commonly missense, followed by nonsense, insertion/deletion, splicing, and other mutations.

Null mutations abolish the protein production or function and cause Typical SCID.

Instead, about 10% of the described *IL2RG* mutations, mainly located in exons 5 and 7 are leaky and associated with phenotypic variants of Atypical SCID, *e.g.* $T^{low}B^+NK^+$, and usually milder immunodeficiency; however, missense mutation exon 5, c.C664T (p.R222C), the most frequent leaky variant, leads to a severe clinical phenotype of Typical SCID [58, 59]. Studies of γc signaling in infant lymphocytes and skewed X-inactivation in maternal lymphocytes may be useful for diagnosis [60].

Janus Associated Kinase-3 (JAK3) Deficiency

Both male and female infants can be affected with JAK3 deficiency, the Autosomal Recessive (AR) T⁻B⁺NK⁻ SCID equivalent of the common γc deficiency X-SCID since the non-receptor tyrosine kinase JAK3 joins to γc in the (IL-2, IL-4, IL-7, IL-9, IL-15, IL-21) - JAK3 - STAT5 signaling pathway; activated STAT5 dimerizes and translocates to the nucleus to promote the transcription of specific target genes [61].

JAK3 gene is located on chromosome 19p13.1, is organized in 23 exons and encodes the 1124-amino acid protein composed of seven Janus homology domains (JH1 - JH7); JH1 is the kinase domain, while the JH4-JH7 domains associate with cytokine receptor chains.

Most JAK3 SCID patients are compound heterozygotes; identified mutations are located on the whole gene and different (missense, nonsense, deletions, insertions, splice-site), and may be both null and leaky, causing respectively Typical and Atypical SCID [62, 63].

Interleukin-7 Receptor α Chain (IL7Rα) Deficiency

ILRA gene, located on chromosome 5p13 and organized in 8 exons, encodes the 459-amino acid α subunit of the IL-7 receptor, a heterodimer composed of this IL7Rα chain and the common γ chain encoded by *IL2RG*.

The receptor for the thymic stromal lymphopoietin (TSLP) also contains the IL7Rα chain, in association with the TSLP receptor chain.

Unlike IL-7 and TSLP, IL-15 function (necessary for NK cell development) is normal, so IL7Rα deficiency causes an AR T⁻B⁺NK⁺ SCID [64, 65], both Typical and Atypical.

Note that, in the beginning, the dosage of IL-7 level in Guthrie card eluate was tested together with TRECs for SCID NBS because in humans, IL-7 produced by stromal cells of lymphoid tissues and by hepatocytes is the true "T cell growth development factor" and blood IL-7 increases "by feedback' if T-cell lymphopenia [66].

SCID Caused by Pre-T Cell Receptor Defects

The pre-T cell receptor (pre-TCR), formed by a TCRβ chain (rearranged TCRβ gene) and by the disulfide-linked invariant pre-TCRα chain (pTα chain, codified by the *PTCRA* gene, located on chromosome 6p21.1 and still a very suspect candidate gene for SCID) is essential during T lymphopoiesis in thymic microenviroment at the stage of large pre-T cell [67].

The pre-TCR also transmits its signal through numerous other molecules common to the TCR (T cell receptor of mature T lymphocytes), mainly: CD3 complex (CD3γ, CD3δ, CD3ε, CD3ζ), protein-tyrosine kinases (*e.g.*, ZAP-70), adaptor proteins (*e.g.*, LAT), protein-phosphotyrosine phosphatases (*e.g.*, CD45) [68].

There are evident similarities with the pre-B cell receptor (pre-BCR) of B lymphopoiesis.

Defects of the pre-BCR ((Immunoglobulin Heavy Constant Mu chain, Igα, Igβ, λ5, p85α, Bruton tyrosine kinase BTK, B cell linker protein BLNK) cause arrest of the development of B lymphocytes at the stage of large pre-B cell and therefore agammaglobulinemia [69];

Defects of the pre-TCR subdivided into

1) defects of V(D)J recombination, and 2) impaired signaling through the pre-T cell receptor (defects of the CD3- TCR complex and of its signaling pathway), cause arrest of the development of T lymphocytes at the stage of large pre-T cell and therefore SCID (Fig. **3**).

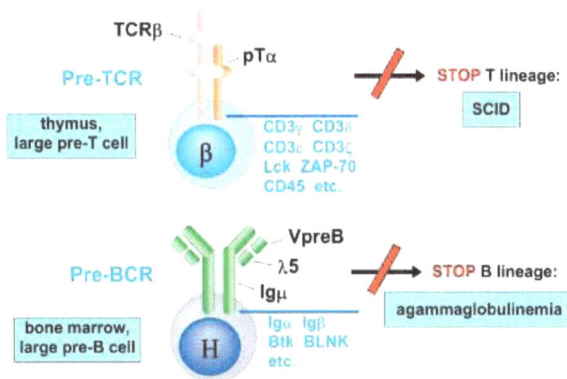

Fig. (3). Pre-TCR and pre-BCR. Schematic drawing of pre-T cell receptor (pre-TCR; thymus, large pre-T cell with rearranged TCRβ gene) and pre-B cell receptor (pre-BCR; bone marrow, large pre-B cell with rearranged IgHμ gene) (Cossu F. Genetics of SCID. Ital J Pediatr 2010; 36: 76).

1) Defects of V(D)J Recombination

The variable antigen-specific regions of the TCRβ chain of pre-TCR, Igμ chain of pre-BCR and then TCR, BCR and Ig chains are encoded by the correspondent gene domains rearranged through the V(D)J recombination of DNA [70].

This recombination occurs in two steps: 1st step specific to T and B lymphocytes (RAG1 and RAG2 "transposases", encoded by the Recombination Activating Genes *RAG1* and *RAG2*); and 2nd step due to the Non-Homologous End-Joining (NHEJ) proteins: Ku70/80, DNA-PKcs, Artemis, DNA ligase IV, XRCC4 and Cernunnos/XLF ("DNA repair genes"), that repairs double-strand breaks in DNA also in all other living cells [36, 71].

Defects of all these molecules cause T⁻B⁻NK⁺ SCID because, unlike T and B lymphocytes, NK cells do not rearrange their germline DNA to produce genes encoding antigen-specific receptors.

In defects of 1st step (RAG1, RAG2), abnormalities are limited to T and B lymphocytes; by contrast, defects of 2nd step (NHEJ) affect all cells and cause problems similar to other syndromes with DNA repair defects: cellular radiosensitivity (radiosensitive RS-SCID), extreme toxicity by pre-HSCT conditioning (especially by alkylating agents and, of course, by irradiation), predisposition to neoplasia, and in some forms (DNA ligase IV deficiency, Cernunnos/XLF deficiency) dysmorphic facies, microcephaly, psychomotor delay [72, 73]. Comet assay is a suitable technique for diagnosing the radiosensitive form of SCID before HSCT, distinguishing between the radioresistant RAG1/RAG2 and the radiosensitive NHEJ (commonly ARTEMIS) SCID infants [74].

RAG1/RAG2 Deficiencies

RAG1 or *RAG2* null mutations are worldwide among the most common causes of Typical SCID (AR T⁻B⁻NK⁺ SCID).

The compact "*RAG* gene locus", apparently a mobile genetic transposable element integrated into the vertebrate genome, located on chromosome 11p13; *RAG1* and *RAG2* are separated, in an unusual tail-to-tail configuration, by only about 8 kb, and both contain only one coding exon. They are convergently transcribed, and RAG1 (1043 amino acids) and RAG2 (527 amino acids) protein chains assemble into a heterotetramer that binds the lymphocyte germline DNA to introduce a double-stranded break at the junction between the recombination signal sequences (RSSs) and the flanking coding segments of the Variable (V), Diversity (D), and Joining (J) genes of the TCR and Ig loci.

RAG genes are expressed and active only in T and B cells rearranging their antigen-receptor genes, while they are inactive in very immature and mature lymphocytes and in all other cells; they are controlled by complex mechanisms, certainly including the enigmatic third gene *NWC* ("Nad Wyraz Ciekawy", which translates from Polish to "extremely interesting") evolutionarily conserved within the *RAG* locus [75 - 77].

More than 150 unique mutations have been identified in *RAG1* gene: missense and then frameshift and nonsense mutations; they are mainly located in the zinc-binding domain (ZBD), nonamer-binding domain (NBD) and C-terminal domain (CTD) of the core region.

More than 60 unique mutations have been identified in the *RAG2* gene: missense and then frameshift and nonsense mutations, mainly in the core region and plant homeodomain (PHD) of the non-core region [36].

As described above in this Chapter, *RAG1* or *RAG2* leaky mutations (often compound heterozygosity and at least one hypomorphic variant allowing a little residual recombinase activity) are the first identified and most commonly mutated genes in infants with Omenn Syndrome.

But, *RAG* mutations may also cause many other highly variable clinical phenotypes, with marked immune deficiency and immune dysregulation [36, 78, 79]:

Atypical $T^{low}B^{low}$ SCID with common autoimmune manifestations, especially cytopenias; Atypical SCID with disseminated cytomegalovirus (CMV) infection, oligoclonal expansion of autologous $\gamma\delta$ T cells, and detectable B cells at risk for lymphoproliferation by Epstein–Barr virus ($\gamma\delta$ $T^{+}B^{+}$SCID); autoimmunity (cytopenias, vitiligo, psoriasis, vasculitis, nephritis, myasthenia gravis and Guillain–Barré syndrome) and extensive granulomas in the skin and internal organs in the "CID-G/AI phenotype", Combined Immune Deficiency with granulomatous disease and treatment-refractory autoimmunity/ hyperinflammation, often so serious as to require prompt HSCT; idiopathic CD4 T cell lymphopenia; Common Variable Immunodeficiency-like phenotype; IgA deficiency; selective deficiency of polysaccharide-specific antibody responses; hyper-IgM syndrome-like phenotype; sterile chronic multifocal osteomyelitis.

Note that Typical or Atypical SCID, Omenn Syndrome or other phenotypes may occur in patients carrying identical *RAG1/RAG2* mutations, even within the same family, suggesting a role for other genetic modifiers and environmental factors [36 - 38].

NHEJ Deficiencies (Defects in DNA Repair Genes)

Radiosensitive AR $T^{-}B^{-}NK^{+}$ SCID due to defects of four Non-Homologous End-Joining (NHEJ) proteins have been identified in humans:

Artemis Deficiency (ART-SCID)

Artemis deficiency, due to mutations of the *DCLRE1C* (DNA cross-link repair protein 1C) gene, is also worldwide among the most common SCIDs (AR T⁻B⁻NK⁺ RS-SCID). Once it was known as "SCIDA", that is SCID of Athabascan-speaking Native Americans (Apache, Navajo), in which because of a founder effect 1 person every 10 is a heterozygote for the mutation exon 8 C576A Artemis Y192X and 1 in 2,000 newborns is affected with, notably, a characteristic frequent presence of noma-like ulcers of the oral mucosa or genitalia [80, 81].

DCLRE1C gene, ubiquitously expressed, locates on chromosome 11p13 with 14 exons and encodes the 692-amino acid protein Artemis, containing a highly conserved catalytic sequence with a metallo-β lactamase homology domain. Artemis is a nuclease, activated (phosphorylated) in the NEJH pathway by DNA-PKcs (DNA-dependent Protein Kinase catalytic subunit), and during V(D)J recombination in T and B cells specifically opens hairpin structures generated at the coding joints by RAG1/RAG2 heterotetramer.

DCLRE1C null mutations causing RS Typical SCID are mainly missense/nonsense mutations located in the β-lactamase domain (exons 1-13), and then large deletions extending into several exons [82].

Patients with *DCLRE1C* hypomorphic mutations may manifest variable clinical phenotypes: Atypical SCID, Omenn Syndrome, hyper-IgM syndrome-like phenotype, T^{low}B^{low} combined immunodeficiency (CID) with autoimmune manifestations, candidiasis, chronic diarrhoea, sinopulmonary infections, bronchiectasis, granulomatous skin lesions, predisposition to lymphoma, and other malignancies during childhood, adolescence or adulthood [83].

DNA-PKcs Deficiency

It has been known for many years that mutations of *PRKDC* (Protein kinase, DNA-activated, catalytic polypeptide) gene, encoding DNA-PKcs (DNA-dependent protein kinase catalytic subunit) cause the naturally occurring SCID in mice, Arabian foals and Jack Russell terriers; so, the defect has been long predicted in human SCID and finally found in a 5-month-old girl from consanguineous parents of Turkish origin, diagnosed with AR T⁻B⁻NK⁺ SCID by homozygous missense mutation (T9185C, L3062R) [84].

PRKDC gene is located on chromosome 8q11.21 with 86 exons and encodes the 4096-amino acid protein DNA-PKcs; RS-SCID by *PRKDC* mutations is very rare, and some patients present with microcephaly, dysmorphic facies, growth failure, neurological disorder and seizures, while hypomorphic mutations lead to autoimmunity/hyperinflammation [85].

DNA ligase IV Deficiency

LIG4 gene is located on chromosome 13q33-q34 and encodes the 911-amino acid protein DNA ligase IV, which forms a complex with XRCC4 (X-ray repair cross-complementing protein 4) and is indispensable for NHEJ and V(D)J recombination.

LIG4 null mutations cause defective neurogenesis and embryonic lethality in mice, and no null mutation has been observed in humans: described only functionally hypomorphic missense mutations or frameshift/nonsense mutations resulting in a truncated protein with impaired interactions and activities.

Phenotypes are very heterogeneous: Typical AR T$^-$B$^-$NK$^+$ RS-SCID, Atypical SCID, Omenn Syndrome, CID, progressive bone marrow failure, normal neurologic development or severe developmental and psychomotor delay, skin and bone anomalies, microcephaly, dysmorphic faces, severe growth retardation ("Ligase IV syndrome") and predisposition, also in heterozygotes, to leukemia and other neoplasia [86, 87].

Cernunnos (XLF) Deficiency

Cernunnos, also named XLF (XRCC4-like factor), interacts with the XRCC4-DNA ligase IV complex during the DNA repair process; it is a 299-amino acid protein, encoded by NEHJ1 (nonhomologous end-joining factor 1) gene located on chromosome 2q35.

NEHJ1 mutations are very rare, and affected patients present with heterogeneous phenotypes similar to those of DNA ligase IV deficiency: AR T$^-$B$^-$NK$^+$ RS-SCID, CID, autoimmunity, bone marrow failure, microcephaly, facial dysmorphism ("birdlike face"), severe growth retardation with small stature, developmental delay [88, 89].

2) Impaired Signaling through the Pre-T cell Receptor

(Defects of the CD3-TCR Complex and of its Signaling Pathway)

The different CD3 subunits, organized as γε, δε and ζ dimers, join to pre-TCR and TCR and are essential for their assemblage in the cell membrane and signal transmission after specific pMHC (peptides bound to MHC molecules) engagement, and therefore for thymic T lymphopoiesis and mature T lymphocyte functions.

Among the main steps in the extremely complex pre-TCR/TCR activation signaling pathway [90], phosphorylated cytoplasmic immunoreceptor tyrosine-based activation motifs (ITAMs) of the CD3 chains transduce signal and activate ZAP70 (Zeta-chain-associated protein kinase 70kDa); ZAP70 then phosphorylates the transmembrane adapter protein LAT (linker of activated T cells); the protein-phosphotyrosine phosphatase CD45 (LCA, Leucocyte Common Antigen) interacts mainly with other protein kinases (*e.g.*, Lck, lymphocyte-specific protein tyrosine kinase, *etc.*) and it is also essential for signaling.

CD3G, *CD3D*, and *CD3E* genes are located on chromosome 11q23.3 and encode CD3γ, CD3δ CD3δ respectively, and CD3ε chains; *CD3Z*, encoding CD3ζ chain, is located on chromosome 1q24.2; *ZAP70* gene is located on chromosome 2q11.2, *LAT* gene on chromosome 16p11.2, and *PTPRC* (protein tyrosine phosphatase, receptor type, C) gene, encoding CD45, on chromosome 1q31.3.

Complete ***CD3δ, CD3ε or CD3ζ deficiencies*** are very rare (about 2% of SCID) and cause AR T⁻B⁺NK⁺ SCID [91 - 93];

CD3γ deficiency is also extremely rare and leads to combined immunodeficiency with early recurrent infections and autoimmunity [94].

LAT deficiency, caused by homozygous mutations in the *LAT* gene, has been reported in two unrelated kindreds with eight patients that presented with variable phenotypes: AR T⁻B⁺NK⁺ SCID, early-onset AR CID, autoimmunity [95, 96].

AR T⁻B⁺NK⁺ SCID due to ***CD45 deficiency*** by *PTPRC* mutations is also very rare: only a few patients after the first child described in 1997 [97]. *PTPRC* gene is very complex, with 34 exons; CD45 constitutes about 10% of the proteins of T and B lymphocyte membrane and exists in multiple isoforms produced by complex alternative splicing of the exons encoding its extracellular domains. The expression of the different CD45 isoforms depends on cell type and state of differentiation and activation: *e.g.*, naïve CD4 CD45RA⁺ T cells, and memory CD4 CD45RO⁺ T cells [98].

ZAP70 deficiency is caused by mutations of the *ZAP70* gene, located on chromosome 2q11.2 with 14 exons and encoding the 619-amino acid ZAP70 tyrosine kinase, associated with the CD3ζ chain.

Typically, patients have a very low number of CD8 T cells, while CD4 T cells are present in normal numbers (with normal to elevated ALC) but fail to respond to mitogens (PHA) and antigens.

Clinical phenotypes are variable: AR T+(CD4+CD8-)B+NK+ SCID, late-onset CID, autoimmunity, non-infectious cutaneous manifestations, enteropathy, failure to thrive, increased risk of lymphoproliferation and malignancy [43]. Most *ZAP70* mutations are missense and located in the kinase domain; null-mutations resulting in SCID phenotype are rare, so in the 2019 IUIS classification (see above) ZAP70 deficiency is found among the "Combined immunodeficiency (CID), generally less profound than SCID" [50]. ZAP70 deficiency is more prevalent in the Mennonite population (included the first three identified patients), in which there is a high frequency of the splice- site mutation c.1624-11G>A (p.K541_K542insLEQ) [99, 100].

SCID Caused by Metabolic Disorders

Reticular Dysgenesis (RD)

Reticular dysgenesis, the most severe form of inborn human immunodeficiency, associates AR T-B-NK- SCID and severe congenital neutropenia: SCID *plus* arrest of myeloid maturation at the promyelocyte stage with total leukocytes <400/μL ("aleukocytosis"), very early bacterial infections with fatal neonatal sepsis, no response to granulocyte colony-stimulating factor (G-CSF), and severe sensorineural deafness.

It is a tissue-specific mitochondriopathy caused by mutations (missense/ nonsense, deletion, splicing) of the *AK2* gene located on chromosome 1p35.1 with 9 exons and encoding the mitochondrial enzyme adenylate kinase 2, AK2 [101, 102].

Adenylate kinases (AKs) catalyze the reversible transfer of a phosphoryl group from adenosine triphosphate to adenosine monophosphate:

2 ADPs < == > ATP + AMP; from bacteria to humans, every cell survives only if ATP/ADP/AMP concentrations are maintained within very narrow and tightly regulated ranges. Nine different AK isozymes have been characterized so far in human cells, with different tissue and subcellular distribution: AK2 is the only isoenzyme identified in bone marrow white blood cells progenitors and cells of *stria vascularis* in the inner ear.

Rare hypomorphic *AK2* mutations result in atypical phenotypes by residual enzymatic activity and variable production of myeloid and lymphoid cells [44, 103].

Adenosine Deaminase-1 Deficiency (ADA-SCID)

Null mutations of *ADA* gene, located on chromosome 20q13.11 with 12 exons and encoding the 363–amino acid single chain adenosine deaminase-1 (ADA-1) cause ADA-SCID, which is among the most common form of SCID [104].

ADA-1 is a purine salvage enzyme and catalyzes the irreversible deamination of adenosine (Ado) and 2-deoxyadenosine (dAdo) to inosine and deoxyinosine, respectively. Its deficiency results in "metabolic poisoning" from an accumulation of Ado, dAdo, and deoxyadenosine triphosphate (dATP): excess intracellular dAdo and dATP cause generalized lymphocyte apoptosis, while excess extracellular Ado acts on specific receptors with further lymphocyte inhibition.

In humans, the highest ADA-1 enzyme activity is found in lymphocytes, particularly in intrathymic immature T cells, but ADA-1 is a ubiquitous "housekeeping" enzyme present in all cell types; therefore, ADA deficiency is a 'systemic' metabolic disorder causing AR T$^-$B$^-$NK$^-$ ADA-SCID as well as several nonimmunological abnormalities: alterations of the ribs (costochondral junctions), vertebral bodies, iliac crests, and other skeletal segments; neonatal hepatitis; renal and lung abnormalities (atypical hemolytic uremic syndrome; pulmonary alveolar proteinosis); sensorineural deafness; neurological anomalies, cognitive, motor, behavioral problems with a poor prognosis also after the correction of the immune defect (Intelligence Quotient IQ < -2 SD correlates with dATP levels at diagnosis). Neutropenia is also frequent.

ADA-1 activity can be measured by various direct or indirect diagnostic methods: enzyme assay of erythrocytes or other cell types (absent or very low, <1% of normal, activity in RBCs with pathognomonic increased dATP level); increased Ado/dAdo/dATP nucleotides in blood, plasma, urine, identified by spectrophotometric, chromatographic or tandem mass spectrometry methods.

This latter identifies early- and, unlike TRECs measurement, also delayed-onset ADA-SCID by an expanded newborn screening of dried blot spots collected at birth [105].

Different *ADA* mutations cause variable impairment of the ADA-1 enzymatic activity with corresponding clinical phenotypes of varying severity:

"early-onset" AR T$^-$B$^-$NK$^-$ ADA-SCID (about 90% of patients);

"delayed-onset" Atypical ADA-SCID (about 5% of patients),

"late- and adult-onset" ADA-1 deficiency (patients over 3 years of age and also adult, diagnosed with lymphopenia, recurrent infections, autoimmunity, chronic lung disease).

Null *ADA* mutations causing ADA-SCID are mainly missense/nonsense or splice-site and located in exons 4, 5, 7 or 10, encoding enzyme regions essential for substrate binding and catalytic activity; there are "hot spots" and "ethnic" founder mutations [106].

Highly effective therapeutic options really exist, but without prompt diagnosis and treatment, ADA-SCID quickly leads to irreversible damages and death due to metabolic poisoning and infections; so, ideally, the affected newborn should be identified when still asymptomatic by NBS or positive family history.

All ADA-SCID infants should immediately receive enzyme replacement therapy (ERT), followed by allogeneic hematopoietic stem cell transplantation (HSCT) or autologous hematopoietic stem cell gene therapy (HSC-GT) (see later in this Chapter) [107].

ERT consists of weekly or twice-weekly intramuscular injection of PEG-ADA (polyethylene-glycol-modified calf intestinal ADA), that protects from metabolic poisoning both lymphocytes (restoring immune function within 2 to 4 months) and other cells, and it is often life-saving therapy at diagnosis.

Patients frequently produce ADA-neutralizing antibodies; in 2018 a recombinant version of bovine ADA conjugated to PEG has been approved and hopefully, it will replace the animal-sourced enzyme after the current multicenter trials.

ERT alone gives an overall 80% probability of surviving in 20 years; in the remaining 20% of patients, early mortality (within 6 months) resulted from serious conditions already present at diagnosis, late mortality from refractory hemolytic anemia, chronic respiratory insufficiency, lymphoproliferative disorders, liver malignancies; also, long-term (8-10 years) PEG-ADA treated patients show a gradual decline of thymic function and T cell counts.

ERT effects should be regularly assessed by metabolic, immune, and clinical testing; however, ERT should be used continuously (and for no more than 6-8 years) only if neither HSCT nor HSC-GT is available or in older patients.

The time to discontinue ERT before, or for a time after, HSCT or HSC-GT is relevant: better immunity by ERT reduces the risk of infections but could increase the risk of graft rejection, especially if no conditioning regimen; low levels of toxic metabolites by ERT are beneficial, especially if conditioning; for γ-retrovirus based HSC-GT ERT is usually discontinued 14 to 21 days before gene therapy, while for lentivirus based HSC-GT ERT is continued during gene therapy until 30 days after infusion [107].

Other SCIDs

Coronin 1A Deficiency

Coronins (1A, 1B, 1C, 2A, 2B, 6, 7) are a highly conserved family of proteins, regulators of cell F-actin structures, cytoskeletal rearrangements and intracellular membrane transport; they, by contrast to WASP (Wiskott-Aldrich Syndrome Protein) antagonize actin polymerization [108].

CORO1A gene, located on chromosome 16p11.2 with 12 exons, encodes the 461-amino acid actin-regulating protein Coronin 1A, mainly expressed in hematopoietic cells.

Coronin 1A deficiency causes defects in T cell migration and survival (accumulation of F-actin, *etc*.) and patients have severe peripheral CD4 and CD8 naïve lymphopenia (despite the presence of a normal-sized thymus), impaired T-cell proliferation, normal B-cell (and NK-cell) counts but impaired antibody response.

In a 13-month-old girl with severe mucocutaneous VZV following attenuated live viral vaccine and a clinical phenotype of AR T⁻B⁺NK⁺ SCID (requiring HSCT) has been identified a complete Coronin 1A deficiency resulting by a *de novo* 600-kb deletion of chromosome 16p11.2 encompassing 24 genes including *CORO1A*, associated in compound heterozygosity to a dinucleotide deletion, resulting in frameshift and premature termination, *CORO1A* c.248_249delCT (p.P83RfsX10).

Hypomorphic *CORO1A* mutations have been then described in three siblings with immunodeficiency and early EBV-associated B-cell lymphoproliferation, and in other siblings with immunodeficiency, molluscum contagiosum, epidermodysplasia verruciformis and granulomatous tuberculoid leprosy [109].

Other "Non-Classical" SCIDs

Other genetic diseases may occasionally cause in infants a SCID-like clinical and immunological phenotype, *e.g.*: **_AR Multiple intestinal atresias with combined immune deficiency_**, by mutation of *TTC7A* (Tetratricopeptide Repeat Domain 7A) gene [110, 111]; **_XL-Hoyeraal-Hreidarsson Syndrome_** by mutation of *DKC1* gene encoding dyskerin, a component of telomerase (Fig. **4**) [112]; **_Hereditary folate malabsorption_** by mutation of *PCFT* gene encoding proton-coupled folate transporter [113]; ___DNMT3B deficiency___ by mutation of *DNMT3B* gene encoding DNA methyltransferase 3 beta, usually mutated in about 50% of patients with ICF, Immunodeficiency, Centromeric instability, and Facial anomalies, syndrome [114].

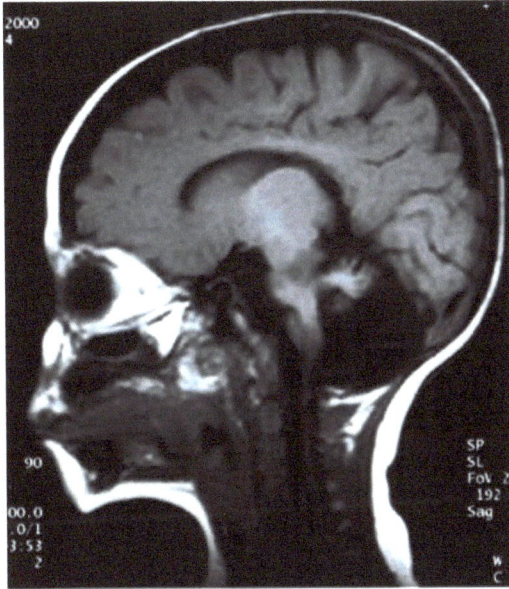

Fig. (4). Cerebellar hypoplasia in a 6-month-old male with T^{low}B$^-$NK$^-$ SCID, missense mutation of *DKC1* gene encoding dyskerin, exon 3 c.113T>C, p.Ile38Thr (X-linked Hoyeraal-Hreidarsson syndrome) (Cossu F. Genetics of SCID. Ital J Pediatr 2010; 36: 76).

Moreover, as well as ___ZAP70 deficiency___, in the 2019 IUIS classification, also other genetic disorders historically included in the SCIDs are now found in other categories [50].

These infants do not completely fulfill the various criteria established to define SCID in 2014 by the Primary Immune Deficiency Treatment Consortium [20], but in several studies published from 2014 until now (also just published) many Authors of that research continue to define "SCID" many disorders of these children.

Nevertheless, all these infants may present with clinical and immunological features of Typical or Atypical SCID (sometimes Omenn Syndrome, *i.e.*, "Omenn SCID"), severe and potentially fatal infections, need for an emergency diagnosis (ideally by newborn screening), and therapy.

Purine Nucleoside Phosphorylase (PNP) Deficiency

Purine nucleoside phosphorylase (PNP) follows ADA in the purine salvage pathway, and PNP deficiency by different mutations of *PNP* gene (chromosome 14q13.1, 6 exons) results in excess deoxyguanosine and deoxyguanosine triphosphate that causes apoptosis of lymphocytes, mainly immature T lymphocytes, and systemic metabolic poisoning.

Variable impairment of the PNP enzymatic activity corresponds to clinical phenotypes of highly varying severity, including AR $T^-B^{-/+}NK^+$ SCID/CID with neurological abnormalities and psychomotor delay [115, 116].

PNP deficient cells do not produce uric acid, that, therefore, is usually low or undetectable in serum.

Complete PNP deficiency has a poor prognosis: enzyme replacement is not available, and gene therapy is still experimental; autoimmunity (hemolytic anemia, autoimmune thrombocytopenia, neutropenia, arthritis, *etc.*) and lymphoma are frequent.

HSCT is the only therapy and sometimes improves the severe neurological problems usually present (hypertonia, hypotonia, ataxia, delay): its efficacy is of course, higher if performed early to correct both immunodeficiency and metabolic poisoning before irreversible damage has occurred.

Similar to ADA-SCID, also delayed-onset PNP deficiency can be identified by tandem mass spectrometry of dried blot spots collected at birth [117].

ORAI1 Deficiency - STIM1 Deficiency (Impaired Calcium Flux)

The variations of intracellular $Ca2^+$ levels are a fundamental mechanism for the signal transduction in all living cells; in T lymphocytes, the activation of the TCR/CD3 complex causes a release of intracellular $Ca2^+$ from the endoplasmic reticulum (ER) stores, followed by a "store-operated $Ca2^+$ entry" (SOCE) that is a conspicuous influx into the cell of other $Ca2^+$ ions from extracellular space because of the opening of the $Ca2^+$ release-activated calcium channels (CRAC) of the cell membrane; a final main effect of intracellular $Ca2^+$ increase is the translocation of NFAT (nuclear factor of activated T cells) into the nucleus, with activation of specific genes.

In rare AR $T^+B^+NK^+$ SCID-like patients have been identified a SOCE-CRAC defect, caused by mutations in genes encoding two highly conserved proteins: ORAI1 (subunit forming pores in CRAC; its name comes from ORAI, the three sisters of Greek mythology), and STIM1 (stromal interaction molecule-1; it is the sensor of Ca2$^+$ levels in ER and the activator of ORAI1-CRAC).

ORAI1 gene is located on chromosome 12q24.31 with 2 exons, *STIM1* gene on chromosome 11p15.5 with 12 exons.

The clinical phenotypes of severe ORAI1 deficiency or STIM1 deficiency are similar [118]: serious AR T$^+$B$^+$NK$^+$ SCID, with normal T, B, and NK cell differentiation and counts but severe T lymphocyte defect of Ca2$^+$ influx and of proliferation after mitogen stimulation, hypergammaglobulinemia but with deficiency of specific antibody production, congenital non-progressive global myopathy (hypotonic infant), ectodermal dysplasia (anhydrosis, defects in the formation of dental enamel). In STIM1 deficiency, there is also CD4 T$_{REG}$ lymphocyte deficiency, with severe autoimmunity (autoimmune thrombocytopenia, hemolytic anaemia), enlarged lymph nodes and hepato-splenomegaly.

MHC II Deficiency

The genes *CIITA* (chromosome 16p13), *RFXANK* (19p12), *RFX5* (1q21) and *RFXAP* (13q14) encode four factors that regulate promoters and transcription of the HLA DR, DP, DQ cluster, localized at 6p21.3.

Mutations of any of these genes cause absence of Major histocompatibility complex class II (MHC II) molecules, normally expressed at cell surface by activated T lymphocytes and by thymic epithelial cells and other cells (B lymphocytes, dendritic cells, monocytes/macrophages) that present antigens to CD4 T cells in the form of specific pMHC (peptides bound to MHC II molecules).

MHC class II deficiency may cause a serious AR T$^+$(CD4$^-$CD8$^+$)B$^+$NK$^+$ SCID-like phenotype, with lymphocyte proliferation to mitogens normal but absent to antigens and low immunoglobulins [119].

It is highly recommended that HSCT be performed in very young children, as early as possible after the diagnosis, before the onset of acute and chronic (especially viral) infections and disease-related organ damage.

Prognosis was poor, but in a recent report, the 3-year overall survival has improved to 94% for children with MHC class II deficiency transplanted since 2008, and no patient had severe acute or chronic Graft *versus* Host Disease (GvHD) [120].

HSCT normalizes lymphocyte proliferation to mitogens and antibody production in response to vaccination, although it does not correct the lack of MHC II expression on thymic epithelial cells, and some patients show persistent CD4 lymphopenia by a defect of thymic function.

Cartilage-hair Hypoplasia (CHH)

Mutations of the highly polymorphic *RMRP* (ribonuclease mitochondrial RNA processing) gene, located on chromosome 9p21-p12 with no introns and encoding not a protein but the 267-nucleotide-long RNA component of the mitochondrial RNA-processing endonuclease (a multiprotein RNA complex with at least ten different proteins), cause defects in mitochondrial DNA replication, ribosomal RNA processing, telomeres, cell replication, and a heterogeneous phenotypic spectrum [121].

Cartilage hair hypoplasia, particularly frequent in the Amish and the Finnish populations (respectively 1:19 and 1:76 individuals carriers of the mutation g.70 A > G, because of a founder effect) is a metaphyseal chondrodysplasia with short-limbed dwarfism, light-colored hypoplastic hair, and variable immunodeficiency [49, 122, 123]: AR T⁻B⁺NK⁺ SCID, also manifested as Omenn syndrome, selective CD8⁺ T lymphopenia, autoimmunity and immune dysregulation, increased risk of lymphoma. Both immunodeficiency and skeletal alterations can occur without each other.

Apart from CHH, mutations of *RMRP* (usually in different nucleotides of the RNA molecule) cause other three skeletal disorders: metaphyseal dysplasia without hypotrichosis (MDWH), kyphomelic dysplasia, and anauxetic dysplasia.

Thymic Disorders (Defect in Thymus Embryogenesis, "Athymia")

Thymocytes cannot develop to normal mature T lymphocytes without cross-talk with thymic epithelial cells (TECs) [124].

TECs derive from the endodermal epithelium of the third pharyngeal pouch, and their early development is controlled by several specific transcription factors, *e.g.*, forkhead box N1 (FOXN1), paired box 1 (PAX1), T-box transcription factor 1 (TBX1), T-box transcription factor 2 (TBX2).

Some "historical" and new forms of SCID recognize a primary embryonic thymic defect with the absence of the thymus (athymia).

Nude/SCID Syndrome (FOXN1 deficiency), the equivalent to the mouse Nude/SCID phenotype, with total congenital alopecia, absence of the thymus and AR T⁻B⁺NK⁺ SCID, is caused by mutations of the *FOXN1* gene (also named

WHN, winged helix naked, gene), located on chromosome 17q11.2 with 8 exons and encoding FOXN1, a transcription factor selectively expressed in skin and thymic epithelia.

The human form has been first identified in two sisters of a small Italian village, Acerno, where because of a founder effect the 6.52% of inhabitants are heterozygous carriers of the mutation exon 5 C792T R255X; so far, only other two mutations have been identified worldwide: exon 6 C987T R320W, and exon 2 c.562delA S188fs [125].

PAX1 deficiency by homozygous null mutations of *PAX1* gene, located on chromosome 20p11.2, may cause athymia and AR T-B+NK+ SCID associated to Otofaciocervical syndrome type 2 (OTFCS2), a rare AR disorder characterized by facial anomalies, cup-shaped low-set ears, preauricular fistulas, hearing loss, branchial defects, skeletal anomalies, and mild intellectual disability [126, 127].

Complete DiGeorge Syndrome is characterized by athymia with consequent T⁻B⁺NK⁺ SCID and variously associated facial dismorphy and palatal abnormalities, neonatal hypocalcemia by a defect of parathyroid glands, congenital heart disease (conotruncal malformations) and multiple additional congenital anomalies.

Note that the vast majority of infants with DiGeorge syndrome have "Partial" DiGeorge Syndrome, *i.e.* some functioning thymus with reduced/normal T cell counts and not SCID.

Complete or Partial DiGeorge Syndrome has different etiologies [128], mainly:

-22q11.2 deletion syndrome (22q11.2DS): microdeletions of approximately 0.7–3 million base pairs, interesting >35 genes, among which the *TBX-1* gene involved in the development of heart, thymus, parathyroid glands, palate, face;

22q11.2DS is the most common human chromosomal microdeletion disorder, with a prevalence of about 1 in 3,000 to 6,000 live births (but, Complete DiGeorge Syndrome with athymia and SCID is present in <1% of 22q11.2DS infants);

-CHARGE association (coloboma, heart defects, atresia choanae, retardated growth and development, genital hypoplasia, ear anomalies/deafness), with in the majority of patients mutation of the *CHD7* gene located on chromosome 8q12.2 and encoding the chromodomain helicase DNA-binding protein-7 [48]; note that 22q11.2 deletion and *CHD7* mutation have autosomal dominant (AD) transmission, with *de novo* mutation in more than 90% of cases; in around 1/3 of

the cases of Complete DiGeorge Syndrome, SCID manifests as Omenn syndrome [46 - 48].

Apart from the other malformations often present, athymia with consequent T⁻B⁺NK⁺ SCID is a life-threatening condition and it is essential to identify these infants as early as possible, ideally by newborn screening for SCID [129].

Athymic newborns need more and more the usual "emergency" intensive treatment of SCID (immediate reverse isolation, antimicrobial drugs, immunoglobulin replacement, supportive treatment, *etc.*). Their unique feature is that they have normal hematopoietic stem cells (so, HSCT would be meaningless), but these cells cannot develop to mature T lymphocytes because of the absence of thymic stroma and epithelium.

Therefore, the specific treatment is "thymus transplant", that is Cultured thymus tissue transplantation (CTTT): thymus tissue is obtained during newborn heart surgery, sectioned in slices and cultured *in vitro* for 2-3 weeks, then about 15-40 slices containing thymic epithelial cells (that are, surprisingly, functionally not HLA-restricted) are implanted each in the single pocket into the quadriceps muscle of the athymic infant.

However, CTTT is a technically very demanding procedure (with a mortality >25%, mostly by viral infections), and only two Center, Duke University Durham USA and, recently, Great Ormond Street Hospital London UK, are currently able to accomplish it [130, 131].

Alternatively, some T cell immunity may be obtained in these children by the adoptive transfer of HLA identical expanding and long-lasting T lymphocytes present in simple peripheral blood of a fully HLA-matched donor; such T cells are present also in non-depleted bone marrow transplant, and this explains some long-lasting efficacy in rare athymic patients (however, with mortality similar to CTTT) [132, 133].

Examples of SCID Cohorts

Also, regarding the controversial definitions of SCID/nonSCID, it is very useful to know the frequency of the mutated genes reported in some SCID cohorts, *e.g.*:

California (USA), no. 49 SCID infants, all identified by newborn screening:

IL2RG no. 14, *ADA 9*, *RAG1* 8, *IL7RA* 6, *JAK3* 3, *RAG2* 3, *RMRP* 1, *BCL11B* (B-cell lymphoma/leukaemia 11B gene) 1, Unknown 4; also identified no. 4 infants with Complete DiGeorge syndrome who received thymus transplants [9, 134].

Canada and USA, no. 250 SCID infants diagnosed by NBS (60%), family history (20%), or clinical signs (20%), with 182 Typical SCID and 68 Atypical SCID (patients with leaky mutations, included Omenn syndrome, and Reticular Dysgenesis):

IL2RG no. 77, *RAG1/RAG2* 48, *ADA* 32, *IL7RA* 19, *JAK3* 13, *RMRP* 9, *DCLRE1C* 8, *AK2* 4, *ZAP70* 4, *CD3 subunit* 3, *PNP* 2, *LIG4* 2, *NHEJ1* 2, *MSN* (Moesin gene) 2, *BCL11B* 1, *ORAI1* 1, *TTC7A* 1, "novel" 4, Unknown 18 [135, 136].

India, no. 57 SCID infants (only 4 patients could undergo HSCT):

JAK3 no. 9 (1 OS), *RAG1* 8 (2 OS), *IL2RG* 8, *ADA* 6, *RAG2* 4 (1 OS), *RFXAP* 3, *DCLRE1C* 2, *ZAP70* 2, *AK2* 1, *IL7RA* 1, *CIITA* 1, *PNP* 1, *PRKDC* 1, *RFXANK* 1, RFX5 1, Unknown 8 [137].

Iran, no. 62 SCID infants:

RAG1 no. 10, *RAG2* 6, *JAK3* 6, *IL2RG* 5, *ADA* 5, *CD3E* 5, *DCLRE1C* 4, *RFXANK* 2, *CD3D* 1, *CIITA* 1, *IL7RA* 1, *IL17RA* 1, *NHEJ1* 1, *ZAP70* 1, *MALT1* (Mucosa-Associated Lymphoid Tissue lymphoma-translocation gene 1) 1, Unknown 12 [138, 139].

Italy (excluded Sardinia), no. 88 SCID infants (66 patients of Italian origin, 22 patients from different geographic areas):

RAG1/RAG2 no. 20, *IL2RG* 19, *ADA* 15, *JAK3* 7, *FOXN1* 2, *LIG4* 2, *TTC7A* 2, *NHEJ1* 1, *CIITA* 1, *DCLRE1C* 1, *IL7RA* 1, *PAX1* 1, *RFXANK* 1, *RFX5* 1, 14qdel 1, 22q11.2DS 1, *NFKBIA* (Nuclear Factor of Kappa light polypeptide gene enhancer in B-cells Inhibitor Alpha) 1, Unknown 11 [140, 141].

Sardinia (Italy), no. 7 SCID infants diagnosed from 1998 to 2019 (in about 250,000 births, thus 1 in about 36,000 births):

DCLRE1C no. 2, *CHD7* (OS) 1, *DKC1* 1, *FOXN1* 1, *RAG2* (OS) 1, Unknown (OS) 1; curiously, the two *DCLRE1C* patients, even if completely unrelated and coming from very distant Sardinian countries, presented the same "novel" null homozygous mutation (and both with heterozygous parents): *DCLRE1C* exon 14 c.1217delT, p.fsPhe396X.

NEWBORN SCREENING FOR SCID

As noted in the introduction to this Chapter, SCID infants have a completely different fate depending on whether or not neonatal screening (NBS) for SCID is available, apart, of course, the availability/unavailability of SCID therapies (HSCT, *etc.*) [10, 12].

NBS for SCID has a very interesting "theoretical basis" [3]:

- even if most newborns with SCID appear normal and healthy at birth, human SCID is always a prenatal disorder of the development of T lymphocytes, already present at birth;

- unlike mice, in which *in utero* exposure to foreign antigens can produce tolerance and neonatal thymectomy can cause SCID [142, 143], normal development of the human immune system starts very early, and it is notably advanced before birth [144]; in the absence of SCID, in human embryos, there is intensive thymic T lymphopoiesis since 9-10 weeks of age, and *in utero* exposure to foreign antigens does activate immunological response and does not produce tolerance apart from that towards non-inherited maternal alloantigens, mediated by specific regulators T lymphocytes $CD4^+CD25^{high}FoxP3^+$ T_{REG}, that represent 15-20% of CD4 T lymphocytes in the peripheral lymphoid organs of the human fetus [145];

- SCID mutations affect human embryos, so SCID is already present at birth and can be identified with TRECs NBS that does not measure enzyme activity or search for mutations; it only counts normal naïve T lymphocytes, already absent or markedly reduced.

T cell receptor excision circles, TRECs, (Fig. **5**) are episomal DNA circles produced in thymocytes by excisional rearrangements of T cell receptor (TCR) genes; they are stable, not duplicated during mitosis, diluted out with each cell division, and therefore higher in thymocytes, recent thymic emigrants (RTEs) and naïve T cells. In newborn dried blood spots, quantitative polymerase chain reaction (qPCR) of coding-joint (cj) δRec ψJα TREC, produced at TCRα/δ locus within chromosome 14 (14q11) by >70% of developing human α:β T cells counts in the peripheral blood naïve α:β T lymphocytes. Inclusion of a quality qPCR control assessing amplification of β-actin or RNaseP gene is mandatory.

Similar to TRECs, qPCR of kappa-deleting recombination excision circles (KRECs), produced during recombination of B cell receptor genes, counts naïve B cells and in some NBS programs is associated to TRECs to identify B⁻ SCID and B cell disorders (Bruton's X-linked Agammaglobulinemia, AR Agammaglobulinemia).

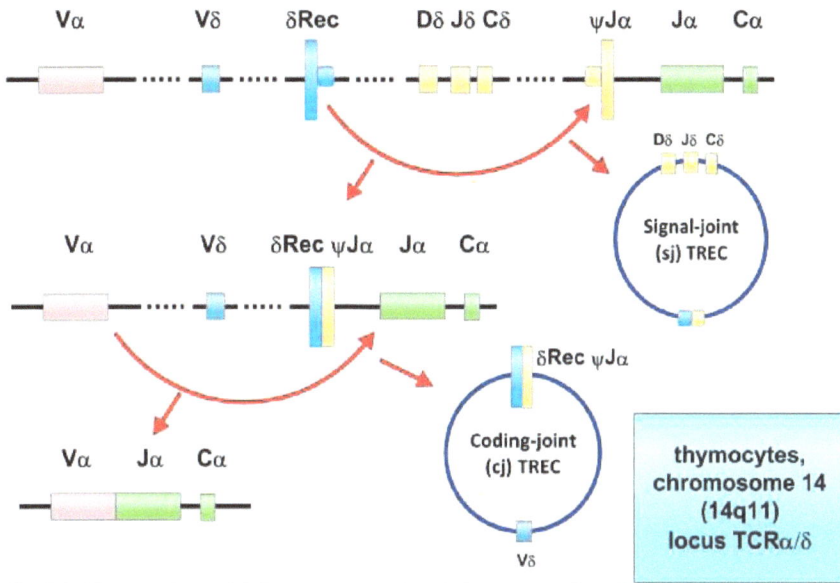

Fig. (5). T cell Receptor Excision Circles (TRECs) (Cossu F. Genetics of SCID. Ital J Pediatr 2010; 36: 76).

In SCID NBS, TREC values are expressed in copies/µL and a positive NBS is defined by TREC levels absent or below the cut-off value (some variable in the different NBS programs) associated with normal amplification of the β-actin or RNaseP qPCR control.

The results of SCID NBS are defined as either normal, abnormal, or borderline:

- if abnormal, the infant should be evaluated by an immunologist as early as possible;

- if borderline, a second dried blood spot should be tested within 24 hours;

- in both cases, families and their physicians should receive all information, instructions and also emotional support regarding appropriate care of the infant while evaluations are being completed [146, 147].

SCID NBS by TRECs is actually a newborn screening for T cell lymphopenia, and it also detects newborns with low total T cells (and therefore low naïve T cells) due to many other conditions that usually require different forms of treatment than those needed for SCID infants [9, 148]: prematurity, especially <32 weeks of gestational age (of course, a SCID infant can also be born prematurely); thymic disorders: Partial DiGeorge Syndrome, but also T⁻B⁺NK⁺ SCID with athymia; syndromes with immunodeficiency: Ataxia-Telangiectasia, Trisomy 21, Wiskott-Aldrich syndrome, Nijmegen syndrome, and many others.

"Idiopathic" T Cell Lymphopenia

Secondary causes of T cell lymphopenia: congenital heart disease, hydrops, chylothorax, maternal use of immunosuppressive drugs, *etc.*

Therefore, it is always of paramount importance to determine as early as possible the presence and precise cause of the T cell lymphopenia and, ultimately, the appropriate treatment.

DIAGNOSIS

In the absence of NBS, the initial diagnostic approach is still on clinical history and examination: as most SCID infants appear normal, without dysmorphic notes, malformations or other nonimmunological manifestations (however to be looked for), the main diagnostic clues are positive family history, recurrent fungal, viral, and bacterial infections with microbiological positivity for unusual opportunistic agents, diarrhea, skin eczematous rashes, failure to thrive, eventually absent tonsils, lack of palpable peripheral lymph nodes, and absent thymic shadow on chest X-ray [15].

Of course, if the newborn screening is available, most SCID infant has only a positive, abnormal NBS with naïve T cell lymphopenia.

As noted above in this Chapter, in most SCID infants, the absence of T lymphocytes (and possibly of B or/and NK cells) causes marked blood lymphopenia, of course, defined by normal for age ranges [21, 22]: in the first few months of life any ALC <2,500/µL is potentially pathogenic and may indicate SCID.

Therefore, in both cases, the next simplest laboratory step is the evaluation of absolute lymphocyte count (ALC/µL) in the complete blood count (CBC) with differential white blood cell counts.

Especially when more expensive exams (including TRECs and flow cytometry) are not possible, during the postpartum hospital stay, this low cost, widely available test is a useful first option to identify newborns with lymphopenia and suspect SCID and in the meantime to withhold BCG vaccine and other live attenuated vaccines [149].

Unfortunately, a normal for age ALC/µL in the CBC counts is not sufficient to rule out SCID diagnosis because many infants with SCID have normal or high

ALS (Atypical SCID by leaky mutations; maternal T cell engraftment; Omenn Syndrome).

So, the necessary next step is the flow cytometric evaluation with a "SCID panel" at least enumerating T cells (CD3, CD4, CD8), naïve *versus* memory T cells (respectively, CD45RA and CD45RO), B cells (CD19, CD20) and NK cells (CD16, CD56) [150].

These cytometric counts, associated with ALC, define the infant T/B/NK profile and, particularly if absent or very low naïve CD45RA T cells with an excess of memory CD45RO T cells, can actually enable highly suspect or definitive diagnosis of SCID in a very few days: always remember that "SCID is a pediatric emergency" [36].

When available, many other laboratory tests with different levels and specificities are very useful or essential in the SCID diagnostic evaluation:

- test for the pathognomonic engraftment of maternal T lymphocytes (HLA typing of infant blood, and maternal DNA in infant blood);

- extended flow cytometric T cell immunophenotyping and surface protein expression studies (TCRαβ/γδ, CD3DR, CD3 chains, CD31, CD27, CD62L, CCR7, IL-2Rγ, IL-7Rα, MHC-II, *etc.*);

- T-cell proliferative response *in vitro* to mitogens (Phytohemagglutinin, Concanavalin A, Pokeweed mitogen, *etc.*) and antigens (recall antigens: Candidin, *etc.*; or alloantigens: mixed-lymphocyte culture, MLC), now performed also by flow cytometric methods without radioactive tritiated thymidine (^{3}H-TdR); response to recall antigens may also be evaluated *in vivo* by delayed-type cutaneous hypersensitivity, DTH, test;

- fluorescence *in situ* hybridization (FISH) or chromosomal microarray for 22q11.2 deletion;

- ADA-1 or PNP enzymatic activity measured by direct or indirect methods;

- Vβ TCR repertoire, by spectratyping or immunophenotype;

- *in vitro* cytokine production;

- radiosensitivity testing (Comet assay).

Finally, when available, genetic testing is, of course, essential to identify the SCID genotype and so the precise, definitive, genetic/clinical diagnosis.

This is essential for prognosis and therapeutic approach (for example, choosing the type of conditioning regimen pre-HSCT) and family counselling.

Several genetic approaches are available with an increasing level of complexity and costs, and each with advantages and disadvantages [151]:

- Sanger sequencing of DNA regions (PCR amplified by specific primers) is the traditional, accurate and still common method used to perform single-gene sequencing: candidate genes, assessment of family members for an identified mutation, confirmation of mutations identified by next-generation sequencing.

- Chromosomal microarray analyses (CMAs), by array comparative genomic hybridization (aCGH) and single nucleotide polymorphism (SNP) array hybridization allow for detection in the entire genome of, respectively.

- Submicroscopic chromosomal unbalanced rearrangements, losses and gains (copy number variants, CNVs).

- Nucleotide variants, and absence of heterozygosity (by consanguinity, identity by descent, uniparental disomy, or hemizygous deletion).

CMAs are very useful when the clinical phenotype appears syndromic (with dysmorphism, multiple congenital anomalies, neurodevelopmental problems) and too nonspecific to suggest a single candidate gene or narrow panel of genes.

- Next-generations sequencing (NGS) approaches:

• targeted gene panels (TGPs) of multiple candidate genes, *e.g.* "SCID panel":

ADA, AK2, CD3D, CD3E, CD3Z, CORO1A, DCLRE1C, IL2RG, IL7RA, JAK3, LIG4, NHEJ1, PNP, PRKDC, PTPRC, RAG1, RAG2, ZAP70;

• whole-exome sequencing (WES): nearly all exons/coding sequences, *i.e.* about 21,000 genes or 1.5% of the entire genome;

• whole-genome sequencing (WGS): nearly all coding and non-coding regions (about 3.2 billion base pairs), so detects also pathogenic variants in gene regulatory regions, polyadenylation signals, deep intronic regions and "junk DNA"; costs and complexity are prohibitive, so it primarily remains a research tool.

Of course, the simple to sometimes extremely challenging interpretation of the genetic results (well known disease-causing mutations *versus* novel gene Variants of Unknown Significance, VUS) requires guidelines associating clinical expertise and computing technology of a large genomic population.

Open-access, searchable databases from different ethnic and geographic backgrounds are available, for example:

- the Human Genome Variation Society, HGVS (https://hgv.figshare.com/),

- ClinVar (https://www.ncbi.nlm.nih.gov/clinvar/),

- gnomAD (https://gnomad.broadinstitute.org),

- OMIM (https://www.omim.org/).

TREATMENT

To prevent infections, infants diagnosed or suspected of having SCID should be kept in reverse isolation as soon as possible, ideally in rooms with HEPA (High-Efficiency Particulate Air filtration) and laminar airflow (LAF).

Supportive treatment (with possibly parenteral nutrition), antiviral, antibacterial and antifungal prophylaxis/therapy (including Sulfamethoxazole/ Trimethoprim against *Pneumocystis jirovecii*), and immunoglobulin replacement to maintain serum IgG levels above 800 mg/dL, need to be started immediately.

Breastfeeding from CMV positive mothers has to be suspended in CMV negative infants, who should also receive only CMV negative (and of course irradiated and preferably WBC-filtered) blood products. Palivizumab is useful as prophylaxis for RSV.

Prophylactic treatment with isoniazid and rifampicin is mandatory for infants who received routine vaccination with *Bacille Calmette-Guérin* (BCG), and anti-tuberculosis treatment including four or more drugs is necessary in systemic, potentially life-threatening BCGitis.

As noted above in this Chapter, Omenn SCID infants also need topical (skin) and systemic steroids and other immunosuppressive drugs (cyclosporine A, *etc.*), which are at even higher risk of invasive bacterial infections due to skin and mucosal breakdown and need intensive supportive treatment.

For athymic $T^-B^+NK^+$ SCID infants (complete DiGeorge syndrome, FOXN1 deficiency), Cultured thymus tissue transplantation, CTTT ("thymus transplant") is the specific treatment;

ADA-SCID newborns should immediately start enzyme replacement therapy (ERT).

Aside from these two exceptions, allogeneic hematopoietic stem cell transplantation (HSCT) is the urgent and curative, life-saving treatment for nearly all SCID infants.

Currently, autologous hematopoietic stem cells gene therapy (HSC-GT) is really available for a few forms of SCID, mainly ADA-SCID.

Hematopoietic Stem Cell Transplantation (HSCT)

Since the first transplant in 1968 [152], thousands of SCID infants have undergone allogeneic HCST; many studies report on HSCT survival and long-term outcome in several hundreds of patients over the last decades, with a success rate ranging from 70-90 percent and varying incidence of side effects, complications, and late effects of disease or treatment [153 - 156].

Main variables influence the HSCT outcome [157, 158]:

- Age and clinical condition at the time of diagnosis.

As evident in a 1997 cardinal paper [159], a much better result is obtained if HSCT is performed in the first months of life (<3.5 months in that study), ideally before clinical presentation with infections and delay of growth.

Of course, again, this now makes the difference between children who receive NBS for SCID and those who do not.

- HSC donor.

Donor has to be found as early as possible, but unfortunately, only a minority of SCID infants have a matched related donor (MRD), *i.e.* an HLA-matched sibling or other family members.

If an MRD is not available, alternative donors is:

• matched unrelated donor, MUD, by World Marrow Donor Association, WMDA: this donor may have variable HLA mismatches, resulting principally in increased GvHD rate;

• $\alpha\beta^+$ T and $CD19^+$ B cell-depleted haploidentical related donor [160 - 162].

Before transplant infusion, it is performed *in vitro* removal of cells respectively responsible for GvHD and post-transplant lymphoproliferative disorder (PTLD), and enrichment of CD34$^+$ hematopoietic stem cells and of $\gamma\delta^+$ T cells and NK cells which facilitate engraftment and provide anti-infective activity; when available, this really ingenious procedure finds a suitable related donor for every child very quickly, and has supplanted the other T depletion methods; disadvantages are an increased rate of viral infections, high costs and high laboratory expertise required;

• cord blood unit: has the known disadvantages of very low total CD34$^+$ count, long engraftment time, high rate of viral infections, and resulting in increased transplant-related mortality.

- No conditioning *versus* conditioning regimen:

HSCT engraftment without any pre-transplant conditioning regimen is theoretically possible in most SCID infants, especially if NK$^-$ SCID (*e.g.*, ADA-SCID, common gamma chain (γc) deficiency, JAK3 deficiency), but with frequently defective donor B cell reconstitution and so persistent B cell deficiency that requires long-term (for the rest of life) immunoglobulin replacement therapy;

reduced-intensity conditioning regimens reduce short- and long-term toxicity and long-term effects on, for example, growth and endocrine system, therefore are probably recommended, if possible, in all these very young (few months of age) children [163, 164].

In SCID infants with generalized DNA repair defect and radiosensitive AR T$^-$B$^-$NK$^+$ SCID due to deficiency of NHEJ proteins (Artemis and, rarely, DNA-PKcs, DNA ligase IV, Cernunnos) the molecular problem causes cellular radiosensitivity and extreme toxicity by "historical" pre-transplant conditioning regimen with alkylating agents: striking differences have been described respect to SCID infants with RAG1/RAG2 deficiency, in which the defect is limited to lymphocytes [165].

- SCID genotype.

It influences the outcome of HSCT not only for the different sensitivity to conditioning regimen, *e.g.*, a better outcome is usual in SCID with common gamma chain (γc) deficiency, JAK3 deficiency (aside from frequent cutaneous HPV) and IL-7Rα deficiency;

on the contrary, a complicated outcome is more frequent in SCID with V(D)J recombination - DNA repair defects: high risk of conditioning toxicity, if not "disease-modulated"; and, also if normal immunologic reconstitution, frequent autoimmunity, gut problems, *etc.*; in ADA-SCID the frequent neurological anomalies (cognitive, motor and behaviour problems) have a poor prognosis also after the correction of the immune defect.

Regularly updated, open-access guidelines for allogeneic HSCT in SCID infants are published by the Inborn Errors Working Party (IEWP) of EBMT (European Group for Blood and Marrow Transplantation) and ESID (European Society for Immune deficiency), and by the Primary Immune Deficiency Treatment Consortium (PIDTC).

Autologous Hematopoietic Stem Cell Gene Therapy (HSC-GT)

HSC-GT is performed with these main steps [166 - 168]:

- the patient follows the same treatments as any HSCT for SCID: reverse isolation in hospital, a central venous catheter (CVC) positioned, supportive care, prophylaxis/therapy of infections which obviously must be absent before the procedure begins;

- patient's autologous haematopoietic CD34$^+$ stem cells are collected by bone marrow harvest or, in a few cases, mobilised peripheral blood (if conditioning pre-gene therapy, this "main" collection is preceded about one month before by a HSC backup harvested and cryopreserved unmanipulated to be used in case of poor engraftment or technical issues);

- in a "Good Manufacturing Practice Laboratory" for *ex vivo* manipulation, CD34$^+$ stem cells are selected and enriched, and through viral vectors derived from γ-retrovirus (γ-RV) or lentivirus (LV) the healthy gene is permanently inserted into their chromosomal DNA: hence, it will function like a cellular gene transcribed to mRNA and translated to produce the therapeutic gene product;

- the patient receives non-myeloablative conditioning to facilitate engraftment, *e.g.* low-dose Busulfan 4 mg/kg adjusted in accordance with pharmacokinetics (pK)–predetermined targets [169];

- modified CD34$^+$ stem cells are formulated for intravenous administration and certified for release criteria and absence of microbial contamination, and are

reinfused in the patient through a central venous catheter (CVC).

The administration of adequate numbers of gene-modified CD34$^+$ stem cells is essential: in HSC-GT for ADA-SCID a minimum dose at infusion of 2×10^6 CD34$^+$ cells/kg with a target of $5\text{-}10 \times 10^6$ CD34$^+$ cells/kg (and corrected HSC levels 1-10%) is recommended.

Therefore, due to the expected cell loss during subsequent procedures, bone marrow harvest for HSC-GT requires collecting a higher number of cells than that usually recommended for conventional unmanipulated transplantation: at least 5-10 x 10^6 CD34$^+$ cells/kg, corresponding to at least 30 mL/kg of bone marrow volumes [170].

γ-RV and LV are viruses of the Retroviridae family and transfer their genome into the chromosomal DNA of the infected cell as a permanently integrated DNA provirus, which produces new viruses and also duplicated and is passed on to progeny cells with cell division [166];

γ-RV and LV vectors are designed and constructed incapable of viral replication by removing all of the viral protein-encoding genes, replaced with the normal, therapeutic, gene sequences; they insert randomly into the genome, with preferential sites depending on vector and cell type; modern γ-RV and LV vectors are SIN (self-inactivating), with long terminal repeat (LTR) deleted and expression of the therapeutic gene controlled by an internal promoter;

(SIN) γ-RV are now preferentially supplanted by new SIN LV vectors: unlike γ-RV vectors, SIN LV vectors also integrate into the cells, not in mitosis (effective gene transfer to human HSC can be accomplished with 1-2 days of culture), do not have as preferential integration site the promoter regions of active, expressed, genes, and their viral enhancer elements that could activate cellular *proto-oncogenes* have been deleted [168, 171].

Since the year 2000, more than 100 ADA-SCID (ADA-1 deficiency) patients received γ-RV or, more recently, LV HSC-GT: all of them are reported to be alive and most with near-normal immunity; 10-20% had to restart ERT or receive subsequent HSCT or HSC-GT; notably, even if more than 50 patients received γ-RV vectors, no patient has been reported the complication of clonal leukemic proliferation because of insertional mutagenesis.

Therefore, for ADA-SCID infants, HSC-GT is currently considered a safe and effective alternative therapeutic option to HSCT [107, 168, 172].

Beginning in 1999 in Paris and in 2001 in London, two European groups performed HSC-GT for Common gamma chain (γc) deficiency (SCIDX-1) in 20 children aged from 1 to 33 months and with no matched sibling donor.

Without any conditioning regimen, γ-RV vectors were used, derived from the Moloney murine leukaemia virus (Paris) or from a gibbon-ape leukaemia virus (London); 18 of 20 children had satisfactory T cell reconstitution, while NK cell and B cell function remained mostly defective.

Unfortunately, between 2.5 years and 15 years post-therapy, at least six patients (of whom one died) developed a vector-driven acute T lymphoblastic leukaemia [167, 168].

T cell leukaemia was caused by complex DNA mutagenesis started with the insertion (insertional mutagenesis) at chromosome 11p13, a few kilobases upstream of protooncogene *LMO2* (LIM domain only 2), of a single copy of the γ-RV vector, containing the normal *IL2RG* gene but also its enhancer; thus, *LMO2* gene was aberrantly transcribed and expressed, followed by several other acquired oncogenic somatic mutations [173].

New *IL2RG* vectors have now been designed and used in three recent studies:

- nine SCIDX-1 infants received a SIN *IL2RG* γ-retroviral vector in which the Moloney murine leukaemia virus LTR U3 enhancer was deleted; two infants received treatment for massive maternal T cell engraftment with respectively fludarabine and rabbit anti-thymocyte globulin, while no conditioning was given to any of the patients; reported follow-up is 12 to 39 months [174];

- five patients aged 7, 10, 16, 22, 23 years, with persistent disease after one or more haploidentical HSCT, received a SIN *IL2RG* LV vector after Busulfan 6 mg/kg; reported follow-up is 6 to 36 months [175];

- eight infants received a SIN *IL2RG* LV vector after low-dose non-myeloablative Busulfan; reported median duration of follow-up is 16.4 months, with range 6 to 24 months [176].

The preliminary results of these studies appear encouraging both for effectiveness and safety (so far not reported leukoproliferative complications), even if follow-up is short and great caution is warranted.

Recently, five ART-SCID (Artemis deficiency) infants, all diagnosed by newborn screening for SCID, have been treated at a median age of 2.6 months (range 2.3-3.7) with HSC-GT using a SIN lentiviral vector containing the human *DCLRE1C* promoter and cDNA, after a very low dose of busulfan; median follow-up is 10.5 months (range 0 -15.6), and 3/3 evaluable patients (≥8 weeks post-HSC-GT) developed multilineage engraftment of transduced cells with reconstitution of T cell immunity and evidence for B cell immune development [177].

In a 2003 report, a single JAK3-deficient patient (2.5-year-old boy, after having previously failed two allogeneic transplant attempts using his mother as a donor) was treated in a HSC-GT trial without benefit [178].

Extensive preclinical studies of HSC-GT in mouse models have been performed or are ongoing to correct defective *RAG1* and *RAG2* genes [179, 180].

CONCLUSION

SCID is a pediatric emergency: essentially every affected infant could be be cured by very early diagnosis, prevention (sterile rooms) and treatment of infections, and timely HSCT or GT. Even if clinically silent in most affected newborns, human SCID is always a prenatal disorder of T lymphocyte development, already present at birth, so it's detected by newborn screening through measurement of TRECs, which counts naïve T lymphocytes, already absent or markedly reduced. The diagnostic approach to SCID and the 'natural history' of SCID infants, their families, and their clinicians are now completely different in these two conditions: NO NBS for SCID (unfortunately the vast majority of newborns worldwide) versus YES NBS for SCID. The IUIS 2019 classification lists only 18 genes whose mutations cause SCID, but this is controversial, and many "Historical" or "Non-Classical" SCIDs are still included in the published SCID cohorts. Typical SCID, caused by null mutations, is a T- SCID (ALC < 500 cells/µL, CD3 T cells > 300/µL) and could also be defined as T0 (zero) SCID; however, many infants with SCID have more than 300 T cells/µL and this T+/++ SCID (SCID with Tlow/normal/high counts) occurs in three conditions: Atypical SCID by leaky mutations, SCID with massive engraftment of transplacentally derived maternal T lymphocytes, and Omenn Syndrome.

PATIENT CONSENT

Written informed consent was obtained from the parents of the infants for publication of images and clinical data in Figs. (**1**, **2** and **4**).

CONSENT FOR PUBLICATION

Not applicable.

CONFLICT OF INTEREST

The author declares no conflict of interest, financial or otherwise.

ACKNOWLEDGEMENTS

I am very grateful to all the Sardinian patients and families for their participation, interest and support in the study of SCID.

I dedicate this work to the memory of my Professor Antonio Cao, an extraordinary researcher and teacher in Pediatrics and Genetics.

REFERENCES

[1]   Le Deist F, Moshous D, Villa A, *et al.* Combined T and B Cell Immunodeficiencies. In: Rezaei N, Aghamohammadi A, Notarangelo LD, Eds. Primary Immunodeficiency Diseases Definition, Diagnosis, and Management. 2nd ed. Berlin: Springer-Verlag 2017; pp. 83-182.
[http://dx.doi.org/10.1007/978-3-662-52909-6_2]

[2]   Candotti F, de Villartay JP, Moshous D, Villa A, Notarangelo LD. Severe combined immune deficiency. In: Sullivan KE, Stiehm ER, Eds. Stiehm's Immune Deficiencies Inborn Errors of Immunity. 2nd ed. London: Elsevier Academic Press 2020; pp. 153-205.
[http://dx.doi.org/10.1016/B978-0-12-816768-7.00007-7]

[3]   Cossu F. Genetics of SCID. Ital J Pediatr 2010; 36(1): 76.
[http://dx.doi.org/10.1186/1824-7288-36-76] [PMID: 21078154]

[4]   Puck JM. Newborn screening for severe combined immunodeficiency and T-cell lymphopenia. Immunol Rev 2019; 287(1): 241-52.
[http://dx.doi.org/10.1111/imr.12729] [PMID: 30565242]

[5]   Al-Mousa H, Al-Saud B. Primary Immunodeficiency Diseases in Highly Consanguineous Populations from Middle East and North Africa: Epidemiology, Diagnosis, and Care. Front Immunol 2017; 8: 678.
[http://dx.doi.org/10.3389/fimmu.2017.00678] [PMID: 28694805]

[6]   Greenberg-Kushnir N, Lee YN, Simon AJ, *et al.* A Large Cohort of RAG1/2-Deficient SCID Patients-Clinical, Immunological, and Prognostic Analysis. J Clin Immunol 2020; 40(1): 211-22.
[http://dx.doi.org/10.1007/s10875-019-00717-1] [PMID: 31838659]

[7]   Kwan A, Hu D, Song M, *et al.* Successful newborn screening for SCID in the Navajo Nation. Clin Immunol 2015; 158(1): 29-34.
[http://dx.doi.org/10.1016/j.clim.2015.02.015] [PMID: 25762520]

[8]   Verbsky J, Thakar M, Routes J. The Wisconsin approach to newborn screening for severe combined immunodeficiency. J Allergy Clin Immunol 2012; 129(3): 622-7.
[http://dx.doi.org/10.1016/j.jaci.2011.12.004] [PMID: 22244594]

[9]   Amatuni GS, Currier RJ, Church JA, *et al.* Newborn Screening for Severe Combined Immunodeficiency and T-cell Lymphopenia in California, 2010-2017. Pediatrics 2019; 143(2): e20182300.
[http://dx.doi.org/10.1542/peds.2018-2300] [PMID: 30683812]

[10]   Quinn J, Orange JS, Modell V, Modell F. The case for severe combined immunodeficiency (SCID) and T cell lymphopenia newborn screening: saving lives...one at a time. Immunol Res 2020; 68(1): 48-53.
[http://dx.doi.org/10.1007/s12026-020-09117-9] [PMID: 32128663]

[11]   Chan A, Scalchunes C, Boyle M, Puck JM. Early *vs.* delayed diagnosis of severe combined immunodeficiency: a family perspective survey. Clin Immunol 2011; 138(1): 3-8.
[http://dx.doi.org/10.1016/j.clim.2010.09.010] [PMID: 21035402]

[12]   Krantz MS, Stone CA Jr, Connelly JA, Norton AE, Khan YW. The effect of delayed and early diagnosis in siblings, and importance of newborn screening for SCID. Ann Allergy Asthma Immunol 2019; 122(2): 211-3.
[http://dx.doi.org/10.1016/j.anai.2018.11.002] [PMID: 30439467]

[13]   Erjaee A, Bagherpour M, Van Rooyen C, *et al.* Primary immunodeficiency in Africa - a review. S Afr Med J 2019; 109(8b): 3-11.
[http://dx.doi.org/10.7196/SAMJ.2019.v109i8b.13820] [PMID: 31662142]

[14]   Stephan JL, Vlekova V, Le Deist F, *et al.* Severe combined immunodeficiency: a retrospective single-center study of clinical presentation and outcome in 117 patients. J Pediatr 1993; 123(4): 564-72.
[http://dx.doi.org/10.1016/S0022-3476(05)80951-5] [PMID: 8410508]

[15]   McWilliams LM, Dell Railey M, Buckley RH. Positive Family History, Infection, Low Absolute Lymphocyte Count (ALC), and Absent Thymic Shadow: Diagnostic Clues for All Molecular Forms of Severe Combined Immunodeficiency (SCID). J Allergy Clin Immunol Pract 2015; 3(4): 585-91.
[http://dx.doi.org/10.1016/j.jaip.2015.01.026] [PMID: 25824440]

[16]   Rosen FS. Severe combined immunodeficiency: a pediatric emergency. J Pediatr 1997; 130(3): 345-6.
[PMID: 9063405]

[17]   Fekrvand S, Yazdani R, Olbrich P, *et al.* Primary Immunodeficiency Diseases and *Bacillus Calmette-Guérin* (BCG)-Vaccine-Derived Complications: A Systematic Review. J Allergy Clin Immunol Pract 2020; 8(4): 1371-86.
[http://dx.doi.org/10.1016/j.jaip.2020.01.038] [PMID: 32006723]

[18]   Rosenfeld L, Mas Marques A, Niendorf S, *et al.* Life-threatening systemic rotavirus infection after vaccination in severe combined immunodeficiency (SCID). Pediatr Allergy Immunol 2017; 28(8): 841-3.
[http://dx.doi.org/10.1111/pai.12771] [PMID: 28815852]

[19]   Saravia J, Chapman NM, Chi H. Helper T cell differentiation. Cell Mol Immunol 2019; 16(7): 634-43.
[http://dx.doi.org/10.1038/s41423-019-0220-6] [PMID: 30867582]

[20]   Shearer WT, Dunn E, Notarangelo LD, *et al.* Establishing diagnostic criteria for severe combined immunodeficiency disease (SCID), leaky SCID, and Omenn syndrome: the Primary Immune Deficiency Treatment Consortium experience. J Allergy Clin Immunol 2014; 133(4): 1092-8.

[21]   Amatuni GS, Sciortino S, Currier RJ, Naides SJ, Church JA, Puck JM. Reference intervals for lymphocyte subsets in preterm and term neonates without immune defects. J Allergy Clin Immunol 2019; 144(6): 1674-83.
[http://dx.doi.org/10.1016/j.jaci.2019.05.038] [PMID: 31220471]

[22]   Fleisher TA, Rosenzweig SD. Lymphocyte reference intervals in the era of newborn screening. J Allergy Clin Immunol 2019; 144(6): 1516-7.
[http://dx.doi.org/10.1016/j.jaci.2019.09.022] [PMID: 31600546]

[23]   Denianke KS, Frieden IJ, Cowan MJ, Williams ML, McCalmont TH. Cutaneous manifestations of maternal engraftment in patients with severe combined immunodeficiency: a clinicopathologic study. Bone Marrow Transplant 2001; 28(3): 227-33.
[http://dx.doi.org/10.1038/sj.bmt.1703128] [PMID: 11535989]

[24]   Müller SM, Ege M, Pottharst A, Schulz AS, Schwarz K, Friedrich W. Transplacentally acquired maternal T lymphocytes in severe combined immunodeficiency: a study of 121 patients. Blood 2001; 98(6): 1847-51.
[http://dx.doi.org/10.1182/blood.V98.6.1847] [PMID: 11535520]

[25]   Shahbazi Z, Parvaneh N, Shahbazi S, *et al.* Graft *versus* host disease and microchimerism in a *JAK3 deficient* patient. Allergy Asthma Clin Immunol 2019; 15(1): 47.
[http://dx.doi.org/10.1186/s13223-019-0361-2] [PMID: 31440277]

[26]   Palmer K, Green TD, Roberts JL, *et al.* Unusual clinical and immunologic manifestations of transplacentally acquired maternal T cells in severe combined immunodeficiency. J Allergy Clin Immunol 2007; 120(2): 423-8.
[http://dx.doi.org/10.1016/j.jaci.2007.02.047] [PMID: 17481714]

[27]   Kobrynski LJ, Abramowsky C. Monoclonal IgA gammapathy due to maternal B cells in an infant with severe combined immunodeficiency (SCID) prior to hematopoietic stem cell transplantation. J Pediatr Hematol Oncol 2006; 28(1): 53-6.
[PMID: 16394896]

[28]   Tezcan I, Ersoy F, Sanal O, *et al.* Long-term survival in severe combined immune deficiency: the role of persistent maternal engraftment. J Pediatr 2005; 146(1): 137-40.
[http://dx.doi.org/10.1016/j.jpeds.2004.09.010] [PMID: 15644840]

[29]   Wahlstrom J, Patel K, Eckhert E, *et al.* Transplacental maternal engraftment and posttransplantation graft-*versus*-host disease in children with severe combined immunodeficiency. J Allergy Clin Immunol 2017; 139(2): 628-633.e10.
[http://dx.doi.org/10.1016/j.jaci.2016.04.049] [PMID: 27444177]

[30]   Omenn GS. FAMILIAL RETICULOENDOTHELIOSIS WITH EOSINOPHILIA. N Engl J Med 1965; 273(8): 427-32.
[http://dx.doi.org/10.1056/NEJM196508192730806] [PMID: 14328107]

[31]   Villa A, Notarangelo LD, Roifman CM. Omenn syndrome: inflammation in leaky severe combined immunodeficiency. J Allergy Clin Immunol 2008; 122(6): 1082-6.
[http://dx.doi.org/10.1016/j.jaci.2008.09.037] [PMID: 18992930]

[32]   Poliani PL, Facchetti F, Ravanini M, *et al.* Early defects in human T-cell development severely affect distribution and maturation of thymic stromal cells: possible implications for the pathophysiology of Omenn syndrome. Blood 2009; 114(1): 105-8.
[http://dx.doi.org/10.1182/blood-2009-03-211029] [PMID: 19414857]

[33]   Cassani B, Poliani PL, Moratto D, *et al.* Defect of regulatory T cells in patients with Omenn syndrome. J Allergy Clin Immunol 2010; 125(1): 209-16.
[http://dx.doi.org/10.1016/j.jaci.2009.10.023] [PMID: 20109747]

[34]   Lee YN, Frugoni F, Dobbs K, *et al.* Characterization of T and B cell repertoire diversity in patients with RAG deficiency. Sci Immunol 2016; 1(6): eaah6109.
[http://dx.doi.org/10.1126/sciimmunol.aah6109] [PMID: 28783691]

[35]   Villa A, Santagata S, Bozzi F, *et al.* Partial V(D)J recombination activity leads to Omenn syndrome. Cell 1998; 93(5): 885-96.
[http://dx.doi.org/10.1016/S0092-8674(00)81448-8] [PMID: 9630231]

[36]   Notarangelo LD, Kim MS, Walter JE, Lee YN. Human *RAG* mutations: biochemistry and clinical implications. Nat Rev Immunol 2016; 16(4): 234-46.
[http://dx.doi.org/10.1038/nri.2016.28] [PMID: 26996199]

[37]   Corneo B, Moshous D, Güngör T, *et al.* Identical mutations in *RAG1* or *RAG2* genes leading to defective V(D)J recombinase activity can cause either T⁻B⁻severe combined immune deficiency or Omenn syndrome. Blood 2001; 97(9): 2772-6.
[http://dx.doi.org/10.1182/blood.V97.9.2772] [PMID: 11313270]

[38]   IJspeert H, Driessen GJ, Moorhouse MJ, *et al.* Similar recombination-activating gene (*RAG*) mutations result in similar immunobiological effects but in different clinical phenotypes. J Allergy Clin Immunol 2014; 133(4): 1124-33.
[http://dx.doi.org/10.1016/j.jaci.2013.11.028] [PMID: 24418478]

[39]   Gruber TA, Shah AJ, Hernandez M, *et al.* Clinical and genetic heterogeneity in Omenn syndrome and severe combined immune deficiency. Pediatr Transplant 2009; 13(2): 244-50.
[http://dx.doi.org/10.1111/j.1399-3046.2008.00970.x] [PMID: 18822103]

[40]   Giliani S, Bonfim C, de Saint Basile G, *et al.* Omenn syndrome in an infant with *IL7RA* gene mutation. J Pediatr 2006; 148(2): 272-4.
[http://dx.doi.org/10.1016/j.jpeds.2005.10.004] [PMID: 16492442]

[41]   Ege M, Ma Y, Manfras B, *et al.* Omenn syndrome due to ARTEMIS mutations. Blood 2005; 105(11): 4179-86.
[http://dx.doi.org/10.1182/blood-2004-12-4861] [PMID: 15731174]

[42]   Grunebaum E, Bates A, Roifman CM. Omenn syndrome is associated with mutations in DNA ligase IV. J Allergy Clin Immunol 2008; 122(6): 1219-20.
[http://dx.doi.org/10.1016/j.jaci.2008.08.031] [PMID: 18845326]

[43]   Turul T, Tezcan I, Artac H, *et al.* Clinical heterogeneity can hamper the diagnosis of patients with ZAP70 deficiency. Eur J Pediatr 2009; 168(1): 87-93.

[http://dx.doi.org/10.1007/s00431-008-0718-x]

[44]   Henderson LA, Frugoni F, Hopkins G, *et al.* First reported case of Omenn syndrome in a patient with reticular dysgenesis. J Allergy Clin Immunol 2013; 131(4): 1227-1230, 1230.e1-1230.e3.
[http://dx.doi.org/10.1016/j.jaci.2012.07.045] [PMID: 23014587]

[45]   Roifman CM, Zhang J, Atkinson A, Grunebaum E, Mandel K. Adenosine deaminase deficiency can present with features of Omenn syndrome. J Allergy Clin Immunol 2008; 121(4): 1056-8.
[http://dx.doi.org/10.1016/j.jaci.2007.12.1148] [PMID: 18243287]

[46]   Markert ML, Alexieff MJ, Li J, *et al.* Complete DiGeorge syndrome: development of rash, lymphadenopathy, and oligoclonal T cells in 5 cases. J Allergy Clin Immunol 2004; 113(4): 734-41.
[http://dx.doi.org/10.1016/j.jaci.2004.01.766] [PMID: 15100681]

[47]   Vu QV, Wada T, Toma T, *et al.* Clinical and immunophenotypic features of atypical complete DiGeorge syndrome. Pediatr Int 2013; 55(1): 2-6.
[http://dx.doi.org/10.1111/j.1442-200X.2012.03722.x] [PMID: 22978387]

[48]   Gennery AR, Slatter MA, Rice J, *et al.* Mutations in *CHD7* in patients with CHARGE syndrome cause T-B + natural killer cell + severe combined immune deficiency and may cause Omenn-like syndrome. Clin Exp Immunol 2008; 153(1): 75-80.
[http://dx.doi.org/10.1111/j.1365-2249.2008.03681.x] [PMID: 18505430]

[49]   Roifman CM, Gu Y, Cohen A. Mutations in the RNA component of RNase mitochondrial RNA processing might cause Omenn syndrome. J Allergy Clin Immunol 2006; 117(4): 897-903.
[http://dx.doi.org/10.1016/j.jaci.2006.01.003] [PMID: 16630949]

[50]   Tangye SG, Al-Herz W, Bousfiha A, *et al.* Human Inborn Errors of Immunity: 2019 Update on the Classification from the International Union of Immunological Societies Expert Committee. J Clin Immunol 2020; 40(1): 24-64.
[http://dx.doi.org/10.1007/s10875-019-00737-x] [PMID: 31953710]

[51]   Williamson AP, Montgomery JR, South MA, Wilson R. A special report: four-year study of a boy with combined immune deficiency maintained in strict reverse isolation from birth. Pediatr Res 1977; 11(1 Pt 2): 63-89.
[http://dx.doi.org/10.1203/00006450-197701000-00001] [PMID: 401538]

[52]   Paschall VL, Brown LA, Lawrence EC, *et al.* Immunoregulation in an isolated 12-year-old boy with congenital severe combined immunodeficiency. Pediatr Res 1984; 18(8): 723-8.
[http://dx.doi.org/10.1203/00006450-198408000-00009] [PMID: 6332299]

[53]   Shearer WT, Ritz J, Finegold MJ, *et al.* Epstein-Barr virus-associated B-cell proliferations of diverse clonal origins after bone marrow transplantation in a 12-year-old patient with severe combined immunodeficiency. N Engl J Med 1985; 312(18): 1151-9.
[http://dx.doi.org/10.1056/NEJM198505023121804] [PMID: 2984567]

[54]   Noguchi M, Yi H, Rosenblatt HM, *et al.* Interleukin-2 receptor gamma chain mutation results in X-linked severe combined immunodeficiency in humans. Cell 1993; 73(1): 147-57.
[http://dx.doi.org/10.1016/0092-8674(93)90167-O] [PMID: 8462096]

[55]   Berg LJ. The "bubble boy" paradox: an answer that led to a question. J Immunol 2008; 181(9): 5815-6.
[http://dx.doi.org/10.4049/jimmunol.181.9.5815] [PMID: 18941168]

[56]   Leonard WJ, Lin JX, O'Shea JJ. The γ_c Family of Cytokines: Basic Biology to Therapeutic Ramifications. Immunity 2019; 50(4): 832-50.
[http://dx.doi.org/10.1016/j.immuni.2019.03.028] [PMID: 30995502]

[57]   Nowak K, Linzner D, Thrasher AJ, Lambert PF, Di WL, Burns SO. Absence of γ-Chain in Keratinocytes Alters Chemokine Secretion, Resulting in Reduced Immune Cell Recruitment. J Invest Dermatol 2017; 137(10): 2120-30.
[http://dx.doi.org/10.1016/j.jid.2017.05.024] [PMID: 28634034]

[58]   Fuchs S, Rensing-Ehl A, Erlacher M, *et al.* Patients with T$^+$/low NK$^+$ IL-2 receptor γ chain deficiency have differentially-impaired cytokine signaling resulting in severe combined immunodeficiency. Eur J Immunol 2014; 44(10): 3129-40.
        [http://dx.doi.org/10.1002/eji.201444689] [PMID: 25042067]

[59]   Lim CK, Abolhassani H, Appelberg SK, Sundin M, Hammarström L. *IL2RG* hypomorphic mutation: identification of a novel pathogenic mutation in exon 8 and a review of the literature. Allergy Asthma Clin Immunol 2019; 15(1): 2.
        [http://dx.doi.org/10.1186/s13223-018-0317-y] [PMID: 30622570]

[60]   Purswani P, Meehan CA, Kuehn HS, *et al.* Two Unique Cases of X-linked SCID: A Diagnostic Challenge in the Era of Newborn Screening. Front Pediatr 2019; 7: 55.
        [http://dx.doi.org/10.3389/fped.2019.00055] [PMID: 31024866]

[61]   Rochman Y, Spolski R, Leonard WJ. New insights into the regulation of T cells by gamma(c) family cytokines. Nat Rev Immunol 2009; 9(7): 480-90.
        [http://dx.doi.org/10.1038/nri2580] [PMID: 19543225]

[62]   Cattaneo F, Recher M, Masneri S, *et al.* Hypomorphic Janus kinase 3 mutations result in a spectrum of immune defects, including partial maternal T-cell engraftment. J Allergy Clin Immunol 2013; 131(4): 1136-45.
        [http://dx.doi.org/10.1016/j.jaci.2012.12.667] [PMID: 23384681]

[63]   Di Matteo G, Chiriaco M, Scarselli A, *et al. JAK3* mutations in Italian patients affected by SCID: New molecular aspects of a long-known gene. Mol Genet Genomic Med 2018; 6(5): 713-21.
        [http://dx.doi.org/10.1002/mgg3.391] [PMID: 30032486]

[64]   Giliani S, Mori L, de Saint Basile G, *et al.* Interleukin-7 receptor alpha (IL-7Ralpha) deficiency: cellular and molecular bases. Analysis of clinical, immunological, and molecular features in 16 novel patients. Immunol Rev 2005; 203: 110-26.

[65]   Leiding JW, Sriaroon P, Ly JM, *et al.* Hypomorphic interleukin-7 receptor α-chain mutations and T-cell deficiency: a delay in diagnosis. Ann Allergy Asthma Immunol 2015; 115(1): 1-3.
        [http://dx.doi.org/10.1016/j.anai.2015.04.024] [PMID: 26123418]

[66]   McGhee SA, Stiehm ER, Cowan M, Krogstad P, McCabe ER. Two-tiered universal newborn screening strategy for severe combined immunodeficiency. Mol Genet Metab 2005; 86(4): 427-30.
        [http://dx.doi.org/10.1016/j.ymgme.2005.09.005] [PMID: 16260163]

[67]   Nemazee D. Receptor editing in lymphocyte development and central tolerance. Nat Rev Immunol 2006; 6(10): 728-40.
        [http://dx.doi.org/10.1038/nri1939] [PMID: 16998507]

[68]   Xu X, Li H, Xu C. Structural understanding of T cell receptor triggering. Cell Mol Immunol 2020; 17(3): 193-202.
        [http://dx.doi.org/10.1038/s41423-020-0367-1] [PMID: 32047259]

[69]   Smith T, Cunningham-Rundles C. Primary B-cell immunodeficiencies. Hum Immunol 2019; 80(6): 351-62.
        [http://dx.doi.org/10.1016/j.humimm.2018.10.015] [PMID: 30359632]

[70]   Schatz DG, Ji Y. Recombination centres and the orchestration of V(D)J recombination. Nat Rev Immunol 2011; 11(4): 251-63.
        [http://dx.doi.org/10.1038/nri2941] [PMID: 21394103]

[71]   Wang XS, Lee BJ, Zha S. The recent advances in non-homologous end-joining through the lens of lymphocyte development. DNA Repair (Amst) 2020; 94: 102874.
        [http://dx.doi.org/10.1016/j.dnarep.2020.102874] [PMID: 32623318]

[72]   Dvorak CC, Cowan MJ. Radiosensitive severe combined immunodeficiency disease. Immunol Allergy Clin North Am 2010; 30(1): 125-42.
        [http://dx.doi.org/10.1016/j.iac.2009.10.004] [PMID: 20113890]

[73] Slatter MA, Gennery AR. Update on DNA-Double Strand Break Repair Defects in Combined Primary Immunodeficiency. Curr Allergy Asthma Rep 2020; 20(10): 57.
[http://dx.doi.org/10.1007/s11882-020-00955-z] [PMID: 32648006]

[74] Fayez EA, Qazvini FF, Mahmoudi SM, Khoei S, Vesaltalab M, Teimourian S. Diagnosis of radiosensitive severe combined immunodeficiency disease (RS-SCID) by Comet Assay, management of bone marrow transplantation. Immunobiology 2020; 225(3): 151961.
[http://dx.doi.org/10.1016/j.imbio.2020.151961] [PMID: 32517885]

[75] Cebrat M, Miazek A, Kisielow P. Identification of a third evolutionarily conserved gene within the RAG locus and its RAG1-dependent and -independent regulation. Eur J Immunol 2005; 35(7): 2230-8.
[http://dx.doi.org/10.1002/eji.200526225] [PMID: 15971274]

[76] Kuo TC, Schlissel MS. Mechanisms controlling expression of the RAG locus during lymphocyte development. Curr Opin Immunol 2009; 21(2): 173-8.
[http://dx.doi.org/10.1016/j.coi.2009.03.008] [PMID: 19359154]

[77] Sniezewski L, Janik S, Laszkiewicz A, Majkowski M, Kisielow P, Cebrat M. The evolutionary conservation of the bidirectional activity of the NWC gene promoter in jawed vertebrates and the domestication of the RAG transposon. Dev Comp Immunol 2018; 81: 105-15.
[http://dx.doi.org/10.1016/j.dci.2017.11.013] [PMID: 29175053]

[78] Bulkhi AA, Dasso JF, Schuetz C, Walter JE. Approaches to patients with variants in *RAG* genes: from diagnosis to timely treatment. Expert Rev Clin Immunol 2019; 15(10): 1033-46.
[http://dx.doi.org/10.1080/1744666X.2020.1670060] [PMID: 31535575]

[79] Delmonte OM, Villa A, Notarangelo LD. Immune dysregulation in patients with RAG deficiency and other forms of combined immune deficiency. Blood 2020; 135(9): 610-9.
[http://dx.doi.org/10.1182/blood.2019000923] [PMID: 31942628]

[80] Kwong PC, O'Marcaigh AS, Howard R, Cowan MJ, Frieden IJ. Oral and genital ulceration: a unique presentation of immunodeficiency in Athabascan-speaking American Indian children with severe combined immunodeficiency. Arch Dermatol 1999; 135(8): 927-31.
[http://dx.doi.org/10.1001/archderm.135.8.927] [PMID: 10456341]

[81] Li L, Moshous D, Zhou Y, *et al.* A founder mutation in Artemis, an SNM1-like protein, causes SCID in Athabascan-speaking Native Americans. J Immunol 2002; 168(12): 6323-9.
[http://dx.doi.org/10.4049/jimmunol.168.12.6323] [PMID: 12055248]

[82] Felgentreff K, Lee YN, Frugoni F, *et al.* Functional analysis of naturally occurring DCLRE1C mutations and correlation with the clinical phenotype of ARTEMIS deficiency. J Allergy Clin Immunol 2015; 136(1): 140-150.e7.
[http://dx.doi.org/10.1016/j.jaci.2015.03.005] [PMID: 25917813]

[83] Lee PP, Woodbine L, Gilmour KC, *et al.* The many faces of Artemis-deficient combined immunodeficiency - Two patients with *DCLRE1C* mutations and a systematic literature review of genotype-phenotype correlation. Clin Immunol 2013; 149(3): 464-74.
[http://dx.doi.org/10.1016/j.clim.2013.08.006] [PMID: 24230999]

[84] van der Burg M, van Dongen JJ, van Gent DC. DNA-PKcs deficiency in human: long predicted, finally found. Curr Opin Allergy Clin Immunol 2009; 9(6): 503-9.
[http://dx.doi.org/10.1097/ACI.0b013e3283327e41] [PMID: 19823081]

[85] Esenboga S, Akal C, Karaatmaca B, *et al.* Two siblings with PRKDC defect who presented with cutaneous granulomas and review of the literature. Clin Immunol 2018; 197: 1-5.
[http://dx.doi.org/10.1016/j.clim.2018.08.002] [PMID: 30121298]

[86] Staines Boone AT, Chinn IK, Alaez-Versón C, *et al.* Failing to Make Ends Meet: The Broad Clinical Spectrum of DNA Ligase IV Deficiency. Case Series and Review of the Literature. Front Pediatr 2019; 6: 426.
[http://dx.doi.org/10.3389/fped.2018.00426] [PMID: 30719430]

[87]   Madhu R, Beaman GM, Chandler KE, *et al.* Ligase IV syndrome can present with microcephaly and radial ray anomalies similar to Fanconi anaemia plus fatal kidney malformations. Eur J Med Genet 2020; 63(9): 103974.
[http://dx.doi.org/10.1016/j.ejmg.2020.103974]

[88]   Buck D, Malivert L, de Chasseval R, *et al.* Cernunnos, a novel nonhomologous end-joining factor, is mutated in human immunodeficiency with microcephaly. Cell 2006; 124(2): 287-99.
[http://dx.doi.org/10.1016/j.cell.2005.12.030] [PMID: 16439204]

[89]   Yazdani R, Abolhassani H, Tafaroji J, *et al.* Cernunnos deficiency associated with BCG adenitis and autoimmunity: First case from the national Iranian registry and review of the literature. Clin Immunol 2017; 183: 201-6.
[http://dx.doi.org/10.1016/j.clim.2017.07.007] [PMID: 28729231]

[90]   Gaud G, Lesourne R, Love PE. Regulatory mechanisms in T cell receptor signalling. Nat Rev Immunol 2018; 18(8): 485-97.
[http://dx.doi.org/10.1038/s41577-018-0020-8] [PMID: 29789755]

[91]   de Saint Basile G, Geissmann F, Flori E, *et al.* Severe combined immunodeficiency caused by deficiency in either the delta or the epsilon subunit of CD3. J Clin Invest 2004; 114(10): 1512-7.
[http://dx.doi.org/10.1172/JCI200422588] [PMID: 15546002]

[92]   Roberts JL, Lauritsen JP, Cooney M, *et al.* T⁻B⁺NK⁺ severe combined immunodeficiency caused by complete deficiency of the CD3zeta subunit of the T-cell antigen receptor complex. Blood 2007; 109(8): 3198-206.
[http://dx.doi.org/10.1182/blood-2006-08-043166] [PMID: 17170122]

[93]   Erman B, Fırtına S, Fışgın T, Bozkurt C, Çipe FE. Biallelic Form of a Known *CD3E* Mutation in a Patient with Severe Combined Immunodeficiency. J Clin Immunol 2020; 40(3): 539-42.
[http://dx.doi.org/10.1007/s10875-020-00752-3] [PMID: 32016651]

[94]   Tokgoz H, Caliskan U, Keles S, Reisli I, Guiu IS, Morgan NV. Variable presentation of primary immune deficiency: two cases with CD3 gamma deficiency presenting with only autoimmunity. Pediatr Allergy Immunol 2013; 24(3): 257-62.
[http://dx.doi.org/10.1111/pai.12063] [PMID: 23590417]

[95]   Keller B, Zaidman I, Yousefi OS, *et al.* Early onset combined immunodeficiency and autoimmunity in patients with loss-of-function mutation in *LAT.* J Exp Med 2016; 213(7): 1185-99.
[http://dx.doi.org/10.1084/jem.20151110] [PMID: 27242165]

[96]   Bacchelli C, Moretti FA, Carmo M, *et al.* Mutations in linker for activation of T cells *(LAT)* lead to a novel form of severe combined immunodeficiency. J Allergy Clin Immunol 2017; 139(2): 634-642.e5.
[http://dx.doi.org/10.1016/j.jaci.2016.05.036] [PMID: 27522155]

[97]   Cale CM, Klein NJ, Novelli V, Veys P, Jones AM, Morgan G. Severe combined immunodeficiency with abnormalities in expression of the common leucocyte antigen, CD45. Arch Dis Child 1997; 76(2): 163-4.
[http://dx.doi.org/10.1136/adc.76.2.163] [PMID: 9068311]

[98]   Tchilian EZ, Beverley PC. Altered CD45 expression and disease. Trends Immunol 2006; 27(3): 146-53.
[http://dx.doi.org/10.1016/j.it.2006.01.001] [PMID: 16423560]

[99]   Arpaia E, Shahar M, Dadi H, Cohen A, Roifman CM. Defective T cell receptor signaling and CD8⁺ thymic selection in humans lacking zap-70 kinase. Cell 1994; 76(5): 947-58.
[http://dx.doi.org/10.1016/0092-8674(94)90368-9] [PMID: 8124727]

[100] Sharifinejad N, Jamee M, Zaki-Dizaji M, *et al.* Clinical, Immunological, and Genetic Features in 49 Patients With ZAP-70 Deficiency: A Systematic Review. Front Immunol 2020; 11: 831.
[http://dx.doi.org/10.3389/fimmu.2020.00831] [PMID: 32431715]

[101] Hoenig M, Lagresle-Peyrou C, Pannicke U, *et al.* Reticular dysgenesis: international survey on clinical

presentation, transplantation, and outcome. Blood 2017; 129(21): 2928-38.
[http://dx.doi.org/10.1182/blood-2016-11-745638] [PMID: 28331055]

[102] Hoenig M, Pannicke U, Gaspar HB, Schwarz K. Recent advances in understanding the pathogenesis and management of reticular dysgenesis. Br J Haematol 2018; 180(5): 644-53.
[http://dx.doi.org/10.1111/bjh.15045] [PMID: 29270983]

[103] Ghaloul-Gonzalez L, Mohsen AW, Karunanidhi A, *et al.* Reticular Dysgenesis and Mitochondriopathy Induced by Adenylate Kinase 2 Deficiency with Atypical Presentation. Sci Rep 2019; 9(1): 15739.
[http://dx.doi.org/10.1038/s41598-019-51922-2] [PMID: 31673062]

[104] Bradford KL, Moretti FA, Carbonaro-Sarracino DA, Gaspar HB, Kohn DB. Adenosine Deaminase (ADA)-Deficient Severe Combined Immune Deficiency (SCID): Molecular Pathogenesis and Clinical Manifestations. J Clin Immunol 2017; 37(7): 626-37.
[http://dx.doi.org/10.1007/s10875-017-0433-3] [PMID: 28842866]

[105] la Marca G, Giocaliere E, Malvagia S, *et al.* The inclusion of ADA-SCID in expanded newborn screening by tandem mass spectrometry. J Pharm Biomed Anal 2014; 88: 201-6.
[http://dx.doi.org/10.1016/j.jpba.2013.08.044] [PMID: 24076575]

[106] Adams SP, Wilson M, Harb E, *et al.* Spectrum of mutations in a cohort of UK patients with ADA deficient SCID: Segregation of genotypes with specific ethnicities. Clin Immunol 2015; 161(2): 174-9.
[http://dx.doi.org/10.1016/j.clim.2015.08.001] [PMID: 26255240]

[107] Kohn DB, Hershfield MS, Puck JM, *et al.* Consensus approach for the management of severe combined immune deficiency caused by adenosine deaminase deficiency. J Allergy Clin Immunol 2019; 143(3): 852-63.
[http://dx.doi.org/10.1016/j.jaci.2018.08.024] [PMID: 30194989]

[108] Pieters J, Müller P, Jayachandran R. On guard: coronin proteins in innate and adaptive immunity. Nat Rev Immunol 2013; 13(7): 510-8.
[http://dx.doi.org/10.1038/nri3465]

[109] Stray-Pedersen A, Jouanguy E, Crequer A, *et al.* Compound heterozygous *CORO1A* mutations in siblings with a mucocutaneous-immunodeficiency syndrome of epidermodysplasia verruciformis-HPV, molluscum contagiosum and granulomatous tuberculoid leprosy. J Clin Immunol 2014; 34(7): 871-90.
[http://dx.doi.org/10.1007/s10875-014-0074-8] [PMID: 25073507]

[110] Notarangelo LD. Multiple intestinal atresia with combined immune deficiency. Curr Opin Pediatr 2014; 26(6): 690-6.
[http://dx.doi.org/10.1097/MOP.0000000000000159] [PMID: 25268403]

[111] Yang W, Lee PP, Thong MK, *et al.* Compound heterozygous mutations in *TTC7A* cause familial multiple intestinal atresias and severe combined immunodeficiency. Clin Genet 2015; 88(6): 542-9.
[http://dx.doi.org/10.1111/cge.12553] [PMID: 25534311]

[112] Cossu F, Vulliamy TJ, Marrone A, Badiali M, Cao A, Dokal I. A novel *DKC1* mutation, severe combined immunodeficiency (T⁻B⁻NK⁻ SCID) and bone marrow transplantation in an infant with Hoyeraal-Hreidarsson syndrome. Br J Haematol 2002; 119(3): 765-8.
[http://dx.doi.org/10.1046/j.1365-2141.2002.03822.x] [PMID: 12437656]

[113] Borzutzky A, Crompton B, Bergmann AK, *et al.* Reversible severe combined immunodeficiency phenotype secondary to a mutation of the proton-coupled folate transporter. Clin Immunol 2009; 133(3): 287-94.
[http://dx.doi.org/10.1016/j.clim.2009.08.006] [PMID: 19740703]

[114] Mehawej C, Khalife H, Hanna-Wakim R, Dbaibo G, Farra C. DNMT3B deficiency presenting as severe combined immune deficiency: A case report. Clin Immunol 2020; 215: 108453.
[http://dx.doi.org/10.1016/j.clim.2020.108453] [PMID: 32360517]

[115] Somech R, Lev A, Grisaru-Soen G, Shiran SI, Simon AJ, Grunebaum E. Purine nucleoside

phosphorylase deficiency presenting as severe combined immune deficiency. Immunol Res 2013; 56(1): 150-4.
[http://dx.doi.org/10.1007/s12026-012-8380-9] [PMID: 23371835]

[116] Fekrvand S, Yazdani R, Abolhassani H, Ghaffari J, Aghamohammadi A. The First Purine Nucleoside Phosphorylase Deficiency Patient Resembling IgA Deficiency and a Review of the Literature. Immunol Invest 2019; 48(4): 410-30.
[http://dx.doi.org/10.1080/08820139.2019.1570249] [PMID: 30885031]

[117] la Marca G, Canessa C, Giocaliere E, *et al.* Diagnosis of immunodeficiency caused by a purine nucleoside phosphorylase defect by using tandem mass spectrometry on dried blood spots. J Allergy Clin Immunol 2014; 134(1): 155-9.
[http://dx.doi.org/10.1016/j.jaci.2014.01.040] [PMID: 24767876]

[118] Lacruz RS, Feske S. Diseases caused by mutations in *ORAI1* and *STIM1*. Ann N Y Acad Sci 2015; 1356(1): 45-79.
[http://dx.doi.org/10.1111/nyas.12938] [PMID: 26469693]

[119] Farrokhi S, Shabani M, Aryan Z, *et al.* MHC class II deficiency: Report of a novel mutation and special review. Allergol Immunopathol (Madr) 2018; 46(3): 263-75.
[http://dx.doi.org/10.1016/j.aller.2017.04.006] [PMID: 28676232]

[120] Lum SH, Anderson C, McNaughton P, *et al.* Improved transplant survival and long-term disease outcome in children with MHC class II deficiency. Blood 2020; 135(12): 954-73.
[http://dx.doi.org/10.1182/blood.2019002690] [PMID: 31932845]

[121] Kavadas FD, Giliani S, Gu Y, *et al.* Variability of clinical and laboratory features among patients with ribonuclease mitochondrial RNA processing endoribonuclease gene mutations. J Allergy Clin Immunol 2008; 122(6): 1178-84.
[http://dx.doi.org/10.1016/j.jaci.2008.07.036] [PMID: 18804272]

[122] Ip W, Gaspar HB, Kleta R, *et al.* Variable phenotype of severe immunodeficiencies associated with *RMRP* gene mutations. J Clin Immunol 2015; 35(2): 147-57.
[http://dx.doi.org/10.1007/s10875-015-0135-7] [PMID: 25663137]

[123] Vakkilainen S, Taskinen M, Mäkitie O. Immunodeficiency in cartilage-hair hypoplasia: Pathogenesis, clinical course and management. Scand J Immunol 2020; 92(4): e12913.
[http://dx.doi.org/10.1111/sji.12913] [PMID: 32506568]

[124] Kadouri N, Nevo S, Goldfarb Y, Abramson J. Thymic epithelial cell heterogeneity: TEC by TEC. Nat Rev Immunol 2020; 20(4): 239-53.
[http://dx.doi.org/10.1038/s41577-019-0238-0] [PMID: 31804611]

[125] Gallo V, Cirillo E, Giardino G, Pignata C. FOXN1 Deficiency: from the Discovery to Novel Therapeutic Approaches. J Clin Immunol 2017; 37(8): 751-8.
[http://dx.doi.org/10.1007/s10875-017-0445-z] [PMID: 28932937]

[126] Paganini I, Sestini R, Capone GL, *et al.* A novel *PAX1* null homozygous mutation in autosomal recessive otofaciocervical syndrome associated with severe combined immunodeficiency. Clin Genet 2017; 92(6): 664-8.
[http://dx.doi.org/10.1111/cge.13085] [PMID: 28657137]

[127] Yamazaki Y, Urrutia R, Franco LM, *et al.* PAX1 is essential for development and function of the human thymus. Sci Immunol 2020; 5(44): eaax1036.
[http://dx.doi.org/10.1126/sciimmunol.aax1036] [PMID: 32111619]

[128] McDonald-McGinn DM, Sullivan KE, Marino B, *et al.* 22q11.2 deletion syndrome. Nat Rev Dis Primers 2015; 1(1): 15071.
[http://dx.doi.org/10.1038/nrdp.2015.71] [PMID: 27189754]

[129] Liao HC, Liao CH, Kao SM, Chiang CC, Chen YJ. Detecting 22q11.2 Deletion Syndrome in Newborns with Low T Cell Receptor Excision Circles from Severe Combined Immunodeficiency

Screening. J Pediatr 2019; 204: 219-224.e1.
[http://dx.doi.org/10.1016/j.jpeds.2018.08.072] [PMID: 30268402]

[130] Markert ML, Devlin BH, McCarthy EA. Thymus transplantation. Clin Immunol 2010; 135(2): 236-46.
[http://dx.doi.org/10.1016/j.clim.2010.02.007]

[131] Davies EG, Cheung M, Gilmour K, *et al.* Thymus transplantation for complete DiGeorge syndrome: European experience. J Allergy Clin Immunol 2017; 140(6): 1660-1670.e16.
[http://dx.doi.org/10.1016/j.jaci.2017.03.020] [PMID: 28400115]

[132] McGhee SA, Lloret MG, Stiehm ER. Immunologic reconstitution in 22q deletion (DiGeorge) syndrome. Immunol Res 2009; 45(1): 37-45.
[http://dx.doi.org/10.1007/s12026-009-8108-7] [PMID: 19238335]

[133] Janda A, Sedlacek P, Hönig M, *et al.* Multicenter survey on the outcome of transplantation of hematopoietic cells in patients with the complete form of DiGeorge anomaly. Blood 2010; 116(13): 2229-36.
[http://dx.doi.org/10.1182/blood-2010-03-275966] [PMID: 20530285]

[134] Punwani D, Zhang Y, Yu J, *et al.* Multisystem Anomalies in Severe Combined Immunodeficiency with Mutant *BCL11B*. N Engl J Med 2016; 375(22): 2165-76.
[http://dx.doi.org/10.1056/NEJMoa1509164] [PMID: 27959755]

[135] Dvorak CC, Haddad E, Buckley RH, *et al.* The genetic landscape of severe combined immunodeficiency in the United States and Canada in the current era (2010-2018). J Allergy Clin Immunol 2019; 143(1): 405-7.
[http://dx.doi.org/10.1016/j.jaci.2018.08.027] [PMID: 30193840]

[136] Lagresle-Peyrou C, Luce S, Ouchani F, *et al.* X-linked primary immunodeficiency associated with hemizygous mutations in the moesin (MSN) gene. J Allergy Clin Immunol 2016; 138(6): 1681-1689.e8.
[http://dx.doi.org/10.1016/j.jaci.2016.04.032] [PMID: 27405666]

[137] Aluri J, Desai M, Gupta M, *et al.* Clinical, Immunological, and Molecular Findings in 57 Patients With Severe Combined Immunodeficiency (SCID) From India. Front Immunol 2019; 10: 23.
[http://dx.doi.org/10.3389/fimmu.2019.00023] [PMID: 30778343]

[138] Shahbazi Z, Yazdani R, Shahkarami S, *et al.* Genetic mutations and immunological features of severe combined immunodeficiency patients in Iran. Immunol Lett 2019; 216: 70-8.
[http://dx.doi.org/10.1016/j.imlet.2019.10.001] [PMID: 31589898]

[139] Frizinsky S, Rechavi E, Barel O, *et al.* Novel *MALT1* Mutation Linked to Immunodeficiency, Immune Dysregulation, and an Abnormal T Cell Receptor Repertoire. J Clin Immunol 2019; 39(4): 401-13.
[http://dx.doi.org/10.1007/s10875-019-00629-0] [PMID: 31037583]

[140] Cirillo E, Cancrini C, Azzari C, *et al.* Clinical, Immunological, and Molecular Features of Typical and Atypical Severe Combined Immunodeficiency: Report of the Italian Primary Immunodeficiency Network. Front Immunol 2019; 10: 1908.
[http://dx.doi.org/10.3389/fimmu.2019.01908] [PMID: 31456805]

[141] Lopez-Granados E, Keenan JE, Kinney MC, *et al.* A novel mutation in *NFKBIA/IKBA* results in a degradation-resistant N-truncated protein and is associated with ectodermal dysplasia with immunodeficiency. Hum Mutat 2008; 29(6): 861-8.
[http://dx.doi.org/10.1002/humu.20740] [PMID: 18412279]

[142] Medawar P. Nobel Lecture 1960.https://www.nobelprize.org/prizes/medicine/1960/medawar/lecture/

[143] Miller JF. Effect of neonatal thymectomy on the immunological responsiveness of the mouse. Proc R Soc Lond B Biol Sci 1962; 156: 410-28.

[144] Park JE, Jardine L, Gottgens B, Teichmann SA, Haniffa M. Prenatal development of human immunity. Science 2020; 368(6491): 600-3.
[http://dx.doi.org/10.1126/science.aaz9330] [PMID: 32381715]

[145] Mold JE, Michaëlsson J, Burt TD, *et al.* Maternal alloantigens promote the development of tolerogenic fetal regulatory T cells in utero. Science 2008; 322(5907): 1562-5.
[http://dx.doi.org/10.1126/science.1164511] [PMID: 19056990]

[146] Buckley RH. SCID: A Pediatric Emergency. N C Med J 2019; 80(1): 55-6.
[http://dx.doi.org/10.18043/ncm.80.1.55] [PMID: 30622209]

[147] Raspa M, Lynch M, Squiers L, *et al.* Information and Emotional Support Needs of Families Whose Infant Was Diagnosed With SCID Through Newborn Screening. Front Immunol 2020; 11: 885.
[http://dx.doi.org/10.3389/fimmu.2020.00885] [PMID: 32435251]

[148] Mandola AB, Reid B, Sirror R, *et al.* Ataxia Telangiectasia Diagnosed on Newborn Screening-Case Cohort of 5 Years' Experience. Front Immunol 2019; 10: 2940.
[http://dx.doi.org/10.3389/fimmu.2019.02940] [PMID: 31921190]

[149] Madkaikar M, Aluri J, Gupta S. Guidelines for Screening, Early Diagnosis and Management of Severe Combined Immunodeficiency (SCID) in India. Indian J Pediatr 2016; 83(5): 455-62.
[http://dx.doi.org/10.1007/s12098-016-2059-5] [PMID: 26920398]

[150] Maecker HT, McCoy JP, Nussenblatt R. Standardizing immunophenotyping for the Human Immunology Project. Nat Rev Immunol 2012; 12(3): 191-200.
[http://dx.doi.org/10.1038/nri3158] [PMID: 22343568]

[151] Chinn IK, Chan AY, Chen K, *et al.* Diagnostic interpretation of genetic studies in patients with primary immunodeficiency diseases: A working group report of the Primary Immunodeficiency Diseases Committee of the American Academy of Allergy, Asthma & Immunology. J Allergy Clin Immunol 2020; 145(1): 46-69.
[http://dx.doi.org/10.1016/j.jaci.2019.09.009] [PMID: 31568798]

[152] Gatti RA, Meuwissen HJ, Allen HD, Hong R, Good RA. Immunological reconstitution of sex- linked lymphopenic immunological deficiency. Lancet 1968; 2(7583): 1366-9.

[153] Pai SY, Logan BR, Griffith LM, *et al.* Transplantation outcomes for severe combined immunodeficiency, 2000-2009. N Engl J Med 2014; 371(5): 434-46.
[http://dx.doi.org/10.1056/NEJMoa1401177] [PMID: 25075835]

[154] Heimall J, Logan BR, Cowan MJ, *et al.* Immune reconstitution and survival of 100 SCID patients post-hematopoietic cell transplant: a PIDTC natural history study. Blood 2017; 130(25): 2718-27.
[http://dx.doi.org/10.1182/blood-2017-05-781849] [PMID: 29021228]

[155] Heimall J, Buckley RH, Puck J, *et al.* Recommendations for Screening and Management of Late Effects in Patients with Severe Combined Immunodeficiency after Allogenic Hematopoietic Cell Transplantation: A Consensus Statement from the Second Pediatric Blood and Marrow Transplant Consortium International Conference on Late Effects after Pediatric HCT. Biol Blood Marrow Transplant 2017; 23(8): 1229-40.
[http://dx.doi.org/10.1016/j.bbmt.2017.04.026] [PMID: 28479164]

[156] Haddad E, Logan BR, Griffith LM, *et al.* SCID genotype and 6-month posttransplant CD4 count predict survival and immune recovery. Blood 2018; 132(17): 1737-49.
[http://dx.doi.org/10.1182/blood-2018-03-840702] [PMID: 30154114]

[157] Horn B, Cowan MJ. Unresolved issues in hematopoietic stem cell transplantation for severe combined immunodeficiency: need for safer conditioning and reduced late effects. J Allergy Clin Immunol 2013; 131(5): 1306-11.
[http://dx.doi.org/10.1016/j.jaci.2013.03.014] [PMID: 23622119]

[158] Gennery AR, Lankester A. Long Term Outcome and Immune Function After Hematopoietic Stem Cell Transplantation for Primary Immunodeficiency. Front Pediatr 2019; 7: 381.
[http://dx.doi.org/10.3389/fped.2019.00381] [PMID: 31616648]

[159] Puck JM. Population-based newborn screening for severe combined immunodeficiency: steps toward implementation. J Allergy Clin Immunol 2007; 120(4): 760-8.

[http://dx.doi.org/10.1016/j.jaci.2007.08.043] [PMID: 17931561]

[160] Bertaina A, Merli P, Rutella S, *et al.* HLA-haploidentical stem cell transplantation after removal of αβ⁻ T and B cells in children with nonmalignant disorders. Blood 2014; 124(5): 822-6.
[http://dx.doi.org/10.1182/blood-2014-03-563817] [PMID: 24869942]

[161] Li Pira G, Malaspina D, Girolami E, *et al.* Selective Depletion of αβ T Cells and B Cells for Human Leukocyte Antigen-Haploidentical Hematopoietic Stem Cell Transplantation. A Three-Year Follow-Up of Procedure Efficiency. Biol Blood Marrow Transplant 2016; 22(11): 2056-64.
[http://dx.doi.org/10.1016/j.bbmt.2016.08.006] [PMID: 27519279]

[162] Sahasrabudhe K, Otto M, Hematti P, Kenkre V. TCR αβ⁺/CD19⁺ cell depletion in haploidentical hematopoietic allogeneic stem cell transplantation: a review of current data. Leuk Lymphoma 2019; 60(3): 598-609.
[http://dx.doi.org/10.1080/10428194.2018.1485905] [PMID: 30187806]

[163] Castagnoli R, Delmonte OM, Calzoni E, Notarangelo LD. Hematopoietic Stem Cell Transplantation in Primary Immunodeficiency Diseases: Current Status and Future Perspectives. Front Pediatr 2019; 7: 295.
[http://dx.doi.org/10.3389/fped.2019.00295] [PMID: 31440487]

[164] Gennery AR, Albert MH, Slatter MA, Lankester A. Hematopoietic Stem Cell Transplantation for Primary Immunodeficiencies. Front Pediatr 2019; 7: 445.
[http://dx.doi.org/10.3389/fped.2019.00445] [PMID: 31737589]

[165] Schuetz C, Neven B, Dvorak CC, *et al.* SCID patients with ARTEMIS *vs* RAG deficiencies following HCT: increased risk of late toxicity in ARTEMIS-deficient SCID. Blood 2014; 123(2): 281-9.
[http://dx.doi.org/10.1182/blood-2013-01-476432] [PMID: 24144642]

[166] Staal FJT, Aiuti A, Cavazzana M. Autologous Stem-Cell-Based Gene Therapy for Inherited Disorders: State of the Art and Perspectives. Front Pediatr 2019; 7: 443.
[http://dx.doi.org/10.3389/fped.2019.00443] [PMID: 31737588]

[167] Cavazzana M, Bushman FD, Miccio A, André-Schmutz I, Six E. Gene therapy targeting haematopoietic stem cells for inherited diseases: progress and challenges. Nat Rev Drug Discov 2019; 18(6): 447-62.
[http://dx.doi.org/10.1038/s41573-019-0020-9] [PMID: 30858502]

[168] Kuo CY, Kohn DB. Overview of the current status of gene therapy for primary immune deficiencies (PIDs). J Allergy Clin Immunol 2020; 146(2): 229-33.
[http://dx.doi.org/10.1016/j.jaci.2020.05.024] [PMID: 32771134]

[169] Bradford KL, Liu S, Krajinovic M, *et al.* Busulfan Pharmacokinetics in Adenosine Deaminase-Deficient Severe Combined Immunodeficiency Gene Therapy. Biol Blood Marrow Transplant 2020; S1083-8791(20): 30413-4.

[170] Tucci F, Frittoli M, Barzaghi F, *et al.* Bone marrow harvesting from paediatric patients undergoing haematopoietic stem cell gene therapy. Bone Marrow Transplant 2019; 54(12): 1995-2003.
[http://dx.doi.org/10.1038/s41409-019-0573-6] [PMID: 31150018]

[171] Lewis PF, Emerman M. Passage through mitosis is required for oncoretroviruses but not for the human immunodeficiency virus. J Virol 1994; 68(1): 510-6.

[172] Cicalese MP, Ferrua F, Castagnaro L, *et al.* Gene Therapy for Adenosine Deaminase Deficiency: A Comprehensive Evaluation of Short- and Medium-Term Safety. Mol Ther 2018; 26(3): 917-31.
[http://dx.doi.org/10.1016/j.ymthe.2017.12.022] [PMID: 29433935]

[173] Howe SJ, Mansour MR, Schwarzwaelder K, *et al.* Insertional mutagenesis combined with acquired somatic mutations causes leukemogenesis following gene therapy of SCID-X1 patients. J Clin Invest 2008; 118(9): 3143-50.
[http://dx.doi.org/10.1172/JCI35798] [PMID: 18688286]

[174] Hacein-Bey-Abina S, Pai SY, Gaspar HB, *et al.* A modified γ-retrovirus vector for X-linked severe

combined immunodeficiency. N Engl J Med 2014; 371(15): 1407-17.
[http://dx.doi.org/10.1056/NEJMoa1404588] [PMID: 25295500]

[175] De Ravin SS, Wu X, Moir S, *et al.* Lentiviral hematopoietic stem cell gene therapy for X-linked severe combined immunodeficiency. Sci Transl Med 2016; 8(335): 335ra57.
[http://dx.doi.org/10.1126/scitranslmed.aad8856] [PMID: 27099176]

[176] Mamcarz E, Zhou S, Lockey T, *et al.* Lentiviral Gene Therapy Combined with Low-Dose Busulfan in Infants with SCID-X1. N Engl J Med 2019; 380(16): 1525-34.
[http://dx.doi.org/10.1056/NEJMoa1815408] [PMID: 30995372]

[177] Cowan MJ, Yu J, Facchino J, *et al.* Early Outcome of a Phase I/II Clinical Trial (NCT03538899) of Gene-Corrected Autologous CD34+ Hematopoietic Cells and Low- Exposure Busulfan in Newly Diagnosed Patients with Artemis-Deficient Severe Combined Immunodeficiency (ART-SCID). Biol Blood Marrow Transplant 2020; 26(3) (Suppl.): S88-9.
[http://dx.doi.org/10.1016/j.bbmt.2019.12.589]

[178] Sorrentino BP, Lu TH, Ihle J, Buckley RH, Cunningham JM. A clinical attempt to treat JAK3-deficient SCID using retroviral-mediated gene transfer to bone marrow CD34+ cells. Mol Ther 2003; 7(5): S449-.

[179] Garcia-Perez L, van Eggermond M, van Roon L, *et al.* Successful Preclinical Development of Gene Therapy for Recombinase-Activating Gene-1-Deficient SCID. Mol Ther Methods Clin Dev 2020; 17: 666-82.
[http://dx.doi.org/10.1016/j.omtm.2020.03.016] [PMID: 32322605]

[180] Capo V, Castiello MC, Fontana E, *et al.* Efficacy of lentivirus-mediated gene therapy in an Omenn syndrome recombination-activating gene 2 mouse model is not hindered by inflammation and immune dysregulation. J Allergy Clin Immunol 2018; 142(3): 928-941.e8.
[http://dx.doi.org/10.1016/j.jaci.2017.11.015] [PMID: 29241731]

CHAPTER 12

Updates on PFAPA- Periodic Fever, Aphthous Stomatitis, Pharyngitis, and Cervical Adenitis Syndrome

Beata Wolska-Kuśnierz[1,*] and **Bożena Mikołuć[2]**

[1] *Immunology Department, Children's Memorial Health Institute, Av. Dzieci Polskich 20, 04-730 Warsaw, Poland*

[2] *Department of Pediatrics, Rheumatology, Immunology and Metabolic Bone Diseases, Medical University of Bialystok, Waszyngtona 17 Str., 15-274 Bialystok, Poland*

Abstract: PFAPA- Periodic Fever, Aphthous Stomatitis, Pharyngitis, and Cervical Adenitis syndrome are the most common autoinflammatory syndromes in children. In this chapter, the characteristic manifestation and clinical criteria of PFAPA, which remain the basis of diagnosis, are presented. The therapeutic options and prognosis are discussed in detail.

Keywords: Adenitis, Anakinra, Aphthous stomatitis, Autoinflammation, Colchicine, Interleukin-1, Interleukin-1 blockers, Marshall syndrome, Periodic fevers, PFAPA, Pharyngitis, Tonsillectomy, Tonsillotomy.

INTRODUCTION

PFAPA syndrome, firstly described in 1987 by Marshall et al., is the most common among the auto-inflammatory diseases of childhood [1, 2]. The name is derived from the first letters of the main clinical symptoms: **P**eriodic **F**ever, **A**phthous stomatitis, **P**haryngitis, and Cervical **A**denitis. Despite the passage of more than 30 years, knowledge about the pathogenesis of the syndrome remains still limited. We currently include PFAPA in the group of autoinflammatory diseases caused by polygenic or complex inheritance of variants in many genes in association with environmental factors. There appears to be no predilection for a particular ethnic or racial group, although male predominance for a particular ethnic group was established [3 - 5]. The concept of auto-inflammation was proposed by Kastner in 1999, and it included genetically determined disorders of

---
* **Corresponding author Beata Wolska-Kuśnierz:** Immunology Department, Children's Memorial Health Institute, Av.Dzieci Polskich 20, 04-730 Warsaw, Poland; Fax: +48 11 815 18 39; Email: b.wolska-kusnierz@ipczd.pl

Nima Rezaei and Noosha Samieefar (Eds.)

the innate immune system, manifested by recurrent fever with a different spectrum of accompanying symptoms. Auto-inflammatory diseases, in contrast to autoimmune disorders, are characterized by seemingly unprovoked, pathological activation of the innate immune system in the absence of autoantibodies or autoreactive T cells [6]. This new group of diseases has been dynamically developing in the last two decades and already covers several dozen disease entities, the number of which is systematically growing every year.

ETIOLOGY

PFAPA syndrome has no established genetic basis, may occur sporadically, but quite often, the family history of patients with recurrent fever, tonsillitis, recurrent streptococcal pharyngitis, tonsillectomy, and recurrent aphthous ulcers indicates the possibility of a genetic predisposition, perhaps of a multigenic nature. Although knowledge about PFAPA pathomechanism is still a puzzle, research indicates impaired functioning of the innate immune system. Similarly, as in other classical auto-inflammatory syndromes, the role of inflammasome over-activation and interleukin-1(Il-1) secretion during episodes of fever is underlined. In the course of relapses, IFN-gamma, IFN-gamma induced proteins (IP 10 also called CXCL10 for chemokine, CXC motif, ligand 10) and proteins induced by gamma interferon (MIG or CXCL9), G-CSF, TNF-alpha, and other proinflammatory cytokines (IL-1 beta, IL-6, IL-18) are elevated [7, 8]. Monocytes isolated from patients during fever secrete greater amounts of IL-1β after stimulation with LPS (lipopolysaccharides) compared to cells collected in the asymptomatic period and from healthy people [8 - 10]. Relapses of fever are accompanied by an increase in the number of neutrophils and monocytes and a decrease in the number of eosinophils and lymphocytes. Probably unknown environmental factors constitute a trigger mechanism to over-run the inflammatory response with activation of the complement and interleukins IL-1β/IL-18, with induction of Th1 response, followed by inhibition of the activated T lymphocytes in peripheral tissues. Long et al. hypothesized that the periodicity of the PFAPA syndrome derives from intermittent expression or suppression of antigens or epitopes of infectious agents or an alteration in the nature or kinetics of immunological response [11]. In spite of its strong familial clustering, the genetic basis and inheritance pattern of PFAFA are still unknown. Results of a relatively large cohort indicate that PFAPA syndrome is unlikely to be a monogenic condition [12]. Some variants of unknown significance in known auto-inflammatory-causing genes have been reported in PFAPA syndrome at higher frequency (also known as burden of variants). Best known examples include p.R121Q(R92Q) in TNF receptor superfamily member 1A (*TNFRSF1A*), heterozygosis or polymorphisms in the familial Mediterranean fever gene *MEFV*, mevalonate kinase *MVK* gene, or NLR family pyrin domain-containing 3 (*NLRP3*) [13].

In the literature, we found information about genetic similarities among PFAPA, recurrent aphthous stomatitis, and Behçet's disease. PFAPA shares risk loci at *IL12A, STAT4, IL10,* and *CCR1-CCR3* with Behçet's disease and recurrent aphthous stomatitis, defining a family of Behçet's spectrum disorders (BSDs). Manthiram and colleagues confirmed new class I and II *HLA* associations for PFAPA distinct from Behçet's disease and recurrent aphthous stomatitis, but HLA-B15 was identified as a risk allele for all of the BSDs [14]. All data suggest that PFAPA results from oligogenic or complex inheritance of variants in multiple disease genes and/or non-genetic factors. Because tonsillectomy is curative in most patients, there is a hypothesis that the palatine tonsils are the primary site of immune dysregulation in children with PFAPA. Tonsils of adult- and pediatric-onset in the asymptomatic PFAPA phase share unique histological features: smaller germinal center areas with a lower percentage of B lymphocytes, a higher percentage of CD8+ cytotoxic T lymphocytes and naïve T cells, and a lower percentage of CD4+ T cells with high expression of the inhibitory molecule PD-1 (programmed cell death 1) in germinal centers compared with controls [15 - 17]. In addition, high expression of T cell chemokines and proinflammatory cytokines in tonsils from patients with PFAPA was found [18].

CLINICAL MANIFESTATIONS

PFAPA is characterized by sudden onset of stereotypical episodes of fever, which persists for 3-6 days, resolves spontaneously, and regularly reoccurs every three to eight weeks; the average is approximately four weeks, alongside at least one of three main symptoms: aphthous stomatitis, cervical adenitis, and pharyngitis. It is an early-onset disease usually starting before the age of 5 years in 90% of patients [19]. The age of fever onset of adult patients with PFAPA is between 20 and 33 years of age. Fever episodes begin abruptly, and a temperature range from 38.5 to 41°C for two to seven days and then abruptly fall to normal. Episodes rarely last for more than seven days. Thus, prolonged fever episodes should prompt consideration of other diagnoses. It is important to confirm that the symptoms with each episode are nearly identical. There is male predominance but no predilection for a particular ethnic group [3]. However, an increasing number of adults with PFAPA have been diagnosed in recent years [4, 5]. Aphthous stomatitis, usually on the inner lips or buccal mucosa, occasionally in the posterior pharynx, is present in about 40-70% of children reported with PFAPA. Patients have had few to several non-clustered, small (<5 mm), shallow ulcers that heal over 5 to 10 days. In opposite to the ulcers of Behçet syndrome, aphthous ulcers in PFAPA are not as large or painful nor do they scar. Prodromal symptoms such as malaise, irritability, and fatigue may manifest during the preceding days. Typically, along with a fever, tonsillitis is observed. Tonsils are red inflammatory exudates with different morphology (photo 1 and 2). Their appearance may suggest both viral infections, including mononucleosis and bacterial, including streptococcal one. Enlarged cervical lymph nodes are moderately tender, rapidly appearing and regressing, but are bilateral, not exceeding 5 cm in diameter, not red or warm, and never fluctuant. Generalized lymphadenopathy or hepatosplenomegaly suggests a diagnosis other than PFAPA syndrome. Less common symptoms include headache, arthralgia, gastrointestinal disturbances: diarrhea, vomiting, abdominal pain. Adult patients with PFAPA are characterized by a wider repertoire of inflammatory signs and more likely to have arthralgias, myalgias, headache, chest pain, rashes and ocular signs, than regular pharyngitis.

DIAGNOSIS

The diagnosis of PFAPA syndrome still faces considerable difficulties. No diagnostic tests for PFAPA syndrome are available at the moment, so the diagnosis is initially based upon clinical history and physical exam findings. Therefore, it is often delayed, and its symptoms are frequently misinterpreted as upper respiratory infections, leading to an inappropriate therapeutic strategy, particularly antibiotic overuse. Nonspecific viral illnesses with fever are common in childhood and may occur as often as 5–10 times per year but are not periodic. In the Costagliola study, in more than half of patients (55%), the clinical phenotype was first interpreted as recurrent respiratory infections, which resulted in otolaryngologic or immunologic consultations [20]. The median time to diagnosis, since first symptoms, was 14.5 months, and 40% of patients received more than 5 cycles of antibiotic/year. The first step to establishing a diagnosis is paying attention to the recurrence and regularity of the observed symptoms. Recurrent fever syndromes, including PFAPA syndrome, can be considered in the differential diagnosis of febrile states only when symptoms are cyclical above 4-6 fever recurrences within 6-12 months 21. The diagnosis of PFAPA syndrome is currently defined according to the clinical criteria proposed by Marshall in 1989 and modified by Thomas et al. in 1999 [21, 22]. The cardinal feature is the child's complete wellness between episodes with no disturbances in growth and development. Duration of PFAPA for years, without progression, weighs heavily against infectious disease as causative. In case of doubts about whether the diagnostic criteria are met, patients should undergo genetic testing for monogenic auto-inflammatory diseases. Clinical manifestations of PFAPA syndrome largely overlap with those of monogenic auto-inflammatory diseases: Familial Mediterranean Fever (FMF), tumor necrosis factor (TNF) receptor-associated periodic syndrome (TRAPS), and mevalonate kinase deficiency (MKD). Moreover, Gattorno et al. found that a significant number of patients with monogenic periodic fevers also meet the diagnostic criteria for PFAPA syndrome, highlighting the poor specificity of the current classification criteria. A diagnostic score has been proposed to select those patients who should be tested for mutations of genes involved in monogenetic auto-inflammatory syndromes [23]. During flares, genetically positive patients had a higher frequency of abdominal pain, diarrhea, vomiting, cutaneous rash, arthralgia, and genetically negative patients had a higher frequency of pharyngitis. Particularly the presence of gastrointestinal manifestations and skin rash in patients fulfilling the current PFAFA criteria should orientate towards the exclusion of monogenic periodic fevers by molecular analysis [24]. In patients with aphthous stomatitis as a leading symptom, Behcet disease should be considered in the differential diagnosis. Aphthous stomatitis is usually the initial symptom of Behçet's disease and can predate other manifestations by years. In laboratory analysis, moderate leukocytosis with neutrophilia, monocytosis, and mild lymphopenia are seen. Erythrocyte sedimentation rate (ESR) and C-reactive protein (CRP) are usually persistently elevated during episodes. Between attacks, all inflammatory parameters normalize, sometimes increased platelets are observed. Procalcitonin concentrations usually do not increase proportionally to the increase in other acute-phase reactants, such as CRP, which may help discriminate PFAPA attacks from acute bacterial infections. Some PFAPA patients had elevated serum concentrations of immunoglobulin D (IgD) during flares but not as high as in the hyper-IgD syndrome (HIDS) [25]. The other immunoglobulin (Ig) levels, IgG, IgM, and IgA, stayed within the normal range. All patients should be screened by serial white blood counts toward cyclic neutropenia. The use of genetic testing can be justified for differential diagnosis in the cases of PFAPA displaying a classical manifestation but without spontaneous remission before adulthood.

TREATMENT

To date, no completely satisfactory treatment options exist. There is no evidence that medical treatment can modify the outcome, but it can be efficacious for treating the episodes. Inducing a rapid remission of episodes is important to improve the quality of life for patients and their families. The use of antibiotics in PFAPA syndrome is ineffective and unjustified. The history of 20-30 courses of antibiotics in patients before a diagnosis is established. The first diagnostic and therapeutic step is to stop antibiotics and show spontaneous remission of the next flares on symptomatic treatment (ibuprofen, paracetamol). Antipyretic drugs and non-steroidal anti-inflammatory drugs do not reduce the duration of fever. The spectacular effect of shortening the duration of symptoms can be achieved after oral corticosteroids. The accompanying aphthous, pharyngitis and / or adenitis may take longer to resolve. Unfortunately, corticosteroids often increase the frequency of fever episodes. Over time with continued prednisone /prednisolone use, the shortened cycles may lengthen [21]. There were no reports on side effects of on-demand usage of steroids 1-2 doses monthly, except for irritability or transitory sleep disturbances [3]. The recommended treatment of the disease flare is a single dose of prednisone at the dosage of 0.5–2 mg/kg or betamethasone at the dosage of 0.1–0.2 mg/kg, although, in some patients, the second dose of corticosteroid could be necessary. Most (>80%) of the patients obtain satisfactory control of the disease flares with corticosteroids. Yazgan et al. did not show any statistical significance in efficacy between a dose of 2 mg/kg/day versus a dose of 0.5 mg/kg/day, respectively, in 40 and 46 PFAPA febrile attacks [26, 27]. Tonsillectomy is an alternative therapeutic option with complete resolution of PFAPA symptoms in 63-100% of patients as reported in several case series and two randomized trials [26, 28, 29]. Adenoidectomy alone, as well as tonsillotomy, is not effective. The role of tonsillectomy in the treatment of PFAPA is still controversial due to the lack of definitive data in literature and case reports of fever relapses several years after surgery. Indeed, it is important to underline that surgery, as an invasive procedure, is associated with some risks such as bleeding, anesthetics side effects, etc. Therefore, since PFAPA syndrome generally evolves towards a spontaneous resolution, tonsillectomy should be considered just in case of intolerance or failure of the standard medical treatment. So far, tonsillectomy (+/- adenoidectomy) is the most effective intervention for long-term resolution of PFAPA symptoms [27]. Colchicine prophylaxis may be beneficial for frequent PFAPA episodes. In case series of nine patient colchicine increased the interval between PFAPA episodes from an average of 1.7 weeks to 8.4 weeks [30]. Interleukin (IL)-1β inhibition recently proved successful in the treatment of resistant PFAPA attacks [31]. Future randomized treatment trials of patients will help to determine the definite role of anakinra in the management of PFAPA.

PROGNOSIS

The prognosis is good because, in the majority of patients, spontaneous remission is observed in a median of 9-10 years without sequelae. Cases of PFAPA that were persistent after adolescence have also been reported, but the episodes are shorter in duration and occur less frequently. There is no report on amyloidosis as a long-term complication.

CONCLUSION

PFAPA syndrome is a complex genetic disease and one of the most common periodic fever syndromes. It is a self-limited disease in both children and adults with no long-term sequelae. PFAPA syndrome is also a perfect example that a carefully collected medical history of a patient and multiple, diligent physical examinations of a child are still the basis for the diagnosis. Despite a benign clinical course, PFAPA syndrome is associated with a significant impact on the quality of life of the patients and their families. There is the necessity of greater awareness and knowledge of the disease among primary care physicians to shorten the diagnostic odyssey and avoid inappropriate treatment.

CONSENT FOR PUBLICATION

Not applicable.

CONFLICT OF INTEREST

The authors declare no conflict of interest, financial or otherwise.

ACKNOWLEDGEMENT

Declared none.

REFERENCES

[1]   Marshall GS, Edwards KM, Butler J, Lawton AR. Syndrome of periodic fever, pharyngitis, and aphthous stomatitis. J Pediatr 1987; 110(1): 43-6.
        [http://dx.doi.org/10.1016/S0022-3476(87)80285-8] [PMID: 3794885]

[2]   Harel L, Hashkes PJ, Lapidus S, *et al.* The First International Conference on Periodic Fever, Aphthous Stomatitis, Pharyngitis, Adenitis Syndrome. J Pediatr 2018; 193: 265-274.e3.
        [http://dx.doi.org/10.1016/j.jpeds.2017.10.034] [PMID: 29246466]

[3]   Vigo G, Zulian F. Periodic fevers with aphthous stomatitis, pharyngitis, and adenitis (PFAPA). Autoimmun Rev 2012; 12(1): 52-5.
        [http://dx.doi.org/10.1016/j.autrev.2012.07.021] [PMID: 22878272]

[4]   Colotto M, Maranghi M, Durante C, Rossetti M, Renzi A, Anatra MG. PFAPA syndrome in a young adult with a history of tonsillectomy. Intern Med 2011; 50(3): 223-5.
        [http://dx.doi.org/10.2169/internalmedicine.50.4421] [PMID: 21297324]

[5]   Padeh S, Stoffman N, Berkun Y. Periodic fever accompanied by aphthous stomatitis, pharyngitis and cervical adenitis syndrome (PFAPA syndrome) in adults. Isr Med Assoc J 2008; 10(5): 358-60.
        [http://dx.doi.org/10.1186/1546-0096-6-S1-P183] [PMID: 18605359]

[6]   McDermott MF, Aksentijevich I, Galon J, *et al.* Germline mutations in the extracellular domains of the 55 kDa TNF receptor, TNFR1, define a family of dominantly inherited autoinflammatory syndromes. Cell 1999; 97(1): 133-44.
        [http://dx.doi.org/10.1016/S0092-8674(00)80721-7] [PMID: 10199409]

[7]   Stojanov S, Lapidus S, Chitkara P, *et al.* Periodic fever, aphthous stomatitis, pharyngitis, and adenitis (PFAPA) is a disorder of innate immunity and Th1 activation responsive to IL-1 blockade. Proc Natl Acad Sci USA 2011; 108(17): 7148-53.
        [http://dx.doi.org/10.1073/pnas.1103681108] [PMID: 21478439]

[8]   Stojanov S, Hoffmann F, Kéry A, *et al.* Cytokine profile in PFAPA syndrome suggests continuous inflammation and reduced anti-inflammatory response. Eur Cytokine Netw 2006; 17(2): 90-7.
        [PMID: 16840027]

[9]   Brown KL, Wekell P, Osla V, *et al.* Profile of blood cells and inflammatory mediators in periodic fever, aphthous stomatitis, pharyngitis and adenitis (PFAPA) syndrome. BMC Pediatr 2010; 10(1): 65.
        [http://dx.doi.org/10.1186/1471-2431-10-65] [PMID: 20819226]

[10]   Gonzalez CT, *et al.* Cytokine genotyping and serum profile in a PFAPA syndrome. Tissue Antigens 2015.

[11]   Long SS. Syndrome of Periodic Fever, Aphthous stomatitis, Pharyngitis, and Adenitis (PFAPA)--what it isn't. What is it? J Pediatr 1999; 135(1): 1-5.
[http://dx.doi.org/10.1016/S0022-3476(99)70316-1] [PMID: 10393593]

[12]   Di Gioia SA, Bedoni N, von Scheven-Gête A, *et al.* Analysis of the genetic basis of periodic fever with aphthous stomatitis, pharyngitis, and cervical adenitis (PFAPA) syndrome. Sci Rep 2015; 5(1): 10200.
[http://dx.doi.org/10.1038/srep10200] [PMID: 25988833]

[13]   Grandemange S, Cabasson S, Sarrabay G, *et al.* Clinical dose effect and functional consequences of R92Q in two families presenting with a TRAPS/PFAPA-like phenotype. Mol Genet Genomic Med 2017; 5(2): 110-6.
[http://dx.doi.org/10.1002/mgg3.229] [PMID: 28361096]

[14]   Manthiram K, Preite S, Dedeoglu F, *et al.* Common genetic susceptibility loci link PFAPA syndrome, Behçet's disease, and recurrent aphthous stomatitis. Proc Natl Acad Sci USA 2020; 117(25): 14405-11.
[http://dx.doi.org/10.1073/pnas.2002051117] [PMID: 32518111]

[15]   Yamahara K, Lee K, Egawa Y, Nakashima N, Ikegami S. Surgical outcomes and unique histological features of tonsils after tonsillectomy in adults with periodic fever, aphthous stomatitis, pharyngitis, and cervical adenitis syndrome. Auris Nasus Larynx 2020; 47(2): 254-61.
[http://dx.doi.org/10.1016/j.anl.2019.08.009] [PMID: 31495531]

[16]   Manthiram K, Correa H, Boyd K, Roland J, Edwards K. Unique histologic features of tonsils from patients with periodic fever, aphthous stomatitis, pharyngitis, and cervical adenitis (PFAPA) syndrome. Clin Rheumatol 2018; 37(5): 1309-17.
[http://dx.doi.org/10.1007/s10067-017-3773-8] [PMID: 28748511]

[17]   Førsvoll J, Janssen EA, Møller I, *et al.* Reduced Number of CD8+ Cells in Tonsillar Germinal Centres in Children with the Periodic Fever, Aphthous Stomatitis, Pharyngitis and Cervical Adenitis Syndrome. Scand J Immunol 2015; 82(1): 76-83.
[http://dx.doi.org/10.1111/sji.12303] [PMID: 25882211]

[18]   Dytrych P, Krol P, Kotrova M, *et al.* Polyclonal, newly derived T cells with low expression of inhibitory molecule PD-1 in tonsils define the phenotype of lymphocytes in children with Periodic Fever, Aphtous Stomatitis, Pharyngitis and Adenitis (PFAPA) syndrome. Mol Immunol 2015; 65(1): 139-47.
[http://dx.doi.org/10.1016/j.molimm.2015.01.004] [PMID: 25656804]

[19]   Hofer M, Pillet P, Cochard MM, *et al.* International periodic fever, aphthous stomatitis, pharyngitis, cervical adenitis syndrome cohort: description of distinct phenotypes in 301 patients. Rheumatology (Oxford) 2014; 53(6): 1125-9.
[http://dx.doi.org/10.1093/rheumatology/ket460] [PMID: 24505122]

[20]   Costagliola G, Maiorino G, Consolini R. Periodic fever, aphthous stomatitis, pharyngitis, and cervical adenitis syndrome (PFAPA): A clinical challenge for primary care physicians and rheumatologists. Front Pediatr 2019; 7: 277.
[http://dx.doi.org/10.3389/fped.2019.00277] [PMID: 31334209]

[21]   Thomas KT, Feder HM Jr, Lawton AR, Edwards KM. Periodic fever syndrome in children. J Pediatr 1999; 135(1): 15-21.
[http://dx.doi.org/10.1016/S0022-3476(99)70321-5] [PMID: 10393598]

[22]   Marshall GS, Edwards KM, Lawton AR. PFAPA syndrome. Pediatr Infect Dis J 1989; 8(9): 658-9.
[http://dx.doi.org/10.1097/00006454-198909000-00026] [PMID: 2797967]

[23]   Gattorno M, Sormani MP, D'Osualdo A, *et al.* A diagnostic score for molecular analysis of hereditary autoinflammatory syndromes with periodic fever in children. Arthritis Rheum 2008; 58(6): 1823-32.
[http://dx.doi.org/10.1002/art.23474] [PMID: 18512793]

[24]   Caorsi R, Meini A, Sormani MP, *et al.* Evidences for the need of new Diagnostic Criteria for PFAPA syndrome. Pediatr Rheumatol Online J 2008; 6(S1): 307.
[http://dx.doi.org/10.1186/1546-0096-6-S1-P181]

[25]   Padeh S, Brezniak N, Zemer D, *et al.* Periodic fever, aphthous stomatitis, pharyngitis, and adenopathy syndrome: clinical characteristics and outcome. J Pediatr 1999; 135(1): 98-101.
[http://dx.doi.org/10.1016/S0022-3476(99)70335-5] [PMID: 10393612]

[26]   Wurster VM, Carlucci JG, Feder HM Jr, Edwards KM. Long-term follow-up of children with periodic fever, aphthous stomatitis, pharyngitis, and cervical adenitis syndrome. J Pediatr 2011; 159(6): 958-64.
[http://dx.doi.org/10.1016/j.jpeds.2011.06.004] [PMID: 21798555]

[27]   Peridis S, Pilgrim G, Koudoumnakis E, Athanasopoulos I, Houlakis M, Parpounas K. PFAPA syndrome in children: A meta-analysis on surgical versus medical treatment. Int J Pediatr Otorhinolaryngol 2010; 74(11): 1203-8.
[http://dx.doi.org/10.1016/j.ijporl.2010.08.014] [PMID: 20832871]

[28]   Garavello W, Romagnoli M, Gaini RM. Effectiveness of adenotonsillectomy in PFAPA syndrome: a randomized study. J Pediatr 2009; 155(2): 250-3.
[http://dx.doi.org/10.1016/j.jpeds.2009.02.038] [PMID: 19464029]

[29]   Renko M, Salo E, Putto-Laurila A, *et al.* A randomized, controlled trial of tonsillectomy in periodic fever, aphthous stomatitis, pharyngitis, and adenitis syndrome. J Pediatr 2007; 151(3): 289-92.
[http://dx.doi.org/10.1016/j.jpeds.2007.03.015] [PMID: 17719940]

[30]   Tasher D, Stein M, Dalal I, Somekh E. Colchicine prophylaxis for frequent periodic fever, aphthous stomatitis, pharyngitis and adenitis episodes. Acta Paediatr 2008; 97(8): 1090-2.
[http://dx.doi.org/10.1111/j.1651-2227.2008.00837.x] [PMID: 18462461]

[31]   Soylu A, Yıldız G, Torun Bayram M, Kavukçu S. IL-1β blockade in periodic fever, aphthous stomatitis, pharyngitis, and cervical adenitis (PFAPA) syndrome: case-based review. Rheumatol Int 2019.
[http://dx.doi.org/10.1007/s00296-019-04389-3] [PMID: 31324971]

CHAPTER 13

Updates on Pediatric Hepatoblastoma

Consolato M. Sergi[1,2,*]

[1] *Division of Anatomic Pathology, Children's Hospital of Eastern Ontario, University of Ottawa, ON, Canada*

[2] *Department of Laboratory Medicine and Pathology, Stollery Children's Hospital, University of Alberta, Edmonton, AB, Canada*

Abstract: The developing human liver is embryologically central in embryogenesis. It plays a significant role as a hematopoietic and endocrine organ. During the development, hepatocytes change their phenotype. They vary from blueish cells to cells with an eosinophilic nuance and decreased nucleus to cytoplasm ratio. Apart from congenital abnormalities of this organ and inflammatory conditions that can populate medical charts in childhood and youth, the liver's neoplastic transformation in childhood and adolescence is a rare event. In children younger than three years, the liver's most dramatic neoplasm is represented by the occurrence of hepatoblastoma. It is an embryologic tumor. It retains the suffix "blastoma," similar to neuroblastoma as any other embryologic tumor. Hepatoblastoma originates presumably from the primitive embryo-fetal progenitors. In this chapter, we update our knowledge of this pediatric tumor, specifically the pathology and the treatment.

Keywords: Advocacy, Anatomy, Beckwith Wiedemann syndrome, Beta-Catenin, Child, Embryology, Familial adenomatous polyposis coli, Genetics, Hepatoblastoma, Liver, Microscopy, Neoplasm, Pathology, Quality Assurance, Radiology, Simpson–Golabi–Behmel syndrome, Sotos syndrome, Trisomy 18 syndrome, Tumor, World Health Organization.

INTRODUCTION

Hepatoblastoma is one of the most dramatic neoplasm of the first three years of life. It is an embryologic tumor of the liver showing several histologic patterns ranging from small round blue cell type morphology to a phenotype. It is quite similar to normal hepatocytes. The developing human liver is embryologically central in embryogenesis. It plays a major role as a hematopoietic and endocrine organ. In terms of development, hepatocytes change their phenotype. They vary

---

[*] **Corresponding author Consolato M. Sergi:** Division of Anatomical Pathology, Children's Hospital of Eastern Ontario (CHEO), University of Ottawa 401 Smyth Road Ottawa, ON K1H 8L1 Canada; Tel: 613-737-7600 x 2427; Fax: 613-738-4837; E-mail: csergi@cheo.on.ca

Nima Rezaei and Noosha Samieefar (Eds.)

from blueish cells to cells with an eosinophilic nuance and decreased or variable nucleus to cytoplasm ratio. Apart from congenital abnormalities of this organ and inflammatory conditions that can populate medical charts in childhood and youth, the liver's neoplastic transformation in childhood and adolescence is a rare event. About two-thirds of liver neoplasms occurring in the pediatric age are malignant. Nearly the same ratio is either hepatoblastoma or hepatocellular carcinoma. The former occurs mainly in the first triennium and the latter in children aged four or older [1 - 4]. This update will highlight the impressive increase in the overall survival of patients suffering from hepatoblastoma.

TUMOR CELL OF ORIGIN

In children younger than three years, the liver's most dramatic neoplasm is represented by the occurrence of hepatoblastoma. This tumor is an embryologic neoplasm. It retains the suffix "blastoma" similar to neuroblastoma or nephroblastoma (Wilms' tumor) that characterizes most of the embryologic tumors [5]. Hepatoblastoma does not originate from primary hepatoblasts, but it seems that less differentiated cells are the culprit in this neoplastic event. The human fetal liver multipotent progenitor cells (hFLMPCs), which are poorly differentiated, can convert into various tissues. These tissues include hepatocytes, bone, fat, or bile ducts. The differences identified in multiple histological patterns of hepatoblastoma would explain its variety. In fact, up to 40% of tumor samples contain both epithelial and mesenchymal components [6]. The beta-catenin pathway is crucial for developing a variety of organs in the human body [7]. It is tightly linked to the Wnt signaling pathway. Wnt is a hybrid name created from the words Wingless and Int-1. In cell physiology, Wnt signaling use either cell-cell (paracrine) or same-cell communication (autocrine). It is so powerful that it is highly evolutionarily conserved in animals, ranging from fruit flies to humans. The canonical Wnt-beta-catenin pathway is a complex, evolutionarily conserved mechanism that regulates essential processes in both physiology and pathology. Among the several aspects, it has been demonstrated that Wnt-beta-catenin signalling controls embryogenesis, maturation and zonation [7]. In the healthy liver of a mature organism, the Wnt-beta-catenin pathway is mostly inactive. However, this pathway becomes active (or better re-active) during cell renewal and/or regenerative processes. These processes include several diseases, pre-malignant abnormalities, and neoplasms. In both hepatocellular carcinoma (HCC) and cholangiocarcinoma (CCA), which are the two most prevalent primary liver tumors in adults, Wnt-beta-catenin signaling is often hyperactivated. It is critical in promoting tumor cell growth and dissemination. Activating mutations have been found in a considerable percentage of both HCC and CCA, although HCC is largely dominant on CCA [8, 9]. Similarly, hepatoblastoma researchers discover Wnt-beta-catenin activation with beta-catenin mutations in most of these embryologic tumors [10]. In a murine transgenic model using floxed beta-catenin (exons 2-6), and mice intercrossed with Albumin-Cre recombinase, Tan *et al.* found beta-catenin redundancy in the liver [11]. Lack of beta-catenin delays liver regeneration, but it does occur in a suboptimal way. In the case of 2/3 of partial hepatectomy, the Ctnnb1(loxp/loxp)-Alb-Cre(+/-) mice were passive in the first three days, but they showed an increase of hepatocyte proliferation after this time [11]. Beta-catenin has recently been demonstrated to cooperate with Yap signaling in the majority of hepatoblastomas [12 - 15].

CLINICAL PRESENTATION

Hepatoblastoma can occur sporadically or in the setting of familial cancer syndromes. These syndromes are Beckwith Wiedemann syndrome, Simpson–Golabi–Behmel syndrome, Sotos syndrome, familial adenomatous polyposis (FAP) coli, and trisomy 18 syndrome. Hepatoblastoma is more often seen in premature babies, with about 60% of a Japanese series affecting infants with birth weight less than 1000g [16]. In about 90% of patients with hepatoblastoma, there is an increase of alpha-fetoprotein (AFP), which may be puzzling because the premature liver contains and secretes a substantial amount of AFP. Other than nonspecific symptoms, including not gain of weight or weight loss associated with loss of appetite or anorexia, the abdominal mass can be discovered by ultrasound examination. It is a hyperechoic solid mass, which can be better delineated by computed tomography (CT) scan. CT scan will highlight the hepatoblastoma as a hypoattenuating mass with a clear boundary between the tumor and surrounding liver tissue.

PATHOLOGY

Hepatoblastoma can be essentially divided into two main categories, which include epithelial and epithelial/mesenchymal or mixed type. A few subtypes have been recognized in the epithelial category. They comprise fetal, embryonal, combined fetal and embryonal, macrotrabecular, and small cell types. The presence of mixed type is characterized by some mesenchymal tissue elements, such as cartilage or osteoid in addition to the epithelial component. In 6-8 weeks of gestation, the human liver shows basophilic cells with a high nucleus to cytoplasm ratio. This feature is seen in embryonal hepatoblastoma (EHB), which is the most often met histology pattern. These cells are approximately 10-15 micrometers in diameter and mostly round. The embryonal hepatoblast joins neighboring cells and grows in sheets. They form acinar (2D) or tubular (3D) structures around a central lumen. The more mature liver cells or fetal hepatoblasts acquire some features similar to more mature hepatocytes. These cells are relatively bigger than embryonal hepatoblasts. The nucleus to cytoplasm ratio is smaller than the large cells because the cytoplasm is more abundant and contains more cytosol and subcellular organelles. Both fetal and embryonal hepatoblasts can be seen in instances of epithelial hepatoblastoma. The concept of anaplasia has been imported from research on nephroblastoma or Wilms' tumor. Anaplasia is not identified with brisk mitotic activity but encompasses an increase of at least three times of normal neighboring tumor cells, atypical multipolar mitotic figures, and hyperchromatism or excessive basophilia. In Wilms' tumor, the anaplastic phenotype is often accompanied by the expression of p53 on immunohistochemistry, and *TP53* gene mutations have been discovered [17, 18]. *TP53* gene mutation has been seen to target patients' survival, overall and event-free. Therefore, it has the potential as an adverse prognostic factor combined with anaplastic morphological features [15]. Dysregulation of the MYCN gene in WTs with anaplastic histology has also been reported to be involved in developing tumors with adverse outcomes (16). A pleomorphic epithelial pattern may be encountered in fetal hepatoblastoma and, more rarely, in embryonal hepatoblastoma. In the pleomorphic component, tumor cells reveal nuclei that harbor coarse chromatin and nucleoli larger and more irregular than normal nucleoli. In about 5% of cases, i.e., one hepatoblastoma in approximately 20 tumors (1/20), hepatoblastoma maintains some very characteristic cell fearures of small round blue cell tumor. Originally, this tumor was labeled as anaplastic, but this term had been used and misused by several classifications. The term "anaplasia" is well characterized in Wilms' tumor, where it has prognostic relevance. Still, it does not seem to have any prognostic relevance in rhabdomyosarcoma, another small round blue cell tumor [19]. The negative labeling of anaplastic is associated with an unfavorable outcome in patients harboring anaplastic rhabdomyosarcoma. A not trivial aspect to consider is that the hepatoblastoma of small cell types may trigger only low AFP levels in serum. A small cell hepatoblastoma histology harbors tiny cytology with cells measuring 7-8 microns, i.e., slightly larger than a normal lymphocyte. The small cell hepatoblastoma exhibits round to oval cell morphology with scant cytoplasm. There is a relatively fine nuclear chromatin, inconspicuous nucleoli. The mitotic activity is just minimal. It differs predominantly with the mitotic activity of a poorly differentiated or undifferentiated neuroblastoma IVS (stage IV, special), which may enter the differential diagnosis in this age group. In hepatoblastoma, the growing pattern is important to be considered because it may deceive the pathologist, and misdiagnosis can be communicated at the time of the intraoperative frozen section. It is imperative at this stage to remind the residents, attending pathologists, and staff, that a diagnosis during an intraoperative frozen section is not mandatory, and deferral to permanent sections may be a good choice. In small cell hepatoblastoma, a diffuse pattern or a glandular pattern may be encountered. Other growth patterns can be recognized, and an organoid pattern can even be identified. In rare cases, highly deceptive growth patterns can be detected. They include a myxoid background and a microcystic pattern, among others. Of course, the microcystic growth pattern reminds the pathologist of a yolk sac tumor, and proper immunohistochemistry investigations are mandatory. Immunohisto-chemistry has become an undebatable partner in helping the pathologists reaching the diagnosis. In small cell hepatoblastoma, there is an immunologic reactivity for keratins 8 and 18 and vimentin, a common mesenchymal marker. Although vimentin is not a predilected marker by pathologists because of the nonspecific positivity in numerous tissues, organs, and tumors, it still harbors a good value because it allows the pathologists to check the immunologic reactivity of the tissue overall. Keratins or (cyto-)keratins are intermediate filaments of the cytoskeleton. The immunohistochemistry comprises an antibody cocktail (primary antibody) against a mixture of cytokeratin epitopes (AE 1-3, Linaris, Camon, Wiesbaden, Germany) or specific antibodies against keratins. AE 1 reacts with specific group A acidic keratins with a molecular weight of 40,000–50,000 (CK 10, 14–16, and 19), while AE 3 recognizes all eight group B basic keratins with a molecular weight of 58,000–67,000 (CK 1–8) [20]. In some cases, the immunohistochemical evaluation of the intraportal vessels may be crucial using an antibody (primary antibody) against factor VIII, an endothelial cell marker (anti-human factor VIII–related antigen, Dako, Hamburg, Germany). Factor VIII is a macromolecular complex consisting of a clot-promoting factor, von Willebrand factor, and the factor VIII–related antigen. This antigen is localized in the cytoplasm of vascular endothelial cells (Weibel-Palade bodies), platelets, megakaryocytes, and various vascular lesions, both inflammatory and neoplastic. A caveat in the diagnosis is that small cell hepatoblastomas do not express AFP or glypican, one of the two major groups of heparan sulfate proteoglycans. The other major family is constituted by the syndecans. Six glypicans have been identified in mammals. They are referred to as GPC1 through GPC6. Abnormal expression of glypicans has been identified in various tumors, including hepatocellular carcinoma, pancreatic carcinoma, ovarian cancer, mesothelioma, glioma, breast cancer, and neuroblastoma. The INI1 (integrase interactor 1) expression is retained, eliminating the possibility of misdiagnosing a malignant rhabdoid tumor. In case the diagnosis of small cell hepatoblastomas is done and, for some reason, INI1 expression is lost, the case should be sent to a molecular biology laboratory for mutation and deletion testing. INI1 is expressed in all cell types and is a protein involved in chromatin remodeling and transcriptional regulation [21]. Other synonyms of INI1 include hSNF5, SMARCB1, and BAF47 [22]. INI1 is a chromatin-remodeling protein, which specifically represses Aurora A, required for rhabdoid tumor cell survival [23]. Additional repression is on basal HIV1 promoter activity [24]. The loss of INI1 expression is usually associated with deletion or mutation of the INI1 gene on

22q11.2, although it is not always the case [25]. It is important to remember that germline INI1 mutations are associated with sporadic schwannomatosis [26] and rhabdoid tumors [27]. Loss of INI1 expression is found in CNS atypical teratoid / rhabdoid tumor [28], epithelioid MPNST (50%), epithelioid sarcoma [29], extraskeletal myxoid chondrosarcomas, myoepithelial carcinoma, and renal medullar carcinoma [30 - 32]. In the Lopez-Terrada *et al* classification, the worldwide most used classification of hepatoblastoma [33], the epithelial subtypes apart from the "pure fetal with low mitotic activity" (Fig. **1**) include the "fetal, mitotically active", embryonal (Fig. **2**), pleomorphic, small cell undifferentiated (INI1-negative and INI1-positive), cholangioblastic, macrotrabecular, and mixed epithelial (any/all above). Also, mixed epithelial and mesenchymal hepatoblastomas are subtyped separately in a group with and another group without teratoid features. Cholangioblastic hepatoblastoma is a particular type of hepatoblastoma evidencing cholangiocyte differentiation. This hepatoblastoma pattern exhibits cholangiocyte differentiation resembling acinar structures seen in the neo-ductlar proliferation of biliary atresia or any other state of prolonged cholestasis [34, 35]. The antibodies against cytokeratins 7 and 19 may be useful in this setting [36 - 39]. The pathology of hepatoblastoma is also key to assess the treatment response following chemotherapy (Fig. **3**). The extension of necrosis should be documented. Pigment-laden macrophages are often seen.

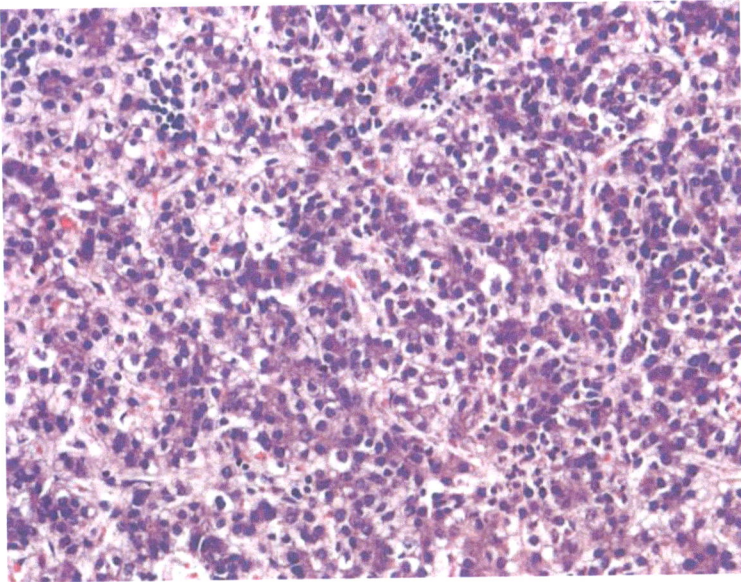

Fig. (1). Microphotograph depicting hepatoblastoma with epithelial fetal and embryonal components (H&E staining 200 x original magnification).

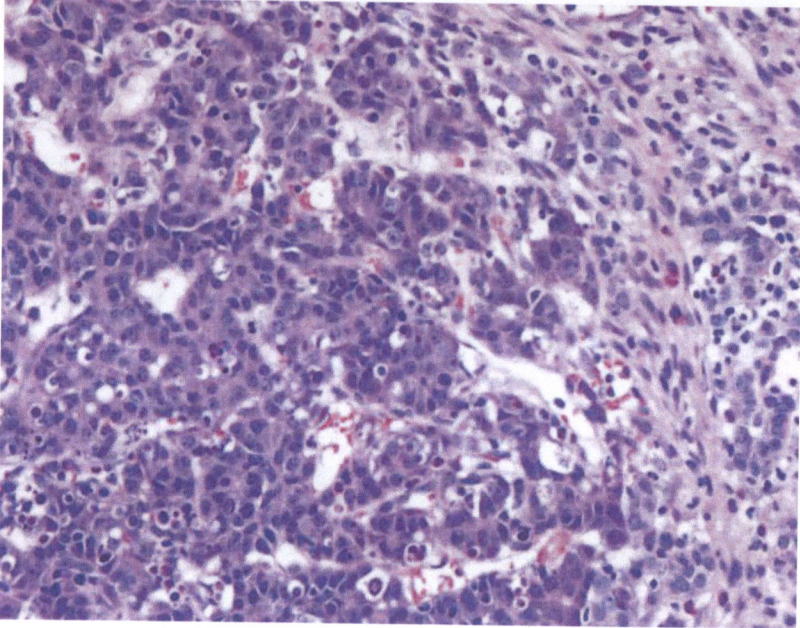

Fig. (2). Microphotograph showing an embryonal epithelial hepatoblastoma (H&E staining 200 x original magnification).

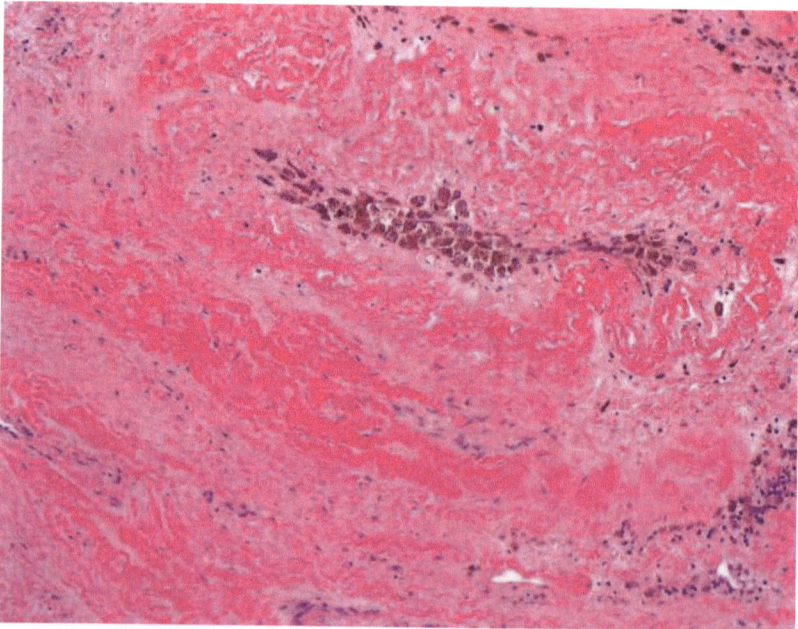

Fig. (3). Microphotograph showing a good chemotherapy response with extensive necrosis (red-pink area) of the tumor cells and pigment-laden macrophages (brown cells) following two cycles of chemotherapy (H&E staining 100 x original magnification).

OUTCOME AND THERAPY

The molecular profiling of hepatoblastoma has identified some groups of this specific liver tumor that may benefit from further stratification. In North America, the Children's Oncology Group (COG), and in Europe and Asia, the International Society of Pediatric Oncology (SIOP) have been important in reaching impressive results for the outcome of this dreadful tumor. In the past three decades, patients affected with hepatoblastoma have survived better than before, showing a change from 30% to 70%. Most of this success rate is due to the better knowledge of tumor cell biology encompassing this rare embryologic tumor. The COG based staging system relies on tumor resectability and perioperative findings. This system is beneficial for treatment protocols that encourage surgery immediately after diagnosis. A decrease in resectability degree connects to higher stages of the disease. In the SIOP based staging system, the PRETEXT staging system is favored. The International Childhood Liver Tumor Strategy Group (SIOPEL) has been influential in reaching remarkable results in terms of the outcome of these patients. The PRETEXT system relies on the Couinaud's system and precisely on the number of contiguous Couinaud's liver sections not involved by neoplasm. The eight liver segments are assembled into four major groups or segments. Segments 2 and 3 consist of the left lateral section, while segments 4a and 4b encompass the left medial section. Also, segments 5 and 8 involve the right anterior section, while segments 6 and 7 encompass the liver's right posterior section. The PRETEXT system is an excellent system with worldwide application in the pediatric oncology setting for hepatoblastoma staging with the updated revision in 2017 [40]. However, disagreement has been identified, particularly from the French Paediatric Liver Tumour Group (i.e., the French members of the SIOPEL). Pariente *et al.* [41] disagree with the recommendation to perform magnetic resonance imaging (MRI) with the injection of a hepatocyte-specific contrast agent at diagnosis and at every time point, rather than CT. A prolonged MRI examination in an infant under general anesthesia needs to be balanced with the risk of ionizing radiation from a CT. Also, the use of a hepatocyte-specific contrast agent would have been based on Towbin's *et al.*'s experience [40] with gadoxetate disodium (Eovist/Primovist; Bayer HealthCare, Whippany, NJ). The recommended agents do not have official pediatric age group marketing approval in various countries. Pariente *et al.* stress the hepatocyte-specific contrast agent, widely available in several countries, gadopentetate dimeglumine (MultiHance; Bracco, Milan, Italy). This contrast agent has a more delayed hepatocyte phase starting at least 40 min after injection, which can significantly lengthen the MRI's duration. The debated arguments also involve the safety of each agent and the annotation factors used. The annotations V (hepatic venous/inferior vena cava involvement), P (portal venous involvement), and M (distant metastases) have been highly modified compared to the definitions used in 2005 PRETEXT [42] and in the database of the Children's Hepatic Tumours International Collaboration [43]. Overall, Towbin's protocol seems to be more aggressive, comparing Pariente *et al.*'s arguments. These latter authors reflect that obliteration of the inferior vena cava should not be considered as an involvement of the tumor. A thrombus seen in only one hepatic vein or only one portal vein branch should not be considered as V+ or P+. This setting is because, in the 2005 PRETEXT, only the thrombus extending to all three hepatic veins or into the IVC or to both portal vein branches or the main portal vein was considered as a high-risk criterion. Finally, some arguments refer to nodules of 3 mm that should not be considered metastases when the outcome was excellent with cisplatin monotherapy in previous trials. There is an obvious interest in decreasing the chemotherapy burden and risk of toxicity for infants who have had fairly good results with standard risk treatment regimes. However, the Towbin's protocol is reiterated, and Pariente *et al.*'s argument is debated [44], underlying the number of subsequent studies supporting their guidelines and indicating that the choice of imaging may rely on the institution. Data from the COG and SIOPEL study groups have pinpointed several factors that are crucial for the outcome of patients affected with hepatoblastoma. These prognostic factors include the age of the patient, PRETEXT stage, vascular involvement, metastatic disease, serologic AFP levels, pathologic type, response to chemotherapy, and surgical resectability. Overall, favorable factors include age less than 1-year, low PRETEXT stage at diagnosis (PRETEXT I, II, and III), and pure fetal histology. On the other hand, age above 6-years, high PRETEXT stage, multifocal disease, unresectable vascular involvement, extrahepatic tumor extension, metastasis at diagnosis, regional lymph node involvement, tumor rupture at the time of diagnosis, small cell morphology, serum AFP 41.2 million or100–1000, positive surgical margin, and surgically unresectable neoplasm. In a nutshell, COG, PRETEXT, and SIOPEL are presented. The COG staging system for hepatoblastoma includes four stages [45]. They include I (neoplasm completely resected), II (grossly resected neoplasm with a microscopic residual disease), III (unresectable or resected neoplasm with a gross residual disease with or without nodal involvement), and IV (presence of distant metastasis, regardless of the extent of liver involvement). The PRETEXT staging system for hepatoblastoma includes four stages, as well [42]. They are I (one section is involved, and adjoining three sections are free), II (one or two sections are involved but adjoining two sections are free), III (two or three sections are involved, and no two adjoining sections are free), and IV (all four sections are involved). The SIOPEL Risk Stratification for Hepatoblastoma [46] emphasizes serum AFP of less than 100 µg/L, PRETEXT IV stage, and additional PRETEXT criteria (E1, E1a, E2, E2a, H1, M1, N1, N2, P2, P2a, V3, V3a) as high risk. At the same time, all other patients are set to a standard risk.

However, the histology remains critical. In particular, hepatoblastoma with pure fetal hepatoblastoma with minimal mitotic activity does substantially well [47]. Recognizing pure, well-differentiated fetal hepatoblastoma that is surgically treatable is paramount. It would decrease chemotherapy burden for the child and the risk of a second neoplasm. It remains clear that a small-cell-undifferentiated hepatoblastoma harbors aggressive biology, and survival is considerably worse than other histology patterns. In the case of PRETEXT I and II, a segmentectomy or lobectomy should be recommended. In PRETEXT III and POSTTEXT I, II, and III neoplasms without vascular involvement undergoing surgical resection, a lobectomy or *tri*-segmentectomy should be proposed. In PRETEXT IV or POSTTEXT III with vascular involvement, radical resection or liver transplantation should be advised. COG protocols include cisplatin, 5-fluorouracil, and vincristine in low-risk patients (PRETEXT I/II with any histology). The addition of doxorubicin is strongly suggested for patients with intermediate-risk (PRETEXT III/IV, small cell undifferentiated) and high risk (metastatic tumor disease, AFP at diagnosis less than 100 µg/mL). COG recommends 2-8 cycles of chemotherapy and tumor resection after accomplishing 2–6 cycles. SIOPEL guidelines support standard-risk patients (PRETEXTI-III, AFP > 100ng/mL) having monotherapy with cisplatin. They obtain 6 courses, and surgical resection is suggested after 4 cycles. High-risk patients (PRETEXT IV, PRETEXT I-III with all hepatic vein involvement, both vein involvement, extrahepatic involvement of neighboring structures, distant metastatic disease, lymph node involvement, serum AFP < 100 ng/mL, and small cell un-differentiated histology) receive cisplatin and doxorubicin. Cisplatin is administered weekly for 8 courses and doxorubicin every 3 weeks for 3 courses. After 8 cycles, surgery is endeavored. The response rate to chemotherapy is crucial, and SIOPEL studies emphasize that the response rate was 97%, resection rate 87%, three-year event-free survival 80%, and three-year (same period) overall survival of 80% [48]. Finally, it is essential to explain to the family and attending physicians and nurses that chemotherapy is associated with side effects that may include mild symptoms (nausea, vomiting, and mucositis). Severe side effects include myelosuppression, oto- and nephrotoxicity, and cardiomyopathy. In case of an unresectable tumor (POSTTEXT III/IV), following neoadjuvant chemotherapy, 49–50, and for tumors with vascular involvement, liver transplantation has been advocated with legitimacy.

CONCLUSION

The liver's neoplastic transformation in childhood and adolescence is a rare event. In children younger than three years, the liver's most dramatic neoplasm is represented by the occurrence of hepatoblastoma. Prognosis is based on many factors. In the past three decades, patients affected with hepatoblastoma survived better than before, showing a change from 30% to 70%. Most of this success rate is due to the better knowledge of tumor cell biology encompassing this rare embryologic tumor.

CONSENT FOR PUBLICATION

Not applicable.

CONFLICT OF INTEREST

Dr. C. Sergi is Section Editor of the Bentham Journal "Recent Patents on Anti-Cancer Drug Discovery" (10.2174/157489281502200923150750) and receives royalties from books published by Springer and Nova publishers. All royalties go to pediatric charities. Dr. C. Sergi has no other conflict of interest to declare with regard to this manuscript.

ACKNOWLEDGMENTS

This research has been funded by the generosity of the Stollery Children's Hospital Foundation and supporters of the Lois Hole Hospital for Women through the Women and Children's Health Research Institute (WCHRI Grant ID #: 2096), Hubei Province Natural Science Funding for Hubei University of Technology (100-Talent Grant for Recruitment Program of Foreign Experts Total Funding: Digital PCR and NGS-based diagnosis for infection and oncology, 2017-2022), Österreichische Krebshilfe Tyrol (Krebsgesellschaft Tirol, Austrian Tyrolean Cancer Research Institute, 2007 and 2009 - "DMBTI and cholangiocellular carcinomas" and "Hsp70 and HSPBP1 in carcinomas of the pancreas"), Austrian Research Fund (Fonds zur Förderung der wissenschaftlichen Forschung, FWF, Grant ID L313-B13), Canadian Foundation for Women's Health ("Early Fetal Heart-RES0000928"), Cancer Research Society (von Willebrand factor gene expression in cancer cells), Canadian Institutes of Health Research (Omega-3 Fatty Acids for Treatment of Intestinal Failure Associated Liver Disease: A Translational Research Study, 2011-2014, CIHR 232514), and the Saudi Cultural Bureau, Ottawa, Canada. The funders had no role in study design, data collection and analysis, decision to publish, or preparation of the manuscript.

REFERENCES

[1]   Xie L, Onysko J, Morrison H. Childhood cancer incidence in Canada: demographic and geographic variation of temporal trends (1992-2010). Health Promot Chronic Dis Prev Can 2018; 38(3): 79-115.
[http://dx.doi.org/10.24095/hpcdp.38.3.01] [PMID: 29537768]

[2]   Khanna R, Verma SK. Pediatric hepatocellular carcinoma. World J Gastroenterol 2018; 24(35): 3980-99.
[http://dx.doi.org/10.3748/wjg.v24.i35.3980] [PMID: 30254403]

[3]   Spector LG, Birch J. The epidemiology of hepatoblastoma. Pediatr Blood Cancer 2012; 59(5): 776-9.

[http://dx.doi.org/10.1002/pbc.24215] [PMID: 22692949]

[4]   Sharma D, Subbarao G, Saxena R. Hepatoblastoma. Semin Diagn Pathol 2017; 34(2): 192-200.
        [http://dx.doi.org/10.1053/j.semdp.2016.12.015] [PMID: 28126357]

[5]   Sergi CM. Pathology of Childhood and Adolescence. An Illustrated Guide. 1st ed. Springer 2020; p.
        1617.
        [http://dx.doi.org/10.1007/978-3-662-59169-7]

[6]   Stiller D, Holzhausen HJ. Congenital hepatoblastoma of mixed type. Light and electron microscopy
        studies. Zentralbl Allg Pathol 1983; 128(5-6): 317-26. https://www.ncbi.nlm.nih.gov/pubmed/6328792

[7]   Perugorria MJ, Olaizola P, Labiano I, *et al.* Wnt-β-catenin signalling in liver development, health and
        disease. Nat Rev Gastroenterol Hepatol 2019; 16(2): 121-36.
        [http://dx.doi.org/10.1038/s41575-018-0075-9] [PMID: 30451972]

[8]   Abuetabh Y, Persad S, Nagamori S, Huggins J, Al-Bahrani R, Sergi C. Expression of E-cadherin and
        beta-catenin in two cholangiocarcinoma cell lines (OZ and HuCCT1) with different degree of
        invasiveness of the primary tumor. Ann Clin Lab Sci 2011; 41(3): 217-3.
        [PMID: 22075503]

[9]   Al-Bahrani R, Abuetabh Y, Zeitouni N, Sergi C. Cholangiocarcinoma: risk factors, environmental
        influences and oncogenesis. Ann Clin Lab Sci 2013; 43(2): 195-210.
        [PMID: 23694797]

[10]   Russell JO, Monga SP. Wnt/β-Catenin Signaling in Liver Development, Homeostasis, and
        Pathobiology. Annu Rev Pathol 2018; 13(1): 351-78.
        [http://dx.doi.org/10.1146/annurev-pathol-020117-044010] [PMID: 29125798]

[11]   Tan X, Behari J, Cieply B, Michalopoulos GK, Monga SP. Conditional deletion of beta-catenin
        reveals its role in liver growth and regeneration. Gastroenterology 2006; 131(5): 1561-72.
        [http://dx.doi.org/10.1053/j.gastro.2006.08.042] [PMID: 17101329]

[12]   Chen X, Kiss A, Schaff Z, *et al.* CDK9 is dispensable for YAP-driven hepatoblastoma development.
        Pediatr Blood Cancer 2020; 67(5): e28221.
        [http://dx.doi.org/10.1002/pbc.28221] [PMID: 32124532]

[13]   Molina L, Yang H, Adebayo Michael AO, *et al.* mTOR inhibition affects Yap1-β-catenin-induced
        hepatoblastoma growth and development. Oncotarget 2019; 10(15): 1475-90.
        [http://dx.doi.org/10.18632/oncotarget.26668] [PMID: 30863496]

[14]   Min Q, Molina L, Li J, *et al.* β-Catenin and Yes-Associated Protein 1 Cooperate in Hepatoblastoma
        Pathogenesis. Am J Pathol 2019; 189(5): 1091-104.
        [http://dx.doi.org/10.1016/j.ajpath.2019.02.002] [PMID: 30794807]

[15]   Sylvester KG, Colnot S. Hippo/YAP, β-catenin, and the cancer cell: a "ménage à trois" in
        hepatoblastoma. Gastroenterology 2014; 147(3): 562-5.
        [http://dx.doi.org/10.1053/j.gastro.2014.07.026] [PMID: 25072176]

[16]   Ikeda H, Hachitanda Y, Tanimura M, Maruyama K, Koizumi T, Tsuchida Y. Development of
        unfavorable hepatoblastoma in children of very low birth weight: results of a surgical and pathologic
        review. Cancer 1998; 82(9): 1789-96.
        [PMID: 9576303]

[17]   Ghanem MA, van Steenbrugge GJ, Nijman RJ, van der Kwast TH. Prognostic markers in
        nephroblastoma (Wilms' tumor). Urology 2005; 65(6): 1047-54.
        [http://dx.doi.org/10.1016/j.urology.2004.12.005] [PMID: 15922430]

[18]   Koshinaga T, Ohashi K, Sugitou K, Ikeda T. Clinical features of solid malignant tumors in childhood.
        Gan To Kagaku Ryoho 2013; 40(7): 825-32.
        [PMID: 23863721]

[19]   Shenoy A, Alvarez E, Chi YY, *et al.* The prognostic significance of anaplasia in childhood

rhabdomyosarcoma: A report from the Children's Oncology Group. Eur J Cancer 2021; 143: 127-33.
[http://dx.doi.org/10.1016/j.ejca.2020.10.018] [PMID: 33302115]

[20] Moll R, Franke WW, Schiller DL, Geiger B, Krepler R. The catalog of human cytokeratins: patterns of expression in normal epithelia, tumors and cultured cells. Cell 1982; 31(1): 11-24.
[http://dx.doi.org/10.1016/0092-8674(82)90400-7] [PMID: 6186379]

[21] Calderaro J, Moroch J, Pierron G, et al. SMARCB1/INI1 inactivation in renal medullary carcinoma. Histopathology 2012; 61(3): 428-35.
[http://dx.doi.org/10.1111/j.1365-2559.2012.04228.x] [PMID: 22686875]

[22] Schaefer IM, Hornick JL. SWI/SNF complex-deficient soft tissue neoplasms: An update. Semin Diagn Pathol 2020.
[http://dx.doi.org/10.1053/j.semdp.2020.05.005] [PMID: 32646614]

[23] Lee S, Cimica V, Ramachandra N, Zagzag D, Kalpana GV. Aurora A is a repressed effector target of the chromatin remodeling protein INI1/hSNF5 required for rhabdoid tumor cell survival. Cancer Res 2011; 71(9): 3225-35.
[http://dx.doi.org/10.1158/0008-5472.CAN-10-2167] [PMID: 21521802]

[24] Boese A, Sommer P, Holzer D, Maier R, Nehrbass U. Integrase interactor 1 (Ini1/hSNF5) is a repressor of basal human immunodeficiency virus type 1 promoter activity. J Gen Virol 2009; 90(Pt 10): 2503-12.
[http://dx.doi.org/10.1099/vir.0.013656-0] [PMID: 19515827]

[25] Haberler C. Intact INI1 gene region with paradoxical loss of protein expression in AT/RT: implications for a possible novel mechanism associated with absence of INI1 protein immunoreactivity. Am J Surg Pathol 2012; 3612: 1903.
[http://dx.doi.org/10.1097/PAS.0b013e31825d53d5]

[26] Rousseau G, Noguchi T, Bourdon V, Sobol H, Olschwang S. SMARCB1/INI1 germline mutations contribute to 10% of sporadic schwannomatosis. BMC Neurol 2011; 11(1): 9.
[http://dx.doi.org/10.1186/1471-2377-11-9] [PMID: 21255467]

[27] Bourdeaut F, Lequin D, Brugières L, et al. Frequent hSNF5/INI1 germline mutations in patients with rhabdoid tumor. Clin Cancer Res 2011; 17(1): 31-8.
[http://dx.doi.org/10.1158/1078-0432.CCR-10-1795] [PMID: 21208904]

[28] Judkins AR, Mauger J, Ht A, Rorke LB, Biegel JA. Immunohistochemical analysis of hSNF5/INI1 in pediatric CNS neoplasms. Am J Surg Pathol 2004; 28(5): 644-50.
[http://dx.doi.org/10.1097/00000478-200405000-00013] [PMID: 15105654]

[29] Raoux D, Péoc'h M, Pedeutour F, Vaunois B, Decouvelaere AV, Folpe AL. Primary epithelioid sarcoma of bone: report of a unique case, with immunohistochemical and fluorescent in situ hybridization confirmation of INI1 deletion. Am J Surg Pathol 2009; 33(6): 954-8.
[http://dx.doi.org/10.1097/PAS.0b013e31819b92d5] [PMID: 19342946]

[30] Kojima Y, Tanabe M, Kato I, et al. Myoepithelioma-like tumor of the vulvar region showing infiltrative growth and harboring only a few estrogen receptor-positive cells: A case report. Pathol Int 2019; 69(3): 172-6.
[http://dx.doi.org/10.1111/pin.12765] [PMID: 30737997]

[31] Hollmann TJ, Hornick JL. INI1-deficient tumors: diagnostic features and molecular genetics. Am J Surg Pathol 2011; 35(10): e47-63.
[http://dx.doi.org/10.1097/PAS.0b013e31822b325b] [PMID: 21934399]

[32] Kohashi K, Oda Y, Yamamoto H, et al. SMARCB1/INI1 protein expression in round cell soft tissue sarcomas associated with chromosomal translocations involving EWS: a special reference to SMARCB1/INI1 negative variant extraskeletal myxoid chondrosarcoma. Am J Surg Pathol 2008; 32(8): 1168-74.
[http://dx.doi.org/10.1097/PAS.0b013e318161781a] [PMID: 18580682]

[33] López-Terrada D, Alaggio R, de Dávila MT, *et al.* Towards an international pediatric liver tumor consensus classification: proceedings of the Los Angeles COG liver tumors symposium. Mod Pathol 2014; 27(3): 472-91.
[http://dx.doi.org/10.1038/modpathol.2013.80] [PMID: 24008558]

[34] Sergi CM. Genetics of Biliary Atresia: A Work in Progress for a Disease with an Unavoidable Sequela into Liver Cirrhosis following Failure of Hepatic Portoenterostomy. In: Tsoulfas G, Ed. Liver Cirrhosis - Debates and Current Challenges. IntechOpen 2019.
[http://dx.doi.org/10.5772/intechopen.85071]

[35] Sergi C, Benstz J, Feist D, Nutzenadel W, Otto HF, Hofmann WJ. Bile duct to portal space ratio and ductal plate remnants in liver disease of infants aged less than 1 year. Pathology 2008; 40(3): 260-7.
[http://dx.doi.org/10.1080/00313020801911538] [PMID: 18428045]

[36] Dorn L, Menezes LF, Mikuz G, Otto HF, Onuchic LF, Sergi C. Immunohistochemical detection of polyductin and co-localization with liver progenitor cell markers during normal and abnormal development of the intrahepatic biliary system and in adult hepatobiliary carcinomas. J Cell Mol Med 2009; 13(7): 1279-90.
[http://dx.doi.org/10.1111/j.1582-4934.2008.00519.x] [PMID: 19292732]

[37] Sergi C, Adam S, Kahl P, Otto HF. The remodeling of the primitive human biliary system. Early Hum Dev 2000; 58(3): 167-78.
[PMID: 10936437]

[38] Sergi C, Kahl P, Otto HF. Contribution of apoptosis and apoptosis-related proteins to the malformation of the primitive intrahepatic biliary system in Meckel syndrome. Am J Pathol 2000; 156(5): 1589-98.
[http://dx.doi.org/10.1016/S0002-9440(10)65031-6] [PMID: 10793071]

[39] Sergi C, Adam S, Kahl P, Otto HF. Study of the malformation of ductal plate of the liver in Meckel syndrome and review of other syndromes presenting with this anomaly. Pediatr Dev Pathol 2000; 3(6): 568-83.
[PMID: 11000335]

[40] Towbin AJ, Meyers RL, Woodley H, *et al.* 2017 PRETEXT: radiologic staging system for primary hepatic malignancies of childhood revised for the Paediatric Hepatic International Tumour Trial (PHITT). Pediatr Radiol 2018; 48(4): 536-54.
[http://dx.doi.org/10.1007/s00247-018-4078-z] [PMID: 29427028]

[41] Pariente D, Franchi-Abella S, Cellier C, *et al.* Another point of view on 2017 PRETEXT. Pediatr Radiol 2018; 48(12): 1817-9.
[http://dx.doi.org/10.1007/s00247-018-4227-4] [PMID: 30109379]

[42] Roebuck DJ, Aronson D, Clapuyt P, *et al.* 2005 PRETEXT: a revised staging system for primary malignant liver tumours of childhood developed by the SIOPEL group. Pediatr Radiol 2007; 37(2): 123-32.
[http://dx.doi.org/10.1007/s00247-006-0361-5] [PMID: 17186233]

[43] Czauderna P, Haeberle B, Hiyama E, *et al.* The Children's Hepatic tumors International Collaboration (CHIC): Novel global rare tumor database yields new prognostic factors in hepatoblastoma and becomes a research model. Eur J Cancer 2016; 52: 92-101.
[http://dx.doi.org/10.1016/j.ejca.2015.09.023] [PMID: 26655560]

[44] Towbin AJ, Meyers RL, Woodley H, *et al.* Another point of view on 2017 PRETEXT: reply to Pariente *et al.* Pediatr Radiol 2018; 48(12): 1820-2.
[http://dx.doi.org/10.1007/s00247-018-4228-3] [PMID: 30112622]

[45] Meyers RL, Rowland JR, Krailo M, Chen Z, Katzenstein HM, Malogolowkin MH. Predictive power of pretreatment prognostic factors in children with hepatoblastoma: a report from the Children's Oncology Group. Pediatr Blood Cancer 2009; 53(6): 1016-22.
[http://dx.doi.org/10.1002/pbc.22088] [PMID: 19588519]

[46]   Maibach R, Roebuck D, Brugieres L, *et al.* Prognostic stratification for children with hepatoblastoma: the SIOPEL experience. Eur J Cancer 2012; 48(10): 1543-9.
[http://dx.doi.org/10.1016/j.ejca.2011.12.011] [PMID: 22244829]

[47]   Weinberg AG, Finegold MJ. Primary hepatic tumors of childhood. Hum Pathol 1983; 14(6): 512-37.
[PMID: 6303939]

[48]   Czauderna P, Lopez-Terrada D, Hiyama E, Häberle B, Malogolowkin MH, Meyers RL. Hepatoblastoma state of the art: pathology, genetics, risk stratification, and chemotherapy. Curr Opin Pediatr 2014; 26(1): 19-28.
[http://dx.doi.org/10.1097/MOP.0000000000000046] [PMID: 24322718]

CHAPTER 14

Updates on Mitochondrial Disorders in Children

Ramesh Bhat Y[1,*]

[1] *Department of Paediatrics, Kasturba Medical College, Manipal Academy of Higher Education University, Manipal-576104, Karnataka, India*

Abstract: Each human cell contains a few hundred mitochondria that are essential for aerobic energy metabolism. Among many fundamental metabolic pathways in mitochondria, the oxidative phosphorylation (OXPHOS) or the respiratory chain (RC) represents the final stage in oxidative metabolism. RC is under the dual control of the mitochondrial genome (mtDNA) and the nuclear genome (nDNA). The proper assembly and functioning of the RC involve many steps. The genetic defects in mtDNA, nDNA, and related functions of mitochondria affect the functioning of RC resulting in insufficient energy production and organ dysfunction.

Mitochondrial disorders are increasingly recognized. The clinical manifestations vary widely, causing a significant diagnostic challenge. Manifestations range from lesions of single tissue or structure to widespread lesions, including myopathies, encephalomyopathies, cardiopathies, neurogastrointestinal form, psychiatric symptoms, or complex multisystem syndromes. Coenzyme Q10 deficiency may present with isolated proximal muscle weakness. Leigh syndrome and MELAS are the most common clinical multisystem syndromes. The age at onset ranges from neonatal to adult life. The mortality remains high, and the median survival for early onset severe disease is 12years. Initial evaluations include blood transaminases, lactate-to-pyruvate ratio, amino acids, acylcarnitine profile, creatine kinase, and organic acids. Genetic tests are needed for confirmation.

Treatment depends on the specific mitochondrial disorder and its severity. In an acute presentation, an infection should be sought and treated promptly. Coenzyme Q10, thiamine, riboflavin, lipoic acid, L-carnitine, Creatine, and L-Arginine are found to be beneficial. Although there are no cures, treatments reduce symptoms or slow the decline in health.

Keywords: Arginine, Carnitine, Coenzyme Q, Encephalopathy, Energy, Lactic acidosis, Leigh syndrome, Magnetic resonance, MELAS, Mitochondrial disorders, Mitochondrial depletion, Mitochondrial membrane, mtDNA, Muscle

* **Corresponding author Ramesh Bhat Y:** Department of Paediatrics, Kasturba Medical College, Manipal Academy of Higher Education University, Manipal- 576104, Karnataka, India; Tel: +91 9448296564; Fax: +91820 2571927; E-mail: docrameshbhat@yahoo.co.in

Nima Rezaei and Noosha Samieefar (Eds.)

biopsy, Myopathy, nDNA, Neuropathy, OXPHOS, Ragged-red fibers, Respiratory chain, Riboflavin, Stroke, Thiamine.

INTRODUCTION

Mitochondria are the cellular organelles responsible for oxidative phosphorylation (OXPHOS) and the production of energy in the form of adenosine triphosphate (ATP). The energy production occurs in the mitochondrial respiratory chain (RC). Mitochondria also perform other tasks such as combating the production of reactive oxygen species and initiating apoptosis. They also house a variety of metabolic reactions such as pyruvate oxidation and metabolism of amino acids, fatty acids, and steroids. The five complexes, complexes I to V, of the mitochondrial RC contain approximately 80 proteins, of which 13 are encoded by mtDNA and the remaining proteins by the nDNA. The nDNA ultimately controls the proper assembly and functioning of the RC involving many steps. The defects of mtDNA and nDNA result in two important categories of mitochondrial disorders. Mutations in mtDNA such as tRNA or rRNA gene mutations and rearrangements may impair the total mitochondrial protein synthesis or may affect one of the 13 respiratory chain subunits encoded by mtDNA [1 - 4].

Mitochondrial disorders are inherited disorders of energy metabolism caused by impairment of the OXPHOS system. Defects in any of the mitochondrial functions can lead to primary mitochondrial disorders. Mitochondrial disorders present with a wide range of clinical expressions. Multisystem involvement is the hallmark of the disorder and is quite disabling. The organ systems that mostly rely on aerobic metabolism are preferentially affected. In patients with predominantly multisystem disorder, there is a variable combination of central and/or peripheral nervous system involvement, ophthalmologic abnormalities, sensorineural hearing loss, gastrointestinal symptoms, cardiac, hepatic and renal disorder, endocrine dysfunction, and short stature. Central nervous system involvement is also common. Single structure involvement may be seen in Leber's hereditary optic neuropathy (LHON) and maternally inherited non-syndromic deafness. Mitochondrial myopathy refers to skeletal muscle involvement either alone or with central nervous system disorder. The major mitochondrial depletion syndromes (MDS) include myopathic (mutations in TK2, RRM2B, and AGK), encephalomyopathic (mutations in SUCLA2, SUCLG1, and RRM2B), hepatocerebral (mutations in GDUOK, MPV17, POLG, and C10ORF2), and/or neurogastrointestinal (TYMP mutations) types. The age of onset of mitochondrial disorders varies from neonatal to adult life. Neonates, too, have severe manifestations. The diagnosis, lab investigation, and treatment depend on the clinical type and severity of the disorder [1, 2, 5, 6].

EPIDEMIOLOGY

The current prevalence of childhood-onset mitochondrial disorders has been predicted to range from 5 to 15 cases per 10,000. Primary genetic mitochondrial disorders are among the most common inborn errors of metabolism, with a minimum incidence of 1: 5,000. The point prevalence in children younger than age 16 years is estimated to be 1 in 21,000. A population-based study from western Sweden from 1984 until 1999 found that the incidence of mitochondrial encephalomyopathies in preschool aged children was 1 in 11,000 [7]. The incidence and prevalence of mitochondrial myopathies are slightly less than those reported for mitochondrial encephalomyopathies. The prevalence of mtDNA point mutations was greater than 1 in 200 individuals among newborns. Due to variable heteroplasmy, some of these mutations will never be clinically expressed. An Australian study estimated the minimal birth prevalence of primary mitochondrial disorders to be 6.2 cases per 100,000 births [8]. The mortality of these disorders in childhood is high, and many children are expected to survive till 3 to 9 years of age. The median survival for children with infantile onset is said to be 12years.

PATHOGENESIS

Mitochondria, the organelles present in each human cell, carry out many fundamental metabolic pathways, including the respiratory chain, fatty acid β-oxidation, and the tricarboxylic acid (TCA) cycle. The much essential aerobic energy metabolism takes place in the mitochondria. The oxidative phosphorylation or the respiratory chain represents the final stage in oxidative metabolism. The respiratory chain is located in the inner mitochondrial membrane and is composed of five intramembrane complexes and two mobile electron carriers, coenzyme Q10 (CoQ10) and cytochrome c. The five multi-subunit enzyme complexes include complex I, or NADH ubiquinone reductase, which re-oxidizes NADH derived from the oxidation of fatty acids, amino acids, and pyruvate; complex II, or succinate-ubiquinone oxidoreductase, which oxidizes $FADH_2$ derived from the TCA cycle; complex III, or ubiquinol-ferricytochrome-c oxidoreductase; complex IV or cytochrome c oxidase, and complex V, or ATP synthase. Complexes I, III, and IV pump protons from the mitochondrial matrix into the intermembrane space and the energy which this creates is harnessed by ATP synthase for the production of ATP from ADP. Both the mitochondrial and nuclear genes contribute proteins to the OXPHOS pathway. Human mtDNA is a 16.569-kb circular, double-stranded molecule, which contains 37 genes: 2 rRNA genes, 22 tRNA genes, and 13 structural genes encoding the respiratory chain subunits. About 13 proteins of RC are encoded by mtDNA, and the remaining proteins by the nDNA. Complex II, coenzyme Q, and cytochrome c are exclusively encoded by nDNA [3, 4].

At fertilization, all mtDNA derive from the oocyte. A mother carrying an mtDNA point mutation will transfer it to both sons and daughters, but only her daughters will transmit it to their progeny. Because of these reasons, the mode of transmission of mtDNA and mtDNA point mutations differs from Mendelian inheritance. The energy production in mitochondria requires a full assembly of functional protein in the inner mitochondrial membrane as well as a bidirectional flow of information between the nuclear genome and the mitochondrial genome to adjust energy production in tissues to different energy demands. Therefore different mutations in mtDNA and nDNA encoding subunits, components, or regulators of the RC functions result in a wide range of OXPHOS disorders. Deleterious mutations of mtDNA usually affect some but not all mtDNA within a cell, a tissue, or an individual. This is known as heteroplasmy. The clinical expression of a pathogenic mtDNA mutation is largely determined by the relative proportion of normal and mutant mtDNA genomes in different tissues. A minimum critical number of mutant mtDNA is required to cause mitochondrial dysfunction in a particular organ or tissue. This is known as the threshold effect. A phenomenon called mitotic segregation explains how certain patients with mtDNA related disorders manifest different mitochondrial disorders at different stages of their lives [4, 9].

Based on the primary genetic defect, the mitochondrial disorders occur due to defects in RC ancillary proteins, mitochondrial RNA translation, mitochondrial inner membrane lipid milieu, depletion of mtDNA, or mitochondrial dynamics. The proteins of the OXPHOS pathway must be translated, imported into the mitochondria, and inserted into the inner mitochondrial membrane. Mutations in genes affecting these processes cause defects in RC ancillary proteins. Defects in the translation of mitochondrial RNA can disrupt multiple OXPHOS processes. The mitochondria are dynamic in nature, and they are constantly moving, fusing, and dividing. An adequate number of mtDNA are required to maintain the key subunits of mitochondrial RC complexes for energy production. Mitochondrial DNA depletion syndromes (MDS) are secondary to defects in mtDNA maintenance caused by mutations in nuclear genes. All these effects ultimately lead to insufficient energy production. Insufficient energy production likely results in organ dysfunction [9 - 12].

MDS are characterized by a significant decrease in mitochondrial DNA affecting multiple tissues. The manifestations usually involve muscle, liver, or both muscle and brain. The major MDS types include myopathic (mutations in TK2, RRM2B, and AGK), encephalomyopathic (mutations in SUCLA2, SUCLG1, and RRM2B), hepatocerebral (mutations in GDUOK, MPV17, POLG, and C10ORF2), and/or neurogastrointestinal (TYMP mutations) types. Coenzyme Q10 deficiency due to nuclear DNA mutations can present with isolated proximal muscle weakness apart from encephalomyopathy, cerebellar ataxia, nephrotic syndrome, and multisystem disorder. Mitochondrial disorders may present as recognized clinical syndromes involving multiple organ systems. Leigh syndrome and MELAS are the most common clinical syndromes affecting multiple organs [4, 5, 13 - 15].

TYPES OF MITOCHONDRIAL DISORDERS

Mitochondrial RC is under the dual control of mtDNA and nDNA. The steps involved in the proper assembly and functioning of the RC are under the control of nDNA. The five complexes of the human RC contain about 80 proteins; 13 of them are encoded by mtDNA and the rest by the nDNA. Therefore, mitochondrial disorders can be classified into two major categories, i.e, disorders due to defects of mtDNA and disorders due to defects of nDNA from the genetic point of view. Mutations in mtDNA can be divided into those that impair total mitochondrial protein synthesis, such as tRNA or rRNA gene mutations and rearrangements, and those that affect one of the 13 respiratory chain subunits. The disorders also could be related to the synthesis of assembly proteins, intergenomic signaling, mitochondrial importation of nDNA-encoded proteins, synthesis of inner mitochondrial membrane phospholipids, and mitochondrial motility and fission [1, 6, 11, 12].

1. Mitochondrial Disorders Due to Defects of mtDNA

A. Defects in Mitochondrial Protein Synthesis

<u>*mtDNA rearrangements*</u>

Single deletions of mtDNA have been associated with three important conditions that are sporadic in nature.

<u>*(a). Pearson syndrome (PS)*</u>

A disorder characterized by sideroblastic anemia and dysfunction of the exocrine pancreas. It is a fatal disorder and common in infants.

<u>*(b). Kearns-Sayre syndrome (KSS)*</u>

A disorder with onset before age 20 characterized by progressive external ophthalmoplegia (PEO), pigmentary retinopathy and heart block. Ataxia, dementia, endocrine problems such as diabetes mellitus, short stature and hypoparathyroidism may be frequently associated with the syndrome. Lactic acidosis, elevated cerebrospinal fluid protein and ragged red fibers in the muscle biopsy are important findings in the laboratory tests.

(c). Progressive External Ophthalmoplegia With or Without Proximal Limb Weakness

A disorder associated with frequent deletion of 5 kb in size. Rarely there may be duplications or deletion of mtDNA in isolation or together. It is a mild disorder often having a normal life span.

ii). mtDNA point mutations

The defect results in a multisystem disorder mostly maternally inherited. Some of them may be sporadic and tissue-specific. Two common syndromes include:

a) Mitochondrial encephalomyopathy, lactic acidosis, and stroke-like episodes (MELAS)

b) Myoclonus epilepsy with ragged red fibers (MERRF)

c) Syndromes associated with tRNA mutations can affect the eye (optic atrophy, retinitis pigmentosa, cataracts); hearing (sensorineural deafness); the endocrine system (short stature, diabetes mellitus, hypoparathyroidism); the heart (hypertrophic cardiomyopathies, heart blocks); the gastrointestinal tract (exocrine pancreas dysfunction, intestinal pseudo-obstruction, gastroesophageal reflux); and the kidney (renal tubular acidosis).

B. Defects of Protein-coding Genes

There are two syndromes due to mutations at nt-8993 of the ATPase6 gene.

1. (a) Neuropathy, ataxia, retinitis pigmentosa (NARP)

A syndrome affecting young adults manifesting with retinitis pigmentosa, dementia, seizures, ataxia, proximal weakness and sensory neuropathy.

(b). Maternally inherited Leigh syndrome (MILS)

Characterized by severe infantile encephalopathy with symmetrical basal ganglia and the brainstem lesions.

2. Leber's Hereditary Optic Neuropathy (LHON)

2.1. Mitochondrial Disorders Due to Mutations in nDNA

There are many disorders due to mutations in nDNA of mitochondria.

A). *Mutations in genes encoding subunits or ancillary proteins of the respiratory chain*

nDNA encodes all subunits of complex II, most subunits of the other four complexes, as well as CoQ10 and cytochrome c. There are direct hits and indirect hits in mutations involving nDNA.

i). *Direct "hits" are mutations*

In the gene encoding RC subunits, including subunits of complex I and complex II.

These disorders are associated mostly with autosomal recessive forms of Leigh syndrome.

A primary CoQ10 deficiency

Can cause three major syndromes, a predominantly myopathic disorder with recurrent myoglobinuria, a predominantly encephalopathic disorder with ataxia and cerebellar atrophy, and a generalized form.

ii) Indirect "hits" are mutations in genes encoding proteins that are needed for the proper assembly and function of RC complexes. Mutations in five ancillary proteins, SURF1, SCO2, SCO1, COX10, and COX15, have been associated with COX-deficient Leigh syndrome or other multisystemic fatal infantile disorders, in which encephalopathy is accompanied by cardiomyopathy (SCO2, COX15), nephropathy (COX10), or hepatopathy (SCO1). Mutations in a complex III assembly protein, BCS1L are associated with Leigh-like syndromes and GRACILE (growth retardation, aminoaciduria, cholestasis, iron overload, lactic acidosis and early death) disorder. A defect of complex V due to mutations in the assembly protein ATP12 is associated with congenital lactic acidosis and a multisystemic disorder involving the brain, liver, heart, and muscle in infants.

B) *Defects of Intergenomic Signaling*

The mtDNA is highly dependent for its proper function and replication on many factors that are encoded by nuclear genes. Mutations in these genes cause qualitative or quantitative alterations of mtDNA. These disorders are Mendelian disorders.

i) Qualitative alterations in mtDNA: autosomal dominant or autosomal recessive multiple deletions of mtDNA, usually manifest as progressive external ophthalmoplegia (PEO) in addition to other symptoms and signs. Four of these conditions have been well characterized.

a) Mutations in the gene for thymidine phosphorylase (TP) are responsible for an autosomal recessive multisystemic syndrome called mitochondrial neurogastrointestinal encephalomyopathy (MNGIE).

b) Mutations in the gene encoding one isoform of the adenine nucleotide translocator (ANT1) have been identified in some patients with autosomal dominant PEO. Both types of mutations affect mitochondrial nucleotide pools.

c) Mutations in a gene Twinkle are associated with autosomal dominant PEO.

d) Mutations in the gene encoding polymerase g (POLG) may cause either autosomal dominant or autosomal recessive PEO, sometimes associated with psychiatric symptoms or parkinsonism.

ii) Quantitative alterations of mtDNA: Severe or partial expressions of mtDNA depletion are usually characterized by congenital or childhood forms of myopathy or hepatopathy that are autosomal recessive in inheritance. The skeletal muscle and liver are the main target organs. The kidney and central nervous system (CNS) are often affected. The CNS involvement may mimic spinal muscular atrophy. Mutations in two genes involved in mitochondrial nucleotide homeostasis have been associated with MDS. Mutations in the gene encoding thymidine kinase 2 (TK2) are often seen in patients with myopathic MDS. Mutations in the gene encoding deoxyguanosine kinase (dGK) predominate in patients with hepatic or multisystemic MDS.

C) Defects of Mitochondrial Protein Importation

Mutations in components of the mitochondrial transport machinery result in two common disorders.

i) The deafness-dystonia syndrome (Mohr-Tranebjaerg syndrome): This is characterized by sensorineural hearing loss, dystonia, cortical blindness and psychiatric symptoms. Mutations in the TIMM8A gene, that encodes the deafness dystonia protein (DDP1), an intermembrane space component of the transport machinery is responsible for this X-linked disorder.

ii) An autosomal dominant form of hereditary spastic paraplegia (HSP): This condition is due to mutations in the chaperonin HSP60.

D) Alterations of the lipid milieu of the inner mitochondrial membrane: Barth syndrome (BTHS) is characterized by myopathy, cardiopathy, growth retardation, and leucopenia. This is an X-linked recessive disorder.

E) Alterations of mitochondrial motility or fission: an autosomal dominant form of optic atrophy resulting in early-onset blindness.

CLINICAL FEATURES

Mitochondrial disorders manifest with a wide range of clinical features and present a significant diagnostic challenge for pediatricians. One of the hallmarks of mitochondrial disorders is multisystem involvement. In children with mitochondrial multisystem disorder, there is a variable combination of central and/or peripheral nervous system involvement, eye abnormalities, sensorineural hearing loss, gastrointestinal symptoms, cardiac, hepatic and renal disorder, endocrine dysfunction, and growth failure. Tissues with high energy requirements such as the brain, heart and skeletal muscle are preferentially affected in mitochondrial disorders [10, 16 - 18]. Mitochondrial myopathy refers to skeletal muscle involvement and mitochondrial encephalomyopathy applies to the brain and skeletal muscle involvement. Mitochondrial encephalomyopathies predominate over mitochondrial myopathies. But in patients with LHON, myopathy predominates over encephalomyopathy.

Mitochondrial DNA depletion syndrome (MDS) refers to a group of conditions characterized by a significant decrease in mitochondrial DNA affecting multiple tissues, with manifestations involving muscle, liver, or both muscle and brain. Psychiatric symptoms may also be observed in patients with mitochondrial disorders, and psychotropic medications can negatively impact mitochondrial functions.

Symptoms related to isolated myopathy in mitochondrial disorders include exercise intolerance, fatigue, muscle weakness, elevated serum creatine kinase (CK), myalgia and rhabdomyolysis [18].The pattern of muscle involvement varies widely. Proximal muscles of limbs are more commonly involved than the distal muscles. The defects of the respiratory chain, ancillary proteins, intergenomic signaling, and the lipid milieu of the inner mitochondrial membrane may present with myopathy. Coenzyme Q10 deficiency due to nDNA mutations can present with encephalomyopathy, cerebellar ataxia, nephrotic syndrome, and multisystem disorder. It can also present with proximal muscle weakness in isolation. A slowly progressive generalized myopathy and a rapidly progressive and predominantly myopathic presentation have been found to be associated with severe mitochondrial DNA depletion of infancy and childhood.

In children, the most frequent clinical features are severe psychomotor delay, generalized hypotonia, lactic acidosis and signs of cardiorespiratory failure. The most common, and well-characterized, early-onset mitochondrial encephalopathy is Leigh syndrome. Mitochondrial disorders can present with epilepsy. The presentation of mitochondrial epilepsy in children can be highly varied from infantile spasms, generalized seizures, focal seizures, myoclonic epilepsy to refractory status epilepticus.

RECOGNISED CLINICAL SYNDROMES

Some of the mitochondrial disorders that manifest as recognized clinical syndromes with multiple organ systems involvements are as follows [1, 3, 19]:

1. Leigh syndrome (subacute necrotizing encephalomyelopathy)

2. Mitochondrial encephalomyopathy with lactic acidosis and stroke-like episodes (MELAS)

3. Myoclonic epilepsy with ragged red fibers (MERRF)

4. The syndrome of myoclonic epilepsy, myopathy, and sensory ataxia (MEMSA)

5. Maternally inherited deafness and diabetes (MIDD)

6. Mitochondrial neurogastrointestinal encephalopathy (MNGIE)

7. Neuropathy, ataxia, and retinitis pigmentosa (NARP)

8. Pearson syndrome (sideroblastic anemia and pancreatic dysfunction)

9. Coenzyme Q10 deficiency

10. Kearns-Sayre syndrome (KSS) refers to the combination of CPEO with pigmentary retinopathy

11. Severe encephalomyopathy of infancy or childhood

12. Barth syndrome (X-linked cardiomyopathy, mitochondrial myopathy, and cyclic neutropenia)

13. Growth retardation, aminoaciduria, cholestasis, iron overload, lactic acidosis and early death (GRACILE)

14. Leber hereditary optic neuropathy (LHON)

1. Leigh syndrome: This subacute necrotizing encephalomyelopathy typically presents in infancy or early childhood. The characteristic clinical features are developmental delay or psychomotor regression, ataxia, dystonia, external ophthalmoplegia, seizures, lactic acidosis, vomiting and weakness. The pathogenic mutations are identified in about 85 genes. The alterations of mitochondrial metabolism occur due to abnormalities of the pyruvate dehydrogenase complex and RC dysfunction due to either nDNA or mtDNA mutations. The pathologic hallmarks of Leigh syndrome are bilateral, symmetric necrotizing lesions with spongy changes and microcysts in the basal ganglia, thalamus, brainstem, and spinal cord. The mammary bodies are spared. The magnetic resonance imaging (MRI) of the brain shows abnormal white matter signal in the putamen, basal ganglia and brainstem on T2 and fluid-attenuated inversion recovery (FLAIR) sequence images. The prognosis is generally poor, and the affected children may survive only a few months after disorder onset [1, 3, 19]

2. MELAS: This syndrome is a maternally inherited multisystem disorder caused by mutations of mtDNA. The hallmark of this syndrome is the occurrence of stroke-like episodes that result in hemiparesis, hemianopia, or cortical blindness. Focal or generalized seizures, recurrent migraine-like headaches, vomiting, short stature, hearing loss, and muscle weakness may be present. A multitude of tRNA mutations can be responsible for MELAS. About 80 percent of cases are related to the m.3243A>G mutation and 10 percent to the m.3271T>C tRNA mutation.

MELAS usually manifests in childhood after a normal early development with a relapsing-remitting course. The stroke-like episodes lead to progressive neurologic dysfunction and dementia. These episodes are characterized by the acute onset of neurologic symptoms and high signal on diffusion-weighted MRI brain images. The brain lesions do not correlate vascular territories and the apparent diffusion coefficient on MRI is not always decreased but may be increased or demonstrate a mixed pattern. The acute MRI signal changes may migrate, fluctuate, or resolve more quickly and more often than those observed in a typical ischemic stroke.

POLG mutations have also been associated with stroke-like episodes in childhood with predominant involvement of the occipital lobes. Seizures and liver dysfunction may be associated with children affected by stroke [1, 3, 19, 20].

3. MERRF: The characteristic manifestations include myoclonus, generalized epilepsy, ataxia, myopathy, dementia, optic atrophy, bilateral deafness, peripheral neuropathy, spasticity, lipomatosis, and/or cardiomyopathy with Wolff-Parkinso-
-White syndrome. Childhood onset after a normal early development is common.

MERRF is caused by mutations in mtDNA (1, 3, 20). About 80 percent of patients having MERRF demonstrate an A to G mutation at nucleotide 8344 in the mitochondrial *MT-TK* gene encoding tRNA (Lys).

4. MEMSA: It is a syndrome of myoclonic epilepsy, myopathy, and sensory ataxia caused by pathogenic variants *POLG*. They do not have ophthalmoplegia [1, 3].

5. MIDD: This disorder of maternally inherited deafness and diabetes is characterized by a defect in insulin secretion and sensorineural hearing loss. MIDD is caused by a mitochondrial DNA A to G mutation at nucleotide position 3243 in a tRNA. The mean age of onset of diabetes and hearing loss is between 30 and 40. Other abnormalities commonly associated with MIDD include macular retinal dystrophy, myopathy, cardiac disorders, gestational diabetes, focal segmental glomerular sclerosis, short stature, and gastrointestinal disorder. Myopathy may be found in 50% cases affecting typically proximal limbs and may be associated with exercise induced cramps and weakness. The features may overlap with those of MELAS (1, 3).

6. MNGIE: This mitochondrial disorder is characterized by progressive, severe gastrointestinal dysmotility, pseudo-obstruction and cachexia, ptosis, ophthalmoplegia without diplopia, symmetric polyneuropathy, and asymptomatic leukoencephalopathy.

The gastrointestinal symptoms include early satiety, nausea, dysphagia, gastroesophageal reflux, postprandial vomiting, intermittent abdominal pain, abdominal distention and diarrhea. The neuropathy symptoms include paresthesia, pain and distal weakness due to predominant demyelinating neuropathy. The age of onset, presentation, and disorder progression are highly variable. In 60 to 75 percent of patients, the disorder begins before age 20 although the onset age ranges from the first to the fifth decades. The long-term prognosis of MNGIE is poor.

MNGIE is an nDNA disorder which is autosomal recessive in inheritance. Most cases are caused by mutations of the *TYMP* gene (*ECGF1*) that encodes thymidine phosphorylase (1, 3, 20).

7. NARP: This mitochondrial disorder is characterized by a variable combination of developmental delay, sensory polyneuropathy, ataxia, pigmentary retinopathy, muscle weakness, epilepsy, and dementia. Onset age is either late childhood or adults. NARP is caused by a T to G mutation at nucleotide 8993 of the mitochondrial ATPase 6 (*MT-ATP6*) gene.

8. Pearson syndrome: Pearson syndrome is a congenital disorder characterized by severe anemia, ring sideroblasts in the bone marrow, neutropenia, thrombocytopenia, and exocrine pancreatic insufficiency. It is usually fatal in infancy. It is caused by mitochondrial DNA deletions ranging from 2 to 10 kilobases in size.

9. Coenzyme Q10 deficiency: Primary CoQ10 deficiency occurs due to defects in CoQ10 biosynthesis. Secondary deficiency occurs when a disorder of the mitochondrial RC reduces CoQ10 levels without a defect in the biosynthesis of CoQ10 pathway. CoQ10 acts as an electron carrier in the mitochondrial RC and an antioxidant. The major clinical manifestations of CoQ10 deficiency include cerebellar ataxia, severe infantile multisystem disorder, nephropathy, isolated myopathy and encephalomyopathy. Clinical heterogeneity is a common feature of CoQ10 deficiency [1, 3].

10. Kearns-Sayre syndrome: This syndrome occurs before the age 20 and manifests as CPEO with pigmentary retinopathy. Other abnormalities such as short stature, cerebellar ataxia, raised cerebrospinal fluid protein, cardiac conduction defects, anemia, diabetes, deafness, and cognitive deficits or mental retardation may be present. The disorder is usually due to large-scale mtDNA rearrangements and rarely due to point mutations [3].

11. Severe encephalomyopathy of infancy or childhood: This mitochondrial disorder has a variable clinical expression and presents at birth with marked hypotonia, feeding difficulty and respiratory muscle weakness requiring mechanical ventilation. They may have associated brain, heart, liver or kidney involvement. Affected infants usually die before reaching one year of age. The cause is usually a mitochondrial DNA depletion syndrome secondary to mutations in the thymidine kinase 2 (TK2) or succinyl-CoA synthetase ligase 2 (SUCLA2) genes. Few children may have associated generalized proximal tubular dysfunction and a deficiency in complex III. CoQ10 deficiency can also cause a rapidly fatal encephalomyopathy of infancy with nephrotic syndrome. Mutations in the TK2 gene or SUCLA2 gene can also present with a childhood onset phenotype reminiscent of muscular dystrophy with elevated serum creatine kinase levels mimicking Duchenne muscular dystrophy [3, 19].

An infantile severe pure myopathy is a rare disorder due to a mitochondrial tRNA mutation without other system involvement. The children with COX subunit deficiency improve spontaneously over the following two years. POLG-related disorders can cause severe encephalopathies of infancy or adulthood. The childhood myocerebrohepatopathy spectrum is characterized by developmental delay, lactic acidosis, myopathy, and failure to thrive. The Alpers-Huttenlocher syndrome is another POLG-related disorder characterized by childhood onset, progressive encephalopathy, intractable epilepsy, and liver failure.

APPROACH TO MITOCHONDRIAL DISORDERS

Clues from Patient History

It is important to note that at the first presentation the clinical phenotype may be incomplete. The history and physical examination findings may suggest multisystem involvement. They include CNS involvement such as stroke-like episodes, seizures, myoclonus, ataxia, developmental delay or regression, dementia, migraine and dystonia; eye involvement such as pigmentary retinopathy, optic atrophy, and cataracts; muscle involvement such as exercise intolerance, myalgia, rhabdomyolysis or myoglobinuria, predominant proximal weakness, hypotonia, ptosis, and extraocular motility disorders with or without diplopia; CVS involvement such as cardiac conduction defects and cardiomyopathy; renal involvement such as proximal nephron dysfunction and glomerulopathy; gastrointestinal involvement such as altered gut motility, pseudo-obstruction, liver disorder, episodes of nausea and vomiting, and exocrine pancreatic dysfunction; endocrine involvement such as diabetes and hypoparathyroidism; skin involvement such as multiple lipomas; hematologic involvement such as sideroblastic anemia and pancytopenia; metabolic acidosis; short stature; neuropathy and dysautonomia or concurrent neuropathy and myopathy in the same patient.

The three generation family history with a history of maternal inheritance may suggest mitochondrial disorder. The mtDNA mutations may be sporadic with no history of affected family members. The disorders due to nDNA mutations may be autosomal dominant or recessive in inheritance.

LABORATORY TESTS

In clinically suspected cases of mitochondrial disorders, the initial tests of blood and urine should include transaminases, lactate-to-pyruvate ratio, amino acids, acylcarnitine profile, creatine kinase and organic acids [3, 21, 22]. Appropriate mitochondrial DNA tests are recommended initially for maternally inherited classic mitochondrial disorders such as MELAS, MERRF, NARP, MIDD and LHON bypassing the metabolic tests and muscle biopsy. Similarly, relevant nDNA tests may be carried out initially for MNGIE and chronic PEO. The Mitochondrial Medicine Society (MMS) developed consensus criteria for the diagnosis of mitochondrial disorders which can be found at https://www.mitoaction.org/wp-content/uploads/2019/09/Mitochondrial-Disorder-Consensus-Criteria.pdf.

Consensus based expert recommendations for the evaluation and diagnosis of mitochondrial disorder published in 2014 suggest the following biochemical tests involving blood, urine and cerebrospinal fluid (CSF): complete blood count, serum creatine kinase (CK) and uric acid, serum transaminases, serum albumin, serum lactate and pyruvate, lactate/pyruvate ratio if serum lactate is elevated,serum amino acids, serum acylcarnitine (low free carnitine and elevated acyl/free carnitine ratio are suggestive of disrupted fatty acid oxidation), serum and urine 3-methylgluticonic acid, quantitative or qualitative urine organic acids (for elevations in Krebs cycle intermediates, methylmalonate, and dicarboxylic acid), CSF analysis for lactate, pyruvate, amino acids, and 5-methyltetrahydrofolate [3, 23, 24].

Serum CK level is usually normal or only slightly elevated. In the context of severe myopathy with a normal plasma CK level, the mitochondrial disorder may be considered.

Elevated lactate levels have a specificity of 34 to 62 percent and a sensitivity of 83 to 100 percent for the diagnosis of mitochondrial disorders. Postprandial lactate levels are more sensitive than fasting lactate levels. Lactate levels are usually elevated during physiologic stress. The serum and CSF lactate/pyruvate ratio is only useful when the lactate level is elevated. Disorders like LHON, Leigh syndrome, Kearns-Sayre syndrome, and *POLG*-associated mitochondrial disorders may have a normal or mild elevation of lactate levels.

Other tests such as fasting blood glucose and glycosylated hemoglobin, renal function tests, electrocardiography, MRI of the brain, electromyography, muscle biopsy, cardiac imaging with echocardiography, eye examination, hearing evaluation, thyroid and parathyroid tests, electroencephalogram in patients with encephalopathy or seizures and exercise testing for patients with predominant exercise intolerance give valuable clues for the diagnosis and the extent of multisystem involvement.

Genetic Studies

The genetic studies identify the causative mutations underlying mitochondrial disorders [3, 21]. The next generation sequencing (NGS) is preferred for sequencing of the mtDNA as it yields the detail and detects the heteroplasmy of even one percent. NGS also detects the deletion and duplication of the mitochondrial genome. If genetics testing in the blood is negative in a strongly suspected mitochondrial disorder testing of affected tissue is recommended. For disorders that demonstrate heteroplasmy, urine, and blood testing is preferred. For MDS, analysis by NGS panel for a group of nuclear genes is a preferred test. The copy number of mitochondrial DNA per cell can best be performed on affected tissue by a real-time quantitative polymerase chain reaction. For nuclear gene defects, NGS of a panel including all known nuclear genes affecting mitochondria is preferred over single-gene testing. If NGS is not providing the diagnosis, whole exome sequencing should be considered.

Neuroimaging

Brain MRI may demonstrate nonspecific delayed myelination pattern in early disorder, symmetric lesions of the deep gray matter specific for Leigh disorder, stroke-like lesions suggestive of MELAS, and cerebral and/or cerebellar atrophy with bilateral deep gray lesions in MDS. Magnetic resonance spectroscopy (MRS) of the brain may be helpful to identify pathological lactate peaks.

Nerve Conduction Studies and Electromyography

In mitochondrial disorder, nerve conduction studies are either normal or consistent with a myopathy and show predominantly low amplitude compound motor unit potentials. An axonal polyneuropathy may be observed. Demyelinating polyneuropathies with conduction velocities as low as 15 m/s have also been reported. The needle electromyography test may be normal or show findings consistent with a myopathy such as short duration, small, polyphasic motor unit potentials with early recruitment. Positive sharp waves and fibrillation potentials are rare. Reduced recruitment and large, polyphasic motor unit potentials suggestive of mild neurogenic changes may be observed [3, 19].

Muscle Biopsy

A muscle biopsy is an important investigation in the diagnosis of mitochondrial disorders. Muscle biopsy is suggested when muscle disorder is the only symptom and when DNA testing cannot confirm the diagnosis. Muscle biopsy is also useful to rule out the immune mediated myopathies. The vastus lateralis muscle is usually chosen for the biopsy. The ragged red fibers are likely to be seen on the muscle histology. On Gomori trichrome stain, subsarcolemmal and intermyofibrillar accumulation of mitochondria in muscle fibers is the hallmark of mitochondrial disorders. MELAS due to mitochondrial DNA mutation m.3243A>G can be confirmed on DNA extracted from leukocytes in peripheral blood and hence muscle biopsy may not be required. However, when hematopoietic tissue is not affected by the mitochondrial disorder, testing on affected tissue is necessary [3, 18, 21].

Biochemical Tests

Biochemical testing is available usually using muscle tissue. The liver, cultured fibroblast, or cells obtained by buccal swab may also be used in certain circumstances. Biochemical analysis of the enzyme activity of the respiratory enzyme complexes is available. Measurement of RC function in the affected tissue is possible because the individual respiratory chain complexes can be separated by electrophoresis. Testing RC function usually requires at least 300mg of snap-frozen muscle tissue. These enzymatic measurements are not considered essential for the diagnosis of mitochondrial dysfunction in the 2014 consensus criteria. Despite the potential pitfalls, testing respiratory complex function may be useful in children. They may diagnose defects secondary to point mutations or micro-deletions in either mtDNA or nDNA that affect only one respiratory chain complex. Single complex abnormalities are more commonly seen in children [24].

TREATMENT

Mitochondrial disorders in children need comprehensive and multidisciplinary care. The care includes symptom-based treatment, maintaining optimal health, using preventive measures to avoid symptom worsening during stress situations such as infection, dehydration or surgery, and avoiding mitochondrial toxins. Supportive measures such as improvement of nutrition, correction of lactic acidosis, treatment of seizures, surgical correction of ptosis and other complications can improve the quality of life. Except for coenzyme Q10 supplementation in primary defects of coenzyme Q10 synthesis and L-arginine for metabolic stroke, there is little evidence to support most pharmacological interventions. The beneficial pharmacological agents include respiratory chain cofactors, antioxidants, agents that decrease lactate and other metabolites that are secondarily decreased in mitochondrial disorders [23 - 26].

Now-a-days, there is more scientific support for the use of vitamin-based and cofactor-based mitochondrial therapies. Such pharmacologic therapies are intended to promote critical enzymatic reactions, reduce harmful accumulation of free radicals, and scavenge toxic acyl coenzyme A (acyl CoA) molecules. Some supplements also may act as alternative energy fuels or may bypass biochemical blocks within the RC, although these mechanisms are debatable. Exercise therapy has been shown to reduce the unhealthy mitochondria, increase the percentage of healthy, non-mutated mtDNA and improve endurance and muscle function. The definitive therapy for halting disorder progression is not yet available and the long-term benefits of available treatment are not well established.

Hospitalization of children affected by mitochondrial disorders should be case-specific. Evaluation of a child suspected of mitochondrial disorder in an emergency unit should include routine chemistries, glucose, transaminases, lactate, a complete blood count, liver function tests, ammonia, glucose and other tests as clinically indicated. The ketosis and lactic acidosis should be monitored and any derangements should be corrected. Potential cardiac and neurologic decompensations in these patients should be kept in mind and assessed according to the situation. Treatment during acute decompensation should include dextrose containing intravenous (IV) fluids, correction of metabolic derangements and stopping any mitochondrial toxic medications. Limited or no dextrose recommended in suspected or confirmed disorders of pyruvate metabolism, if the patient is on a ketogenic diet, or earlier history of adverse response to high glucose delivery. Outpatient mitochondrial therapies should be continued when possible. Hydration and substrate therapy involves providing 5% or 10% dextrose containing IV fluids, given at 1.25 to 1.5 times the maintenance rate. Fluids should be weaned based on laboratory parameters, oral intake, and resolution of the underlying metabolic stressor. Avoid lactated Ringer's solution. If there is metabolic acidosis with pH < 7.22 or bicarbonate level < 14 mM, sodium bicarbonate as a bolus (1 mEq/kg) followed by a continuous infusion may be given. Hyperammonemia due to secondary inhibition of the urea cycle may diminish as treatment for the metabolic decompensation proceeds. A level of more than 200 μM may require salvage therapy or dialysis. Consider dextrose delivery with D10 or D20 if fluids containing 5% dextrose are not correcting acidosis or metabolic derangements. In such instances, insulin of 0.05 to 0.1 U/kg per hour may be initiated and titrated further. As soon as the initial crisis subsides, enteral feeding should be started. Once the patient's laboratory parameters begin to normalize, restarting the patient's home-based diet is advised. L-Carnitine therapy intravenously at a dosage of at least 100 mg/kg per day during acute illness may be beneficial. Doses of up to 300 mg/kg per day may be used. CoQ10 and other antioxidants such as vitamins C and E can also be given. IV L-arginine therapy should be considered for a patient with a possible metabolic stroke as it helps by nitric oxide mediated vasodilation.

For anesthesia, sevoflurane is preferred over isoflurane or halothane. The use of propofol in mitochondrial disorder is being debated although it has been used routinely without any problems in many patients for brief periods of sedation lasting less than 30–60minutes. During preoperative and postoperative fasting, catabolism can be prevented by using dextrose containing IV fluids [22, 25, 26].

Stroke-like episodes in primary mitochondrial disorder typically have correlating visible abnormalities on MRI of the brain. An urgent IV arginine hydrochloride administration has been recommended in the acute setting of a stroke-like episode associated with the MELAS m.3243A >G mutation in the MTTL1 gene and other primary mitochondrial cytopathies. Patients should be reassessed after 3 days of continuous IV therapy. Subsequently, the use of daily oral arginine supplementation to prevent strokes should be considered in MELAS. Repeat neuroimaging of the brain should be considered in any mitochondrial patient with an acute change in neurologic status.

Infection should be sought and treated promptly as it may be a precipitating factor for the acute deterioration or a treatable differential diagnosis. In patients with pressor refractory hypotension, empiric administration of stress dose steroids should be considered. Nutritional support must be provided with enteral feeds if tolerated or with peripheral or central parenteral nutrition. Hypoglycemia, hypoalbuminemia, or coagulopathy must be excluded if liver dysfunction is suspected. Mitochondrial patients should take precautions to prevent entering catabolism, especially when exposed to medical stressors. Prolonged fasting should be avoided and dextrose containing IV fluids should be considered before, during, and after procedures and surgeries.

Therapies using vitamins and cofactors are beneficial, but the choice of these agents and the doses prescribed are debatable. Many studies report significant clinical responses to such pharmacologic interventions. A therapeutic trial of coenzyme Q10 along with other antioxidants known as mitochondrial cocktail should be attempted for their synergistic effect.

There are no cures for mitochondrial disorders, but the available treatment can help reduce symptoms or slow the decline in health. Treatment varies from patient to patient and depends on the specific mitochondrial disorder and its severity. There are no ways to predict the response to treatment or the long-term prognosis. The practice of mitochondrial medicine remains challenging due to a paucity of high-quality evidence to guide clinical patient care and management. The consensus recommendations by MMS help to begin the process of standardization of care. These recommendations create more awareness in mitochondrial disorder and aid in the diagnosis, management, and monitoring of comorbid conditions. Consensus guidelines are not meant to apply to all cases or conditions and they should be used with the clinical judgment.

Nutrition, exercise and pharmacological treatment are all important in the treatment of mitochondrial disorders. Pharmacological treatment includes vitamins and supplements.

Nutrition, Ketogenic Diet, Avoiding Toxins and Exercise

Nutrition

Children with mitochondrial disorders have different calorie needs. Caloric supplementation, enteral feeding, avoiding fasting, frequent meals and intravenous nutrition are all potential therapeutic options. Treating swallowing dysfunction, abnormal gut motility, behavioral feeding issues and gastroesophageal reflux is recommended to allow for optimal nutritional intake. Extreme malnutrition, including anorexia, starvation, and illness-related cachexia cause secondary mitochondrial dysfunction. Optimizing the caloric needs in these children will improve mitochondrial health.

Ketogenic Diet

The ketogenic diet with high-fat content may be beneficial in optimizing mitochondrial functions although there is limited evidence. The ketogenic diet is the standard of care for pyruvate dehydrogenase deficiency, but it is contraindicated in patients with known fatty acid oxidation disorders and pyruvate carboxylase deficiency.

Avoiding Mitochondrial Toxins

Some medications and environmental toxins impair mitochondrial functions. Such substances may inhibit the electron transport chain directly, increase reactive oxygen species, impair mitochondrial protein transport or inhibit mtDNA replication. The drugs in this category include valproic acid, topiramate, vigabatrin, statins, metformin, high dose acetaminophen, and selected antibiotics such as aminoglycosides, linezolid, tetracycline, azithromycin and erythromycin. These drugs should be avoided in mitochondrial disorders or should be used with caution and closely monitored. Valproic acid should be avoided as a treatment, especially in POLG disorder.

Exercise

Mitochondrial disorders can lead to exercise intolerance even with activities of daily living. A planned exercise not only improves mitochondrial functions but also decreases the burden of unhealthy mitochondria. Before beginning an exercise regimen, a 12-lead electrocardiogram should be obtained.

Very low intensity and brief duration exercise should be started initially and it should progress gradually. A simple carbohydrate containing drink or meal prior to exercise helps to increase endurance. Exercises including endurance exercises and resistance/strength training exercises increase muscle size and strength. Endurance exercises include walking, running, swimming, dancing, cycling and others. Resistance/strength training exercises include sit-ups, arm curls, knee extensions, weight lifting and others. Endurance exercises are considered better than resistance exercises. Graded endurance exercise can improve exercise tolerance further. Resistance exercise such as using weights can increase muscle strength. Use of a recumbent exercise, bicycle and/or pool therapy may be better tolerated than other regimens in those with gait instability or excessive fatigue [22, 24 - 26].

Pharmacologic Treatment

The pharmacological agents for the treatment of mitochondrial disorders include Coenzyme Q10, B complex vitamins, especially thiamine (B1) and riboflavin (B2), Alpha lipoic acid, L-carnitine, Creatine and L-Arginine. Coenzyme Q10, riboflavin and idebenone are the agents that enhance electron transport at different levels of mitochondrial RC.

Coenzyme Q10

CoQ10 found in all cell and organelle membranes participates in redox shuttling. It has an important intracellular signaling role, as well as both antioxidant and prooxidant roles. CoQ10 is endogenously synthesized in the mitochondria and is an integral component of the mitochondrial electron transport chain, shuttling electrons from complexes I or II and a number of other electron donors, including electron transfer factor, which moves electrons from fatty acid beta oxidation. CoQ10 modulates the mitochondrial permeability transition pore involved in apoptosis and activates uncoupling proteins.

CoQ10 biosynthetic defects underlie several different phenotypes of a human mitochondrial disorder. These defects include neonatal encephalopathy with nephropathy (COQ2), Leigh syndrome, lactic acidosis, and nephropathy (PDSS2), infantile nephropathy, hepatopathy, retardation (PDSS1), and recessive ataxia, cerebellar atrophy with or without retardation, lactic acidosis, and exercise intolerance (ADCK3). These disorders respond to exogenous CoQ10 administration.

CoQ10 is insoluble in water. Powder formulations of CoQ10 have poor intestinal absorption. Bioavailability has been improved with the use of nanoparticles in suspension. The ubiquinol form is three to five times better absorbed than the oxidized form of CoQ, ubiquinone. The plasma half-life of CoQ10 is about 36 hours. Ubiquinol is used in doses of 2 to 8 mg/kg per day in two divided doses with meals. Ubiquinone is used in doses of 5 to 30 mg/kg per day in two divided doses daily with meals.

Co Q analog, Idebenone in the doses of 90 to 270 mg/day shown to be effective in improving recovery after the onset of vision loss in Leber's hereditary optic neuropathy.

Riboflavin

This vitamin B2 that serves as a flavoprotein precursor, is a key building block in complex I and II and, a cofactor in other enzymatic reactions involving fatty acid oxidation and the Krebs cycle. Riboflavin is useful in treating complex I and/or complex II disorder and multiple acyl CoA dehydrogenase deficiency (MADD). It is used in the dosage of 50–400 mg/day. The average dose is 100 mg/day.

L-Carnitine

L-Carnitine plays a critical role in the mitochondrial β-oxidation of fatty acids and the esterification of free fatty acids. Carnitine transfers long chain fatty acids across the mitochondrial inner membrane as acylcarnitine esters. These esters are oxidized to acetyl CoA, which enters the Krebs cycle and results in the subsequent generation of ATP via oxidative phosphorylation. Carnitine prevents CoA depletion and removes toxic acyl compounds. Patients with RC defects tend to have lower than average free carnitine levels in plasma and increased esterified carnitine levels. This shift may reflect partial β-oxidation impairment. L-carnitine supplementation for mitochondrial disorders restores free carnitine levels and removes toxic acyl compounds. The dosage is 20 to 100 mg/kg/day divided into two or three doses orally or 50 to 100 mg/kg/d divided every 4 to 6 hours, to a maximum of 300 mg/kg/d intravenously.

L-Arginine

Arginine is involved in growth, detoxification of urea and creatine synthesis. L-arginine produces nitric oxide, which has neurotransmitter and vasodilator properties. A loading dose of IV L-arginine of 500mg/kg/dose quickly decreases the severity of stroke-like symptoms, enhances microcirculation, and reduces tissue injury from ischemia in MELAS. The IV dose may be continued for 1 to 3 days. Maintenance and prophylactic oral L-arginine in the dosage of 150 to 300mg/kg/day divided every 8-12 hours decreases clinical severity and frequency of stroke-like episodes.

L-creatine

Creatine combines with phosphate in the mitochondria to form phosphocreatine. It serves as a source of high-energy phosphate during anaerobic metabolism. It also acts as an intracellular buffer for ATP and as an energy shuttle for the movement of high energy phosphates from mitochondrial sites of production to cytoplasmic sites of utilization. Creatine treatment in mitochondrial encephalomyopathies is said to increase in high intensity, isometric, and aerobic muscle power. The dose is 0.1 g/kg per day given in two doses.

Redox and Other Agents

Thiamine (B1), vitamins C and E, and alpha lipoic acid have been used in mitochondrial disorders as an antioxidant cocktail. Thiamine enhances pyruvate dehydrogenase activity, thereby increasing the availability of pyruvate for oxidation. Thiamine has been used in doses up to 900 mg/day. Vitamin C is used at 5 mg/kg/ day orally. Vitamin E dosage is 1 to 2 IU/kg/day per orally. Lipoic acid is found naturally within the mitochondria and is an essential cofactor for pyruvate dehydrogenase and ketoglutarate dehydrogenase. It acts as a potent antioxidant and used in the dosage of 50 to 200 mg/day. Dichloroacetate (DCA) is a potent lactate lowering drug that activates the pyruvate dehydrogenase complex by inhibiting the activity of pyruvate dehydrogenase kinase, which normally phosphorylates and inhibits the enzyme. DCA is used at a dose of 25 mg/kg/day in two divided doses.

Folinic Acid

Folinic acid or vitamin B9 is involved as a cofactor in multiple metabolic reactions. It is the natural transport form of folate across the blood brain barrier. Cerebral folate deficiency occurs in mitochondrial disorder especially in patients with Kearns-Sayre syndrome. The dosage of folinic acid is 0.5 to 2.5 mg/kg daily, given once or twice a day [22 - 26].

Treatment of Epilepsy in Mitochondrial Disorder

In general, the treatment of epilepsy in mitochondrial disorders is the same as that of epilepsy with other etiology with certain exceptions. Mitochondrial epilepsy can present as seizure of any type. Mitochondrial dysfunction leads to neuronal hyperexcitability by reducing sodium, potassium ATPase activity, disruption of intracellular calcium homeostasis and glutamate disturbances. This can lead to a destructive positive feedback loop in conditions such as POLG and MELAS. Myoclonic and focal seizures are most common with a significant risk of either generalized or focal status epilepticus. Respiratory chain defects have also been identified in epileptic encephalopathies including Ohtahara syndrome, West syndrome, Lennox-Gastaut syndrome and Landau-Kleffner syndrome.

A combination of sodium channel drugs and benzodiazepines with the addition of topiramate or levetiracetam usually controls the seizures. Carbamazepine was reported to gradually control electroclinical status in a patient with MELAS. Lamotrigine is found to increase the production of ATP with potential neuroprotective effects. Levetiracetam may be a reasonable first-line drug for MERRF. Valproate is contraindicated in POLG related disorders due to the risk of hepatic failure. POLG testing may be considered prior to starting valproate treatment in any patient who develops intractable epilepsy and has a history of developmental delay. Valproate may also worsen MELAS. Ketogenic diet likely to be beneficial in the treatment of epilepsy related to mitochondrial disorder as this diet may partially bypass complex I. Folinic acid may be useful in Kearns-Sayre syndrome. Ketamine may be used for status epilepticus refractory to benzodiazepines, thiopental, phenytoin and propofol. POLG mutation related disorder and PDHE1α gene mutation related Leigh syndrome with epilepsy may benefit from sodium pyruvate at 0.5 g/kg/day. L-arginine infusion or a cocktail of folic acid, riboflavin and CoQ10 may be helpful for status epilepticus associated with MELAS [24 - 26].

Cardiomyopathy Monitoring, Cardiac Pacemakers and Defibrillators

Cardiac conduction defects with or without cardiomyopathy are observed in some mitochondrial disorders, especially in Kearns-Sayre syndrome. Cardiac manifestations may also occur in patients with mtDNA disorders, fatty acid oxidation defects, and disorders due to nuclear genes, such as Friedreich's ataxia and Barth syndrome. A 24 to 48 hours ECG monitoring should be obtained every 1 to 2 years for all patients at high risk of preexcitation syndrome or conduction disorder, patients with severely impaired left ventricular systolic function with ejection fraction <35%, patients with paroxysmal symptoms suggestive of cardiac involvement such as palpitations and patients with left ventricular systolic or diastolic dysfunction.

Ablation should be considered in supraventricular tachycardia, Wolf-Parkinso--White or any arrhythmias potentially treatable by this technique. A low threshold for pacemaker implantation is needed to prevent cardiac death. Pacemakers can be combined with an implantable defibrillator if needed. An implantable cardioverter defibrillator is needed in patients at risk of sudden death when the left ventricle wall thickness is > 30mm, and in patients with ventricular tachycardia. In the setting of end stage heart failure, transplantation may be an option. The newer automatic internal cardiac defibrillators (AICD) are implantable medical devices with benefits as pacemaker and a synchronized cardioversion. Other less sophisticated external devices may also be used as a bridge to AICD [24 - 26].

Role of Organ Transplant

The transplantation of a single organ is not an option in mitochondrial disorders as these disorders mostly involve multiple organ systems. Certain disorders like electron transport chain deficiencies and MDS patients having the hepatocerebral syndrome produced by mutations in deoxyguanosine kinase are currently considered for liver transplants. Mitochondrial disorder with cardiomyopathy may benefit from cardiac transplantation. In the MNGIE, stem cell transplantation may replete the missing enzyme activity and result in long term clinical improvement.

Cochlear Implants

Sensorineural hearing loss is associated with many nDNA and mtDNA related disorders. Children with specific mtDNA mutations such as A1555G mutation have extreme susceptibility to hearing loss upon aminoglycoside exposure. The A3243G mutation in MELAS and the mtDNA deletions in Kearns-Sayre syndrome are associated with spontaneous hearing loss. These are the children for potential cochlear implants.

Newer Therapies

Sirtuin compounds modulate histone deacetylases which affect the activity of multiple metabolic enzymes via stimulation of the peroxisome proliferator activated receptor (PPAR) family, the PPAR-γ coactivator 1α (PGC-1α), and insulin signaling pathway. PPAR signaling regulates gene expression of multiple metabolic pathways, including gluconeogenesis, metabolism of fatty acids, adipocyte differentiation, cell survival, and ubiquitination. Bezafibrate, a PPAR pan agonist was found to improve lifespan and ameliorate muscle manifestations by increasing mitochondrial biogenesis and tissue ATP levels in a skeletal muscle in animal models. Bezafibrate is known to induce mitochondrial biogenesis and to control the expression of antioxidant enzymes and uncoupling proteins. No clinical trials have been completed to guide their use or determine their risks and benefits in primary mitochondrial disorder. It may be a promising therapeutic agent for the treatment of a neurodegenerative disorder associated with mitochondrial dysfunction.

SIRT-1 agonists are currently being developed for a variety of conditions including mitochondrial disorder.

Resveratrol

Resveratrol is an antioxidant, an apoptosis inhibitor, and an SIRT-1 agonist that has role in the treatment of diabetes, cardiovascular disorder, neurodegenerative disorder, cancer, obesity, and aging. Its utility in primary mitochondrial disorder is being explored.

Gene Therapy

Mitochondrial gene delivery by Adeno-associated virus-mediated gene therapy (AAV) is found to be achievable. The introduction of modified genes or gene products into mitochondria via the protein import machinery and inhibition of replication of mutant mtDNA by sequence specific antigenomic peptide-nucleic acids are being explored [24, 26].

CONCLUSION

Mitochondria in human cells participate mainly in oxidative phosphorylation and energy production. The genetic defects in mtDNA, nDNA and related functions of mitochondria result in insufficient energy production and organ dysfunction. Mitochondrial disorders cause significant morbidity and mortality in children. The clinical manifestations vary widely and multisystem involvement is common. Treatment depends on the specific mitochondrial disorder and its severity. At present, there are no cures for these disorders but treatments could reduce symptoms or slow the decline in health. Coenzyme Q10, thiamine, riboflavin, lipoic acid, L-carnitine, Creatine and L-Arginine are found to be beneficial. In future, gene therapy may be available for these disorders.

CONSENT FOR PUBLICATION

Not applicable.

CONFLICT OF INTEREST

The author declares no conflict of interest, financial or otherwise.

ACKNOWLEDGEMENT

Declared none.

REFERENCES

[1]   DiMauro S. Mitochondrial diseases. Biochimica et Biophysica Acta (BBA)-. Biochim Biophys Acta Bioenerg 2004; 1658(1-2): 80-8.
[http://dx.doi.org/10.1016/j.bbabio.2004.03.014]

[2]   Di Donato S. Disorders related to mitochondrial membranes: pathology of the respiratory chain and neurodegeneration. J Inherit Metab Dis 2000; 23(3): 247-63.
[http://dx.doi.org/10.1023/A:1005684029429] [PMID: 10863941]

[3]   Schmiedel J, Jackson S, Schäfer J, Reichmann H. Mitochondrial cytopathies. J Neurol 2003; 250(3): 267-77.
[http://dx.doi.org/10.1007/s00415-003-0978-3] [PMID: 12638015]

[4]   Spinazzola A, Ed. Mitochondrial DNA mutations and depletion in pediatric medicine. Seminars in Fetal and Neonatal Medicine. Seminars in Fetal and Neonatal Medicine. Elsevier 2011.

[5]   Mancuso M, Filosto M, Choub A, *et al.* Mitochondrial DNA-related disorders. Biosci Rep 2007; 27(1-3): 31-7.
[http://dx.doi.org/10.1007/s10540-007-9035-2] [PMID: 17484046]

[6]   Lee YM, Kim HD. Mitochondrial disorders. Hanyang Med Rev 2005; 25(3): 12-8.

[7]   Darin N, Oldfors A, Moslemi AR, Holme E, Tulinius M. The incidence of mitochondrial

encephalomyopathies in childhood: clinical features and morphological, biochemical, and DNA abnormalities. Ann Neurol 2001; 49(3): 377-83.
[http://dx.doi.org/10.1002/ana.75] [PMID: 11261513]

[8]   Skladal D, Halliday J, Thorburn DR. Minimum birth prevalence of mitochondrial respiratory chain disorders in children. Brain 2003; 126(Pt 8): 1905-12.
[http://dx.doi.org/10.1093/brain/awg170] [PMID: 12805096]

[9]   Janssen RJ, van den Heuvel LP, Smeitink JA. Genetic defects in the oxidative phosphorylation (OXPHOS) system. Expert Rev Mol Diagn 2004; 4(2): 143-56.
[http://dx.doi.org/10.1586/14737159.4.2.143] [PMID: 14995902]

[10]   De Vivo DC. The expanding clinical spectrum of mitochondrial diseases. Brain Dev 1993; 15(1): 1-22.
[http://dx.doi.org/10.1016/0387-7604(93)90002-P] [PMID: 8338207]

[11]   Ghezzi D, Zeviani M. Assembly factors of human mitochondrial respiratory chain complexes: physiology and pathophysiology. Mitochondrial Oxidative Phosphorylation. Springer 2012; pp. 65-106.

[12]   Greaves LC, Reeve AK, Taylor RW, Turnbull DM. Mitochondrial DNA and disease. J Pathol 2012; 226(2): 274-86.
[http://dx.doi.org/10.1002/path.3028] [PMID: 21989606]

[13]   DiMauro S, Moraes CT. Mitochondrial encephalomyopathies. Arch Neurol 1993; 50(11): 1197-208.
[http://dx.doi.org/10.1001/archneur.1993.00540110075008] [PMID: 8215979]

[14]   Pagniez-Mammeri H, Rak M, Legrand A, Bénit P, Rustin P, Slama A. Mitochondrial complex I deficiency of nuclear origin II. Non-structural genes. Mol Genet Metab 2012; 105(2): 173-9.
[http://dx.doi.org/10.1016/j.ymgme.2011.10.001] [PMID: 22099533]

[15]   Wallace DC. Mitochondrial defects in neurodegenerative disease. Ment Retard Dev Disabil Res Rev 2001; 7(3): 158-66.
[http://dx.doi.org/10.1002/mrdd.1023] [PMID: 11553931]

[16]   Zeviani M, Antozzi C. Defects of mitochondrial DNA. Brain Pathol 1992; 2(2): 121-32.
[http://dx.doi.org/10.1111/j.1750-3639.1992.tb00680.x] [PMID: 1341953]

[17]   Arnaiz SL, Travacio M, Llesuy S, Boveris A. Hydrogen peroxide metabolism during peroxisome proliferation by fenofibrate. Biochim Biophys Acta 1995; 1272(3): 175-80.
[http://dx.doi.org/10.1016/0925-4439(95)00084-4] [PMID: 8541349]

[18]   Schon EA. Mitochondrial disorders in muscle. Curr Opin Neurol Neurosurg 1993; 6(1): 19-26.
[PMID: 8428062]

[19]   Thyagarajan D, Byrne E. Mitochondrial disorders of the nervous system: clinical, biochemical, and molecular genetic features. Int Rev Neurobiol 2002; 53: 93-144.
[http://dx.doi.org/10.1016/S0074-7742(02)53005-1] [PMID: 12512338]

[20]   Wong L-JC. Diagnostic challenges of mitochondrial DNA disorders. Mitochondrion 2007; 7(1-2): 45-52.
[http://dx.doi.org/10.1016/j.mito.2006.11.025] [PMID: 17276740]

[21]   Wong L-JC, Boles RG. Mitochondrial DNA analysis in clinical laboratory diagnostics. Clin Chim Acta 2005; 354(1-2): 1-20.
[http://dx.doi.org/10.1016/j.cccn.2004.11.003] [PMID: 15748595]

[22]   Parikh S, Goldstein A, Karaa A, *et al.* Patient care standards for primary mitochondrial disease: a consensus statement from the Mitochondrial Medicine Society. Genet Med 2017; 19(12): 1380-97.
[http://dx.doi.org/10.1038/gim.2017.107] [PMID: 28749475]

[23]   Avula S, Parikh S, Demarest S, Kurz J, Gropman A. Treatment of mitochondrial disorders. Curr Treat Options Neurol 2014; 16(6): 292.

[http://dx.doi.org/10.1007/s11940-014-0292-7] [PMID: 24700433]

[24]   Parikh S, Goldstein A, Koenig MK, *et al.* Diagnosis and management of mitochondrial disease: a consensus statement from the Mitochondrial Medicine Society. Genet Med 2015; 17(9): 689-701.
[http://dx.doi.org/10.1038/gim.2014.177] [PMID: 25503498]

[25]   Parikh S, Saneto R, Falk MJ, *et al.* A modern approach to the treatment of mitochondrial disease. Curr Treat Options Neurol 2009; 11(6): 414-30.
[http://dx.doi.org/10.1007/s11940-009-0046-0] [PMID: 19891905]

[26]   Zhang L, Zhang Z, Khan A, Zheng H, Yuan C, Jiang H. Advances in drug therapy for mitochondrial diseases. Ann Transl Med 2020; 8(1): 17.
[http://dx.doi.org/10.21037/atm.2019.10.113] [PMID: 32055608]

SUBJECT INDEX

A

Abdominal 13, 14, 15, 46, 87, 93, 290, 310, 311, 315, 317, 318, 342, 431, 432
  angina 46
  cramping 290
  pain 13, 14, 15, 87, 93, 310, 311, 315, 317, 318, 342, 431, 432
Abnormalities 26, 101, 152, 156, 157, 172, 190, 196, 202, 204, 206, 211, 214, 216, 218, 235, 262, 393, 397, 437, 438, 453, 462, 463, 464, 469
  chromosomal 214
  congenital 26, 437, 438
  coronary artery 101
  cortical migration 202
  genetic 262
  liver function 196
  lung 393
  metabolic 172, 190
  neurological 397
  ophthalmologic 453
Absolute lymphocyte count (ALC) 336, 337, 378, 379, 405, 406, 414
Acalculous cholecystitis 99, 101
Acanthosis nigricans 82
ACE inhibitors 91
Acids 205, 216, 217, 218, 223, 262, 263, 285, 312, 346, 353, 354, 387, 393, 397, 452, 453, 454, 465, 466, 471, 474, 475, 477
  amino 387, 393, 452, 453, 454, 465, 466
  deoxyribonucleic 346
  dicarboxylic 466
  folic 223, 475
  homovanillic 205
  lipoic 452, 474, 477
  mycophenolic 353, 354
  pyrrolidine carboxylic 262
  sialic 312
  tricarboxylic 454
  uric 397, 466
  urocanic 262

  valproic 216, 217, 218, 471
  peptide-nucleic 477
  sphingomyelinase 262, 263
Activated macrophages 126
Acute 10, 11, 17, 25, 43, 231, 233, 234, 235, 236, 239, 241, 245, 246, 247, 249, 251, 252
  disseminated encephalomyelitis (ADEM) 231, 233, 234, 235, 236, 239, 241, 245, 246, 247, 249, 251, 252
  pancreatitis (AP) 17
  post streptococcal glomerulonephritis (APSGN) 25
  recurrent pancreatitis (ARP) 17
  respiratory distress syndrome (ARDS) 10
  rheumatic fever (ARF) 11, 43
Addison's disease 19
Adenoidectomy 433
Adenosine deaminase 107
Adenylate kinases (AKs) 392
Agammaglobulinemia 378, 384, 386
Agents 66, 84, 105, 113, 239, 240, 248, 286, 290, 353, 468, 470, 472, 474
  antimalarial 353
  effective topical antipruritic 286
  immunomodulatory 239
  multiple antihypertensive 113
Aicardi-Goutières syndrome (AGS) 328, 330, 357
Alanine amino-transferase 47
Albumin-Cre recombinase 439
Aleukocytosis 392
Alexander's disease 250
Alkaline phosphatase 47
Allergic rhinitis 27, 92, 146, 260, 266, 272, 277
  and adenotonsillar hypertrophy 146
Alloantigens 403, 406
  non-inherited maternal 403
Alveolar 93, 148
  bone condensation 148
  hemorrhage 93